BIOLOGICAL and BIOMEDICAL COATINGS HANDBOOK

Processing and Characterization

BIOLOGICAL and BIOMEDICAL COATINGS HANDBOOK

Processing and Characterization

Edited by
Sam Zhang

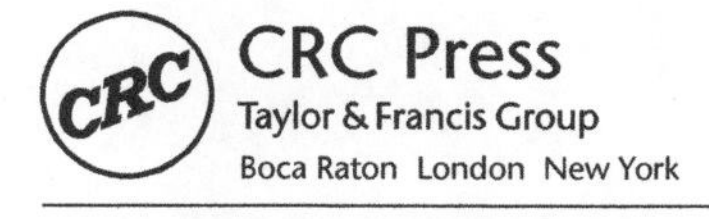

CRC Press is an imprint of the
Taylor & Francis Group, an **informa** business

CRC Press
Taylor & Francis Group
6000 Broken Sound Parkway NW, Suite 300
Boca Raton, FL 33487-2742

First issued in paperback 2019

ISBN-13: 978-1-4398-4995-8 (hbk)
ISBN-13: 978-0-367-38270-4 (pbk)

Visit the Taylor & Francis Web site at
http://www.taylorandfrancis.com

and the CRC Press Web site at
http://www.crcpress.com

Contents

Series Preface

Advances in Materials Science and Engineering

Series Statement

Materials form the foundation of technologies that govern our everyday life, from housing and household appliances to handheld phones, drug delivery systems, airplanes, and satellites. Development of new and increasingly tailored materials is key to further advancing important applications with the potential to dramatically enhance and enrich our experiences.

The ***Advances in Materials Science and Engineering*** series by CRC Press/Taylor & Francis is designed to help meet new and exciting challenges in Materials Science and Engineering disciplines. The books and monographs in the series are based on cutting-edge research and development, and thus are up-to-date with new discoveries, new understanding, and new insights in all aspects of materials development, including processing and characterization and applications in metallurgy, bulk or surface engineering, interfaces, thin films, coatings, and composites, just to name a few.

The series aims at delivering an authoritative information source to readers in academia, research institutes, and industry. The Publisher and its Series Editor are fully aware of the importance of Materials Science and Engineering as the foundation for many other disciplines of knowledge. As such, the team is committed to making this series the most comprehensive and accurate literary source to serve the whole materials world and the associated fields.

As Series Editor, I'd like to thank all authors and editors of the books in this series for their noble contributions to the advancement of Materials Science and Engineering and to the advancement of humankind.

Sam Zhang

Preface

As the clock of history ticks into the twenty-first century, "life sciences" has become one of the buzzwords of the time. Various nanotechnologies are mobilized to serve this field, the field of understanding life, the field of prevention of disease and cure, the field of enhancing quality of life. This two-volume handbook, *Biological and Biomedical Coatings*, comes at the right time to help meet these needs.

Volume 1 has nine chapters focusing on process and characterization of biological and biomedical coatings through sol–gel method, thermal spraying, hydrothermal and physical or chemical vapor deposition, and so forth. These chapters are "Bone-Like Mineral and Organically Modified Bone-Like Mineral Coatings," "Synthesis and Characterization of Hydroxyapatite Nanocoatings by Sol–Gel Method for Clinical Applications," "Hydroxyapatite and Other Biomedical Coatings by Electrophoretic Deposition," "Thermal Sprayed Bioceramic Coatings: Nanostructured Hydroxyapatite (HA) and HA-Based Composites," "Nanostructured Titania Coatings for Biological Applications: Fabrication and Characterization," "Hydrothermal Crystallization with Microstructural Self-Healing Effect on Mechanical and Failure Behaviors of Plasma-Sprayed Hydroxyapatite Coatings," "Bioceramic Coating on Titanium by Physical and Chemical Vapor Deposition," "Coating of Material Surfaces with Layer-by-Layer Assembled Polyelectrolyte Films," and "Bioactive Glass-Based Coatings and Modified Surfaces: Strategies for the Manufacture, Testing, and Clinical Applications for Regenerative Medicine."

Volume 2 contains 10 chapters centering on coating applications in the medical field such as implant and implanted devices, drug release, biosensing, and so forth. These chapters are "Sol–Gel Derived Hydroxyapatite Coatings on Metallic Implants: Characterization, *In Vitro* and *In Vivo* Analysis," "Amorphous Carbon Coatings for Biological Applications," "Biomedical Applications of Carbon-Based Materials," "Impedance Spectroscopy on Carbon-Based Materials," "Control of Drug Release from Coatings: Theories and Methodologies," "Release-Controlled Coatings," "Orthopedic and Dental Implant Surfaces and Coatings," "Piezoelectric Zinc Oxide and Aluminum Nitride Films for Microfluidic and Biosensing Applications," "Medical Applications of Sputter-Deposited Shape Memory Alloy Thin Films," and "Bioactive Coatings for Implanted Devices."

A striking feature of these handbooks is the consideration of both novice and experts: the chapters are written in such a way that, for newcomers in the relevant field, the handbooks serve as an introduction and a stepping stone for them to enter the field with less confusion, whereas for experts, the books provide up-to-date information through figures, tables, and images that will assist their research. I sincerely hope this aim is achieved.

The chapter authors come from different regions all over the globe: Australia, China, France, Hong Kong, Japan, Singapore, Taiwan, the United Kingdom, and the United States. As top researchers in the forefront of their relevant research fields, naturally they all are very busy. As the editor of these volumes, I am very grateful that they all made a special effort to ensure timely response and progress of their respective chapters. I am extremely indebted to many people who accepted my request and acted as reviewers for all the chapters. Since these volumes aim to cater to both novice and experts, the chapters are inevitably lengthy; many were more than 100 pages in the manuscript stage. To ensure the highest quality, close to 50 reviewers (at least two and sometimes three per chapter) painstakingly went through the chapters and came out with sincere and frank criticism and modification suggestions that helped make the chapters what they are today. I would like to take this opportunity to say a big "thank you" to all of them. Last but not least, I would like to register my gratitude to many CRC Press staff, especially Ms. Allison Shatkin, Miss Kari A. Budyk, and Miss Andrea Dale at Taylor & Francis Group for the invaluable assistance they have rendered to me throughout the entire endeavor, which made the smooth publication of these volumes a reality.

Sam Zhang

Editor

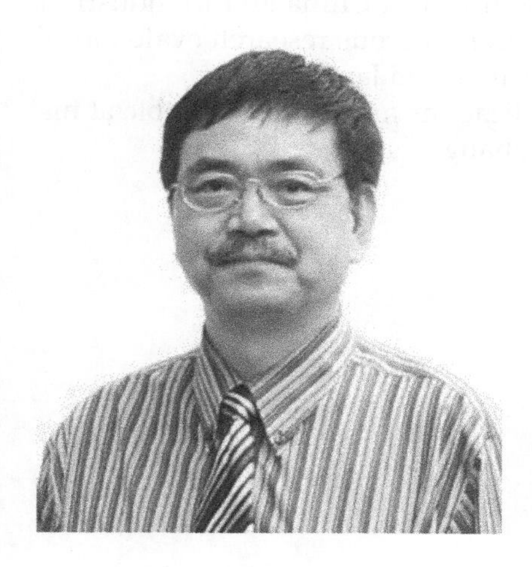

Sam Zhang Shanyong, better known as **Sam Zhang**, received his B. Eng. in materials in 1982 from Northeastern University (Shenyang, China), his M. Eng. in materials in 1984 from the Central Iron and Steel Research Institute (Beijing, China), and his Ph.D. in ceramics in 1991 from the University of Wisconsin–Madison (Madison, WI). He has been a full professor since 2006 at the School of Mechanical and Aerospace Engineering, Nanyang Technological University, Singapore.

Professor Zhang serves as editor-in-chief for *Nanoscience and Nanotechnology Letters* (United States) and principal editor for *Journal of Materials Research* (United States), among his other editorial involvements in international journals. Much of his career has been devoted to processing and characterization of thin films and coatings—from hard coatings to biological coatings and from electronic thin films to energy films and coatings—for the past almost 20 years. He has authored/coauthored more than 200 peer-reviewed papers (published in international journals) and 15 book chapters, and guest-edited 11 journal volumes in *Surface and Coatings Technology*, *Thin Solid Films*, etc. Including this handbook, so far he has published seven books: *CRC Handbook of Nanocomposite Films and Coatings:* Vol. 1. *Nanocomposite Films and Coatings: Mechanical Properties*, Vol. 2. *Nanocomposite Films and Coatings: Functional Properties*, Vol. 3. *Organic Nanostructured Film Devices and Coatings for Clean Energy*, and *Advanced Characterization Techniques* (Sam Zhang, Lin Li, Ashok Kumar, CRC Press/Taylor & Francis Group, 2008), *Nanocomposite Films and Coatings—Processing, Properties and Performance* (edited by Sam Zhang and Nasar Ali, Imperial College Press, UK, 2007), and this *Biological and Biomedical Coatings Handbook* two-volume set (CRC Press/Taylor & Francis Group): *Biological and Biomedical Coatings Handbook: Processing and Characterization* (vol. 1) and *Biological and Biomedical Coatings Handbook: Applications* (vol. 2).

Professor Zhang is currently serving as president of the Thin Films Society, and is a fellow of the Institute of Materials, Minerals and Mining (UK); an honorary professor of the Institute of Solid State Physics, Chinese Academy of Sciences; guest professor at Zhejiang University and Harbin Institute of Technology; and distinguished professor at the Central Iron and Steel Research Institute. He was featured in the first edition of *Who's Who in Engineering Singapore* (2007), and featured in the 26th and 27th editions of *Who's Who in the World* (2009 and 2010, respectively). Since 1998, he has been frequently invited to deliver plenary keynote lectures at international conferences including those held in Japan, the United States, France, Spain, Germany, China, Portugal, New Zealand, Russia, etc. He is also frequently invited by industries and universities to conduct short courses and workshops in Singapore, Malaysia, Portugal, the United States, and China.

Professor Zhang has been actively involved in organizing international conferences: 11 conferences as chairman, 13 conferences as member of the organizing committee, and six conferences as member of the scientific committee. The "Thin Films" conference series

(International Conference on Technological Advances of Thin Films & Surface Coatings), initiated and chaired by Professor Zhang, has grown from its inauguration in 2002 with 70 attendees to 800 strong since 2008. The Thin Films conference series has been a biannual focus in the field of films and coatings in the world.

Professor Zhang served as consultant to a city government in China and to industrial organizations in China and Singapore. He also served in numerous research evaluation/advisory panels in Singapore, Israel, Estonia, China, Brunei, and Japan.

Other details of Professor Zhang's research and publications are easily accessible at his personal Web site, http://www.ntu.edu.sg/home/msyzhang.

Contributors

B. Ben-Nissan
Faculty of Science
University of Technology
Sydney, NSW, Australia

A. Bendavid
Commonwealth Scientific and Industrial Research Organisation
Materials Science and Engineering
Lindfield, NSW, Australia

Thomas Boudou
Grenoble-INP
LMGP-MINATEC
CNRS UMR 5628
Grenoble, France

A. H. Choi
Faculty of Science
University of Technology
Sydney, NSW, Australia

J. Chou
Faculty of Science
University of Technology
Sydney, NSW, Australia

Paul K. Chu
Department of Physics and Materials Science
City University of Hong Kong
Hong Kong, China

Thomas Crouzier
CNRS UMR 5235
Université de Montpellier 2
Montpellier, France

Takashi Goto
Institute for Materials Research
Tohoku University
Sendai, Japan

D. W. Green
Queensland Eye Institute
South Brisbane, QLD, Australia
and
Australian Institute of Bioengineering and Nanotechnology and School of Life Sciences
The University of Queensland
Brisbane, QLD, Australia

David H. Kohn
Department of Biomedical Engineering and Department of Biologic and Materials Sciences
University of Michigan
Ann Arbor, Michigan

B. A. Latella
Commonwealth Scientific and Industrial Research Organisation
Process Science and Engineering
Waterford, WA, Australia

Hua Li
Biology Department
Brookhaven National Laboratory
Upton, New York

Truan-Sheng Lui
Department of Materials Science and Engineering
National Cheng Kung University
Tainan, Taiwan

Jason Maroothynaden
Leilak Biosystems
European Space Agency BIC
Noordwijk, The Netherlands

Takayuki Narushima
Department of Materials Processing
Tohoku University
Sendai, Japan

Timothy C. Palmer
School of Materials Science and Engineering
University of New South Wales
Sydney, NSW, Australia

Fei Peng
Materials Science and Engineering Program
Department of Chemical, Materials and Biomolecular Engineering
University of Connecticut
Storrs, Connecticut

Catherine Picart
Grenoble-INP
LMGP-MINATEC
CNRS UMR 5628
Grenoble, France

Harsha Ramaraju
Department of Biomedical Engineering
University of Michigan
Ann Arbor, Michigan

Janani Ramaswamy
Department of Biomedical Engineering
University of Michigan
Ann Arbor, Michigan

Kefeng Ren
Grenoble-INP
LMGP-MINATEC
CNRS UMR 5628
Grenoble, France

Charles C. Sorrell
School of Materials Science and Engineering
University of New South Wales
Sydney, NSW, Australia

Hariati Taib
School of Materials Science and Engineering
University of New South Wales
Sydney, NSW, Australia

Kyosuke Ueda
Department of Materials Processing
Tohoku University
Sendai, Japan

Mei Wei
Materials Science and Engineering Program
Department of Chemical, Materials and Biomolecular Engineering
University of Connecticut
Storrs, Connecticut

Zengmin Xia
Materials Science and Engineering Program
Department of Chemical, Materials and Biomolecular Engineering
University of Connecticut
Storrs, Connecticut

Yunchang Xin
Department of Physics and Materials Science
City University of Hong Kong
Hong Kong, China
and
School of Materials Science and Engineering
Chongqing University
Chongqing, China

Chung-Wei Yang
Department of Materials Science and Engineering
National Formosa University
Yunlin, Taiwan

1

Bone-Like Mineral and Organically Modified Bone-Like Mineral Coatings

Janani Ramaswamy, Harsha Ramaraju, and David H. Kohn

CONTENTS

Introduction: Cell–Matrix Interactions

Cells interact with their environment, namely, the extracellular matrix (ECM), continuously at each stage of cellular life from embryonic development until death. The ECM is an interconnected network consisting primarily of different types of collagens, proteoglycans, and matricellular proteins, such as fibronectin, laminin, and vitronectin, and in some tissues inorganic mineral (Plopper 2007). This complex matrix is secreted by the cells and serves as a specialized niche microenvironment, providing the specific cues necessary to control the function of each tissue type. The cells respond to these cues by altering their biological activity and, in turn, remodeling their surrounding ECM to reflect this altered activity, resulting in a well-orchestrated feedback system. For instance, the cells in bone (osteoblasts) produce a mineralized matrix during development and form the mature bone tissue, which is then remodeled by osteoclast-mediated resorption and new matrix formation by osteoblasts in response to changes in diet, exercise, and age (Baron 2003).

One of the most important functions of the ECM is to mediate cellular adhesion and consequent differentiation (Ruoslahti, Hayman, and Pierschbacher 1985). Most cell types need to be attached to a matrix in order to survive, grow, and differentiate. Cell adhesion occurs via heterodimeric receptors found in the plasma membrane, known as integrins, which recognize and bind to specific domains found in adhesive ECM proteins. The specific type of integrin receptor involved depends on the cell type and the composition of the ECM. A single cell usually expresses several types of integrin receptors during its lifetime, depending on the type of signals it receives from its environment. These integrins form a part of focal adhesion complexes, linking the ECM molecules to the cell cytoskeleton thus controlling cell adhesion. Furthermore, integrins are also capable of triggering specific cell signaling pathways and thus effectively modulating a variety of cellular functions including cell growth and migration, and differentiation and suppression of apoptosis (Plopper 2007; Ruoslahti, Hayman, and Pierschbacher 1985; Lebaron and Athanasiou 2000; Ruoslahti 1996). Once adhered, cells proliferate and differentiate into a specific lineage with the aid of growth factors and other signaling molecules that are sequestered by the ECM and released during the various stages of cellular activity. Hence, the cell–matrix system is dynamic and complex in nature.

Disruption of cell–cell and/or cell–matrix connections causing either lack of communication or the wrong type of communication to occur between the cells and their surroundings results in abnormal cell activity, manifested in the form of diseased tissues/organs. The fields of tissue engineering and biomimetics employ concepts from biological sciences and engineering to regenerate healthy tissues to replace diseased or damaged ones. Biomimetic materials derive inspiration from naturally occurring systems by imitating aspects of their structural and functional complexity. The main goals of these mimetic biomaterials are to facilitate cellular adhesion and production of ECM by replicating normally occurring cell–matrix interactions in order to control tissue formation.

Biomaterials to be used in bone tissue engineering applications should meet both physical requirements such as mechanical support, surface and bulk material properties and architecture, and biological requirements such as supporting cellular differentiation into osteoblasts. Biomimetic precipitation of calcium phosphate mineral onto biomaterial surfaces facilitates integration of the surface into host bone as well as allows for the incorporation of bioactive moieties under physiological conditions. This chapter focuses on the use of biomimetic apatite coatings to bond to native bone and recreate cell–matrix interactions in vitro and in vivo. The cellular and ECM components present in bone are briefly presented first, followed by a summary of the important material requirements needed to recreate cellular microenvironments in prosthetic and tissue engineering systems. The concept of biomimetic apatite formation and the use of these coatings on metals, ceramics, and polymers are then explored. Finally, a discussion of the use of biomineralization techniques to synthesize organic/inorganic hybrid (bone-like mineral (BLM) integrated with biologically active molecules) coatings that allow for mimicry of cell–matrix interactions is presented.

Engineering Cellular Microenvironments

Before designing any material system to be placed in vivo, it is important to understand the biology of the targeted tissue. Knowledge of the type of cells present, their surrounding matrix, and the type of interactions that occur at the cell–matrix interface is required to design biomaterials that simulate the natural environment in which these materials will be implanted.

Cellular and Matrix Components of Bone

Osteoblasts are derived from mesencyhmal stem cells under the influence of growth factors such as bone morphogenetic proteins (BMPs) and fibroblast growth factors (FGFs) on preosteoblastic cells (Baron 2003). Osteoblasts are mainly responsible for secreting the collagen and ground substance matrix (osteoid), which then undergoes calcification to form bone. Osteoblast–matrix interactions occur largely through β1 integrins, which mediate binding to collagens and other noncollagenous proteins found in the secreted matrix and cause activation of the mitogen-activated protein kinase (MAPK) cell signaling pathway, resulting in osteoblastic differentiation and osteogenesis (Lian, Stein, and Aubin 2003). After producing the osteoid matrix that calcifies, osteoblasts get trapped in the calcified bone tissue where they then function as osteocytes. Osteocytes are found in lacunae in the bone and interact with osteoblasts and other osteocytes, as well as the ECM via gap junctions found at the end of long cytoplasmic processes. Loss of these interactions leads to osteocyte cell death and consequent loss of bone (Baron 2003).

Osteoclasts are derived from the mononuclear/phagocytic cell lineage and are involved in bone resorption and turnover, and indirectly in the maintenance of plasma calcium and phosphate levels. Bone remodeling occurs during development and growth (determines shape and size of bones) as well as in adult bones, where the bone structure is maintained locally by replacement of old bone by new bone (Baron 2003; Martin 1989). The main events that occur during remodeling are (1) osteoclast activation and bone resorption, (2) osteoclast apoptosis, (3) preosteoblast chemotaxis, proliferation, and differentiation, and (4) formation of new bone and cessation of osteoblastic activity (Mundy, Chin, and Oyajobi 2003). The exact mechanisms involved in the coupling of osteoclastic resorption to osteoblastic bone formation are not completely understood, and several theories have been suggested to explain this phenomenon. It is thought that coupling is regulated by local and systemic chemical factors such as parathyroid hormone, 1,25-dihydroxyvitamin D, RANK ligand and its receptors, transforming growth factor (TGFβ), BMPs, and FGFs. Another theory is that once osteoclastic resorption is completed, osteoblasts present normally in the bone repopulate and reline the resorbed area without the action of any humoral factors, probably by detection of the resorption site via cell surface molecules (Mundy, Chin, and Oyajobi 2003). Imbalances in this coupling, where resorption is not followed by an equivalent amount of formation, leads to bone loss, seen in diseases such as osteoporosis. New bone formation can also occur in surfaces that have not been resorbed, such as in cases of prolonged fluoride therapy and in osteoblastic metastases (Baron 2003; Lian, Stein, and Aubin 2003; Mundy, Chin, and Oyajobi 2003; Martin 1989).

The ECM in bone is comprised of 50% to 70% inorganic mineral matrix, 20% to 40% organic matrix, 5% to 10% water, and less than 3% lipids. The inorganic matrix is composed of a hydroxyapatite mineral [$Ca_{10}(PO_4)_6(OH)_2$]. The mineral component contributes to structural support of the skeletal system. Bone mineral is a nonstoichiometric, semicrystalline, calcium, and hydroxide deficient analog of hydroxyapatite. Table 1.1 shows a variety of hydroxyapatite analogs found in bone. Most calcium phosphate precipitates containing calcium/phosphorous ratio between 1.33 to 2.0 result in a diffraction pattern resembling that of an apatite crystal. The apatite crystal size in bone is much smaller (~200 Å in the smallest dimension) than its geologic analog (Robey and Boskey 2003). This size disparity

TABLE 1.1
Calcium-Phosphate Phases with Corresponding Ca/P Ratios

Name	Formula	Ca/P Ratio
Hydroxyapatite (HA)	$Ca_{10}(PO_4)_6(OH)_2$	1.67
Fluorapatite	$Ca_{10}(PO_4)_6F_2$	1.67
Chlorapatite	$Ca_{10}(PO_4)_6Cl_2$	1.67
A-type carbonated apatite (unhydroxylated)	$Ca_{10}(PO_4)_6CO_3$	1.67
B-type carbonated hydroxyapatite (dahllite)	$Ca_{10-x}[(PO_4)_{6-2x}(CO_3)_{2x}](OH)_2$	≥1.67
Mixed A- and B-type carbonated apatites	$Ca_{10-x}[(PO_4)_{6-2x}(CO_3)_{2x}]CO_3$	≥1.67
HPO_4 containing apatite	$Ca_{10-x}[(PO_4)_{6-x}(HPO_4)_x](OH)_{2-x}$	≤1.67
Monohydrate calcium phosphate (MCPH)	$Ca(H_2PO_4)_2H_2O$	0.50
Monocalcium phosphate (MCP	$Ca(H_2PO_4)_2$	0.50
Dicalcium phosphate dihydrate (DCPD)	$Ca(HPO_4)2H_2O$	1.00
Tricalcium phosphate (TCP)	α- and β-$Ca_3(PO_4)_2$	1.50
Octacalcium phosphate (OCP)	$Ca_8H(PO_4)_65H_2O$	1.33

Source: Segvich et al., in *Biomaterials and Biomedical Engineering*, Ahmed et al. (eds.), TTP, Switzerland, pp. 327–373, 2008. With permission.

can arise from lattice substitutions of calcium, phosphate, and hydroxide groups with magnesium and carbonate ions. These substitutions can also give rise to altered solubility of the mineral phase. Since bone mineral contains calcium and alkali reserves, this enhanced solubility can buffer systemic changes in Ca^{2+}, H_3PO_4, and CO_2 (Neuman and Neuman 1957). For instance, during acidosis, the mineral can give up a carbonate ion for a hydronium ion to supplement blood buffers. The crystalline phase contains carbonate lattice substitutions that account for 2 to 7 wt.% of biological apatite (Segvich, Luong, and Kohn 2008). The consensus is that carbonate substitutes directly into the lattice through a type B (Table 1.1) substitution that is most commonly found in biological apatite (LeGeros 2002). The organic matrix is predominantly comprised of collagen, of which type I collagen is the major component, with trace amounts of other collagen isoforms present during certain developmental stages. Noncollagenous proteins comprise the remaining 10% to 15% of total bone protein content and include proteoglycans, glycosylated proteins, and γ-carboxylated proteins. These noncollagenous proteins are involved in directing organic matrix assembly, maintaining structural integrity of the tissue, sequestering and interacting with growth factors, and regulating bone metabolism and mineralization.

Bone ECM also functions as a reservoir of growth factors that are secreted by the cells (Biondi et al. 2008). Growth factors are a major class of hormones that mediate growth, division, and proliferation, and can be involved in endocrine, autocrine, and paracrine signaling (Silverthorn 2003). Cell stimulation by growth factors is influenced by concentration gradients and stage of development at which the active molecules are present. For instance, the role of TGF-β1 in osteogenesis and bone remodeling varies with concentration. TGF-β1 is present in high concentrations during early fracture repair process, but levels off in later stages (Allori, Sailon, and Warren 2008). In the early stages of repair, TGF-β1 promotes division of fibroblasts, osteoblast recruitment, and differentiation. TGF-β1 also inhibits osteoclast proliferation and differentiation. In later stages of wound healing, TGF-β1 promotes osteoclastogenesis. Similarly, BMP2 promotes chemotaxis and cell proliferation at low concentrations and cell differentiation and bone formation at high concentrations (Allori, Sailon, and Warren 2008).

Engineering Biomaterial Surfaces

A range of materials used for both prosthetic and regenerative therapies attempts to emulate some of the compositional, structural, and/or functional characteristics of the native bone microenvironment. Whether biomaterials are designed to function in vivo in a transient or permanent manner, they should integrate with host tissue and not lead to fibrous encapsulation. Clinical success rates of prostheses correlate with implant integration with surrounding tissue. Successful implant integration with host bone is characterized by a bone-like interface that integrates the implant surface with surrounding bone. This interface contains mineral, collagen, and cellular components and functions as a site for bone formation and resorption. This nanometer-thick interface is observed on implant surfaces that are conducive to osteogenic cell attachment, proliferation, and differentiation.

Implant and scaffold materials are designed to promote osteoconduction and/or osteoinduction, thereby improving osseointegration (Albrektsson and Johansson 2001). Osteoconduction refers to the propensity of a surface to allow bone growth. An osteoconductive material implanted at the defect site allows osteogenic precursor migration, adhesion, proliferation, and differentiation (Alsberg, Hill, and Mooney 2001). Conductive materials support adhesion of cells migrating from surrounding host tissue or may be used as a carrier to transplant osteogenic precursors. Therefore, the conductive properties of a substrate surface do not guarantee osseointegration but simply allow it to take place. Integration into host tissue is governed by additional factors that direct cells and organic components to mineralize and form new bone. Therefore, osteoconduction is necessary, but not sufficient for osseointegration.

Osteoinduction refers to the process by which osteogenesis is induced. More specifically, this is the process by which osteogenic precursor cells are actively guided to develop into differentiated osteogenic cells (Albrektsson and Johansson 2001). These differentiated cells partake in the restructuring of the extracellular matrix and the subsequent formation of new bone. Osteoinduction is typically achieved via the incorporation of growth factors, peptides, and/or DNA that interact with cell surface receptors and trigger signal transduction pathways to recruit and direct cell infiltration into the defect site from the surrounding tissue or transplanted donor cells. Osteoinductive materials, functionalized with biomolecules, actively engage in cell recruitment and direction to enhance the quality, amount, and rate of bone formation compared to osteoconductive materials alone (Hirano and Mooney 2004). An osteoinductive material is implicitly osteoconductive since a biofunctionalized nonconductive material surface would negate the inductive effects that would have lead to bone formation. Both osteoinductive and osteoconductive properties of the material play an integral role in osseointegration.

Although bulk properties of a material provide structural stability for both prosthetic and regenerative therapies, surface characteristics play an equally important role in regulating conduction and integration (Mitragotri and Lahann 2009; Murphy et al. 2000b; Liu, de Groot, and Hunziker 2005; Liu, de Groot, and Hunziker 2004). Surface chemistry, surface roughness, and elasticity can affect biological responses to implanted materials (Temenoff and Mikos 2008).

Surface chemistry. Atoms at the surface of a material are not bound on all sides like they are in the bulk. Unbound surface atoms have unfilled valence electrons resulting in surface-free energy also referred to as surface tension. When implanted into the host, proteins migrate toward the implant surface to reduce this surface free energy. Two other factors that regulate protein adsorption or foreign body response are surface charge and surface hydrophilicity (Temenoff and Mikos 2008). Hydrophilic surfaces demonstrate enhanced surface wettability by water. Wettability is the relative adhesion of a fluid to a solid surface. In the case of biomaterials and immiscible fluids, wettability refers to the ability of water to spread or adhere on an implant surface. A wettable surface has surface free energy 10 dyn/cm greater than the surface tension of the liquid. Hydrophilic surfaces that exhibit enhanced wettability can improve osteoconductivity by providing energetically favorable binding sites for integrins (Kilpadi and Lemons 1994; Rupp et al. 2006). Hydrophilic surfaces that exhibit enhanced wettability can improve osteoconductivity by providing energetically favorable binding sites for integrins (Kilpadi and Lemons 1994; Rupp et al. 2006).

An implant's surface charge resulting from dissociating ions can also have an effect on biointegration. With more dissociating surface ionic groups, oppositely charged biomolecules become electrostatically attracted to the surface. For instance, the spontaneously formed TiO_2 film on titanium implants reacts with water to form acidic and basic hydroxyl groups at the surface that enhance surface charge and protein adsorption (Kilpadi and Lemons 1994). Increasing the hydrophilicity improves osteoconduction by increasing osteoblastic cluster formation compared to unmodified titanium surfaces (Rupp et al. 2006).

Surface topography. Cells interact with the ECM through transmembrane focal adhesion kinases that allows them to transduce external cues through the cytoskeleton into the nucleus to induce transcription. Transduction of external mechanical cues elicits specific biochemical signals controlling cell cycle, proliferation, migration, and differentiation. Surface topography and elasticity are key factors that can control and direct this cellular response (Ingber 2006, 1997).

Implant surface topography has been extensively studied to identify correlations between surface structures and fixation to bone. Despite the heterogeneity in experimental methods, there is a positive relationship between surface roughness and bone to implant contact (Shalabi et al. 2006). Several approaches to modify surface roughness at the micron level have been utilized, among which sandblasting, acid etching, and sodium hydroxide treatments are the most widely used (Bollen, Lambrechts, and Quirynen 1997). For instance, osteoblasts cultured on sandblasted implants exhibit enhanced mineralization compared to osteoblasts grown on smooth surfaces (Marchisio et al. 2005). However, there is an upper limit to roughness for improving tissue integration or inducing an enhanced cellular response on the order of R_a = 4 μm (Rønold, Lyngstadaas, and Ellingsen 2003). Roughness is therefore an important design parameter to consider when altering surface characteristics to enhance osteointegration.

Surface chemistry and surface topography are also co-optimized to enhance osseointegration. For instance, sandblasted acid etched implants are contaminated by hydrocarbons minutes after exposure to air, making their surface chemistry hydrophobic. These implants are processed with nitrogen gas and stored in NaCl solution to decrease contamination and increase hydrophilicity. This surface modification procedure results in improved osseointegration (Rupp et al. 2006).

Micro- and nanostructuring techniques are also used to control molecular-level interactions between cells and the environment: soft-lithography, photolithography, sputtering, self-assembling nanostructures, and physical and chemical vapor deposition modify surface topography at the micro- and nanoscales and control cell behavior (Tan and Saltzman 2004; Martinez et al. 2009; Dalby et al. 2007, Dalby et al. 2004; Xia and Whitesides 1998). Surface micro- and nanotopography regulate cell orientation, morphology, and cytoskeletal rearrangement and promote cell adhesion, proliferation, and differentiation (Martinez et al. 2009). For instance, to identify the role of surface topography in directing osteogenic differentiation, human mesenchymal stem cells were grown on 120-nm grooves created by electron beam lithography on polymethylmethacrylate (PMMA). Cells grown on these nanostructures engaged in osteogenic differentiation and bone mineral formation without the addition of osteogenic factors to the culture media (Dalby et al. 2007; Dalby et al. 2004).

Substrate elasticity. Substrate elasticity also plays an important role in cell adhesion, proliferation, and differentiation, thereby enhancing osteoconduction and osseointegration. Advances in materials engineering offer a variety of polymer substrates with elasticities that may be tuned to match the stiffness of specific tissues (Thompson et al. 2005; Kloxin, Benton, and Anseth 2010; Lo et al. 2000; Discher, Mooney, and Zandstra 2009). These tunable polymers are used to observe effects of substrate compliance on adhesion and proliferation independent of surface chemistry and topographical effects.

A variety of cells, including fibroblasts, epithelial cells, myocytes, and osteoblasts, show increased adhesion and proliferation on stiffer substrates (Mitragotri and Lahann 2009; Griffin et al. 2004). For example, kidney epithelial cells grown on polyelectrolyte multilayers show increased adhesion with increasing modulus between 50 and 500 kPa (Kocgozlu et al. 2010). Mesenchymal cells show markers for neurogenic, myogenic, and osteogenic differentiation when cultured on polyacrylamide gels with stiffness analogous to native brain, muscle, and osteoid, respectively (Engler et al. 2006). Therefore, material stiffness can be a useful parameter to direct osteoconduction and osseointegration. However, it is important to consider the integrated roles of surface chemistry, surface topography, and elasticity to amplify osteoconductive effects of a biomaterial surface.

One way to incorporate the desired surface properties into an implant or scaffolding material is to use coating techniques wherein the chemistry of the coatings can be controlled to provide the required roughness, elasticity, and crystallinity. Hydroxyapatite coatings are the most commonly used inorganic coatings on bone implants and in regenerative therapies, and can be used to increase modify the microtopography of substrate surfaces. Hydroxyapatite coatings with surface roughness (R_a) values in the range of 0.7–4.8 show significantly increased human bone marrow stromal cell adhesion and proliferation with increasing R_a (Deligianni et al. 2001).

HA coatings with low crystallinity show increased dissolution compared to highly crystalline coatings (Lee et al. 2009). In addition to varying crystallinity, crystallite size can also be varied by altering processing temperatures. Coatings with larger crystallite size exhibit lower dissolution and improved stability of the crystallographic lattice (Zhang et al. 2003).

In addition to affording control over dissolution and surface roughness, crystallinity is reported to improve osseointegration. For example, fibroblasts cultured on 98% crystalline HA coatings exhibit enhanced adhesion and proliferation compared to 65% crystalline, 25% crystalline, and uncoated titanium surfaces after 14 days of culture (Chou, Marek, and Wagner 1999). In vivo, canine femoral implants having 98% crystalline HA coatings showed greater integration with surrounding bone 3 months postimplantation compared to implants with 50% crystalline HA coatings (Xue et al. 2004).

However, other studies show no significant increase in osseointegration with changes in crystallinity. For example, no difference in bone formation was observed between 50%, 70%, and 90% crystalline coatings at 4, 12, and 24 weeks (Lacefield 1999). Similar studies using 100% and 40% crystalline HA coatings also resulted in no discernable difference in osseointegration (Frayssinet et al. 1994). Further research is required to more thoroughly elucidate the role of crystallinity in osseointegration. Although crystallinity maintains the osteoconductive properties of a material while providing control over coating delamination (Lacefield 1999), an osteoconductive material is not always osseointegrative. Therefore, although osteogenic precursors are still able to adhere and grow on implants with higher crystallinity, this does not translate to an osseointegrative response.

Apatite coatings create surface chemistries more analogous to native bone. Different calcium-phosphate phases present in native bone, such as octacalcium phosphate and carbonated apatite, enhance cell adhesion and osteoconduction (Le Guehennec et al. 2007; Müller et al. 2007; Wang et al. 2004). Altering the phases of the apatite coating can have significant effects on the degree of crystallinity, surface roughness, and solubility of the coating (Barrere et al. 2003a). Apatite coatings therefore afford increased control over surface chemistry and/or topography while maintaining the elastic characteristics of the biomaterial surface. Gaining further control over surface chemistry and topography will enhance the ability to reconstruct cellular microenvironments, thereby improving osseointegration. Apatite coatings also increase the stiffness of soft substrates, providing control over cytoskeletal organization (Murphy et al. 2000b; Leonova et al. 2006). There are several approaches to depositing apatite coatings with controlled composition, topography, and/or stiffness for enhancing conduction. The subsequent sections discuss processing and applications of a biomimetically applied BLM coating precipitated from a supersaturated salt solution and how controlling biomimetic processing, composition, and structure can control biological responses in vitro and in vivo.

Biomimetic Precipitation of Mineral

Implants that do not integrate into host tissue become isolated from the surrounding tissue, limiting the efficiency of load transfer (Jacobs, Gilbert, and Urban 1998). Bioactive materials such as Bioglass 45S5 and A-W glass ceramics form a layer of apatite on the surface when placed in vivo, which is vital for implant/tissue integration (Ducheyne 1985; Nakamura et al. 1985). It is possible to simulate this apatite coating in vitro and thus provide bioactivity to non-bioactive materials using coating techniques such as plasma spraying, electrophoretic deposition, sol–gel deposition, hot isostatic pressing, frit enameling, ion-assisted deposition, pulsed laser deposition, electrochemical deposition, and sputter coating (Liu and Hunziker 2009). Each one of these methods has its own advantages and disadvantages (Table 1.2), and not all techniques can be used with all classes of materials (Table 1.3). Of these methods, the most widely used technique commercially for metals is plasma spraying. Plasma spraying, however, is not ideal with small implants and complex shapes. It requires a coating thickness of 40 to 50 μm to achieve uniform deposition, and is clinically challenged by delamination issues due to variations in the phases that constitute the coating (Le Guehennec et al. 2007). Other methods such as dynamic mixing and hot isostatic pressing are limited by the uniformity of coating that they generate as well (Wie, Hero, and Solheim 1998; Yoshinari, Ohtsuka, and Dérand 1994). However, there are a number of coating methods that deposit mineral uniformly: sputter coating, pulsed laser deposition, sol–gel deposition, and electrophoretic deposition are better suited for uniform coating on complex structures (Wolke et al. 1994; Zeng and Lacefield 2000; Li, De Groot, and Kokubo 1996). However, the use of high processing temperatures in some of these methods results in the formation of apatite that differs from the composition of natural bone apatite, and is also not amenable to soft materials such as polymers (Abe, Kokubo, and Yamamuro 1990). Among these methods, sol–gel deposition is the only other method that can achieve uniform mineral coatings at low processing temperatures, but

TABLE 1.2
Hydroxyapatite Coating Produced Using Various Deposition Technologies

Technique	Thickness	Advantages	Disadvantages	References
Thermal spraying	30–200 μm	High deposition rates; low cost	Line-of-sight technique; high temperatures induce decomposition; rapid cooling produces amorphous coatings	Gross and Berndt 1998; Gross, Berndt, and Herman 1998; Li, Khor, and Cheang 2002; Yang and Ong 2003; Zyman et al. 1993; Tao, Heng, and Chuanxian 2000; Weng et al. 1993; Chen, Wolke, and de Groot 1994; Zyman et al. 1994; Roome and Adam 1995
Sputter coating	0.5–3.0 μm	Uniform coating thickness on flat substrates; dense coating	Line of sight technique; expensive; time-consuming; produces amorphous coating	Ding 2003; Ding, Ju, and Lin 1999; Wolke et al. 2003; Massaro et al. 2001; Ong and Lucas 1994; Ong et al. 1994; Wolke et al. 1994; van Dijk et al. 1996; van Dijk et al. 1995
Pulsed laser deposition	0.05–5.0 μm	Coating with crystalline and amorphous; coating with dense and porous	Line-of-sight technique	Clèries et al. 2000; Fernández-Pradas et al. 2001; Zeng and Lacefield 2000
Dynamic mixing method	0.05–1.30 μm	High adhesive strength	Line-of-sight technique; expensive; produces amorphous coating	Yoshinari, Ohtsuka, and Dérand 1994
Dip coating	0.05–5.0 mm	Inexpensive; coating applied quickly; can coat complex substrates	Requires high sintering techniques; thermal expansion mismatch	Wenjian and Baptista 1998; Choi et al. 2003; Shi, Jiang, and Bauer 2002; Jiang and Shi 1998; Campbell et al. 2000

(continued)

TABLE 1.2 (Continued)

Hydroxyapatite Coating Produced Using Various Deposition Technologies

Technique	Thickness	Advantages	Disadvantages	References
Sol–gel	<1 μm	Can coat complex shapes; low processing temperatures; relatively inexpensive as coating is very thin	Some processes require controlled atmosphere processing; expensive raw materials	Li, De Groot, and Kokubo 1996; Manso et al. 2002; Liu, Yang, and Troczynski 2002; Chai, Gross, and Ben-Nissan 1998
Electrophoretic deposition	0.1–2.0 mm	Uniform coating thickness; rapid deposition rates; can coat complex substrates	Difficult to produce crack-free coatings; requires high sintering temperatures	Ducheyne et al. 1986; Han et al. 1999; Han et al. 2001; Zhu, Kim, and Jeong 2001; Agata De Sena et al. 2002; Ma, Wan, and Peng 2003; Nie et al. 2001; Manso et al. 2000
Biomimetic coating	<30 μm	Low processing temperatures; can form bone-like apatite; can coat complex shapes; can incorporate bone growth stimulating factors	Time-consuming; requires replenishment and constant pH of simulated body fluid	Habibovic et al. 2002; Oliveira et al. 1999; Li et al. 1992
Hot isostatic pressing	0.2–2.0 mm	Produces dense coatings	Cannot coat complex substrates; high temperature required; thermal expansion mismatch; elastic property differences; expensive; removal/interaction of encapsulation material	Wie, Hero, and Solheim 1998

Source: Ong et al. 2009, with kind permission from Springer Science + Business Media.

TABLE 1.3
Classes of Materials That Can Be Coated with Different Calcium-Phosphate Coating Techniques

Coating Technique	Metals	Ceramics	Polymers	Examples
Plasma spraying	×			de Groot et al. 1987; Klein et al. 1991
Sputter coating	×		×	Ong and Lucas 1994; Feddes et al. 2004
Pulsed laser deposition	×	×	×	Baeri et al. 1992; Antonov et al. 1998; Honstu et al. 1997
Electrophoretic deposition	×	×		Ducheyne et al. 1990; Yamashita et al. 1998
Sol–gel	×		×	Kaneko et al. 2009; Montenero et al. 2000
Hot isostatic pressing	×	×		Herø et al. 1994; Li, Liao, and Hermansson 1996
Dynamic mixing method	×			Yoshinari, Ohtsuka, and Dérand 1994
Biomimetic coating	×	×	×	Tanahashi et al. 1994; Habibovic et al. 2002; Abe, Kokubo, and Yamamuro 1990

this method is expensive. A promising alternate technique is biomimetic precipitation of apatite onto implant surfaces using supersaturated salt solutions known as simulated body fluids (SBFs) (Abe, Kokubo, and Yamamuro 1990). These SBFs have similar ionic constitutions to blood plasma and form carbonated apatites at physiologic temperatures, similar to those found in bone (Table 1.4). Commonly used SBF coating regimens for different material applications are listed in Table 1.5.

The mechanism of formation of BLM can be generally outlined as (1) functionalization of the substrate to obtain a negatively charged surface, (2) nucleation by chelation of precursor Ca^{2+} ions to these negatively charged groups, and (3) growth of the BLM layer (Murphy, Kohn, and Mooney 2000a). Surface functionalization can be achieved by several methods, such as grafting functional groups, alkaline treatments, aqueous hydrolysis, heat treatments, and glow discharge treatment in oxygen (Murphy, Kohn, and Mooney 2000a; Segvich et al. 2008; Kokubo 1996; Tanahashi et al. 1995; Luong et al. 2006; Tanahashi and Matsuda 1997). The heterogeneous precipitation of biomineral from solution occurs when the precursor–substrate interfacial energy is lower than the precursor–solution energy,

TABLE 1.4
Chemical Composition (in mM) of Different Types of SBFs

Type of SBF	Na^+	K^+	Mg^{2+}	Ca^{2+}	Cl^-	HCO^{3-}	HPO_4^{2-}	SO_4^{2-}	Reference
1× SBF	142.0	5.0	1.5	2.5	148.8	4.2	1.0	0.5	Abe, Kokubo, and Yamamuro 1990
Revised SBF (r-SBF)	142.0	5.0	1.5	2.5	103.0	27.0	1.0	0.5	Oyane et al. 2003
Newly improved SBF (n-SBF)	142.0	5.0	1.5	2.5	103.0	4.2	1.0	0.5	Takadama et al. 2004
1× mSBF	145.2	6.0	1.5	5.0	157.0	4.2	2.0	0.5	Luong et al. 2006
2× SBF	282.0	10.0	3.0	5.0	304.0	8.4	2.0	1.0	Shin, Jayasuriya, and Kohn 2007
5× SBF	710.0	25.0	12.7	7.7	739.7	21.0	5.0	2.5	Chen et al. 2008
Human plasma	142.0	5.0	2.5	1.5	103.0	27.0	1.0	0.5	Abe, Kokubo, and Yamamuro 1990

TABLE 1.5

Commonly Used SBF Treatment Applications

Application	SBF Treatment	Reference
Metals	1. 5× SBF for 24 h at 37°C 2. 5× mSBF for 24 h at 50°C	Barrere et al. 2003
	1. 5× SBF for 24 h at 37°C 2. 5× mSBF for 48 h at 50°C	Habibovic et al. 2005
Ceramics	1. SBF 4 days at 37°C	Liu, Ding, and Chu 2004
PLGA films	1. 2× mSBF at 37°C	Luong et al. 2006
PLGA scaffolds	1. 4× mSBF for 12 h at 37°C 2. SBF change every 6 h 3. 2× mSBF for 108 h at 37°C 4. SBF change every 8 h	Segvich, Luong, and Kohn 2008; Segvich et al. 2008

Source: Ong et al., in Thin Calcium Phosphate Coatings for Medical Implants, Leon and Jansen (eds.), Springer, pp. 175–198, 2009. With permission.

resulting in the formation of an apatite coating on the substrate. In the absence of this thermodynamically favorable situation, homogeneous precipitation can occur (Bunker et al. 1994). The thickness, morphology, and composition of the BLM formed are dependent on several factors, such as the incubation time and temperature, ionic concentration, composition, and pH of SBF and method of surface functionalization. For example, apatite formed from SBFs with low ionic products is more crystalline compared to apatite formed from SBFs with higher ionic products. Also, the Ca/P ratios of BLM vary inversely with SBF solution ionic activity—higher ionic products lead to lower Ca/P ratios (Shin, Jayasuriya, and Kohn 2007).

Characterization of biomimetic apatite to quantify and understand its properties can be achieved using several methods (Figure 1.1). Fourier transform infrared spectroscopy (FTIR) is useful in determining chemical composition by measuring carbonate and phosphate band intensities and ratios, and presence of any organic constituents. X-ray diffraction (XRD) and transmission electron diffraction (TED) allow the measurement of the lattice parameters of the crystallographic peaks and thereby assess the degree of crystallinity. Scanning electron microscopy (SEM) can be used to observe surface morphology and, when used along with energy dispersive x-ray spectrometry (EDX), can provide a qualitative measure of elemental composition. N-SEM, which is another form of SEM, can be used to characterize surface morphology with high natural contrast but at the cost of resolution. Microcomputed tomography (μCT) generates images of 3-D mineralized scaffolds from which total mineral content, volumetric mineral density, and distribution of mineral can be quantified (Segvich, Luong, and Kohn 2008).

The use of SBF to prepare apatite coatings on prosthetic metal and ceramic implants has been extended to soft resorbable materials used in bone tissue engineering to create a new class of osteoconductive biomaterials. Since biomimetic apatite precipitation occurs at ambient temperatures, it is possible to coat temperature-sensitive scaffold materials such as polymers with a layer of uniform mineral. The use of processing techniques based on biomineralization also allows the incorporation of biologically active molecules such as growth factors, proteins, and nucleic acids into the mineral layer without any loss of bioactivity due to high temperatures (Segvich et al. 2008; Luong et al. 2006; Luong, McFalls, and Kohn 2009). Moreover, since porosity is important for tissue infiltration and vascularization to induce biological fixation, polymer scaffolds can be coated with a spatially uniform

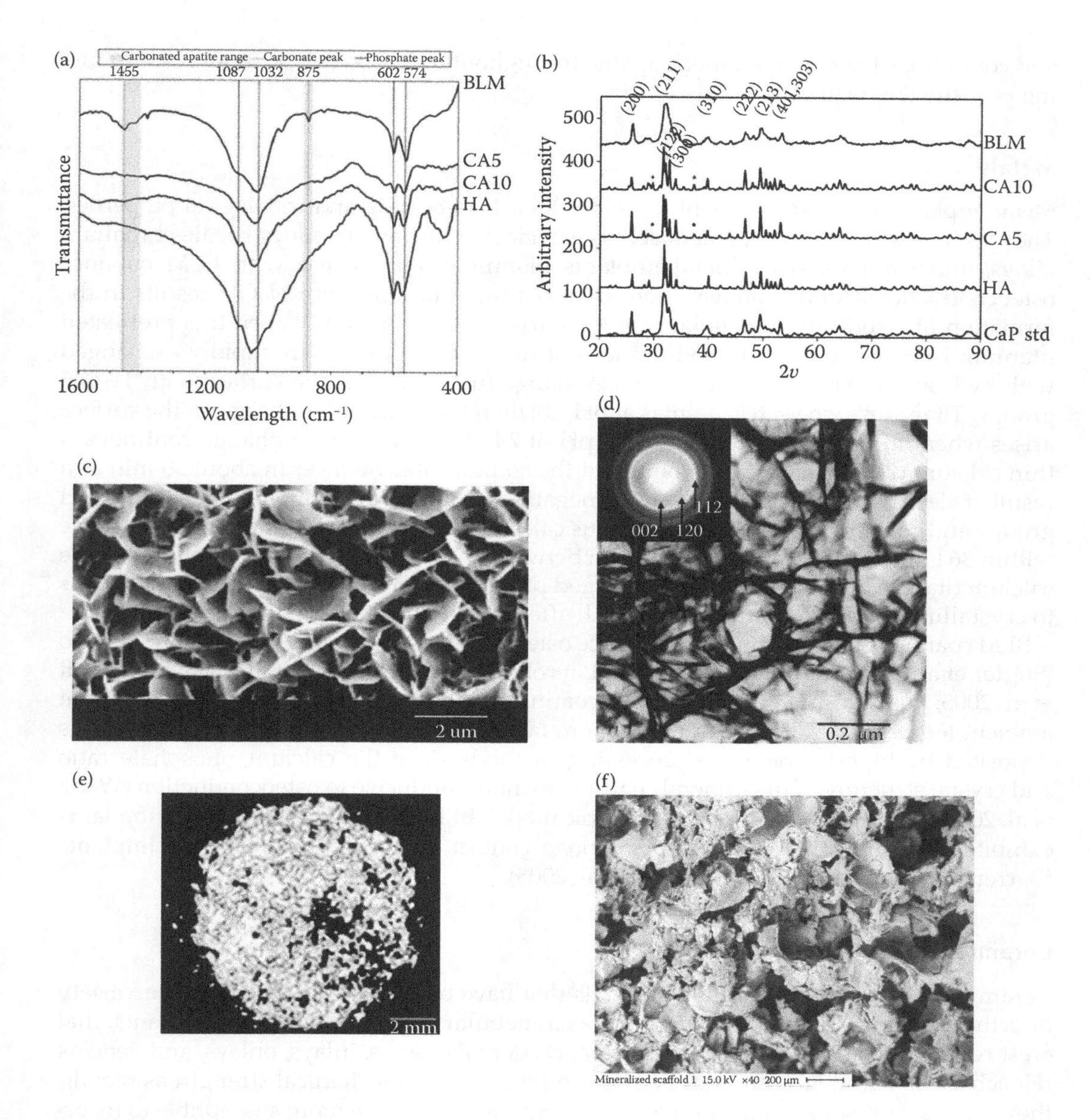

FIGURE 1.1
Different methods of characterization of bone-like mineral (BLM). (a) FTIR spectra for BLM, sintered disks from 5.6% (CA5), and 10.5% (CA10) carbonated apatite powder, sintered disks from hydroxyapatite powder (HA); (b) XRD patterns for BLM, CA5, CA10, HA, and a calcium phosphate standard (CaP std); (c) SEM image of BLM coating on PLGA film (magnification 10,000×); (d) TEM image and diffraction pattern of BLM crystals on PLGA film; (e) micro-CT image of top cross section of BLM coated on PLGA scaffold; (f) N-SEM image of top cross section of BLM coating on PLGA scaffold. (Reprinted from: (a, b) Segvich et al., *Biomaterials*, 30, 1287–1298, 2009, with permission from Elsevier; (c, d) Luong et al., *Biomaterials*, 27(7), 1175–1186, 2006, with permission from Elsevier; (e) Segvich et al., *Journal of Biomedical Materials Research B*, 84B(2), 340–349, 2008, with permission from Wiley.)

and continuous layer of biomimetic apatite throughout the thickness, without compromising porosity (Segvich et al. 2008).

Metals

Metal implants are most commonly used for their load-bearing and tribological properties. The most prevalent metal implant materials include titanium and its alloys, cobalt–chromium alloys, and stainless steel. Metal implants biomimetically coated with BLM enhance osteoconduction and osseointegration. Heat treating titanium with NaOH results in the formation of a sodium titanate layer at the surface of the implant. When this pretreated titanium is immersed in SBF, sodium ions at the titanate surface are rapidly exchanged with hydronium ions in the fluid. This exchange functionalizes the surface with Ti–OH groups. Titanium's isoelectric point is at pH 5.8; therefore, a negative charge on the surface arises when immersed in SBF that has a pH of 7.4. As sodium ion exchange continues, a thin calcium titanate layer forms on top of the sodium titanate layer in about 30 min as a result of electrostatic interaction between negatively charged units of repolymerized TiOH groups and calcium in the SBF. Amorphous calcium phosphate precipitates on the surface within 36 h due to electrostatic interaction between the increasingly positive charge of the calcium titanate layer and negatively charged phosphate ions in SBF. This interaction leads to crystalline apatite formation within 48 h after immersion (Takadama et al. 2001).

BLM coatings on metal implants enhance osteointegrative properties in vitro and in vivo (Stigter et al. 2004; Stigter, de Groot, and Layrolle 2002; Schliephake et al. 2006; Bernhardt et al. 2005; Fujibayashi et al. 2004). BLM coatings deposited on implants from solution at ambient temperature and pressure are more favorable for osteoconduction than coatings deposited by high-temperature processing methods since the calcium/phosphate ratio and crystal structure of the mineral coating are more conducive to osteoconduction (Wang et al. 2004). For instance, in a goat orthotopic model, BLM-coated Ti_6Al_4V femoral implants exhibited significantly greater implant/bone contact compared to noncoated implants (Barrere et al. 2003a, 2003b; Habibovic et al. 2005).

Ceramics

Ceramics are another class of biomaterials that have been successfully used in a variety of orthopedic and dental implants, such as acetabular cups, extracochlear implants, ilial crest replacement, alveolar ridge maintenance, dental crowns, inlays, onlays, and veneers (Hench 1991). Although ceramics do not exhibit the same mechanical strength as metals, they are ideal for some bone microenvironments since they are more susceptible to incorporation into the surrounding tissue while their degradative byproducts are biologically tolerable.

Bioactive glasses improve integration and fixation with host bone tissue. When immersed in SBF, dissolution of calcium and silicate from these bioactive glasses plays an important role in mineralization. Ceramic surfaces, such as metal surfaces, exchange hydronium ions for cations, thereby functionalizing the surface to present nucleation sites for mineralization (Abe, Kokubo, and Yamamuro 1990; Takadama et al. 2001). These functionalized Si–OH surface groups drive the deposition of calcium and phosphate ions, resulting in BLM formation and a subsequent depletion of phosphate ions from the media. Bioglass 45S5, Ceravital-type glass ceramic, glass ceramic A-W, sintered HA, apatite/β-tricalcium phosphate, and calcium sulfate exchange Ca^+ ions with the solution resulting in BLM formation at the surface (Kokubo and Takadama 2006). Nonbioactive glass ceramics do not dissolve these initial calcium and silicate ions nor do they form a BLM layer unless their surfaces are functionalized before immersion (Kokubo 1991). As with metals, the osseointegration of BLM coated ceramics occurs more rapidly than on noncoated surfaces due to the enhanced conductive properties of the mineral layer (Liu, Ding, and Chu 2004).

Polymers

Biomineralized metals, glasses, and glass ceramics bond well to bone and serve as good implant materials. However, these materials possess high elastic moduli compared to bone, which can cause resorption of the host bone tissue (Kokubo 1996; Nagano et al. 1996). Furthermore, metals and many ceramics can only be used as prosthetic implants since they are not bulk biodegradable and thus do not allow replacement of the material by new tissue over time. Polymers are good tissue engineering substitutes and possess advantages such as biodegradability, improved flexibility in controlling structure, composition, and properties, as well as the ability to be molded into different shapes to fit the wound or defect site.

Natural polymers are readily available, inexpensive, and nontoxic. Raw silk, fibrinogen, and collagen have been incubated in SBF solutions to obtain mineralized biopolymers that can be used as biomimetic bone analogs (Takeuchi et al. 2003; Wei et al. 2008; Girija, Yokogawa, and Nagata 2002). However, since these polymers are protein-based, they may elicit undesired immunological responses when placed in vivo. Alternative natural materials are polysaccharide-based systems, several of which have been developed and used as biomineralization templates. Chitosan microparticles functionalized with Si–OH groups are made bioactive by soaking in SBF and can be used as injectable biomaterials and protein/drug delivery systems (Leonor et al. 2008). Another example is a cornstarch–ethylene vinyl alcohol (SEVA-C) polymer blend that is made bioactive by its ability to induce bone-like apatite formation in SBF after the introduction of carboxylic acid functional groups on the surface (Leonor et al. 2007).

While synthetic polymers possess most of the same advantages as biopolymers, they also offer more control in tailoring their synthesis and degradation properties to suit specific applications. Biodegradable synthetic polymers such as poly-L-lactic acid (PLLA), poly-glycolic acid (PGA) and poly-lactic-*co*-glycolic acid (PLGA) break down into nontoxic natural acid metabolites over time (Murphy, Kohn, and Mooney 2000a). Apatite coatings or polymer/apatite composite materials can compensate for this acidic release by the dissolution of basic calcium phosphate and maintain pH within physiological ranges (Linhart et al. 2001).

BLM coatings have been produced on a variety of polymers including polyvinyl chloride, poly(tetrafluoroethylene), nylon 6, poly(ethylene terephthalate), alkanethiols, and polyhydroxyalkanoates (Tanahashi and Matsuda 1997; Tanahashi et al. 1994; Misra et al. 2006). Biomimetic mineral layers formed on electrospun nanofiber poly(ε-caprolactone) meshes support proliferation of Saos-2 osteogenic sarcoma cells up to 2 weeks in culture, demonstrating potential to regenerate bone ECM (Araujo et al. 2008). Continuous and uniform BLM layers can be produced throughout the porous structure of 3-D PLGA scaffolds (Murphy, Kohn, and Mooney 2000a; Segvich et al. 2008). These mineralized scaffolds exhibit superior mechanical properties, as seen by a 5-fold increase in compressive modulus (Murphy, Kohn, and Mooney 2000a). They also support higher bone marrow stromal cell adhesion through well-distributed fibrillar contacts, and when used to transplant bone marrow stromal cells, form a higher bone volume fraction in comparison to nonmineralized polymer scaffolds (Leonova et al. 2006; Kohn et al. 2005). Other in vivo studies using polyethersulfone (PES) coated with bone-like apatite also show bonding of the implant to native bone, accompanied by remodeling and complete resorption of the apatite layer after 30 weeks (Nagano et al. 1996). Thus, a variety of biomimetically mineralized polymer scaffolds have utility in bone tissue engineering.

While these BLM coatings mimic the mineral component of bone, they can be altered to include biomolecules such as proteins, growth factors, enzymes, and nucleic acids within the biomineral layer, resulting in organic/inorganic hybrid biomaterials that have the potential to dictate cellular events in an even more controlled manner.

Organic/Inorganic Hybrids

Native bone is a composite material consisting of both inorganic and organic phases. The organic components play important roles in the nucleation and formation of mineral, while influencing osteogenic growth and differentiation. Incorporation of organic molecules such as proteins, growth factors, and DNA into BLM coatings gives rise to a new class of organic/inorganic hybrid materials. These composites are capable of influencing mineral growth and are also able to enhance cell attachment and direct these adhering cells toward osteogenic differentiation. Using different combinations of biomolecules and mineralization regimens, it is possible to mimic physiologic spatial and temporal gradients of bioactive molecules to modulate cellular function and bone formation during development, repair, and regeneration. Other applications of organic/inorganic hybrids include

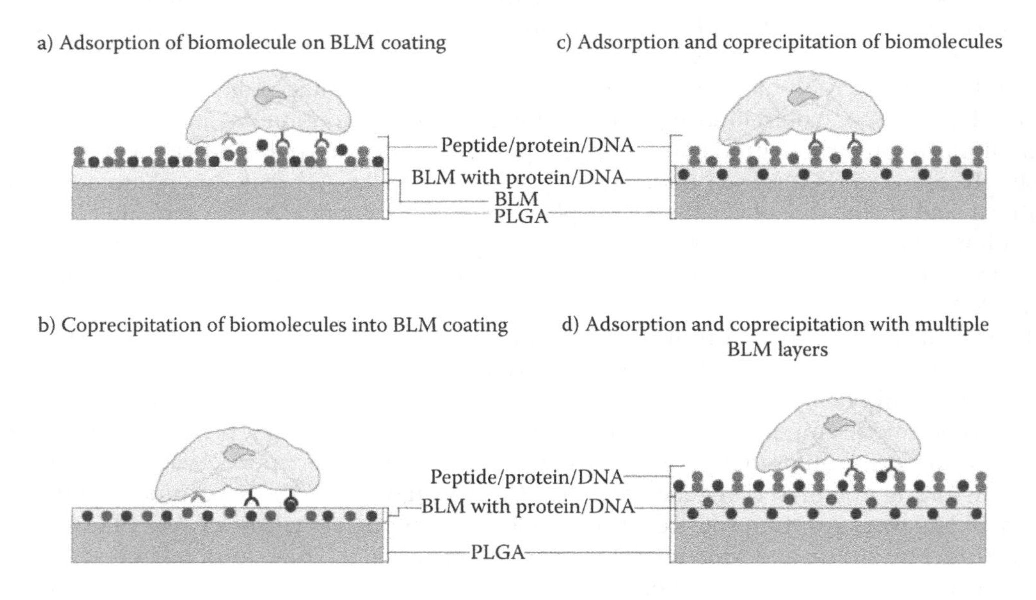

FIGURE 1.2
Schematic representation of cell substrate interactions with several variations of organic/inorganic hybrid constructs. (a, c) Cells binding to biomolecules that have been adsorbed, (b, d) demonstrate cellular interactions with adsorbed and/or coprecipitated moieties. Peptides in panels a, c, d aim to anchor the cells to the substrate surfaces while exposing basal surface for uptake of growth factors and DNA.

creating bone mimics that attempt to recreate the structural hierarchy of natural bone and can be also be used to elucidate the roles of organic molecules in biomineralization.

There are several approaches to create calcium phosphate–organic hybrids. The two main methods to produce organic/BLM hybrids with bioactive molecules discussed in this section are adsorption and coprecipitation. For materials intended as protein delivery systems, each of these approaches has advantages depending on the release profile desired. Adsorption can be used when a quick transient release of the biomolecule is desired, or to recruit cells to the material surface initially. Coprecipitation is more useful in creating gradual release profiles, where the desired molecule is needed over a longer period (Figure 1.2).

Adsorption of Proteins to BLM Surfaces

Adsorption of proteins to mineral surfaces is the simplest method of forming organic/inorganic hybrids containing biologically active molecules and involves incubating the mineralized substrate in a protein solution, allowing the protein to associate itself with the mineral. The mechanism of adsorption is thought to be via electrostatic interactions between the protein and the apatite, and hence the protein–mineral bond created by adsorption is not strong compared to the covalent attachment of proteins to apatite created by other techniques. Adsorption of protein onto biomimetic apatite does not cause any change in the morphology of the mineral (Luong et al. 2006; Liu et al. 2001), since adsorption is a surface phenomenon and does not result in protein integration into the mineral structure (Figure 1.3).

Coating substrates with BLM enhances specificity of protein adsorption. For example, apatite formed on titanium from saturated Ca–P solutions selectively adsorbs proteins from serum and in higher amounts compared to plasma-sprayed hydroxyapatite coatings (Wen, Hippensteel, and Li 2005). Similarly, bioactive glass coated with BLM specifically adsorbs high molecular weight proteins such as fibronectin when incubated in serum (El-Ghannam, Ducheyne, and Shapiro 1999). This enhanced specific adsorptive capability has been attributed to the highly nanoporous structure and high surface area and surface roughness of BLM coatings (Wen, Hippensteel, and Li 2005; Murphy et al. 2005). Increased surface adsorption of proteins onto BLM is especially advantageous for in vivo applications since the adsorbed serum protein layer that forms on implants is vital for cell migration and attachment.

Generally, the release kinetics of an adsorbed protein from a material surface involve a burst profile typified by a fast initial spike in release followed by a more gradual release over time. The amount of protein adsorbed and subsequently released is dependent on the characteristics of the protein (most importantly charge and conformation) and the mineral (surface area, charge). Depending on charge, size, and electrostatic interaction with the BLM surface, different proteins exhibit different affinities to, and therefore different release kinetics from BLM coatings. While TGF-β, Nell-1 and osteocalcin are released gradually over time, BSA exhibits a more characteristic burst release profile (Lee et al. 2009; Wen, Hippensteel, and Li 2005; Krout et al. 2005). BLM coatings may reduce the extent of burst release that occurs with some adsorbed proteins, making BLM coatings more useful therapeutic agent carriers. However, it is important to fully characterize the protein being used to understand the influence of its properties on adsorption and release.

Coprecipitation of proteins along with the mineral is another way to control burst release as the protein is physically incorporated into the mineral and distributed spatially throughout the mineral layer, as compared to surface localization seen with adsorption.

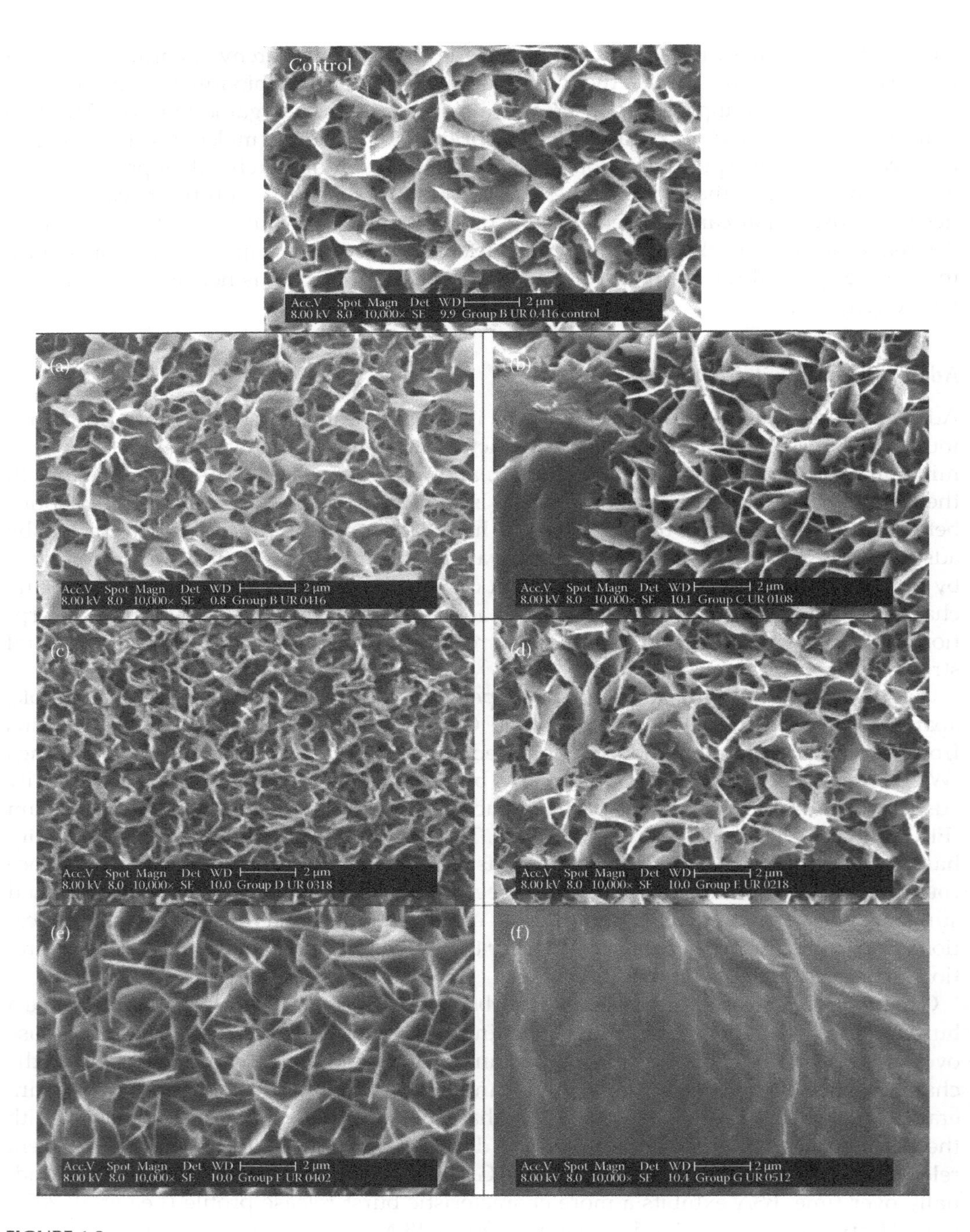

FIGURE 1.3
SEM images of representative samples examined from each of the following groups (magnification 10,000×): (Control) 6-day mineralization, (a) 6-day coprecipitation, (b) 3-day mineralization, 3-day adsorption, (c) 3-day mineralization, 3-day coprecipitation, (d) 3-day mineralization, 2-day adsorption, 1-day mineralization, (e) 3-day mineralization, 2-day coprecipitation, 1-day mineralization, (f) 3-day mineralization, 3-day acid etched adsorption. BSA incorporation via coprecipitation leads to changes in the platelike mineral structure that is observed in the control, whereas BSA adsorption does not change the mineral morphology. (Reprinted from Luong et al., *Biomaterials*, 27, 7, 1175–1186, 2006, with permission from Elsevier.)

For instance, BMP-2 adsorbed on a titanium implant coated with BLM shows a transient release up to 1 week and a sporadic osteogenic response over a 5-week period (Liu, de Groot, and Hunziker 2005).

Surface Adsorption of Peptides to BLM to Enhance Cellular Attachment

Immediately after placing an implant in the body, a protein layer is adsorbed from the surrounding body fluids onto the implant surface, and this protein layer is largely responsible for recruiting cell populations to its surface and mediating all subsequent cellular events (Horbett 2004). An approach that utilizes this adsorbed protein coating to dictate cellular events at the implant surface involves adsorption of adhesive proteins found in the natural bone ECM onto biomaterials, thus attempting to mimic the cell–matrix interactions occurring in vivo. Recognition of specific domains/motifs found within these proteins causes the cells to activate signaling pathways, ultimately resulting in cell proliferation, differentiation, and new bone formation. However, the use of recombinant human and animal proteins in vivo has several disadvantages, including adverse immune responses, enzymatic degradation, and changes in conformation arising from protein–material interactions. Also, proteins usually contain several domains that may be involved in mediating attachment of different types of cells, leading to the possibility of nonspecific cell binding.

Synthetically designed peptides that mimic specific portions of these proteins are able to overcome many of these drawbacks. Table 1.6 provides a list of peptides used in bone tissue engineering. Apart from being cheaper to produce and easier to characterize, peptides are smaller in length (typically 12–30 amino acids) and are less likely to form secondary and tertiary structures, and hence are not affected by changes in conformation. Also, peptides can be engineered to contain domains that are specific to the desired type of cell surface

TABLE 1.6

Examples of Peptides Used in Bone Tissue Engineering Applications

Peptide Sequence	Source/Derived from	Function	Reference
EEEEEEEPRGDT	Bone sialoprotein	Enhances osteoblast adhesion and differentiation	Fujisawa et al. 1997; Itoh et al. 2002
VTKHLNQISQSY	Phage display	Specific affinity toward bone-like mineral (BLM)	Segvich, Smith, and Kohn 2009
KIPKASSVPTELSAISTLYL	BMP2, osteocalcin	Promotes osteogenic differentiation of human mesenchymal stem cells	Lee, Lee, and Murphy 2009
RGDG13PHSRN	Fibronectin	Enhances osteoblast adhesion and differentiation	Benoit and Anseth 2005
KRSR	Heparin	Enhances osteoblast adhesion	Dee, Andersen, and Bizios 1998
DVDVPDGRGDSLAYG	Osteopontin	Enhances osteoblast attachment and differentiation	Shin et al. 2004a, 2004b
SVSVGMKPSPRP	Phage display	Specific affinity toward hydroxyapatite	Roy et al. 2008
(DSS)n	Dentin phosphoprotein	Specific affinity toward calcium phosphate	Yarbrough et al. 2010

Source: Segvich and Kohn 2009, with kind permission from Springer Science + Business Media.

receptors, increasing the likelihood of cell-specific responses (Lebaron and Athanasiou 2000; Segvich, Smith, and Kohn 2009; Hersel, Dahmen, and Kessler 2003).

Noncollagenous proteins found in bone, such as osteopontin, osteonectin, and bone sialoprotein, bind strongly to hydroxyapatite and are thought to be involved in nucleation and growth of crystals during mineralization in vivo (Hunter, Kyle, and Goldberg 1994; Hunter and Goldberg 1994; Fujisawa et al. 1997). These proteins are made up of several regions of acidic amino acids, which are believed to interact with hydroxyapatite crystals. Peptides designed to adhere to hydroxyapatite-based materials have been inspired by these acidic amino acid regions. Peptides consisting of consecutive glutamic acid residues derived from osteonectin bind strongly to hydroxyapatite. The type of acidic amino acid present in these peptides affects mineralization in vitro. For example, polyglutamic acid residues (Glu6) enhanced mineralization, whereas polyaspartic acid residues (Asp6) had an inhibitory effect (Fujisawa et al. 1996). Hence, during the peptide designing process, it is important to understand the contribution of each amino acid to the entire peptide's properties.

ECM proteins are usually multifunctional, containing several domains, allowing them to influence attachment to both materials and cells. Peptidomimetics capable of mediating binding to both hydroxyapatite and cells have been designed using bone sialoprotein as a model. This peptide (EEEEEEEPRGDT) contains a glutamic acid-rich (E7) sequence and the ubiquitous cell binding Arg-Gly-Asp (RGD) domain and binds well to hydroxyapatite, as well as mediates osteoblast attachment and osteogenesis in vitro (Fujisawa et al. 1997; Itoh et al. 2002).

Peptide sequences capable of binding specifically to BLM have recently been identified using a unique combination of phage display and computational modeling techniques (Segvich, Smith, and Kohn 2009) (Figure 1.4). Phage display is a powerful tool as it allows for a wide range of peptides (~10^9) to be panned against any substrate, including natural

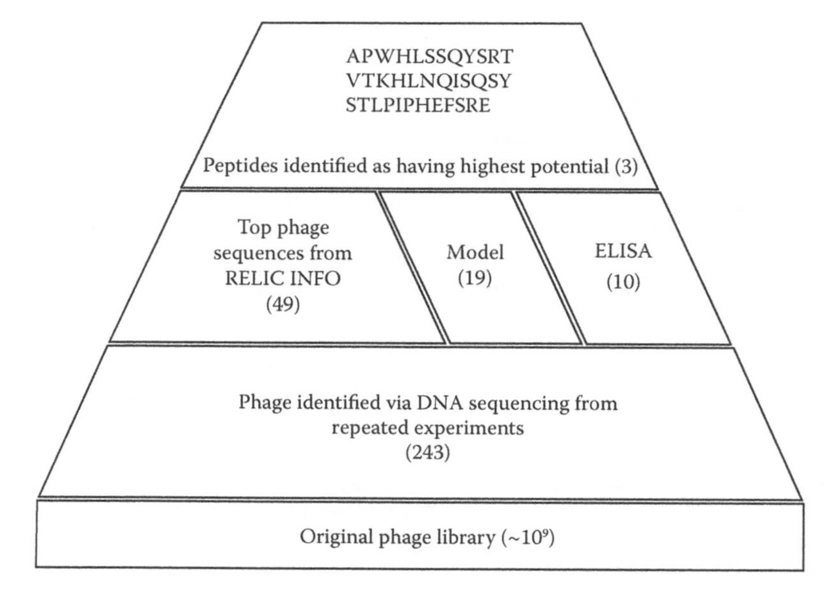

FIGURE 1.4
Schematic displaying the trifold analysis approach used to identify peptides that preferentially bind to BLM and HA. (Reprinted from Segvich, H.J., Smith, H.C., and Kohn, D.H., *Biomaterials*, Vol. 30, pp. 1287–1298, 2009, with permission from Elsevier.)

and synthetic materials, cells, proteins, and viruses, leading to the identification of a few highly specific amino acid sequences. This technique along with ELISA, peptide adsorption assays, and computer modeling were used to discover the peptide VTKHLNQISQSY (VTK), which binds with specific affinity to BLM and HA. An interesting fact is that the VTK peptide has no acidic amino acids, contrary to previously designed HA-binding peptides and therefore is unlikely to have been identified without phage panning.

The same techniques can also be applied to identify cell-specific sequences, allowing for the development of dual functioning peptides that are capable of modulating both mineral-binding and cell adhesion. Multifunctional peptides, whose sequences are inspired by known ECM proteins and growth factors, have also been designed. "Modular" peptides consisting of hydroxyapatite-binding domains derived from osteocalcin and biologically active BMP-2 derived domains bind well to BLM coatings and are capable of directing human mesencyhmal stem cells down osteoblast lineages (Lee, Lee, and Murphy 2009).

The use of protein engineering allows for the development of a new class of biomaterials that are capable of tailoring cellular attachment and function on BLM coatings. The addition of peptides with different charges and conformations into SBF solutions can be used to study nucleation and growth of mineral to gain insight into mineralization processes. Also, peptides can be modified to incorporate important posttranslational modifications such as phosphorylation and glycosylation of certain amino acid residues and can be studied for their effects on mineral formation and cellular differentiation.

Adsorption of DNA to Mineral

Gene therapy may overcome the drawbacks of bioavailability, systemic toxicity, in vivo clearance rate, and manufacturing costs associated with protein delivery (Park, Jeong, and Kim 2006). Design considerations for gene therapy include choosing an effective gene and an efficient and safe delivery system that protects from gene degradation while facilitating transfer to target cells. There are two general methods of gene administration: viral and nonviral.

Viral techniques utilize an adenoviral, retroviral, or lentiviral construct to deliver the gene of interest to the target cell. Disadvantages of using viral gene therapy include mutation risk, induction of immunogenic response, size limitation of DNA construct, and toxicity at high dosages to several tissues (Stigter, de Groot, and Layrolle 2002).

Nonviral delivery methods include naked DNA adsorption, adsorption of conjugated DNA, and coprecipitation of conjugated DNA. Nonviral plasmid DNA conjugation with cationic polymers and liposomal vectors reduces degradation and allows targeting specific cell types; however, surface aggregation and interaction with the biomaterial can reduce transfection efficiency (Luong, McFalls, and Kohn 2009; Shen, Tan, and Saltzman 2004; Park et al. 2003; Jang and Shea 2003; Kofron and Laurencin 2004). Many of the same methods that were used with growth factors can be used to incorporate DNA onto the surface of the mineral coating. Similar to growth factor delivery, adsorption of both naked DNA and DNA lipoplexes results in a burst release of nucleic acid.

Coprecipitation of Proteins and Mineral

An important requirement of a delivery system for sustained release of bioactive molecules is the ability to control the spatial and temporal localization of the molecules across the thickness of the substrate. Such control, along with the degradation and diffusion properties of the carrier will enable the release kinetics to be tailored to achieve a desired biological response. Adsorption, being largely a surface phenomenon and characterized by weak binding forces and burst release, is not useful in producing spatial distributions and/or gradients of biomolecules. Coprecipitation involves adding the protein into the saturated calcium–phosphate solution, resulting in a heterogeneous matrix consisting of both mineral and protein being simultaneously precipitated onto the substrate. It is possible to distribute single or multiple molecules over sections or the entire thickness of the coating by varying the time periods of mineralization and coprecipitation, thus producing gradients of bioactive molecules within the biomaterial (Luong et al. 2006) (Figure 1.5). Further, since the precipitation occurs at ambient temperatures, loss in biological activity of the protein can be minimized.

Effect of Protein Addition on BLM Formation

Bovine serum albumin (BSA) is often used as a model protein to understand the influence of proteins on mineral nucleation and growth. Addition of BSA to SBF causes a delay in the mineral nucleation and growth, indicating that BSA inhibits these processes (Luong

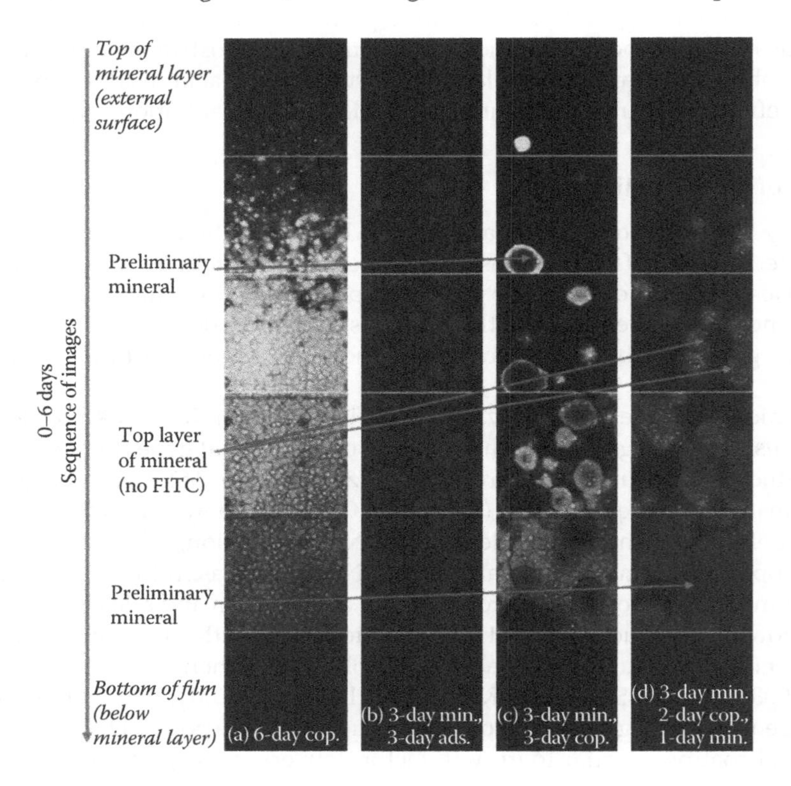

FIGURE 1.5
Images through the thickness of the mineral layer containing FITC-labeled BSA taken using confocal microscopy. Spatial distribution of the protein through the thickness of the mineral layer is exhibited for the following incorporation techniques: (a) 6-day coprecipitation, (b) 3-day mineralization, 3-day adsorption, (c) 3-day mineralization, 3-day coprecipitation, (d) 3-day mineralization, 2-day coprecipitation, 1-day mineralization. Fluorescence can be seen where coprecipitation or adsorption has occurred. Control over the spatial distribution of the protein is shown by the presence of fluorescence through the thickness of the mineral for the different coprecipitation groups. (Reprinted from Luong et al., *Biomaterials*, 27(7), 1175–1186, 2006, with permission from Elsevier.)

et al. 2006). These inhibitory effects are stronger when the BSA is in solution as compared to being preadsorbed onto the substrate (Areva et al. 2002). Also, the stage at which the protein is included affects the extent of inhibition in a concentration-dependent manner. Increasing BSA concentration causes an increase in induction periods for apatite nucleation. Addition of low concentrations of BSA (<10 g/l) during the growth phase causes an increase in the growth rate of the crystals, whereas higher concentrations (>10 g/l) inhibit the growth rate (Combes, Rey, and Freche 1999). Although the exact mechanism by which coprecipitation occurs is not completely understood and may differ from protein to protein, these results suggest that proteins may modulate apatite formation by adsorbing to the initially formed nuclei and stabilizing them by causing a decrease in interfacial energy between the crystal and solution. At low concentrations, there is no sufficient protein to coat the entire mineral surface, allowing the nuclei to grow quickly. At higher concentrations due to coverage of the mineral surface by the protein molecules, growth is prevented (Combes and Rey 2002).

Mineral crystals nucleated in the presence of BSA are smaller in size and less crystalline compared to mineral formed in the absence of BSA (Liu et al. 2001; Combes and Rey 2002). The morphology of the mineral is also affected; protein-free SBF forms sharp platelike mineral crystals that are rounded in the presence of BSA (Luong et al. 2006; Liu et al. 2001) (Figure 1.2). Coprecipitating BSA onto a premineralized surface causes higher quantities of BSA to be loaded, which has been attributed to ability of the negatively charged BSA to interact with the positively charged Ca^{2+} ions. The BSA is attracted to the Ca^{2+} ions in the preliminary mineral layer, causing it to be incorporated into the mineral, which then attracts the Ca^{2+} ions from solution, resulting in a cyclical growth process (Luong et al. 2006; Liu et al. 2001). This interaction of BSA with Ca^{2+} ions is confirmed by slower release of Ca^{2+} ions from coatings formed by coprecipitation with BSA as compared to that in the absence of BSA (Liu et al. 2003).

The above findings show that coprecipitation can be used to integrate proteins into the mineral layer, with their subsequent release being dependent primarily on the rate of dissolution of the mineral. The interaction of each protein with different types of mineral is dependent on several factors including the size, concentration, and charge of the protein, and its influence on the mineral characteristics such as size and crystallinity.

Applications of Protein Coprecipitation in Bone Tissue Engineering

Coprecipitation has been used to incorporate ECM proteins, enzymes, and drugs into biomimetic calcium phosphate coatings. Bone analogs have been produced by coprecipitation of collagen I and mineral onto PLLA substrates using a highly concentrated SBF solution such as 5XSBF. These coatings are capable of enhancing proliferation and differentiation of Saos-2 cells (human osteosarcoma cell line) in vitro (Chen et al. 2008). Coprecipitation has also been used to incorporate enzymes such as amylase and lysozyme into BLM coatings on starch-based polymers (Leonor et al. 2003). These materials can be potentially used as stimulus-responsive scaffolds, undergoing gradual degradation by the incorporated enzyme over time (Martins et al. 2009). Antibiotics such as tobramycin have also been integrated into biomimetic Ca–P coatings on titanium implants and hinder bacterial growth. Biomimetically coated implants that are coprecipitated with antibiotics not only possess the osteoconductive properties of BLM coatings, but are also capable of preventing postoperative infections (Stigter, de Groot, and Layrolle 2002).

Cell–matrix interactions in the natural bone environment orchestrate complex growth factor release profiles that help control bone resorption and formation. TGF-β1 is present in high concentrations during early fracture repair processes, but levels off in later stages, eliciting specific responses resulting from these concentration changes. For instance, in the early stages of repair, TGF-β1 promotes division of fibroblasts, osteoblast recruitment, and differentiation, whereas in later stages, it promotes osteoclastogenesis. Therefore, a temporally graded administration of TGF-β1 would enhance the repair and regeneration process. Similarly, BMP2 promotes chemotaxis and cell proliferation at low concentrations and cell differentiation and bone formation at high concentrations (Allori, Sailon, and Warren 2008). Likewise, a pulsatile delivery of BMP2 may be optimal for tissue regeneration strategies.

Coprecipitation can tailor the administration of growth factors and bioactive molecules to control their release kinetics and the rate of tissue regeneration. For example, rat bone marrow cells cultured on titanium alloys coated with biomimetically precipitated BLM and BMP-2 showed a significant increase in bone formation compared to adsorption (Hunter and Goldberg 1994). This method of growth factor incorporation into the mineral matrix allowed for a sustained release over a period of 5 weeks as compared to the 1-week burst release of adsorbed growth factor that only produced a sporadic osteogenic response. Although the same amount of BMP-2 was used for both methods, BMP incorporated via coprecipitation showed more of a sustained osteogenic response (Liu, de Groot, and Hunziker 2004). Similarly, insulin-like growth factor-1 (IGF-1) coprecipitated with BLM on PLGA scaffolds showed a sustained and linearly increasing release profile over a 30-day period (Jayasuriya and Shah 2008).

A complex biological response such as tissue regeneration is a result of the coordinated cellular events involving the sequential secretion of multiple growth factors. Coprecipitation and surface immobilization could be used to customize and mimic these coordinated events. For example, TGF-β1 also regulates gene expression of other growth factors such as VEGF. In a rat mandibular orthotopic model, TGF-β and VEGF mRNA transcription increased 2.5-fold only 3 h after surgery and TGF-β and VEGF expression increased 3-fold compared to baseline levels for 4 weeks after wound healing commenced (Allori, Sailon, and Warren 2008). Incorporation of multiple growth factors into a single construct has the potential to enhance bioactivity. For example, the delivery of TGF-β and BMP-2 delivery from alginate gels resulted in greater bone tissue formation after 6 weeks, but no significant changes were observed even 22 weeks after implantation when they were administered alone (Simmons et al. 2004).

Coprecipitation provides the flexibility to tailor release profiles since the concentrations of different growth factors could be graded separately through the thickness of the coating. A similar coordinated response can be achieved by coupling coprecipitation of proteins with surface immobilization methods; the adsorbed molecule could be released in a burst profile and the coprecipitated molecule could be delivered in a sustained fashion.

Coprecipitation of DNA and Mineral

DNA coprecipitation allows the incorporation of nucleic acids into the biomimetically precipitated mineral layer at physiological conditions (Figure 1.6). Similar to growth factors, coprecipitation with mineral can be used to control the spatial distribution of DNA through the thickness of the coating. As the mineral layer degrades in physiological conditions, DNA will be released in a spatially and temporally controlled manner. Coprecipitation of mineral also improves the stiffness of soft substrate surfaces, which improves cellular uptake of DNA (Kong et al. 2005).

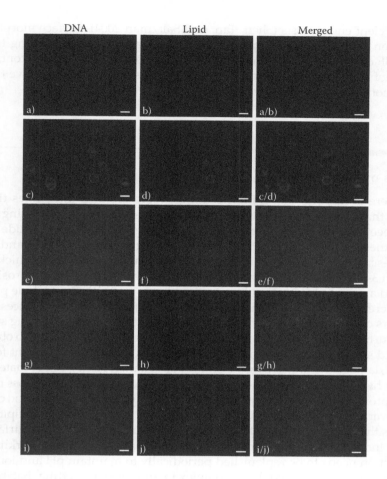

FIGURE 1.6
Fluorescence images of DNA and lipid agent components from representative samples from each of the following groups. (a–b) Mineralized controls, (c–d) plasmid DNA incorporated into PLGA, (e–f) plasmid DNA coprecipitated with mineral, (g–h) plasmid DNA-lipoplex adsorbed to mineralized films, (i–j) plasmid DNA-lipoplex coprecipitated with mineral. Distribution of both the plasmid DNA and the lipid transfection agent on the bone-like mineral was demonstrated by the colocalization of the fluorescent staining in the adsorption and coprecipitation groups and the absence of staining in the mineralized controls. Scale bars represent 100 um. (Reprinted from Luong et al., *Biomaterials*, 30(36), 6996–7004, 2009, with permission from Elsevier.)

The method of DNA application affects transfection efficiency. For example, adsorbed lipoplexes and coprecipitated lipoplexes show significantly different transfection efficiencies. Encapsulation of DNA in a calcium phosphate precipitate improves cellular uptake and produces an enhanced cellular response compared to lipoplexing techniques (Jordan 1996). DNA-lipoplexes coprecipitated with BLM show higher transfection efficiency compared to adsorbed lipoplexes, and coprecipitated naked DNA. This improved transfection efficiency arises from enhanced cellular uptake and protection from degradation as a result of cationic lipid complexation, along with the higher availability of apatite at the surface controlling the rate of release (Luong, McFalls, and Kohn 2009).

Transfection efficiency can also be improved by altering the ionic concentrations of SBF. For instance, removing Mg ions from the solution improves DNA incorporation and facilitates efficient endocytosis (Shen, Tan, and Saltzman 2004). Surface morphology and DNA retention at the mineral surface play an important role in improving transfection efficiency. SBF concentrations and coprecipitation time can be altered to control the dissolution rate of the mineral layer and subsequent release of DNA to improve transfection efficiency (Luong, McFalls, and Kohn 2009).

Drawbacks of Using BLM

Although there is merit to using BLM coatings, there are also difficulties that may be encountered that need to be acknowledged. Challenges that arise when using SBF to coat implants, especially porous and porous-coated implants and scaffolds, include controlling coating thickness, preserving substrate stability during functionalization, and translation to industrial-scale processes. As with all apatite coating techniques, the thickness of the BLM layer on 3-D scaffolds needs to be controlled to maintain sufficient porosity for mass transport and angiogenesis. An implant coating that is too thick can occlude pores, which would interfere with tissue perfusion and vascular infiltration in vivo. Excessively thick mineral layers can result in delamination of the coating from the underlying substrate.

Substrate surface functionalization is carried out before incubation in SBF to obtain a negatively charged surface for calcium nucleation. However, prolonged treatment for functionalization can damage the underlying substrate. For instance, PLGA/PLLA materials etched with sodium hydroxide can undergo considerable hydrolysis resulting in loss of structure, thereby compromising mechanical stability. The necessity for functionalization creates some limitations over the types of substrates that can be used for biomimetic precipitation (Table 1.2) as well as the types of methods that could be used to functionalize the surface.

Achieving industrial-scale batch processing could be a problem when working with SBF. The SBF solution needs to be replenished periodically to maintain pH and ion concentrations near saturation, which would be complex in an industrial setting. Batch processing implants in large volumes of liquid under sterile conditions to prevent contamination can also prove to be difficult.

One main disadvantage of using coprecipitation to create organic/inorganic hybrid materials is the low efficiency of biomolecule incorporation. Although biomolecule retention on BLM is higher with coprecipitation than with adsorption, only about 10% loading can be achieved with coprecipitation. Therefore coprecipitation requires large concentrations of biomolecules to elicit a desired response, which becomes expensive for growth factor administration.

Conclusions

Bone is a complex and dynamic composite tissue that consists of both inorganic and organic phases, supporting cellular adhesion, proliferation, and differentiation. The technique of biomimetic calcium phosphate precipitation attempts to simulate aspects of this complexity by forming a BLM coating on the surface of natural and synthetic substrates. This mineral layer makes a biomaterial more osteoconductive, as well as enhances mechanical strength and stiffness, which are important requirements for load-bearing implants. Inductivity can be integrated into this conductive approach by the incorporation of biomolecules such as proteins, peptides, and DNA to generate inorganic/organic hybrids that are capable of facilitating and enhancing cell–matrix interactions.

These hybrids can be synthesized using adsorption or coprecipitation techniques, or a combination of both depending on the type of response desired. Protein engineering can be utilized to recruit bone cell populations initially to implant surfaces, by designing peptides that bind specifically with strong affinity to both BLM materials and cells. These peptides mimic naturally found bone ECM adhesive proteins, such as osteopontin and bone sialoprotein, and mediate cell adhesion to apatite. Coprecipitating mineral and biomolecules can provide the signaling cues required for cell proliferation and differentiation, leading to new bone formation. Coprecipitation also provides control over spatial and temporal release of the biomolecules, allowing for multiple growth factor delivery during different stages of cellular differentiation, a concept similar to growth factor sequestration by the ECM in vivo. A blend of both adsorption and coprecipitation, in conjunction with biomimetically precipitated apatite, can be utilized to develop bone analogs that mimic the natural environment with greater precision, thereby ensuring controlled and uniform tissue regeneration.

References

Abe, Y., Kokubo, T., and Yamamuro, T. 1990, Apatite Coating on Ceramics, Metals and Polymers Utilizing a Biological Process, *Journal of Materials Science: Materials in Medicine*, Vol. 1, pp. 233–238.

Agata De Sena, L., Calixto De Andrade, M., Malta Rossi, A., and de Almeida Soares, G. 2002, Hydroxyapatite Deposition by Electrophoresis on Titanium Sheets with Different Surface Finishing, *Journal of Biomedical Materials Research*, Vol. 60, No. 1, pp. 1–7.

Albrektsson, T., and Johansson, C. 2001, Osteoinduction, Osteoconduction and Osseointegration, *European Spine Journal: Official Publication of the European Spine Society, the European Spinal Deformity Society, and the European Section of the Cervical Spine Research Society*, Vol. 10, Suppl. 2, pp. S96–S101.

Allori, A.C., Sailon, A.M., and Warren, S.M. 2008, Biological Basis of Bone Formation, Remodeling, and Repair—Part I: Biochemical Signaling Molecules, *Tissue Engineering Part B, Reviews*, Vol. 14, No. 3, pp. 259–273.

Alsberg, E., Hill, E.E., and Mooney, D.J. 2001, Craniofacial Tissue Engineering, *Critical Reviews in Oral Biology & Medicine*, Vol. 12, No. 1, pp. 64–75.

Antonov, E.N., Bagratashvilli, V.N., Popov, V.K., Sobol, E.N., Howdle, S.M., Joiner, C., Parker, K.G., Parker, T.L., Doktorov, A.A., Likhanov, V.B., Volozhin, A.I., Alimpiev, S.S., and Nikiforov, S.S. 1998, Biocompatibility of Laser-Deposited Hydroxylapatite Coatings on Titanium and Polymer Implant Materials, *Journal of Biomedical Optics*, Vol. 3, No. 4, pp. 423–428.

Araujo, J.V., Martins, A., Leonor, I.B., Pinho, E.D., Reis, R.L., and Neves, N.M. 2008, Surface controlled Biomimetic Coating of Polycaprolactone Nanofiber Meshes to Be Used as Bone Extracellular Matrix Analogues, *Journal of Biomaterials Science—Polymer Edition*, Vol. 19, No. 10, pp. 1261–1278.

Areva, S., Peltola, T., Sailynoja, E., Laajalehto, K., Linden, M., and Rosenholm, J.B. 2002, Effect of Albumin and Fibrinogen on Calcium Phosphate Formation on Sol–Gel Derived Titania Coatings in Vitro, *Chemistry of Materials*, Vol. 14, pp. 1614–1621.

Baeri, P., Torrisi, L., Marino, N., and Foti, G. 1992, Ablation of Hydroxyapatite by Pulsed Laser Irradiation, *Applied Surface Science*, Vol. 54, pp. 210–214.

Baron, R. 2003, General Principles of Bone Biology, in *Primer on the Metabolic Bone Diseases and Disorders of Mineral Metabolism*, American Society for Bone and Mineral Research, Washington D.C., pp. 1–8.

Barrere, F., van der Valk, C.M., Dalmeijer, R.A., van Blitterswijk, C.A., de Groot, K., and Layrolle, P. 2003a, In Vitro and in Vivo Degradation of Biomimetic Octacalcium Phosphate and Carbonate Apatite Coatings on Titanium Implants, *Journal of Biomedical Materials Research. Part A*, Vol. 64, No. 2, pp. 378–387.

Barrere, F., van der Valk, C.M., Meijer, G., Dalmeijer, R.A., de Groot, K., and Layrolle, P. 2003b, Osteointegration of Biomimetic Apatite Coating Applied onto Dense and Porous Metal Implants in Femurs of Goats, *Journal of Biomedical Materials Research. Part B, Applied Biomaterials*, Vol. 67, No. 1, pp. 655–665.

Benoit, D.S.W., and Anseth, K.S. 2005, The Effect on Osteoblast Function of Colocalized RGD and PHSRN Epitopes on PEG Surfaces, *Biomaterials*, Vol. 26, pp. 5209–5220.

Bernhardt, R., van den Dolder, J., Bierbaum, S., Beutner, R., Scharnweber, D., Jansen, J., Beckmann, F., and Worch, H. 2005, Osteoconductive Modifications of Ti-Implants in a Goat Defect Model: Characterization of Bone Growth with SR μCT and Histology, *Biomaterials*, Vol. 26, No. 16, pp. 3009–3019.

Biondi, M., Ungaro, F., Quaglia, F., and Netti, P.A. 2008, Controlled Drug Delivery in Tissue Engineering, *Advanced Drug Delivery Reviews*, Vol. 60, No. 2, pp. 229–242.

Bollen, C.M., Lambrechts, P., and Quirynen, M. 1997, Comparison of Surface Roughness of Oral Hard Materials to the Threshold Surface Roughness for Bacterial Plaque Retention: A Review of the Literature, *Dental Materials: Official Publication of the Academy of Dental Materials*, Vol. 13, No. 4, pp. 258–269.

Bunker, B.C., Rieke, P.C., Tarasevich, B.J., Campbell, A.A., Fryxell, G.E., Graff, G.L., Song, L., Liu, J., Virden, J.W., and McVay, G.L. 1994, Ceramic Thin-Film Formation on Functionalized Interfaces Through Biomimetic Processing, *Science*, Vol. 264, pp. 48–55.

Campbell, A.A., Song, L., Li, X.S., Nelson, B.J., Bottoni, C., Brooks, D.E., and DeJong, E.S. 2000, Development, Characterization, and Anti-Microbial Efficacy of Hydroxyapatite-Chlorhexidine Coatings Produced by Surface-Induced Mineralization, *Journal of Biomedical Materials Research*, Vol. 53, No. 4, pp. 400–407.

Chai, C.S., Gross, K.A., and Ben-Nissan, B. 1998, Critical Ageing of Hydroxyapatite Sol–Gel Solutions, *Biomaterials*, Vol. 19, No. 24, pp. 2291–2296.

Chen, J., Wolke, J.G.C., and de Groot, K. 1994, Microstructure and Crystallinity in Hydroxyapatite Coatings, *Biomaterials*, Vol. 15, No. 5, pp. 396–399.

Chen, Y., Mak, A.F.T., Wang, M., Li, J.S., and Wong, M.S. 2008, In Vitro Behavior of Osteoblast-Like Cells on PLLA Films with a Biomimetic Apatite or Apatite/Collagen Composite Coating, *Journal of Materials Science: Materials in Medicine*, Vol. 19, pp. 2261–2268.

Choi, J., Bogdanski, D., Köller, M., Esenwein, S.A., Müller, D., Muhr, G., and Epple, M. 2003, Calcium Phosphate Coating of Nickel–Titanium Shape-Memory Alloys. Coating Procedure and Adherence of Leukocytes and Platelets, *Biomaterials*, Vol. 24, No. 21, pp. 3689–3696.

Chou, L., Marek, B., and Wagner, W.R. 1999, Effects of Hydroxylapatite Coating Crystallinity on Biosolubility, Cell Attachment Efficiency and Proliferation In Vitro, *Biomaterials*, Vol. 20, No. 10, pp. 977–985.

Clèries, L., Martínez, E., Fernández-Pradas, J.M., Sardin, G., Esteve, J., and Morenza, J.L. 2000, Mechanical Properties of Calcium Phosphate Coatings Deposited by Laser Ablation, *Biomaterials*, Vol. 21, No. 9, pp. 967–971.

Combes, C., and Rey, C. 2002, Adsorption of Proteins and Calcium Phosphate Materials Bioactivity, *Biomaterials*, Vol. 23, pp. 2817–2823.

Combes, C., Rey, C., and Freche, M. 1999, *In Vitro* Crystallization of Octacalcium Phosphate on Type I Collagen: Influence of Serum Albumin, *Journal of Materials Science: Materials in Medicine*, Vol. 10, pp. 153–160.

Dalby, M.J., Gadegaard, N., Tare, R., Andar, A., Riehle, M.O., Herzyk, P., Wilkinson, C.D., and Oreffo, R.O. 2007, The Control of Human Mesenchymal Cell Differentiation Using Nanoscale Symmetry and Disorder, *Nature Materials*, Vol. 6, pp. 997–1003.

Dalby, M.J., Riehle, M.O., Sutherland, D.S., Agheli, H., and Curtis, A.S.G. 2004, Use of Nanotopography to Study Mechanotransduction in Fibroblasts—Methods and Perspectives, *European Journal of Cell Biology*, Vol. 83, No. 4, pp. 159–169.

De Groot, K., Geesink, R., Klein, C.P.A.T., and Serekian, P. 1987, Plasma Sprayed Coatings of Hydroxylapatite, *Journal of Biomedical Materials Research,* Vol. 21, pp. 1375–1381.

Dee, K.C., Andersen, T.T., and Bizios, R. 1998, Design and Function of Novel Osteoblast-Adhesive Peptides for Chemical Modification of Biomaterials, *Journal of Biomedical Materials Research,* Vol. 40, pp. 371–377.

Deligianni, D.D., Katsala, N.D., Koutsoukos, P.G., and Missirlis, Y.F. 2001, Effect of Surface Roughness of Hydroxyapatite on Human Bone Marrow Cell Adhesion, Proliferation, Differentiation and Detachment Strength, *Biomaterials,* Vol. 22, No. 1, pp. 87–96.

Ding, S.J., Ju, C.P., and Lin, J.H. 1999, Characterization of Hydroxyapatite and Titanium Coatings Sputtered on Ti-6Al-4V Substrate, *Journal of Biomedical Materials Research,* Vol. 44, No. 3, pp. 266–279.

Ding, S. 2003, Properties and Immersion Behavior of Magnetron-Sputtered Multi-Layered Hydroxyapatite/Titanium Composite Coatings, *Biomaterials,* Vol. 24, No. 23, pp. 4233–4238.

Discher, D.E., Mooney, D.J., and Zandstra, P.W. 2009, Growth Factors, Matrices, and Forces Combine and Control Stem Cells, *Science,* Vol. 324, No. 5935, pp. 1673–1677.

Ducheyne, P., Radin, S., Heughebaert, M., and Heughebaert, J.C. 1990, Calcium phosphate Ceramic Coatings on Porous Titanium: Effect of Structure and Composition on Electrophoretic Deposition, Vacuum Sintering and *In Vitro* Dissolution, *Biomaterials,* Vol. 11, pp. 244–254.

Ducheyne, P. 1985, Bioglass Coatings and Bioglass Composites as Implant Materials, *Journal of Biomedical Materials Research,* Vol. 19, pp. 273–291.

Ducheyne, P., Van Raemdonck, W., Heughebaert, J.C., and Heughebaert, M. 1986, Structural Analysis of Hydroxyapatite Coatings on Titanium, *Biomaterials,* Vol. 7, No. 2, pp. 97–103.

El-Ghannam, A., Ducheyne, P., and Shapiro, I.M. 1999, Effect of Serum Proteins on Osteoblast Adhesion to Surface-Modified Bioactive Glass and Hydroxyapatite, *Journal of Orthopaedic Research,* Vol. 17, pp. 340–345.

Engler, A.J., Sen, S., Sweeney, H.L., and Discher, D.E. 2006, Matrix Elasticity Directs Stem Cell Lineage Specification, *Cell,* Vol. 126, No. 4, pp. 677–689.

Feddes, B., Vredenburg, A.M., Wolke, J.G.C., and Jansen, J.A. 2004, Bulk Composition of RF Magnetron Sputter Deposited Calcium Phosphate Coatings on Different Substrates (Polyethylene, Polytetrafluoroethylene, Silicon), *Surface Coatings and Technology,* Vol. 185, pp. 346–355.

Fernández-Pradas, J.M., Clèries, L., Martínez, E., Sardin, G., Esteve, J., and Morenza, J.L. 2001, Influence of Thickness on the Properties of Hydroxyapatite Coatings Deposited by KrF LASER Ablation, *Biomaterials,* Vol. 22, No. 15, pp. 2171–2175.

Frayssinet, P., Tourenne, F., Rouquet, N., Conte, P., Delga, C., and Bonel, G. 1994, Comparative Biological Properties of HA Plasma-Sprayed Coatings Having Different Crystallinities, *Journal of Materials Science: Materials in Medicine,* Vol. 5, No. 1, pp. 11.

Fujibayashi, S., Neo, M., Kim, H., Kokubo, T., and Nakamura, T. 2004, Osteoinduction of Porous Bioactive Titanium Metal, *Biomaterials,* Vol. 25, No. 3, pp. 443–450.

Fujisawa, R., Mizuno, M., Nodasaka, Y., and Kuboki, Y. 1997, Attachment of Osteoblastic Cells to Hydroxyapatite by a Synthetic Peptide (Glu7-Pro-Arg-Gly-Asp-Thr) Containing Two Functional Sequences of Bone Sialoprotein, *Matrix Biology,* Vol. 16, pp. 21–28.

Fujisawa, R., Wada, Y., Nodasak, Y., and Kuboki, Y. 1996, Acidic Amino Acid-Rich Sequences as Binding Sites of Osteonectin to Hydroxyapatite Crystals, *Biochimica et Biophysica Acta,* Vol. 1292, pp. 53–60.

Girija, E.K., Yokogawa, Y., and Nagata, F. 2002, Bone-Like Apatite Formation on Collagen Fibrils by Biomimetic Method, *Chemical Letters,* pp. 702–703.

Griffin, M.A., Sen, S., Sweeney, H.L., and Discher, D.E. 2004, Adhesion-Contractile Balance in Myocyte Differentiation, *Journal of Cell Science,* Vol. 117, No. 24, pp. 5855–5863.

Gross, K.A., and Berndt, C.C. 1998, Thermal Processing of Hydroxyapatite for Coating Production, *Journal of Biomedical Materials Research,* Vol. 39, No. 4, pp. 580–587.

Gross, K.A., Berndt, C.C., and Herman, H. 1998, Amorphous Phase Formation in Plasma-Sprayed Hydroxyapatite Coatings, *Journal of Biomedical Materials Research,* Vol. 39, No. 3, pp. 407–414.

Habibovic, P., Barrère, F., Blitterswijk, C.A., Groot, K., and Layrolle, P. 2002, Biomimetic Hydroxyapatite Coating on Metal Implants, *Journal of the American Ceramic Society,* Vol. 85, No. 3, pp. 517–522.

Habibovic, P., Li, J., van der Valk, C.M., Meijer, G., Layrolle, P., van Blitterswijk, C.A., and de Groot, K. 2005, Biological Performance of Uncoated and Octacalcium Phosphate-Coated Ti_6Al_4V, *Biomaterials,* Vol. 26, No. 1, pp. 23–36.

Han, Y., Fu, T., Lu, J., and Xu, K. 2001, Characterization and Stability of Hydroxyapatite Coatings Prepared by an Electrodeposition and Alkaline-Treatment Process, *Journal of Biomedical Materials Research,* Vol. 54, No. 1, pp. 96–101.

Han, Y., Xu, K., Lu, J., and Wu, Z. 1999, The Structural Characteristics and Mechanical Behaviors of Nonstoichiometric Apatite Coatings Sintered in Air Atmosphere, *Journal of Biomedical Materials Research,* Vol. 45, No. 3, pp. 198–203.

Hench, L.L. 1991, Bioceramics: From Concept to Clinic, *Journal of the American Ceramic Society,* Vol. 74, No. 7, pp. 1487–1510.

Herø, H., Wie, H., Jørgensen, R.B., and Ruyter, I.E. 1994, Hydroxyapatite Coatings on Ti Produced by Hot Isostatic Pressing, *Journal of Biomedical Materials Research,* Vol. 28, No. 3, pp. 343–348.

Hersel, U., Dahmen, C., and Kessler, H. 2003, RGD Modified Polymers: Biomaterials for Stimulated Cell Adhesion and Beyond, *Biomaterials,* Vol. 24, pp. 4385–4415.

Hirano, Y., and Mooney, D. 2004, Peptide and Protein Presenting Materials for Tissue Engineering, *Advanced Materials,* Vol. 16, No. 1, pp. 17–25.

Honstu, S., Matsumotu, T., Ishii, J., Nakamori, M., Tabata, H., and Kawai, T. 1997, Electrical Properties of Hydroxyapatite Thin Films Grown by Pulsed Laser Deposition, *Thin Solid Films,* Vol. 295, pp. 214–217.

Horbett, T.A. 2004, The Role of Adsorbed Proteins in Tissue Response to Biomaterials, in *Biomaterials Science: An Introduction to Materials in Medicine,* B.D. Ratner, A.S. Hoffman, F.J. Schoen, and J.E. Lemons (eds.), 2nd Edition, Elsevier, San Diego, pp. 237–246.

Hunter, G.K., Kyle, L.C., and Goldberg, H.A. 1994, Modulation of Crystal Formation by Bone Phosphoproteins: Structural Specificity of the Osteopontin-Mediated Inhibition of Hydroxyapatite Formation, *Biochemical Journal,* Vol. 300, pp. 723–728.

Hunter, G.K., and Goldberg, H.A. 1994, Modulation of Crystal Formation by Bone Phosphoproteins: Role of Glutamic Acid-Rich Sequences in the Nucleation of Hydroxyapatite by Bone Sialoprotein, *Biochemical Journal,* Vol. 302, pp. 175–179.

Ingber, D.E. 2006, Cellular Mechanotransduction: Putting All the Pieces Together Again, *The FASEB Journal: Official Publication of the Federation of American Societies for Experimental Biology,* Vol. 20, No. 7, pp. 811–827.

Ingber, D.E. 1997, Tensegrity: The Architectural Basis of Cellular Mechanotransduction, *Annual Review of Physiology,* Vol. 59, No. 1, pp. 575–599.

Itoh, D., Yoneda, S., Kuroda, S., Kondo, H., Umezawa, A., Ohya, K., Ohyama, T., and Kasugai, S. 2002, Enhancement of Osteogenesis on Hydroxyapatite Surface Coated with Synthetic Peptide (EEEEEEEPRGDT), *In Vitro, Journal of Biomedical Materials Research,* Vol. 62, pp. 292–298.

Jacobs, J.J., Gilbert, J.L., and Urban, R.M. 1998, Corrosion of Metal Orthopaedic Implants, *The Journal of Bone and Joint Surgery. American Volume,* Vol. 80, No. 2, pp. 268–282.

Jang, J.H., and Shea, L.D. 2003, Controllable Delivery of Non-Viral DNA from Porous Scaffolds, *Journal of Controlled Release: Official Journal of the Controlled Release Society,* Vol. 86, No. 1, pp. 157–168.

Jayasuriya, A.C., and Shah, C. 2008, Controlled Release of Insulin-Like Growth Factor-1 and Bone Marrow Stromal Cell Function of Bone-Like Mineral Layer-Coated Poly(Lactic-*co*-Glycolic Acid) Scaffolds, *Journal of Tissue Engineering and Regenerative Medicine,* Vol. 2, No. 1, pp. 43–49.

Jiang, G., and Shi, D. 1998, Coating of Hydroxyapatite on Highly Porous Al_2O_3 Substrate for Bone Substitutes, *Journal of Biomedical Materials Research,* Vol. 43, No. 1, pp. 77–81.

Jordan, M. 1996, Transfecting Mammalian Cells: Optimization of Critical Parameters Affecting Calcium–Phosphate Precipitate Formation, *Nucleic Acids Research,* Vol. 24, No. 4, pp. 596–601.

Kaneko, A., Hirai, S., Tamada, Y., and Kuzuya, T. 2009, Evaluation of Calcium Phosphate-Coated Silk Fabric Produced by Sol–Gel Processing as a Wound Cover Material, *Sen'i Gakkaishi,* Vol. 65, No. 3, pp. 97–102.

Kilpadi, D.V., and Lemons, J.E. 1994, Surface Energy Characterization of Unalloyed Titanium Implants, *Journal of Biomedical Materials Research,* Vol. 28, No. 12, pp. 1419–1425.

Klein, Christel P. A. T., Patka, P., van der Lubbe, H. B. M., Wolke, J.G.C., and de Groot, K. 1991, Plasma-Sprayed Coatings of Tetracalcium Phosphate, Hydroxyl-Apatite and Alpha-TCP on Titanium Alloy: An Interface Study, *Journal of Biomedical Materials Research*, Vol. 25, No. 53, p. 65.

Kloxin, A.M., Benton, J.A., and Anseth, K.S. 2010, In Situ Elasticity Modulation with Dynamic Substrates to Direct Cell Phenotype, *Biomaterials*, Vol. 31, No. 1, pp. 1–8.

Kocgozlu, L., Lavalle, P., Koenig, G., Senger, B., Haikel, Y., Schaaf, P., Voegel, J.C., Tenenbaum, H., and Vautier, D. 2010, Selective and Uncoupled Role of Substrate Elasticity in the Regulation of Replication and Transcription in Epithelial Cells, *Journal of Cell Science*, Vol. 123, No. Pt 1, pp. 29–39.

Kofron, M.D., and Laurencin, C.T. 2004, Development of a Calcium Phosphate Co-Precipitate/Poly(Lactide-*co*-Glycolide) DNA Delivery System: Release Kinetics and Cellular Transfection Studies, *Biomaterials*, Vol. 25, No. 13, pp. 2637–2643.

Kohn, D.H., Shin, K., Hong, S., Jayasuriya, C.A., Leonova, E.V., Rossello, R.A., and Krebsbach, P.H. 2005, Self-Assembled Mineral Scaffolds as Model Systems for Biomineralization and Tissue Engineering, W.J. Landis, and J. Sodek (eds.), University of Toronto Press, Toronto.

Kokubo, T. 1991, Bioactive Glass Ceramics: Properties and Applications, *Biomaterials*, Vol. 12, No. 2, pp. 155–163.

Kokubo, T. 1996, Formation of Biologically Active Bone-Like Apatite on Metals and Polymers by a Biomimetic Process, *Thermochimica Acta*, Vol. 280/281, pp. 479–490.

Kokubo, T., and Takadama, H. 2006, How Useful Is SBF in Predicting In Vivo Bone Bioactivity?, *Biomaterials*, Vol. 27, No. 15, pp. 2907–2915.

Kong, H.J., Liu, J., Riddle, K., Matsumoto, T., Leach, K. and Mooney, D.J. 2005, Non-Viral Gene Delivery Regulated by Stiffness of Cell Adhesion Substrates, *Nature Materials*, Vol. 4, No. 6, pp. 460–464.

Krout, A., Wen, H.B., Hippensteel, E., and Li, P. 2005, A Hybrid Coating of Biomimetic Apatite and Osteocalcin, *Journal of Biomedical Materials Research A*, Vol. 73A, pp. 377–387.

Lacefield, W.R. 1999, Biomechanical and Morphometric Analysis of Hydroxyapatite-Coated Implants with Varying Crystallinity, *Journal of Oral and Maxillofacial Surgery*, Vol. 57, No. 9, pp. 1108–1109.

Le Guehennec, L., Soueidan, A., Layrolle, P., and Amouriq, Y. 2007, Surface Treatments of Titanium Dental Implants for Rapid Osseointegration, *Dental Materials: Official Publication of the Academy of Dental Materials*, Vol. 23, No. 7, pp. 844–854.

Lebaron, R.G., and Athanasiou, K.A. 2000, Extracellular Matrix Cell Adhesion Peptides: Functional Applications in Orthopedic Materials, *Tissue Engineering*, Vol. 6, No. 2, pp. 85–103.

Lee, J.S., Lee, J.S., and Murphy, W.L. 2009, Modular Peptides Promote Human Mesenchymal Stem Cell Differentiation on Biomaterial Surfaces, *Acta Biomaterialia*, Vol. 6, No. 1, pp. 21–28.

Lee, M., Li, W., Siu, R.K., Whang, J., Zhang, X., Soo, C., Ting, K., and Wu, B.M. 2009, Biomimetic Apatite-Coated Alginate/Chitosan Microspheres as Osteogenic Protein Carriers, *Biomaterials*, Vol. 30, pp. 6094–6101.

LeGeros, R.Z. 2002, Properties of Osteoconductive Biomaterials: Calcium Phosphates, *Clinical Orthopaedics and Related Research*, Vol. 395, pp. 81–98.

Leonor, I.B., Azevedo, H.S., Alves, C.M., and Reis, R.L. 2003, Effects of the Incorporation of Proteins and Active Enzymes on Biomimetic Calcium–Phosphate Coatings, *Key Engineering Materials*, Vol. 240–242, pp. 97–100.

Leonor, I.B., Baran, E.T., Kawashita, M., Reis, R.L., Kokubo, T., and Nakamura, T. 2008, Growth of a Bonelike Apatite on Chitosan Microparticles after a Calcium Silicate Treatment, *Acta Biomaterialia*, Vol. 4, No. 5, pp. 1349–1359.

Leonor, I.B., Kim, H.M., Balas, F., Kawashita, M., Reis, R.L., Kokubo, T., and Nakamura, T. 2007, Alkaline Treatments to Render Starch-Based Biodegradable Polymers Self-Mineralizable, *Journal of Tissue Engineering and Regenerative Medicine*, Vol. 1, No. 425, p. 435.

Leonova, E.V., Pennington, K.E., Krebsbach, P.H., and Kohn, D.H. 2006, Substrate Mineralization Stimulates Focal Adhesion Contact Redistribution and Cell Motility of Bone Marrow Stromal Cells, *Journal of Biomedical Materials Research A*, Vol. 79A, pp. 263–270.

Li, P., De Groot, K., and Kokubo, T. 1996, Bioactive $Ca_{10}(PO_4)_6(OH)_2$–TiO_2 Composite Coating Prepared by Sol–Gel Process, *Journal of Sol–Gel Science and Technology*, Vol. 7, No. 1, pp. 27–34.

Li, H., Khor, K.A., and Cheang, P. 2002, Titanium Dioxide Reinforced Hydroxyapatite Coatings Deposited by High Velocity Oxy-Fuel (HVOF) Spray, *Biomaterials,* Vol. 23, No. 1, pp. 85–91.

Li, J., Liao, H., and Hermansson, L. 1996, Sintering of Partially-Stabilized Zirconia and Partially-Stabilized Zirconia—Hydroxyapatite Composites by Hot Isostatic Pressing and Pressureless Sintering, *Biomaterials,* Vol. 17, No. 18, pp. 1787–1790.

Li, P., Ohtsuki, C., Kokubo, T., Nakanishi, K., Soga, N., Nakamura, T., and Yamamuro, T. 1992, Apatite Formation Induced by Silica Gel in a Simulated Body Fluid, *Journal of the American Ceramic Society,* Vol. 75, No. 8, pp. 2094–2097.

Lian, J.B., Stein, G.S., and Aubin, J.E. 2003, Bone Formation: Maturation and Functional Activities of Osteoblast Lineage Cells, in *Primer on the Metabolic Bone Diseases and Disorders of Mineral Metabolism,* American Society for Bone and Mineral Research, pp. 13–28.

Linhart, W., Peters, F., Lehmann, W., Schwarz, K., Schilling, F.A., Amling, M., Rueger, J.M., and Epple, M. 2001, Biologically and Chemically Optimized Composites of Carbonated Apatite and Polyglycolide as Bone Substitution Materials, *Journal of Biomedical Materials Research,* Vol. 54, No. 2, pp. 166–171.

Liu, Y., and Hunziker, E.B. 2009, Biomimetic Coating and their Biological Functionalization, in *Thin Calcium Phosphate Coatings for Medical Implants,* eds. B. Leon and J. Jansen, 1st Edition, Springer, New York, NY, pp. 301–314.

Liu, D., Yang, Q., and Troczynski, T. 2002, Sol–Gel Hydroxyapatite Coatings on Stainless Steel Substrates, *Biomaterials,* Vol. 23, No. 3, pp. 691–698.

Liu, X., Ding, C., and Chu, P.K. 2004, Mechanism of Apatite Formation on Wollastonite Coatings in Simulated Body Fluids, *Biomaterials,* Vol. 25, No. 10, pp. 1755–1761.

Liu, Y., de Groot, K., and Hunziker, E.B. 2005, BMP-2 Liberated from Biomimetic Implant Coatings Induces and Sustains Direct Ossification in an Ectopic Rat Model, *Bone,* Vol. 36, No. 5, pp. 745–757.

Liu, Y., de Groot, K., and Hunziker, E.B. 2004, Osteoinductive Implants: The Mise-en-Scene for Drug-Bearing Biomimetic Coatings, *Annals of Biomedical Engineering,* Vol. 32, No. 3, pp. 398–406.

Liu, Y., Hunziker, E.B., Randall, N.X., de Groot, K., and Layrolle, P. 2003, Proteins Incorporated into Biomimetically Prepared Calcium Phosphate Coatings Modulate Their Mechanical Strength and Dissolution Rates, *Biomaterials,* Vol. 24, pp. 65–70.

Liu, Y., Layrolle, P., de Bruijn, J., van Blitterswijk, C., and de Groot, K. 2001, Biomimetic Coprecipitation of Calcium Phosphate and Bovine Serum Albumin on Titanium Alloy, *Journal of Biomedical Materials Research,* Vol. 57, pp. 327–335.

Lo, C., Wang, H., Dembo, M., and Wang, Y. 2000, Cell Movement Is Guided by the Rigidity of the Substrate, *Biophysical Journal,* Vol. 79, No. 1, pp. 144–152.

Luong, L.N., Hong, S.I., Patel, R.J., Outslay, M.E., and Kohn, D.H. 2006, Spatial Control of Protein within Biomimetically Nucleated Mineral, *Biomaterials,* Vol. 27, No. 7, pp. 1175–1186.

Luong, L.N., McFalls, K.M., and Kohn, D.H. 2009, Gene Delivery via DNA Incorporation within a Biomimetic Apatite Coating, *Biomaterials,* Vol. 30, No. 36, pp. 6996–7004.

Ma, J., Wang, C., and Peng, K.W. 2003, Electrophoretic Deposition of Porous Hydroxyapatite Scaffold, *Biomaterials,* Vol. 24, No. 20, pp. 3505–3510.

Manso, M., Langlet, M., Jiménez, C., and Martínez-Duart, J.M. 2002, Microstructural Study of Aerosol–Gel Derived Hydroxyapatite Coatings, *Biomolecular Engineering,* Vol. 19, No. 2–6, pp. 63–66.

Manso, M., Jiménez, C., Morant, C., Herrero, P., and Martínez-Duart, J. 2000, Electrodeposition of Hydroxyapatite Coatings in Basic Conditions, *Biomaterials,* Vol. 21, No. 17, pp. 1755–1761.

Marchisio, M., Di Carmine, M., Pagone, R., Piattelli, A., and Miscia, S. 2005, Implant Surface Roughness Influences Osteoclast Proliferation and Differentiation, *Journal of Biomedical Materials Research. Part B, Applied Biomaterials,* Vol. 75, No. 2, pp. 251–256.

Martin, T.J. 1989, Bone Cell Physiology, *Endocrinology and Metabolism Clinics of North America,* Vol. 18, No. 4, pp. 833–858.

Martinez, E., Engel, E., Planell, J.A., and Samitier, J. 2009, Effects of Artificial Micro- and Nano-Structured Surfaces on Cell Behaviour, *Annals of Anatomy—Anatomischer Anzeiger: Official Organ of the Anatomische Gesellschaft,* Vol. 191, No. 1, pp. 126–135.

Martins, A.M., Pham, Q.P., Malafaya, P.B., Raphael, R.M., Kasper, K.F., Reis, R.L., and Mikos, A.G. 2009, Natural Stimulus Responsive Scaffolds/Cells for Bone Tissue Engineering: Influence of Lysozyme upon Scaffold Degradation and Osteogenic Differentiation of Cultured Marrow Stromal Cells Induced by CaP Coatings, *Tissue Engineering: Part A*, Vol. 15, No. 00, pp. 1–11.

Massaro, C., Baker, M.A., Cosentino, F., Ramires, P.A., Klose, S., and Milella, E. 2001, Surface and Biological Evaluation of Hydroxyapatite-Based Coatings on Titanium Deposited by Different Techniques, *Journal of Biomedical Materials Research*, Vol. 58, No. 6, pp. 651–657.

Misra, S.K., Valappil, S.P., Roy, I., and Boccaccini, A.R. 2006, Polyhydroxyalkanoate (PHA)/Inorganic Phase Composites for Tissue Engineering Applications, *Biomacromolecules*, Vol. 7, No. 8, pp. 2249–2258.

Mitragotri, S., and Lahann, J. 2009, Physical Approaches to Biomaterial Design, *Nature Materials*, Vol. 8, No. 1, pp. 15–23.

Montenero, A., Gnappi, G., Ferrari, F., Cesari, M., Salvioli, E., Mattogno, L., Kaciulis, S., and Fini, M. 2000, Sol–Gel Derived Hydroxyapatite Coatings on Titanium Substrate, *Journal of Materials Science*, Vol. 35, No. 11, pp. 2791–2797.

Müller, L., Conforto, E., Caillard, D., and Müller, F.A. 2007, Biomimetic Apatite Coatings—Carbonate Substitution and Preferred Growth Orientation, *Biomolecular Engineering*, Vol. 24, No. 5, pp. 462–466.

Mundy, G.R., Chin, D., and Oyajobi, B. 2003, Bone Remodeling, in *Primer on the Metabolic Bone Diseases and Disorders of Mineral Metabolism*, American Society for Bone and Mineral Research, Washington D.C., pp. 46–58.

Murphy, W.L., Hsiong, S., Richardson, T.P., Simmons, C.A., and Mooney, D.J. 2005, Effects of a Bone-Like Mineral Film on Phenotype of Adult Human Mesenchymal Stem Cells In Vitro, *Biomaterials*, Vol. 26, No. 3, pp. 303–310.

Murphy, W.L., Kohn, D.H., and Mooney, D.J. 2000a, Growth of Continuous Bonelike Mineral within Porous Poly(Lactide-*co*-Glycolide) Scaffolds *In Vitro*, *Journal of Biomedical Materials Research*, Vol. 50, pp. 50–58.

Murphy, W.L., Peters, M.C., Kohn, D.H., and Mooney, D.J. 2000b, Sustained Release of Vascular Endothelial Growth Factor from Mineralized Poly(Lactide-*co*-Glycolide) Scaffolds for Tissue Engineering, *Biomaterials*, Vol. 21, No. 24, pp. 2521–2527.

Nagano, M., Kitsugi, T., Nakamura, T., Kokubo, T., and Tanahashi, M. 1996, Bone Bonding Ability of an Apatite-Coated Polymer Produced Using a Biomimetic Method: A Mechanical and Histological Study, *In Vivo, Journal of Biomedical Materials Research*, Vol. 31, pp. 487–291.

Nakamura, T., Yamamuro, T., Higashi, S., Kokubo, T., and Itoo, S. 1985, A New Glass-Ceramic for Bone Replacement: Evaluation of Its Bonding to Bone Tissue, *Journal of Biomedical Materials Research*, Vol. 19, pp. 685–698.

Neuman, W.F., and Neuman, M.W. 1957, Emerging Concepts of the Structure and Metabolic Functions of Bone, *The American Journal of Medicine*, Vol. 22, No. 1, pp. 123–131.

Nie, X., Leyland, A., Matthews, A., Jiang, J.C., and Meletis, E.I. 2001, Effects of Solution pH and Electrical Parameters on Hydroxyapatite Coatings Deposited by a Plasma-Assisted Electrophoresis Technique, *Journal of Biomedical Materials Research*, Vol. 57, No. 4, pp. 612–618.

Oliveira, A.L., Elvira, C., Reis, R.L., Vâzquez, B., and San Român, J. 1999, Surface Modification Tailors the Characteristics of Biomimetic Coatings Nucleated on Starch-Based Polymers, *Journal of Materials Science: Materials in Medicine*, Vol. 10, No. 12, pp. 827–835.

Ong, J.L., and Lucas, L.C. 1994, Post-Deposition Heat Treatments for Ion Beam Sputter Deposited Calcium Phosphate Coatings, *Biomaterials*, Vol. 15, No. 5, pp. 337–341.

Ong, J.L., Lucas, L.C., Raikar, G.N., Weimer, J.J., and Gregory, J.C. 1994, Surface Characterization of Ion-Beam Sputter-Deposited Ca–P Coatings after In Vitro Immersion, *Colloids and Surfaces A: Physicochemical and Engineering Aspects*, Vol. 87, No. 2, pp. 151–162.

Ong, J.L., Yang, Y., Oh, S., Appleford, M., Chen, W., Liu, Y., Kim, K., Park, S., Bumgardner, J., Haggard, W., Agrawal, C.M., Carner, D.L., and Oh, N. 2009, Calcium Phosphate Coating Produced by a Sputter Deposition Process, in *Thin Calcium Phosphate Coatings for Medical Implants*, B. León, and J.A. Jansen (eds.), 1st edn, Springer Science, New York, pp. 175–198.

Oyane, A., Kim, H., Furuya, T., Kokubo, T., Miyazaki, T., and Nakamura, T. 2003, Preparation and Assessment of Revised Simulated Body Fluids, *Journal of Biomedical Materials Research A*, Vol. 65A, No. 2, pp. 188–195.

Park, J., Ries, J., Gelse, K., Kloss, F., von der Mark, K., Wiltfang, J., Neukam, F.W., and Schneider, H. 2003, Bone Regeneration in Critical Size Defects by Cell-Mediated BMP-2 Gene Transfer: A Comparison of Adenoviral Vectors and Liposomes, *Gene Therapy*, Vol. 10, No. 13, pp. 1089–1098.

Park, T.G., Jeong, J.H., and Kim, S.W. 2006, Current Status of Polymeric Gene Delivery Systems, *Advanced Drug Delivery Reviews*, Vol. 58, No. 4, pp. 467–486.

Plopper, G. 2007, The Extracellular Matrix and Cell Adhesion, in *Cells*, B. Lewin, V.R. Lingappa, and G. Plopper (eds.), 1st edn, Jones and Bartlett, Ontario, pp. 645–702.

Robey, G.P., and Boskey, A.L. 2003, Extracellular Matrix and Biomineralization of Bone, in *Primer on the Metabolic Bone Diseases and Disorders of Mineral Metabolism*, American Society for Bone and Mineral Research, Washington D.C., pp. 38–46.

Rønold, H.J., Lyngstadaas, S.P., and Ellingsen, J.E. 2003, Analysing the Optimal Value for Titanium Implant Roughness in Bone Attachment Using a Tensile Test, *Biomaterials*, Vol. 24, No. 25, pp. 4559–4564.

Roome, C.M., and Adam, C.D. 1995, Crystallite Orientation and Anisotropic Strains in Thermally Sprayed Hydroxyapatite Coatings, *Biomaterials*, Vol. 16, No. 9, pp. 691–696.

Roy, M.D., Stanley, S.K., Amis, E.J., and Becker, M.L. 2008, Identification of a Highly Specific Hydroxyapatite-binding Peptide using Phage Display, *Advanced Materials*, Vol. 20, No. 10, pp. 1830–1836.

Ruoslahti, E. 1996, RGD and Other Recognition Sequences for Integrins, *Annual Review of Cell and Developmental Biology*, Vol. 12, No. 697, p. 715.

Ruoslahti, E., Hayman, E.G., and Pierschbacher, M.D. 1985, Extracellular Matrices and Cell Adhesion, *Arteriosclerosis*, Vol. 5, No. 6, pp. 581–594.

Rupp, F., Scheideler, L., Olshanska, N., de Wild, M., Wieland, M., and Geis-Gerstorfer, J. 2006, Enhancing Surface Free Energy and Hydrophilicity Through Chemical Modification of Microstructured Titanium Implant Surfaces, *Journal of Biomedical Materials Research Part A*, Vol. 76A, No. 2, pp. 323–334.

Schliephake, H., Scharnweber, D., Roesseler, S., Dard, M., Sewing, A., and Aref, A. 2006, Biomimetic Calcium Phosphate Composite Coating of Dental Implants, *The International Journal of Oral and Maxillofacial Implants*, Vol. 21, No. 5, pp. 738–746.

Segvich, S.J., Luong, L.N., and Kohn, D.H. 2008, Biomimetic Approaches to Synthesize Mineral and Mineral/Organic Biomaterials, in *Biomaterials and Biomedical Engineering*, W. Ahmed, N. Ali, and A. Ochsner (eds.), TTP, Switzerland, pp. 327–373.

Segvich, S., Smith, H.C., Luong, L.N., and Kohn, D.H. 2008, Uniform Deposition of Protein Incorporated Mineral Layer on Three-Dimensional Porous Polymer Scaffolds, *Journal of Biomedical Materials Research B*, Vol. 84B, No. 2, pp. 340–349.

Segvich, S.J., Smith, H.C., and Kohn, D.H. 2009, The Adsorption of Preferential Binding Peptides to Apatite-Based Materials, *Biomaterials*, Vol. 30, pp. 1287–1298.

Shalabi, M.M., Gortemaker, A., Hof, M.A.V., Jansen, J.A., and Creugers, N.H.J. 2006, Implant Surface Roughness and Bone Healing: A Systematic Review, *Journal of Dental Research*, Vol. 85, No. 6, pp. 496–500.

Shen, H., Tan, J., and Saltzman, W.M. 2004, Surface-Mediated Gene Transfer from Nanocomposites of Controlled Texture, *Nature Materials*, Vol. 3, No. 8, pp. 569–574.

Shi, D., Jiang, G., and Bauer, J. 2002, The Effect of Structural Characteristics on the In Vitro Bioactivity of Hydroxyapatite, *Journal of Biomedical Materials Research*, Vol. 63, No. 1, pp. 71–78.

Shin, H., Zygourakis, K., Farach-Carson, M.C., Yaszemski, M.J., and Mikos, A.G. 2004a, Attachment, Proliferation, and Migration of Marrow Stromal Osteoblasts Cultured on Biomimetic Hydrogels Modified with an Osteopontin-Derived Peptide, *Biomaterials*, Vol. 25, pp. 895–906.

Shin, H., Zygourakis, K., Farach-Carson, M.C., Yaszemski, M.J., and Mikos, A.G. 2004b, Modulation of Differentiation and Mineralization of Marrow Stromal Cells Cultured on Biomimetic

Hydrogels Modified with Arg-Gly-Asp Containing Peptides, *Journal of Biomedical Materials Research A*, Vol. 69, pp. 535–543.

Shin, K., Jayasuriya, A., and Kohn, D.H. 2007, Effect of Ionic Activity Products on the Structure and Composition of Mineral Self Assembled on Three-Dimensional Poly(Lactide-*co*-Glycolide) Scaffolds, *Journal of Biomedical Materials Research A*, Vol. 83, No. 4, pp. 1076–1086.

Silverthorn, D.U. 2003, *Human Physiology: An Integrated Approach with Interactive Physiology*, Third Edition, Benjamin Cummings, San Francisco.

Simmons, C.A., Alsberg, E., Hsiong, S., Kim, W.J., and Mooney, D.J. 2004, Dual Growth Factor Delivery and Controlled Scaffold Degradation Enhance In Vivo Bone Formation by Transplanted Bone Marrow Stromal Cells, *Bone*, Vol. 35, No. 2, pp. 562–569.

Stigter, M., Bezemer, J., de Groot, K., and Layrolle, P. 2004, Incorporation of Different Antibiotics into Carbonated Hydroxyapatite Coatings on Titanium Implants, Release and Antibiotic Efficacy, *Journal of Controlled Release: Official Journal of the Controlled Release Society*, Vol. 99, No. 1, pp. 127–137.

Stigter, M., de Groot, K., and Layrolle, P. 2002, Incorporation of Tobramycin into Biomimetic Hydroxyapatite Coating on Titanium, *Biomaterials*, Vol. 23, pp. 4143–4153.

Takadama, H., Hashimoto, M., Mizuno, M., and Kokubo, T. 2004, Round-Robin Test of SBF for In Vitro Apatite-Forming Ability of Synthetic Materials, *Phosphorus Research Bulletin*, Vol. 17, pp. 119–125.

Takadama, H., Kim, H.M., Kokubo, T., and Nakamura, T. 2001, TEM-EDX Study of Mechanism of Bonelike Apatite Formation on Bioactive Titanium Metal in Simulated Body Fluid, *Journal of Biomedical Materials Research*, Vol. 57, No. 3, pp. 441–448.

Takeuchi, A., Ohtsuki, C., Miyazaki, T., Tanaka, H., Yamazaki, M., and Tanihara, M. 2003, Deposition of Bone-Like Apatite on Silk Fiber in a Solution That Mimics Extracellular Fluid, *Journal of Biomedical Materials Research A*, Vol. 65A, pp. 283–289.

Tan, J., and Saltzman, W.M. 2004, Biomaterials with Hierarchically Defined Micro- and Nanoscale Structure, *Biomaterials*, Vol. 25, No. 17, pp. 3593–3601.

Tanahashi, M., and Matsuda, T. 1997, Surface Functional Group Dependence on Apatite Formation on Self-Assembled Monolayers in a Simulated Body Fluid, *Journal of Biomedical Materials Research*, Vol. 34, pp. 305–315.

Tanahashi, M., Yao, T., Kokubo, T., Minoda, M., Miyamoto, T., Nakamura, T., and Yamamuro, T. 1994, Apatite Coating on Organic Polymers by a Biomimetic Process, *Journal of the American Ceramic Society*, Vol. 77, No. 11, pp. 2805–2808.

Tanahashi, M., Yao, T., Kokubo, T., Minoda, M., Miyamoto, T., Nakamuro, T., and Yamamuro, T. 1995, Apatite Coated on Organic Polymers by Biomimetic Process: Improvement in Its Adhesion to Substrate by Glow-Discharge Treatment, *Journal of Biomedical Materials Research*, Vol. 29, pp. 349–357.

Tao, S., Heng, J., and Chuanxian, D. 2000, Effect of Vapor-Flame Treatment on Plasma Sprayed Hydroxyapatite Coatings, *Journal of Biomedical Materials Research*, Vol. 52, No. 3, pp. 572–575.

Temenoff, J.S., and Mikos, A.G. 2008, *Biomaterials: The Intersection of Biology and Materials Science*, 1st Edition, Prentice Hall, New Jersey.

Thompson, M.T., Berg, M.C., Tobias, I.S., Rubner, M.F., and Van Vliet, K.J. 2005, Tuning Compliance of Nanoscale Polyelectrolyte Multilayers to Modulate Cell Adhesion, *Biomaterials*, Vol. 26, No. 34, pp. 6836–6845.

van Dijk, K., Schaeken, H.G., Wolke, J.C., Maree, C.H., Habraken, F.H., Verhoeven, J., and Jansen, J.A. 1995, Influence of Discharge Power Level on the Properties of Hydroxyapatite Films Deposited on Ti_6Al_4V with RF Magnetron Sputtering, *Journal of Biomedical Materials Research*, Vol. 29, No. 2, pp. 269–276.

van Dijk, K., Schaeken, H.G., Wolke, J.G.C., and Jansen, J.A. 1996, Influence of Annealing Temperature on RF Magnetron Sputtered Calcium Phosphate Coatings, *Biomaterials*, Vol. 17, No. 4, pp. 405–410.

Wang, J., Layrolle, P., Stigter, M., and de Groot, K. 2004, Biomimetic and Electrolytic Calcium Phosphate Coatings on Titanium Alloy: Physicochemical Characteristics and Cell Attachment, *Biomaterials*, Vol. 25, No. 4, pp. 583–592.

Wei, G., Reichert, J., Bossert, J., and Jandt, K.D. 2008, Novel Biopolymeric Template for the Nucleation and Growth of Hydroxyapatite Crystals Based on Self-Assembled Fibrinogen Fibrils, *Biomacromolecules,* Vol. 9, No. 3258, p. 3267.

Wen, H.B., Hippensteel, E.A., and Li, P. 2005, Protein Adsorption Property of a Biomimetic Apatite Coating, *Key Engineering Materials,* Vol. 284–286, pp. 403–406.

Weng, J., Liu, X., Zhang, X., Ma, Z., Ji, X., and Zyman, Z. 1993, Further Studies on the Plasma-Sprayed Amorphous Phase in Hydroxyapatite Coatings and Its Deamorphization, *Biomaterials,* Vol. 14, No. 8, pp. 578–582.

Wenjian, W., and Baptista, J.L. 1998, Alkoxide route for Preparing Hydroxyapatite and Its Coatings, *Biomaterials,* Vol. 19, No. 1–3, pp. 125–131.

Wie, H., Hero, H., and Solheim, T. 1998, Hot Isostatic Pressing-Processed Hydroxyapatite-Coated Titanium Implants: Light Microscopic and Scanning Electron Microscopy Investigations, *The International Journal of Oral and Maxillofacial Implants,* Vol. 13, No. 6, pp. 837–844.

Wolke, J.G., van Dijk, K., Schaeken, H.G., de Groot, K., and Jansen, J.A. 1994, Study of the Surface Characteristics of Magnetron-Sputter Calcium Phosphate Coatings, *Journal of Biomedical Materials Research,* Vol. 28, No. 12, pp. 1477–1484.

Wolke, J.G.C., van der Waerden, J.P.C.M., Schaeken, H.G., and Jansen, J.A. 2003, In Vivo Dissolution Behavior of Various RF Magnetron-Sputtered Ca–P Coatings on Roughened Titanium Implants, *Biomaterials,* Vol. 24, No. 15, pp. 2623–2629.

Xia, Y., and Whitesides, G.M. 1998, Soft Lithography, *Annual Review of Materials Science,* Vol. 28, No. 1, pp. 153–184.

Xue, W., Tao, S., Liu, X., Zheng, X., and Ding, C. 2004, In Vivo Evaluation of Plasma Sprayed Hydroxyapatite Coatings Having Different Crystallinity, *Biomaterials,* Vol. 25, No. 3, pp. 415–421.

Yamashita, K., Yonehara, E., Ding, X., Nagai, M., Umegaki, T., and Matsuda, M. 1998, Electrophoretic Coating of Multilayered Apatite Composite on Alumina Ceramics, *Journal of Biomedical Materials Research (Applied Biomaterials),* Vol. 43, pp. 46–53.

Yang, Y., and Ong, J.L. 2003, Bond Strength, Compositional, and Structural Properties of Hydroxyapatite Coating on Ti, ZrO_2-Coated Ti, and TPS-Coated Ti Substrate, *Journal of Biomedical Materials Research. Part A,* Vol. 64, No. 3, pp. 509–516.

Yarbrough, D.K., Hagerman, E., Eckert, R., He, J., Choi, H., Cao, N., Le, K., Hedger, J., Qi, F., Anderson, M., Rutherford, B., Wu, B., Tetradis, S., and Shi, W. 2010, Specific Binding and Mineralization of Calcified Surfaces by Small Peptides, *Calcified Tissue International,* Vol. 86, pp. 58–66.

Yoshinari, M., Ohtsuka, Y., and Dérand, T. 1994, Thin Hydroxyapatite Coating Produced by the Ion Beam Dynamic Mixing Method, *Biomaterials,* Vol. 15, No. 7, pp. 529–535.

Zeng, H., and Lacefield, W.R. 2000, The Study of Surface Transformation of Pulsed Laser Deposited Hydroxyapatite Coatings, *Journal of Biomedical Materials Research,* Vol. 50, No. 2, pp. 239–247.

Zhang, Q., Chen, J., Feng, J., Cao, Y., Deng, C., and Zhang, X. 2003, Dissolution and Mineralization Behaviors of HA Coatings, *Biomaterials,* Vol. 24, No. 26, pp. 4741–4748.

Zhu, X., Kim, K., and Jeong, Y. 2001, Anodic Oxide Films Containing Ca and P of Titanium Biomaterial, *Biomaterials,* Vol. 22, No. 16, pp. 2199–2206.

Zyman, Z., Weng, J., Liu, X., Li, X., and Zhang, X. 1994, Phase and Structural Changes in Hydroxyapatite Coatings under Heat Treatment, *Biomaterials,* Vol. 15, No. 2, pp. 151–155.

Zyman, Z., Weng, J., Liu, X., Zhang, X., and Ma, Z. 1993, Amorphous Phase and Morphological Structure of Hydroxyapatite Plasma Coatings, *Biomaterials,* Vol. 14, No. 3, pp. 225–228.

2

Synthesis and Characterization of Hydroxyapatite Nanocoatings by Sol–Gel Method for Clinical Applications

B. Ben-Nissan, A.H. Choi, D.W. Green, B.A. Latella, J. Chou, and A. Bendavid

CONTENTS

Introduction

Nanostructured materials are associated with a diversity of uses within the medical field, for instance, in drug-delivery systems, regenerative medicine, formation of surgical tools, medical devices, and diagnostic systems.

It has long been established that porous bulk hydroxyapatite (HAp) cannot be used for load-bearing applications due to its unfavorable mechanical properties. As a result, HAp has been used instead as a coating in orthopedic surgery on metallic alloys, metals giving the support required. Of the metallic alloys used, titanium-based and cobalt chromium alloys are the preferred materials for these HAp coatings for orthopedic and maxillofacial implants (Figure 2.1).

Nanocoatings present the possibility of altering the surface properties of medical-grade materials to achieve improvements in biocompatibility, reliability, and performance.

The bone mineral is composed of nanocrystals, or more accurately, nanoplatelets originally described as hydroxyapatite and similar to the mineral dahllite. It is now agreed that bone apatite can be better described as carbonate hydroxyapatite (CHA) and approximated by the formula $(Ca,Mg,Na)_{10}(PO_4CO_3)_6(OH)_2$. The composition of commercial CHA is similar to that of bone mineral apatite. Bone pore sizes range from 1 to 100 nm in normal cortical bone and from 200 to 400 nm in trabecular bone tissue, and the pores are interconnected.

The chemical structure and nanocrystallinity of replacement materials determines the success of tissue-implant interactions and long-term reliability. It is well known that the bone consists of nanosized platelike crystals of HAp grown in intimate contact with an organic matrix rich in collagen fibers. Reconstruction of bone tissue using nanocrystalline bone grafts with structure, composition, physicochemical, biomechanical, and biological features that mimic the natural bone is a goal to be pursued. A novel way of fabricating nanocrystalline bone grafts using strategies found in nature has recently received much attention and is perceived to be beneficial over conventional methods.

The current focus is on the manufacture of new nanoceramics and nanocoatings that are appropriate for a wide range of applications, including implantable surface-modified

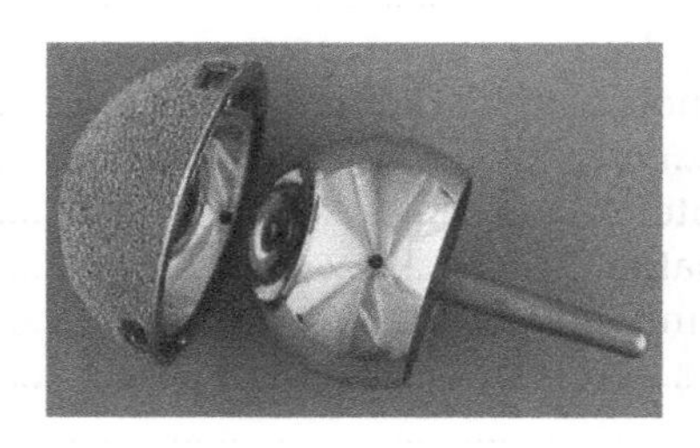

FIGURE 2.1
Hydroxyapatite plasma coated metallic hip resurfacing implant. Plasma coated material is on the acetabulum component and coated on metallic beads for better mechanical interlocking.

medical devices for better hard- and soft-tissue attachment, increased bioactivity for tissue regeneration and engineering; cancer treatment, drug and gene delivery, treatment of bacterial and viral infections, delivery of oxygen to damaged tissues, imaging, targeted slow drug delivery, and devices for minimally invasive surgery. A more futuristic view, which could in fact become reality within less than two decades, includes nanorobotics, nanobiosensors, and micronanodevices for a wide range of biomedical applications.

For clinical applications, four general conventional industrial coating methods have been proposed during the past 30 years for the production of bioactive coatings. For the first method, Hench, Ducheyne, and colleagues developed spray coating that uses relatively thick calcium phosphate coatings (100 µm to 2 mm) for bone ingrowth (Ducheyne et al. 1990); for the second, Hench and colleagues developed thick bioglass coatings for surface bioactivity (Hench and West 1990); the third method, developed in the early 1990s by Kokubo and colleagues, was based on self-assembly by precipitation in a simulated body fluid (SBF) solution (Kokubo et al. 2000). Although thick bioglass coatings and coatings based on self-assembly are effective, spray coating is the only coating method that has been applied commercially to orthopedic implants.

A fourth, newer, and very promising method involves dipping in sol–gel derived HAp solutions to produce strong nanocoatings (Ben-Nissan and Chai 1995).

Advances in nanometric scale inorganic synthesis has helped create novel techniques for the production of bonelike synthetic coatings of HAp. Nanocrystalline HAp has been instrumental in generating new opportunities in the design of superior biocompatible coatings for implants.

Thermal spraying is a term that covers processes such as high-velocity oxygen flame spraying, plasma spraying, detonation gun spraying, and flame spraying. Plasma spraying can be conducted under vacuum (vacuum plasma spraying), under controlled atmospheres, or in an ambient atmosphere (atmospheric plasma spraying). Plasma spraying employs a direct current arc to generate gas plasma, although other sources, such as radiofrequency-generated plasmas, can be used. Each is capable of fabricating coating thicknesses from a few microns to a few millimeters (Berndt et al. 1990). By far, the most popular thermal-spraying technique for the deposition of HAp coatings is plasma spraying. Plasma spraying is the only widely used coating process to fabricate medical implants on a commercial scale. It uses an electrical discharge to convert a carrier gas, such as argon, into plasma (Tjong and Chen 2004). Rapid gas expansion induces speeds of up to 800 m/s. The plasma heats the powder and propels it toward the substrate. An excellent review on the plasma spraying is given by LeGeros et al. (2011).

Problems related to dissociation of HAp have been at least partially solved with the modification of powder composition, additional treatment methods after coating, new generation plasma spraying and coating operational conditions, and coating on macrotextured modified metal surfaces such as beads and wires (Figure 2.2).

At present, the most common materials in clinical use are those selected from a handful of well-characterized and available biocompatible ceramics, metals, polymers, and their combinations as composites or hybrids. These unique production techniques, together with the development of new enabling technologies such as nanoscale bioinspired fabrication (biomimetics) and surface modification methods, have the potential to drive at an unprecedented rate the design and development of new implants (Figure 2.3).

By definition, a biomaterial is a nondrug substance that is suitable for inclusion in systems that augment or replace the function of bodily organs or tissues. When these synthetic materials are placed within the human body, the tissues react toward the implant in a variety of ways. The mechanism of tissue interaction at a nanoscale level is dependent

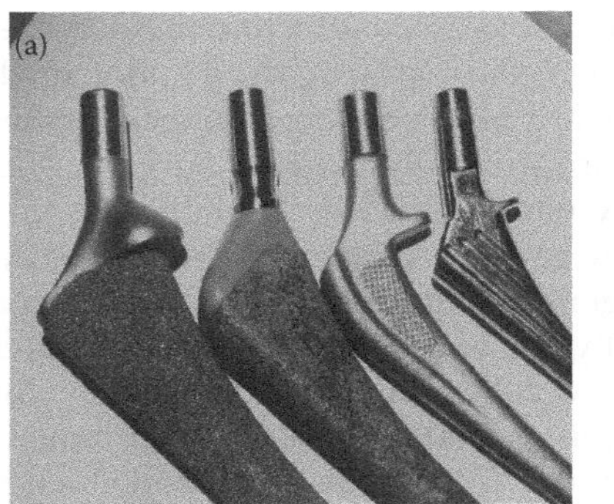

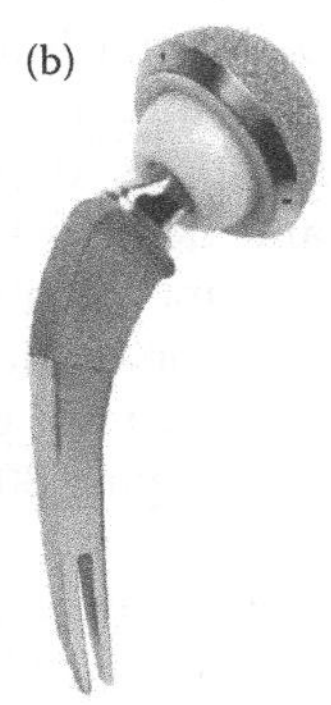

FIGURE 2.2
(a) Four macro-textured total hip replacement implant femoral components prior to hydroxyapatite coating, and (b) a new macro-textured and hydroxyapatite coated advanced TSI stem design total hip replacement implant licensed to Omni Life Science by CDD, LLC, Chagrin Falls, Ohio, USA.

on the response to the implant surface, and during the past 40 years three terms have been defined, which describe a biomaterial with respect to the tissues' responses: bioactive, bioinert, and bioresorbable (Hulbert et al. 1970; Heimke and Griss 1980; Oonishi et al. 1988; Hench 1991; LeGeros 1991).

Bioactive refers to a material which, upon being placed within the human body, interacts with the surrounding bone and, in some cases, even soft tissue. Bioinert refers to any material which, once placed within the human body, has a minimal interaction with its surrounding tissue; examples include stainless steel, titanium, alumina, partially stabilized zirconia, and ultrahigh molecular weight polyethylene. Bioresorbable refers to a material which, upon placement within the human body, begins to dissolve or to be resorbed and slowly replaced by the advancing tissues (e.g., bone).

The main factors in the clinical success of any biomaterial are its biofunctionality and biocompatibility, both of which are related directly to tissue/implant interface interactions. This approach is currently being explored in the development of a new generation of nanobioceramics with a widened range of medical applications (Dorozhkin 2009).

The improvement of interface bonding by nanoscale coatings, based on biomimetics, has been of worldwide interest during the past decade, and today several companies are in early commercialization stages of new-generation, nanoscale-modified implants for orthopedic, tissue regeneration, targeted slow drug delivery, ocular, and maxillofacial surgery.

The aim of this chapter is to provide a brief background on currently used coating methods and further detailed information relating to our choice of sol–gel derived nanohydroxyapatite coatings for medical applications.

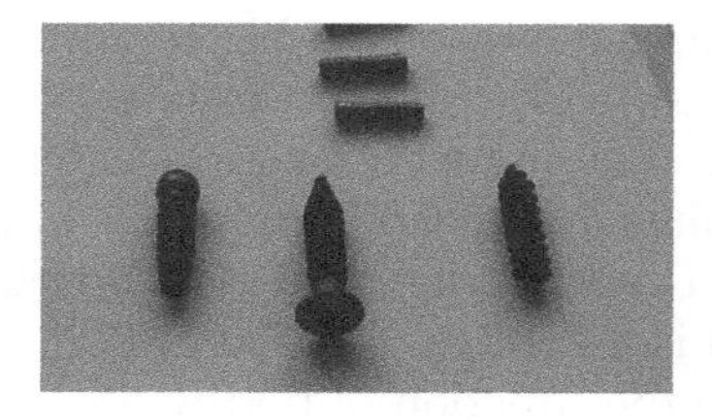

FIGURE 2.3
Carbonate hydroxyapatite-nanocoated dental (top) implants and ACL fixation screws.

Thick- and Thin-Film Coating Methods

Although other oxides and mixed oxides were trialed, hydroxyapatite nanocoatings research and development did not initiate until the early 1990s (Ben-Nissan and Chai 1995).

Coatings offer the possibility of modifying the surface properties of surgical-grade materials to achieve improvements in performance, reliability, and biocompatibility. Techniques such as physical vapor deposition (PVD), chemical vapor deposition (CVD), thermal and electron beam evaporation, plasma metalorganic chemical vapor deposition (MOCVD), electrochemical vapor deposition, thermal or diffusion conversion electrophoretic coating, simulated body fluid (SBF), and sol–gel processing, have been used to produce both macro- and nanocoatings. Except for a few specific sol–gel compositions, all these methods have problems regarding their stoichiometry and chemical composition control and their dissolution within the physiological environment due to the production methods and high-temperature heat treatments used.

In the context of biomedical applications, the definitions of macro-, micro-, thin film, and nanothickness, or more generally, thin films, have been used interchangeably and/or wrongly, the authors of this chapter believe that coatings greater than 1000 μm should be considered thick or macrocoatings, 1 to 1000 μm should be considered thin-film coatings or microcoatings, and below 1 μm should be considered nanocoatings.

Taking into account that most of these coating methods are well covered within this book and a large number of excellent review papers have appeared during the past two decades, only a brief summary of the SBF and biomimetic approach is covered in the next section.

Biomimetics and SBF Hydroxyapatite

Biomimetics Approach

The technology of coating can benefit from the study of the natural world, as a model for biomimicry or as a source of inspiration for new designs. One of the ways the study of nature could augment strategies in thin film coating is by mimicking the growth of bioceramics in ambient conditions in water.

Nature is a consummate problem solver. We see exquisite, almost perfect designs all around us. There are now systematic ways of harnessing these designs for all sorts of challenges in regenerative medicine. A vital part of making regenerative medicine more of a future clinical success is the production of highly proficient scaffolds that function at many different levels: the nanoscale, microscopic, and macroscopic. It can be envisaged that these proficient scaffolds incorporated with biogenic additives such as BMP and MSC will generate macro structures that can pull cells into the hard tissue and in nanoscale release encapsulated chemical signals in a targeted way, and convey them into the body. Why not reverse engineer the structural fabric of human tissues and faithfully copy them artificially? This is not only improbably difficult but is also too time-consuming a task. Instead we extract the key essence of what we are trying to reassemble. There are abundant sources of structures and materials that can be used for a different function to their evolved intended one. The simplest strategy is to select a predesigned, preformed structure but modify it in a directed way specifically for its new intended function. In other strategies we pull out inventive principles to solve a similar problem we are faced with guided by a systematic database amassed from nature but also human technology through patents. Lastly, we study nature and try to faithfully copy the vital components and reinvent this in the laboratory.

SBF Hydroxyapatite

Artificial materials implanted into bone defects might be encapsulated from time to time by fibrous tissue, leading to their isolation from the surrounding bone. Improvement of bone implant bonding to the tissues requires the right implant surface morphology and chemistry to generate mechanical interlock and good surface activity. Interactions between the bone and the implant will be controlled with appropriate biological interactions.

In the past three decades a large number of investigators have proposed that the essential requirement for an artificial material to bond to living bone is the formation of bonelike apatite on its surface when implanted in the living body. In 1991, Kokubo et al. (1992) proposed that in vivo apatite formation on the surfaces of many biomedical materials can be reproduced in SBF with ion concentrations nearly equal to those of human blood plasma. In essence, this means that the in vivo bone bioactivity of a material can be predicted from the apatite formation on its surface in SBF.

Hydroxyapatite layers can be easily produced on various organic and inorganic substrates when submerged in simulated body fluid. In 1989, Kokubo and Takadama (2006) showed that after immersion in SBF, a wide range of biomaterial surfaces initiated very fine crystallites of carbonate ion-containing apatite, and since then a large number of studies have shown that osteoblasts can proliferate and differentiate on this apatite layer.

Since then, SBFs have been produced in order to provide insight into the reactivity of the inorganic component of blood plasma, and predict the bioactivity of implants and bone scaffolds, as well as other novel biomaterials. Kokubo et al. in a number of follow-up studies (Kokubo et al. 2000; Kokubo and Takadama 2006) warned that physiological environments contain not only the inorganic components but organics and dissolved gases and investigators should be careful with the results obtained within the SBF.

SBF solutions are shown to induce apatitic calcium phosphate formation on metals, ceramics, or polymers soaked in them. SBF solutions, in close resemblance to the Hanks' balanced salt solution (HBSS) are prepared with the aim of simulating the ion concentrations present in human plasma. To mimic human plasma, SBF solutions are prepared to have relatively low calcium and phosphate ion concentrations, namely, 2.5 and 1.0 mM, respectively. Furthermore, to mimic human plasma, the pH value of SBF solutions was

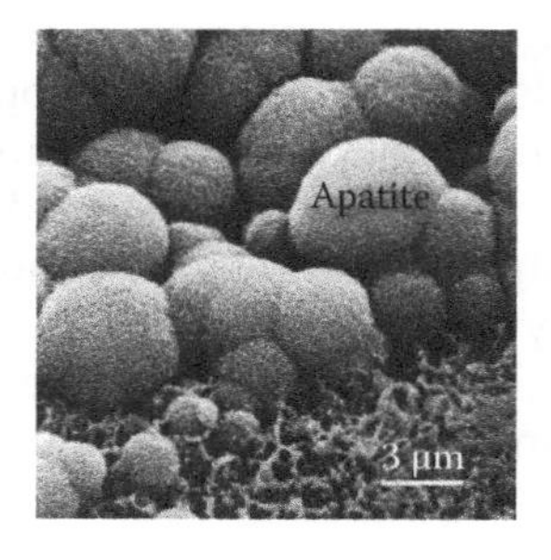

FIGURE 2.4
SBF coating on a porous surface (Kokubo et al. 2000).

adjusted to the physiological value of 7.4 by using organic buffers such as Tris3 or Hepes. These compounds are not present in human plasma (Kokubo et al. 2000; Kokubo and Takadama 2006) (Figure 2.4).

SBF has ionic concentrations of 142.0 mM Na^+, 5.0 mM K^+, 1.5 mM Mg^{2+}, 2.5 mM Ca^{2+}, 147.8 mM Cl^-, 4.2 mM HCO^{3-}, 1.0 mM HPO_4^{2-}, and 0.5 mM SO_4^{2-} and a pH of 7.40, nearly equal to those in human blood plasma at 36.5°C. The SBF is usually prepared by dissolving reagent-grade chemicals of NaCl, $NaHCO_3$, KCl, $K_2HPO_4{\cdot}3H_2O$, $MgCl_2{\cdot}6H_2O$, $CaCl_2$, and Na_2SO_4 into distilled water and buffering at pH 7.40 with tris (hydroxymethyl) aminomethane ($(CH_2OH)_3CNH_3$) and 1.0 M hydrochloric acid at 36.5°C.

With their ionic compositions more or less similar to that of human blood plasma, HBSS or SBF formulations have only limited power with regard to the precipitation of apatitic calcium phosphates. As a direct consequence, nucleation and precipitation of calcium phosphates from HBSS or SBF solutions are rather slow. To obtain total surface coverage of a 10 × 10 × 1 mm titanium or titanium alloy substrate immersed into a 1.5 or 2 × SBF solution, one typically needs to wait for 2 to 3 weeks, with frequent (every 36–48 h) replenishment of the solution (Tas and Bhaduri 2004).

Among the metallic oxide gels prepared using a sol-gel method, those consisting of SiO_2, TiO_2, ZrO_2, and Ta_2O_5 were found to have apatite formation on their surfaces in SBF. These results indicated that Si–OH, Ti–OH, Zr–OH, and Ta–OH groups on the surfaces of these gels are effective for inducing apatite formation on their surfaces in the body environment (Kokubo et al. 2000).

Work has been conducted using SBF solutions to deposit apatite on both 2-D and 3-D scaffolds. Wu et al. (2007) developed a novel bioactive, degradable, and cytocompatible bredigite ($Ca_7MgSi_4O_{16}$) scaffold with a biomimetic apatite layer for bone-tissue engineering. Porous bredigite scaffolds were prepared using the polymer sponge method. The bredigite scaffolds with biomimetic apatite layer were obtained by soaking bredigite scaffolds in SBF (pH 7.40) at 37°C for 10 days, and the ratio of solution volume to scaffold mass was 200 ml/g. After soaking, the scaffolds were dried at 120°C for 1 day and the bredigite scaffolds with biomimetic apatite layer (BTAP) were obtained. Their results showed that the prepared bredigite scaffolds possess a highly porous structure with large pore size (300–500 μm). Cromme et al. (2007) investigated the activation of regenerated cellulose 2-D model thin films and 3-D fabric templates with calcium hydroxide, $Ca(OH)_2$. The Langmuir–Blodgett (LB) film technique was applied for manufacturing of the model thin films using a trimethylsilyl derivative of cellulose (TMS cellulose). Regenerated cellulose films were obtained by treating the TMS cellulose LB films with hydrochloric acid vapors. For 3-D templates, regenerated cellulose fabrics were used.

Kim et al. (2006) identified that bonelike apatite was more efficiently coated onto the scaffold surface by using polymer/ceramic composite scaffolds instead of polymer scaffolds and by using an accelerated biomimetic process to enhance the osteogenic potential of the scaffold. The creation of bonelike, apatite-coated polymer scaffold was achieved by incubating the scaffolds in SBF. The apatite growth on the porous poly(D,L-lactic-*co*-glycolic acid)/nanohydroxyapatite (PLGA/HAp) composite scaffolds was significantly faster than on the porous PLGA scaffolds. In addition, the distribution of coated apatite was more uniform on the PLGA/HAp scaffolds than on the PLGA scaffolds. It was reported that when seeded with osteoblasts, the apatite-coated PLGA/HAp scaffolds exhibited significantly higher cell growth, alkaline phosphatase (ALP) activity, and mineralization in vitro compared to the PLGA scaffolds coated only with hydroxyapatite.

The SBF method was used by Kolos et al. (2006) for fabricating calcium phosphate fibers for biomedical applications. Natural cotton substrate was pretreated with phosphorylation and a $Ca(OH)_2$ saturated solution. The pretreated samples were then soaked in SBF of two different concentrations, 1.5 times and 5.0 times the ion concentration of blood plasma. The cotton was then burnt out via sintering of the ceramic coating at 950°C, 1050°C, 1150°C, and 1250°C. Hollow calcium phosphate fibers approximately 25 μm in diameter and with a 1-μm wall thickness were successfully manufactured. 5.0 × SBF produced a thicker and more crystalline coating of greater uniformity.

Although in micron size rather than nanosize, a bioactive CHA layer on cellulose fabrics was developed by Hofmann et al. (2006). Nonwoven cellulose (regenerated, oxidized) fabrics were coated with CHA using a procedure based on the SBF method. SBF with a high degree of supersaturation (5 × SBF) was applied to accelerate the biomimetic formation of bonelike apatite on the cellulose fabrics. After creating calcium phosphate nuclei on the cellulose fibers in an initial 5 × SBF with high Mg^{2+} and HCO_3^- concentrations, the cellulose fabrics were additionally soaked in a second 5 × SBF that was optimized with regard to accelerated crystal growth by reduced Mg^{2+} and HCO_3^- concentrations. The carbonated apatite layer thickness increased from 6 μm after 4 h of soaking in the latter solution, to 20 μm after 48 h. The amount of CO_3^{2-} substituting PO_4^{3-} in the hydroxyapatite (HAp) lattice of the precipitates can be varied by changing the soaking time.

The Sol–Gel Process

Sol–gel processing is a versatile and attractive technique since it can be used to fabricate ceramic coatings from solutions by chemical means. The sol–gel process is relatively easy to perform and complex shapes can be coated, and it has also been demonstrated that the nanocrystalline grain structure of sol–gel coatings produced results in improved mechanical properties (Kirk and Pilliar 1999; Chen and Lacefield 1994; Anast et al. 1992; Roest et al. 2004; Roest 2010).

The sol–gel process goes back to the genesis of chemistry. It was first identified in 1846 as an application technology, when Ebelmen (1846) observed the hydrolysis and polycondensation of tetraethylorthosilicate (TEOS). In 1939, the first sol–gel patent was published covering the preparation of SiO_2 and TiO_2 coatings (Geffcken and Berger 1939). Roy and Roy (1954) recognized the potential for producing high-purity glasses using methods not possible with traditional ceramic-processing techniques. In doing so, they generated the first report on the use of sol–gel technology to produce homogeneous multicomponent glasses.

Schroeder reported the first investigation conducted by Schott Glass involving sol–gel synthesized coatings (Schroeder 1965). Mixed-oxides coatings were developed although they were mainly interested in single-oxide optical coatings of SiO_2 and TiO_2.

During the late 1980s and 1990s, sol–gel technology also found applications in a number of technology fields, such as biomedical applications (Ben-Nissan and Chai 1995; Chai et al. 1998), in optoelectronics, smart windows, electronic materials, for stabilization of radioactive isotopes (Bartlett and Woolfrey 1990), the laser industry (Yoldas 1984; Floch et al. 1995), and a range of electronic and optoelectronic applications (Anast 1996).

A number of excellent review articles, book chapters, and books cover the science and technology of the basics of sol–gel technology for various ceramic oxide systems (Mazdiyasni 1982; Sakka et al. 1984; Yoldas 1984; Roy 1987; Klein 1988; Scriven 1988; Brinker et al. 1988; Brinker and Scherer 1990; Hench and West 1990).

By definition, a sol is a suspension of colloidal particles in a liquid (Floch et al. 1995). A sol differs from a solution in that a sol is a two-phase, solid-liquid system, whereas a solution is a single-phase system. Colloidal particles can be in the approximate size range of 1 to 1000 nm; for this reason, gravitational forces on these colloidal particles are negligible and interactions are dominated by short-range forces such as van der Waals forces and surface charges. Diffusion of the colloids by Brownian motion leads to a low-energy arrangement, thus imparting stability to the system (Brinker and Scherer 1990).

The stability of the sol particles can be modified by reducing their surface charge. If the surface charge is significantly reduced, then gelation is induced and the resultant product is able to maintain its shape without the assistance of a mould. Gels are regarded as composites, since gels consist of a solid skeleton or network that encloses a liquid phase or excess of solvent. Depending on their chemistry, gels can be soft and have a low elastic modulus, usually obtained through controlled polymerization of the hydrolyzed starting compound. In this case, a three-dimensional network forms, resulting ultimately in a high molecular weight polymeric gel. The resultant gel can be thought of as a macroscopic molecule that extends throughout the solution. The gelation point is the time taken for the last bond in this network to form. This gelation can be used to produce a nanostructured monolith or nanosized coatings, depending on the process applied.

Advantages and Disadvantages

Sol–gel processing is unique in that it can be used to produce different forms, for example coatings, fibers, powders, platelets, and monoliths of the same composition, simply by varying the chemistry, viscosity, and other factors of a given solution. In addition, the range of different compositions that can be produced includes pure single oxides, mixed oxides, and nonoxides, such as borides, chlorides, and nitrides.

The advantages of the sol–gel process are numerous:

1. It is of the nanoscale.
2. It has the ability to produce uniform fine-grained structures.
3. High purity can be maintained as grinding can be avoided.
4. It results in a stoichiometric, homogeneous, and pure product owing to mixing on the molecular scale.
5. It allows reduced firing or sintering temperatures due to its small particle sizes with high surface areas.
6. It allows the use of different chemical routes (alkoxide or aqueous-based).
7. It is easily applied to complex shapes with a range of coating techniques, including dip, spin, and spray deposition.

In addition, sol–gel coatings have the added advantage that the costs of precursors are relatively unimportant, owing to small amounts of material requirements. Shrinkage in coatings, depending on the chemistry, is fairly uniform perpendicular to the substrate and the coating can normally dry without cracking. Shrinkage-generated cracking is an important issue in monolith production and thicker than 500-nm multilayered coatings.

Sol–gel film deposition also offers the significant advantage over other film deposition techniques such as CVD, PVD, and sputtering, in that properties such as surface area, pore volume, and size can be carefully controlled by chemistry. These are particularly important in engineering, biomedical, and optical applications such as in the field of antireflective coatings (Pettie et al. 1988) and on medical porous membranes such as artificial liver or retinal implants.

Precursors

Although it is loosely used, sol–gel process methods can be categorized as alcohol- or aqueous-based. As the name suggest, alcohol-based systems generally exclude water buildup until the hydrolysis stage, whereas aqueous-based systems are carried out in the presence of water. However, there are also nonhydrolytic sol–gel processes that do not require the presence of solvents at all. Similarly, sol–gel precursors can be classified as either alkoxides or nonalkoxides. While alkoxides are the preferred precursors for sol–gel production owing to their volatility, other compounds, such as metal salts, can also be used. This is often the case for Group I and II elements whose alkoxides are solid, nonvolatile, and in many cases have a low solubility (Percy et al. 2000).

The preparation of sol solutions involves the use of solvents. These solvents are usually organic alcohols. While the main objective of the solvent is to dissolve solid precursors, they are also used to dilute liquid precursors and minimize the effect of concentration gradients. The particular solvent employed can influence factors such as particle morphology (Harris et al. 1988) and crystallization temperatures (de Kambilly and Klein 1989).

Alkoxide Precursors

Metal alkoxides are probably the best starting materials in sol–gel preparations (Schroder 1966). All metals are capable of forming metal alkoxides of the form $M(OR)_x$, where M is a metal, R is an alkyl group, and x is the valence state of the metal. Another type of alkoxide that exists is the double alkoxide, which has the general formula $M_x'M_y(OR)_z$, where M′ and M are metals, R is an alkyl group, and x, y, and z are the valence states of the metals. Double alkoxides have the added advantage of retaining their stoichiometry (Thomas 1988).

While the organic group influences the stability of the alkoxide, precursors should also be selected so they have adequate volatility to enable a clean break of the M–OR and MO–R bonds to produce materials free from organics (Mazdiyasni 1982; Eichorst and Payne 1988). Most metal alkoxides are sensitive to heat, light, and moisture. Sensitivity to moisture can be attributed to the electronegative alkoxy groups, which renders the metal atom prone to nucleophilic attack (Bradley et al. 1978).

While alkoxides are the most favorable sol–gel precursor, there are two exceptions to this rule. These are the alkoxides of silicon and phosphorus. Silicon alkoxides require an acid or base catalyst for hydrolysis, and even with such an addition, hydrolysis is very slow. In the same way, trialkylphosphates are very stable and difficult to hydrolyze, and as a result they are generally not used widely as phosphorus precursors in sol–gel production (Thomas 1988).

Nonalkoxide Precursors

Metal salts provide an ideal alternative to alkoxides if they can be transformed readily into their respective oxide by thermal or oxidative decomposition. It is also preferable for such salts to be soluble in organic solvents. Candidates are salts produced from organic acids, such as acetates, formats, and citrates. Nitrates are the most suitable inorganic salts, as chlorides and sulfates are more thermally stable and may be difficult to remove (Wallace and Hench 1984; Schwart et al. 1986). On the other hand, the use of nitrates in amounts greater than a few hundred grams should be avoided, as nitrates are very strong oxidizing agents and can lead to uncontrollable exothermic reactions and even explosions during drying (Thomas 1988). Acetates are a suitable alternative to nitrates, eliminating the possibility of explosions; however, they do not thermally degrade as readily as nitrates, often leaving behind organic residues.

Other Organic Additives

Owing to the large quantity of organic material required in the processing of sol–gel derived forms, cracking during the production stages can be a problem. Shrinkage during drying is common in the case of monoliths. Cracking in thicker coatings is often due to phenomena such as inhomogeneities resulting from phase separation, thermal mismatch with the substrate used, or a number of other factors related to the drying process.

Modification of sols through the addition of organics, sometimes referred to as drying control chemical additives or DCCA, can lessen these problems through the control of evaporation rates of volatile species, which in turn, control hydrolysis rates. They also influence properties such as micro- and nanoporosity (Orcel and Hench 1986; Schmidt et al. 1988). Examples include glycol, acetylacetone, carboxylic acids, or β-diketones.

Process

Sol synthesis involves preparation of a solution from alkoxides, metal salts, or other suitable precursors. Coatings are produced by a number of deposition methods from the solutions. The coated substrate is then exposed to water for hydrolysis. During this process, hydroxides or hydrated oxides form and gelation occurs to form a three-dimensional network. Control of this gelation and the three-dimensional structure determines the final densification and the shape of the product (Figure 2.5). Further heat treating of the resultant gel removes residual organic material and induces conversion to the oxide state under oxidizing conditions (Hench and West 1990; Ben-Nissan et al. 1994; Chai and Ben-Nissan 1999).

Gelation

The simplest picture of gelation is that clusters grow by condensation of polymers or aggregation of particles until the clusters collide. Links then develop between the clusters to generate a single giant cluster that is referred to as a gel (Figure 2.6a and b). The gel point can only be estimated by an increase in viscosity as no latent heat is released. The gel is composed of a solid skeleton surrounding a continuous liquid phase.

There are a number of factors that decreases the gel time:

1. Increasing the concentration and pH of the solution
2. Increasing the gelling temperature
3. Increasing the water/alkoxide ratio
4. Decreasing the size of the alkoxyl groups

In essence, it means appropriate control of the material chemistry (Gottardi et al. 1984; Colby et al. 1988).

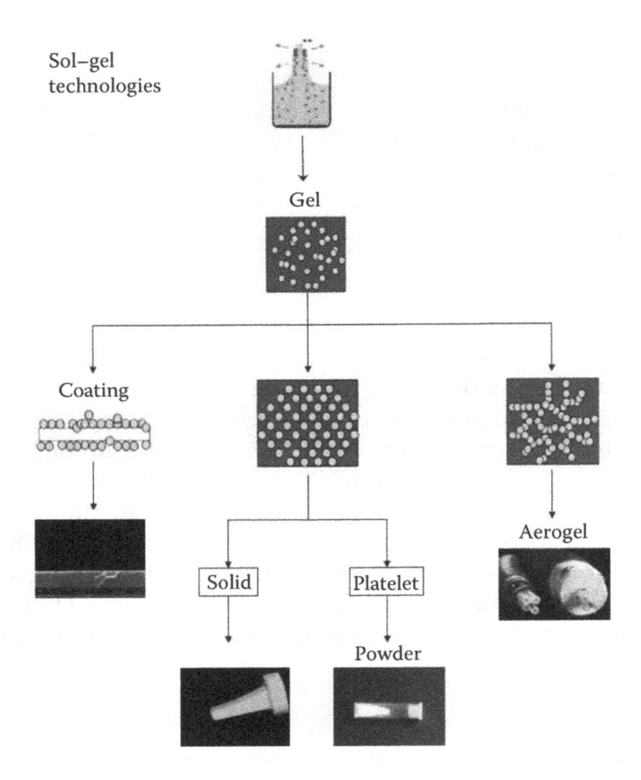

FIGURE 2.5
Sol–gel processing methods and related products, nanocoatings, aerogels, solid ceramics, platelets and powders.

To produce homogeneous gels from a liquid, which is a pertinent requirement to produce homogeneous coatings and powders, it is essential to avoid precipitation. This becomes increasingly important in multicomponent systems. In alkoxide systems, precipitation can be induced by physical agglomeration or by chemical reaction (Zheng et al. 1988).

Chemical precipitation from sol–gel solutions is a result of the alkoxide reacting with water or a chelating agent to form an insoluble product such as a hydroxide or organic salt. Factors affecting precipitation include alkoxide precursor chemistry, temperature of the environment, and water concentration.

Another important factor to be considered on gelation is the gelation environment that influences the reaction rate. If gelation takes place under tightly capped controlled environments, the resultant gel retains all solvents and reaction products remains within the gel. When it is under open conditions, it produces a material called xerogel with less solvent molecules in it. Both structures behave differently in further processing, like sintering, to yield dried gels or sintered gels with different properties (Figure 2.5).

The chemical reactions involved in a sol–gel process are hydrolysis and polymerization. Figure 2.6a and b shows the processes involved with the production of a thin film coating via the sol–gel process. At high temperatures, the rate of polymerization is greater than the rate of hydrolysis, and precipitates such as hydroxides do not have a chance to form. When the rate of hydrolysis is less than the rate of polymerization, that is, when the temperature is low, hydroxides form by nucleation and growth. This general rule applies for neutral solutions, but can be overshadowed by changes in pH to acidic or basic solutions.

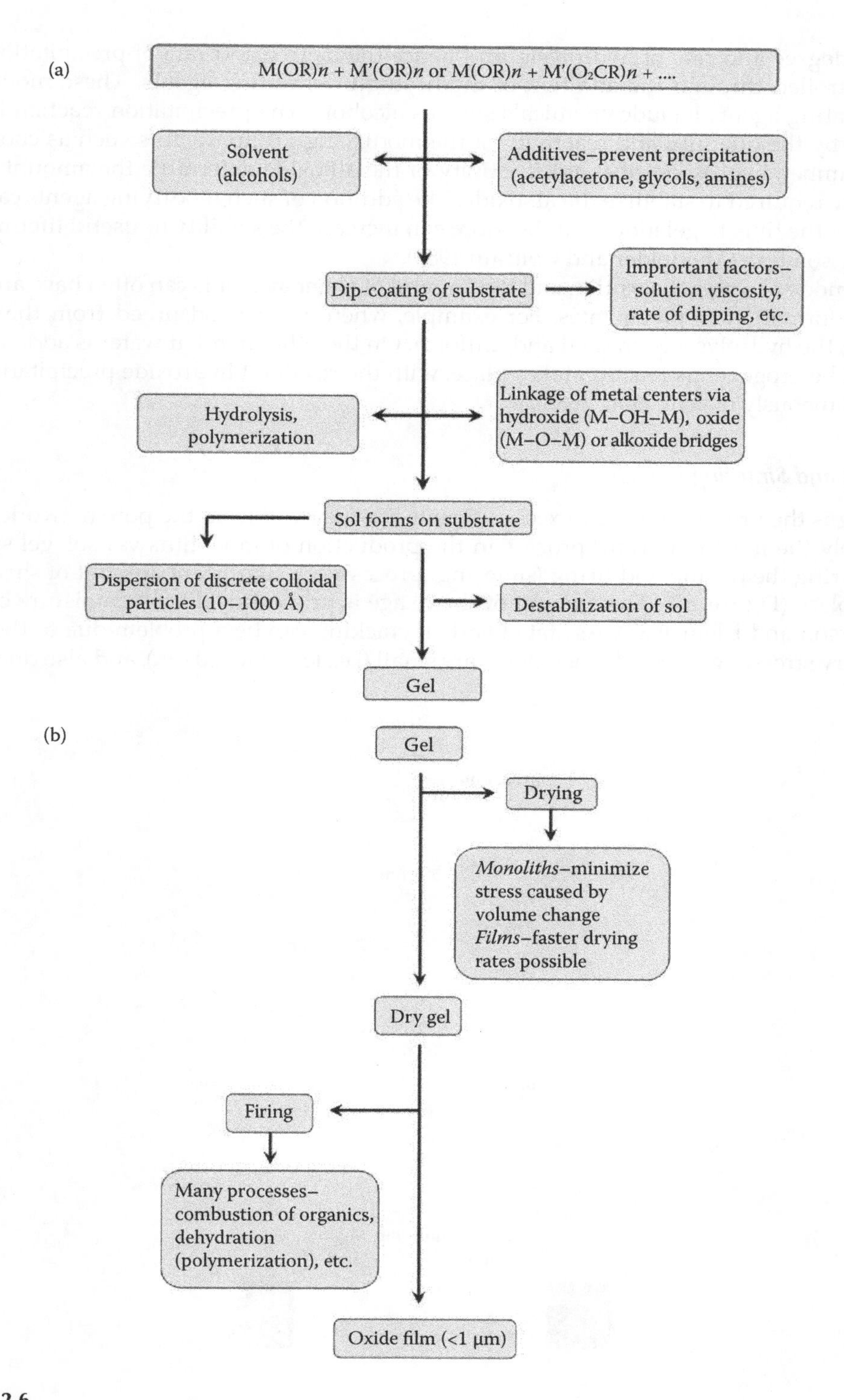

FIGURE 2.6
(a) Chemistry of sol–gel process based on alkoxide route, (b) process covering the process from gel formation to the final oxide nanocoating.

The degree and rate of hydrolysis, and hence the degree and rate of precipitation, can be controlled through the addition of modifying or chelating agents. These modifying or chelating agents include chemicals such as alcohols. The precipitation reaction is controlled by the quantity and reactivity of the modifying group. Factors such as coordination number, hygroscopicity, and reactivity of the alkoxide determine the amount of the additive required to stabilize the alkoxide. The addition of such modifying agents can also increase the time to gelation, and therefore can increase the stability or useful lifetime of a coating solution (Melpolder and Coltrain 1988).

The mode of water absorption and the amount of water available can often have an effect on the formation of precipitates. For example, when water is adsorbed from the atmosphere, the hydrolysis is gradual and uniform. On the other hand, if water is added dropwise, a heterogeneous reaction takes place, with the resultant hydroxide precipitating out instantaneously (Zheng et al. 1988).

Drying and Sintering of Gels

Drying is the process whereby excess solvents are removed from the pore network and is probably the most important process in the production of monoliths via sol–gel synthesis. During the drying and firing (sintering) processes, a significant amount of shrinkage takes place (Figure 2.7). The amount of shrinkage is proportional to the moisture content (Anderson and Klein 1987). As stated earlier, cracking can be a problem due to the large capillary stresses generated when pores are small (i.e., less than 20 nm), and also due to the

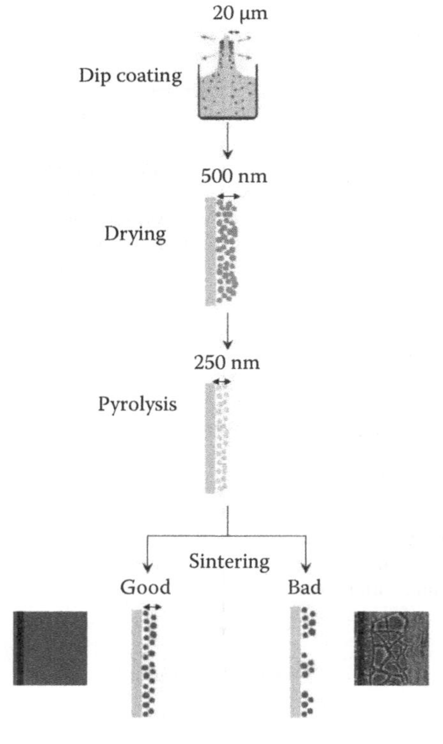

FIGURE 2.7
Schematic diagram showing the drying and sintering stages of gels.

large volume of material that is lost, and therefore the corresponding shrinkage that takes place (Hench and West 1990). This can be avoided through the use of drying control chemical additives (DCCA), careful control of drying conditions, and schedules and increasing the degree of cross-linking. However, the drying of sol–gel derived nanofilms is not such a problem compared with that of monoliths, as they are constrained in the plane of the substrate and all shrinkage takes place normal to the substrate (Pettit et al. 1988). Coatings less than 400 to 500 nm thick can be dried at controlled rates, to minimize the potential for cracking. However, when thickness of the films exceed approximately 500 nm, cracking becomes difficult to avoid (Sakka et al. 1984; Strawbridge and James 1986; Dislich 1988; Gan and Ben-Nissan 1997; Aksakal and Hanyaoglu 2008). The critical thickness for cracking or debonding to occur in coatings is defined (Hu and Evans 1989) as:

$$h = \frac{2E\gamma}{\sigma^2} \tag{2.1}$$

where h is the film thickness, E is the plain strain (Young's modulus) of the film, γ is the fracture energy to create new surface, and σ is the stress in the film.

Firing or sintering is the final stage in the production of ceramic materials via the sol–gel process. By heating dried gels to elevated temperatures, usually approximately 600°C, any remaining organic materials are combusted (Figure 2.7). Due to the small grain sizes obtained in this process, sintering temperatures are between 400°C and 800°C. Some specific chemistry allows lower temperatures such as 90°C. By controlling the atmosphere during the firing process, gel can be converted to oxides (Yoldas 1984; Anast 1996), nitrides (Jimenez and Langlet 1994; Kraus et al. 1996; Gao et al. 1997; Cassidy et al. 1997), carbides (Raman et al. 1995; Hasegawa 1997), and mixtures thereof (Gabriel and Riedel 1997).

The Sol–Gel Process: Coating Techniques

There are two major coating techniques: dip and spin coating.

Dip Coating

Dip coating is primarily used for the fabrication of coatings on items such as flat glass substrates. However, dip coating can also be used for coating complex shapes such as rods, pipes, tubes, and fibers. The dip coating process has the advantage of being capable of producing multilayered coatings with a high degree of thickness uniformity up to 1000 nm thick. In addition multilayered coatings can be manufactured with specific optical characteristics and are used commercially (Dislich 1988).

The film thickness of a single layer is determined by the withdrawal speed for a given solution (Figure 2.8). On the other hand, the thickness can also be modified by altering the physical properties of the solution, for example, viscosity, as well as the number of layers deposited (Turner 1991; Lee et al. 1993; Paterson et al. 1998). The film thickness can be estimated from the following (Scriven 1988):

$$h = c\left(\frac{\eta U}{\rho g}\right)^{1/2} \tag{2.2}$$

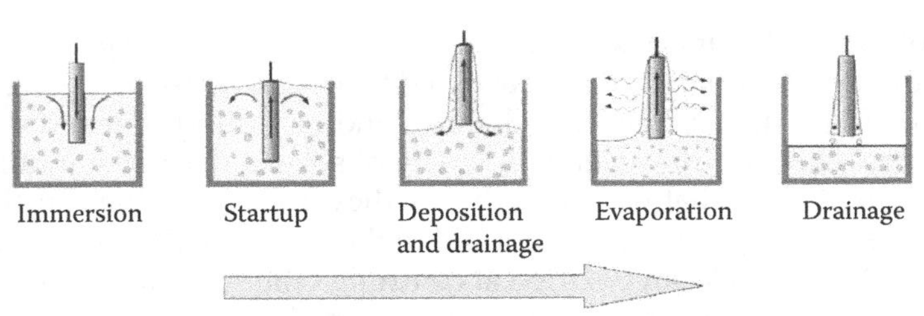

FIGURE 2.8
Schematic diagram of the five stages of dip coating process.

where c is a constant and is about 0.8 for Newtonian liquids, η is the sol viscosity, U is the withdrawal speed, ρ is the density, and g is the acceleration due to gravity.

The dip coating process is normally a batch process but can be adapted to coat long flexible sheets and wires (Scriven 1988). The overall process can be broken up into five stages:

1. Immersion
2. Startup
3. Deposition and drainage
4. Evaporation
5. Drainage

The first two stages are always sequential; the third and fourth may take place concomitantly throughout the entire process, unless the necessary precautions are taken (Figure 2.8).

When substrates are dip-coated, the thickness of the film will be different at the edges. This might generate cracks during firing. Faster pullout rates generate thicker coatings due to less drainage and evaporation during pullout. By proper control of pullout rate we can produce about 70- to 100-nm thick crack-free coatings if all other factors are adequate.

Spin Coating

Spin coating is a process suited to flat shapes such as disks and plates. Similar to dip coating, spin coating can be separated into four stages and evaporation can take place throughout the entire coating process.

The first stage of spin coating involves delivering excess liquid to the substrate while it is stationary or spinning. During the second stage, rotation causes the liquid to move radially outward due to centrifugal forces. This may occur while the substrate is being accelerated to maximum speed. In the third stage, excess liquid flows to the perimeter and is detached in the form of droplets. If the substrate has a central hole, drainage takes place in the same manner as in the dip coating process. The film thins down to a fairly uniform thickness, apart for the edges, which is effected due to the surface tension changes. As the film thins, the flow decreases as drag forces increase. The thinner films are affected more by evaporation, which raises the solution viscosity by concentrating nonvolatiles. Evaporation becomes the dominant process once spinoff has ceased. Film thickness will reach uniformity provided that its viscosity is insensitive to shear rate (Newtonian behavior). Uniformity will occur when viscous forces balance centrifugal forces. The final thickness of a spin coated film is given by Scriven (1988):

$$h = \left(\frac{\rho}{\rho_0}\right)\left(\frac{3\eta e}{2\rho_0 \omega}\right)^{1/3} \tag{2.3}$$

where ρ_0 is the initial solvent volume fraction, ρ is the solvent volume fraction in the film, η is the viscosity of the solution, ω is the angular velocity, and e is the evaporation rate. This equation shows that the film thickness can be controlled by adjusting the viscosity and solids content of the solution and the deposition conditions (spin speed).

Sol–Gel Synthesis of Nanohydroxyapatite

Nanocrystalline hydroxyapatite can be produced by a number of production methods to be used as nanocoatings, monolithic solid ceramic products, or as nanosized powders and platelets for a number of applications (Figure 2.5).

To prepare nanocrystalline apatites, methods of wet chemical precipitation, sol–gel synthesis, coprecipitation, hydrothermal synthesis, mechanochemical synthesis, mechanical alloying, ball milling, radio frequency induction plasma, vibromilling of bones, flame spray pyrolysis, liquid–solid–solution synthesis, electrocrystallization, microwave processing, hydrolysis of other calcium orthophosphates, double step stirring, emulsion-based, or solvothermal syntheses and several other techniques are known. Continuous preparation procedures are also available. Furthermore, nanodimensional HAp might be manufactured by a laser-induced fragmentation of HAp microparticles in water and in solvent-containing aqueous solutions, while dense nanocrystalline HAp films might be produced by radio frequency magnetron sputtering (Dorozhkin 2009). A comparison between the sol–gel synthesis and wet chemical precipitation technique has been performed and both methods appear to be suitable for synthesis of nanocrystalline apatite.

Over the past 40 years, synthetic production methods of crystalline monolithic hydroxyapatite have been extensive, especially once it was discovered that hydroxyapatite has nearly the same mineral component as bone and that it can be implemented as a bone substitute material (Hulbert et al. 1970; Heimke and Griss 1980; LeGeros 1991; Hench 1991; Liu et al. 2003).

Most published information on hydroxyapatite is classified under calcium phosphate, to which hydroxyapatite belongs. As a result, the chemical properties will be viewed from the standpoint that hydroxyapatite is a calcium phosphate, even though it has different reactivity and solubility to other calcium phosphates within the physiological environment.

Calcium phosphates are characterized by particular solubilities, for example when bonding to the surrounding tissue, and their ability to degrade and be replaced by advancing bone growth. The solubilities of various calcium phosphates can be shown as (LeGeros 1991; LeGeros 1993):

amorphous calcium phosphate (ACP) > dibasic calcium phosphate (DCP) > tetracalcium phosphate (TTCP) > α-tricalcium phosphate (α-TCP) > β-tricalcium phosphate (β-TCP) > hydroxyapatite

The sol–gel process offers an improved alternative technique for producing bioactive surfaces for better bone attachment owing to its nanocrystalline characteristics, homogeneity, and bioreactivity (Ben-Nissan and Chai 1995; Gross et al. 1998).

Various sol–gel routes have been employed for the production of synthetic hydroxyapatite powders since the early 1990s. A number of excellent studies have been conducted on a range of precursors to produce pure nanocrystalline apatite powders, solid products, or coatings for medical and engineering applications (Choi and Ben-Nissan 2007). The major ones are calcium acetate, calcium alkoxide, calcium chloride, calcium hydroxide, calcium nitrate, and dicalcium phosphate dihydrate and are shown in Table 2.1. It has been reported by some of the investigators that the thickness of the sol–gel derived hydroxyapatite coatings produced are in the 70 to 100 nm range (Ben-Nissan and Chai 1995; Anast et al. 1996).

TABLE 2.1

Some of the Published Work Showing Nanohydroxyapatite and Related Material Production Based on a Number of Different Sol–Gel Synthesis Methods

Calcium and Phosphorus Precursor		Investigators
Calcium Acetate	$Ca(CH_3COO)_2 \cdot H_2O$ / $(NH_4)_2HPO_4$	Bogdanoviciene et al. (2006)
	$Ca(CH_3COO)_2$ / H_3PO_4 / P_4O_{10}	Balamurugan et al. (2006)
	$Ca(CH_3COO)_2$	Cihlar and Castkova (1998)
Calcium Alkoxide	$Ca(OEt)_2$ / $P(OC_2H_5)_3$	Masuda et al. (1990)
	$Ca(OEt)_2$ / $(C_2H_5O)_2P(O)H)$	Ben-Nissan and Chai (1995) Chai et al. (1995) Gross et al. (1998) Milev et al. (2003)
	$Ca(OEt)_2$ / (H_3PO_4)	Layrolle and Lebugle (1994) Layrolle et al. (1998)
Calcium Chloride	$CaCl_2 \cdot 2H_2O$ / $Na_2HPO_4 \cdot 2H_2O$	Andersson et al. (2005)
	$CaCl_2$ / NaH_2PO_4	Sarig and Kahana (2006)
Calcium Hydroxide	$Ca(OH)_2$ – PVA / H_3PO_4	Wang et al. (2005)
	$Ca(O_2C_8H_{15})_2)$ / $C_{16}H_{35}O_4P$	Tkalcec et al. (2001)
Calcium Nitrate	$Ca(NO_3) \cdot 4H_2O$ / $(NH_4)_2HPO_4$ / Citric Acid	Han et al. (2004)
	$Ca(NO_3) \cdot 4H_2O$ / $PO(OH)_{3-x}(OEt)_x$ / Citric Acid	Weng et al. (2002)
	$Ca(NO_3)$ / $P(OC_2H_5)_3$	Balamurugan et al. (2006)
	$Ca(NO_3)_2 \cdot 4H_2O$ / $P(OC_2H_5)_3$	Kim et al. (2005)
	$Ca(NO_3)_2 \cdot 4H_2O$ / $(NH_4)_3PO_4 \cdot 3H_2O$	Stoch et al. (2005)
	$Ca(NO_3)_2 \cdot 4H_2O$ / P_2O_5	Yang et al. (2005)
	$Ca(NO_3)_2 \cdot 4H_2O$ / $P(OC_2H_5)_3$ & $Ca(NO_3)_2 \cdot 4H_2O$ / $(NH_4)_3PO_4 \cdot 3H_2O$	Gan and Pilliar (2004)
	$Ca(NO_3)_2 \cdot 4H_2O$ / P_4O_{10} & NH_4PF_6 &	Cheng et al. (2001)
	$Ca(NO_3)_2$ / $(NH_4)_3HPO_4$	Bose and Saha (2003)
	$Ca(NO_3)_2 \cdot 4H_2O$ / $(C_2H_5O)_3PO$	Hsieh et al. (2002)
	$Ca(NO_3)_2 \cdot 4H_2O$ / H_3PO_4	Lim et al. (2001)
Calcium Phosphate	$CaHPO_4 \cdot 2H_2O$ / $CaCO_3$	Shin et al. (2004)

Calcium Alkoxide

Masuda et al. (1990) studied nanohydroxyapatite powder production using the alkoxide-based system containing calcium diethoxide, triethyl phosphite, ethanediol, and ethanol, modified with water and acetic acid. Within this system, they synthesized powders and found that the determining factor for the composition of the resultant powder was the solution's pH. This was the first systematic approach on controlling the chemistry for pure nanohydroxyapatite production. No attempts were made to produce monolithic materials or coatings.

Based on the basic chemistry of Matsuda et al. (1990), Ben-Nissan et al. (Ben-Nissan and Chai 1995; Chai et al. 1998; Gross et al. 1998; Ben-Nissan et al. 2001), and Green et al. (2001) employed a modified alkoxide process to synthesize HAp powders and coatings via the sol–gel technique. In a further modified technique, Milev et al. (Milev et al. 2002, 2003; Ben-Nissan et al. 2001) used multinuclear NMR spectroscopy to monitor the synthesis of carbonate-containing HAp for powder, nanoplatelets and nanocoating productions (Figure 2.9).

Layrolle and Lebugle (1994) developed a synthesis route of different calcium phosphates, using anhydrous ethanol as solvent and calcium diethoxide ($Ca(OEt)_2$) and orthophosphoric acid (H_3PO_4) as reagents. In a systematic approach using a simple variance of the ratio of reagents, calcium phosphates of various chemical compositions $Ca_x(HPO_4)_y(PO_4)_z$ were precipitated in the ethanol. The solids that formed were characterized by different physicochemical and thermal analyses. The results revealed that the different solid calcium phosphates are amorphous and of the nanoscale and have large specific surface areas and high reactivities.

Layrolle et al. (1998) also described the production of a nanosized, amorphous, and carbonate-containing calcium phosphate powder synthesized from calcium diethoxide and phosphoric acid in ethanol via a sol–gel method. They concluded that after sintering, the decomposition of carbonated HAp generated a microporous ceramic with an average pore size of 0.2 μm and an open porosity of 15.5% and that this microporous bioceramic can be used as bone filler.

Roest et al. (Roest et al. 2001, 2004; Roest 2010) developed carbonate nanohydroxyapatite coatings on anodized titanium and titanium alloy (Ti–6Al–4V) by dip and spin coating methods successfully. Similar methods were used to coat a range of substrates with zirconia nanocoatings.

Zreiqat et al. (2005) compared the effect of surface chemistry modification of titanium alloy (Ti–6Al–4V) with zinc, magnesium, and alkoxide-derived hydroxy carbonate apatite

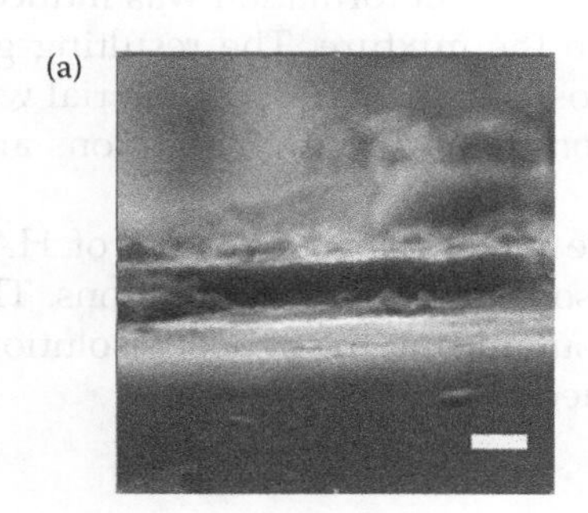

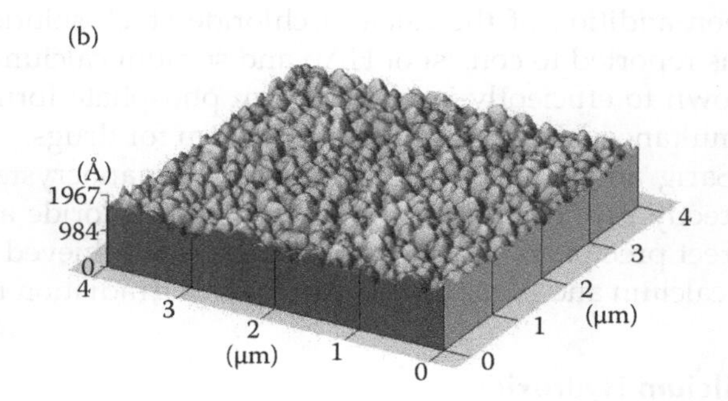

FIGURE 2.9
(a) SEM of nanohydroxyapatite coating (scale 100 nm), (b) AFM image of the same nanohydroxyapatite coating.

produced by Roest et al. 2001, on the regulation of key intracellular signaling proteins in human bone-derived stem cells (HBDC) cultured on these modified Ti–6Al–4V surfaces. They concluded that the surface modification with carbonate apatite coated or Mg incorporated apatite may contribute to successful osteoblast function and differentiation at the skeletal tissue-device interface.

Calcium Acetate

Aqueous sol–gel chemistry routes based on ammonium hydrogen phosphate as the phosphorus precursor and calcium acetate monohydrate as the source of calcium ions have been developed by Bogdanoviciene et al. (2006) to prepare hydroxyapatite powder samples with different morphological properties. In the sol–gel processes, an aqueous solution of ethylenediaminetetraacetic acid (EDTA) or tartaric acid (TA) as complexing agents was added to the reaction mixture. It was reported that the monophasic $Ca_{10}(PO_4)_6(OH)_2$ samples were obtained by calcination of precursor gels for 5 h at 1000°C. They demonstrated that the proposed aqueous sol–gel methods are very simple, inexpensive, and thus appropriate for the large-scale fabrication of calcium hydroxyapatite powders and ceramics.

Cihlar and Castkova (1998) examined the synthesis of calcium phosphates from methyl-, ethyl, *i*-propyl, and *n*-butyl phosphates and calcium acetate in acidic and basic water–alcoholic solutions. A mixture of HAp and beta-tricalcium phosphate (β-TCP) was achieved through the reaction of all alkylphosphates with calcium acetate in an acidic solution. Calcium pyrophosphate was achieved when the reaction proceeded in the presence of ammonium hydroxide. HAp with an admixture of calcium pyrophosphate or β-TCP was prepared by means of monoethanolamine or diethanolamine catalysts.

Calcium Chloride

Andersson et al. (2005) developed a degradable, hierarchically porous apatite composite material from a simple low-temperature synthesis. HAp was produced through a sol–gel method at near room temperature conditions. They used $CaCl_2{\cdot}2H_2O$, $Na_2HPO_4{\cdot}2H_2O$, cetyltrimethylammonium bromide ($C_{16}TAB$), ammonia solution, and tetraethoxysilane (TEOS) as starting material for this investigation. Two stock solutions were prepared from $Na_2HPO_4{\cdot}2H_2O$ and $CaCl_2{\cdot}2H_2O$, using distilled and deionized water. $C_{16}TAB$ was dissolved in phosphate-containing stock solution, after which ammonia was added. The mixture was kept under constant stirring in a closed beaker. Gel formation was induced upon addition of the calcium chloride stock solution to the mixture. The resulting gel was reported to consist of HAp and sodium calcium phosphate. The hybrid material was shown to efficiently induce calcium phosphate formation under in vitro conditions and simultaneously work as a carrier system for drugs.

Sarig and Kahana (2002) synthesized nanocrystalline plate-shaped particles of HAp directly precipitated from dilute calcium chloride and sodium phosphate solutions. The direct precipitation of hydroxyapatite was achieved by submitting the aqueous solutions of calcium and phosphate to microwave irradiation immediately after mixing.

Calcium Hydroxide

Sol–gel inorganic–organic hybrid material coated on glassy carbon electrode used for the immobilization and study of double-stranded DNA with redox-active molecules was developed by Wang et al. (2005). They produced a hybrid material coating consisting of nanohydroxyapatite (HAp)–polyvinyl alcohol (PVA). The hybrid was prepared from phosphoric acid solution and saturated calcium hydroxide solution, while the PVA was dissolved in distilled water. They discovered that mixing a suitable quantity of PVA in HAp sol can prevent the HAp coating from cracking and enhance its stability. The properties of the nano-HAp-PVA hybrid were affected by the concentration of PVA.

HAp and tricalcium phosphate (TCP) powders and coatings were synthesized by Tkalcec et al. (2001) via the sol–gel technique to examine the formation mechanism of crystalline phases in the firing processes of coatings with different Ca/P molar ratios. Calcium hydroxide was suspended in ethanol and ethylhexanoic acid (EHA) was added dropwise to this suspension. The solution was then filtered by pressure filtering to obtain a clear solution of calcium 2-ethylhexanoate ($Ca(O_2C_8H_{15})_2$). Calcium 2-ethylhexanoate and 2-ethyl-hexyl-phosphate were used as calcium and phosphorus precursors, respectively. Coatings were deposited on Si–wafer and Ti–alloy substrates by dipping the substrates into sols at room temperature. The results from the work showed that dip-coating and sintering in two cycles yielded a homogeneous and dense coated film with a thickness of 250 nm.

Calcium Nitrate

Calcium nitrate ($Ca(NO_3)_2$) has been a popular calcium precursor for the synthesis of hydroxyapatite.

The citric acid sol–gel combustion method has been employed by Han et al. (2004) for the synthesis of nanocrystalline HAp powders from calcium nitrate, diammonium hydrogen phosphate, and citric acid. HAp powder was used to sinter a monolithic ceramic product in order to illustrate its sinterability, open porosity, flexural strength, and structural rigidity. Microscopy revealed that there were many pores in the micropore sizes ranging between 1 and 5 μm of irregular shape. Although the open porosity of the resulting ceramic was about 19%, the pore size is not good for bone ingrowth. After sintering at 1200°C, the grain size is about 3 μm.

Weng et al. (2002) also examined the effect on the addition of citric acid on the formation of sol–gel derived HAp. In order to improve the gelation in the sol–gel preparation of HAp by using $Ca(NO_3)_2$ and $PO(OH)_{3-x}(OEt)_x$ as precursors, citric acid was selected as an enhancing gelation additive. HAp derived from the mixed precursor solutions with citric acid showed a different reaction path from that without citric acid. They suggest that citric acid plays a role in enhancing gelation through the strong coordination ability of Ca ions with citrate groups. They have also concluded that the addition of citric acid can provide a way to synthesize a pure oxy-HAp or an apatite with carbonated HAp, HAp, and minor β-TCP, which might have good bioactivity.

Balamurugan et al. (2006) developed a different sol–gel technique for the synthesis phase of pure HAp powder. Triethyl phosphite and calcium nitrate were used as phosphorus and calcium precursors. The powders obtained were dried and calcined at different temperatures up to 900°C. X-ray diffraction analysis and Raman spectra were reported to show the presence of pure HAp.

Kim et al. (2005) coated hydroxyapatite composites with titania (TiO_2) on titanium (Ti) substrate by a sol–gel route, and the mechanical and biological properties of the coating systems were examined. Calcium nitrate tetrahydrate ($Ca(NO_3)_2{\cdot}4H_2O$) and triethyl phosphite ($P(OC_2H_5)_3$) were hydrolyzed together with ethanol and distilled water. Ammonium hydroxide (NH_4OH) was added stepwise to the mixture. To produce a TiO_2 sol, titanium propoxide ($Ti(OCH_2CH_2CH_3)_4$) was hydrolyzed within an ethanol-based solution containing diethanolamine ($(HOCH_2CH_2)_2NH$) and distilled water. The prepared HAp and TiO_2 sols were mixed together and stirred vigorously to obtain HAp–TiO_2 composite sols. Coatings were produced under a controlled spinning and heat treatment process. The HAp–TiO_2 composite coating layers were homogeneous and highly dense, with a thickness of about 800 to 900 nm. The adhesion strength of the coating layers with regard to the Ti substrate increased with increasing TiO_2 addition. The osteoblast-like cells were tried and reported that they grew and spread actively on all the composite coatings. They concluded that the sol–gel derived HAp–TiO_2 composite coatings possess excellent properties for hard tissue applications.

HAp coatings on titanium and its alloy were synthesized by Stoch et al. (2005) for facilitating and shortening the processes towards osseointegration. HAp coatings were obtained by the sol–gel method with sol solutions prepared from calcium nitrate tetrahydrate and triammonium phosphate trihydrate as the calcium and phosphorous sources. Two types of gelatin were added to the sol: agar–agar or animal gelatine. Both were found to enhance the formation and stability of amorphous HAp using soluble salts as the sources of calcium and phosphate. The biological activity of phosphate coatings was observed in the SBF. They found that the chemical composition and structure of HAp coatings depends on the pH and final thermal treatment of the layer.

Sol–gel synthesis and template preparation of nanomaterials to yield a new general route for fabricating highly ordered HAp nanowire arrays were fabricated by Yang et al. (2005) using a porous anodic aluminum oxide (AAO) template from a sol–gel solution containing P_2O_5 and $Ca(NO_3)_2$. The AAO template membrane was immersed into this sol for the desired amount of time and allowed to dry in air. Excess sol on the membrane surface was carefully wiped off and then heat-treated in an open furnace. HAp nanowire arrays were formed inside the pores of the AAO template. Various characterization techniques such as TEM, SEM, XRD, and XPS were applied to examine the structure of HAp nanowires. HAp nanowires had a uniform length and diameter and form highly ordered arrays, which are determined by the pore diameter and the thickness of the applied AAO template. They have reported that their novel method of preparing highly ordered HAp nanowires with a large area might be very important in many biomedical applications. No attempts were made to use the wires as nanocomposite coatings.

Thin sol–gel formed calcium phosphate (Ca–P) films were produced on sintered porous-surfaced implants as an approach to increase the rate of bone ingrowth by Gan and Pilliar (2004). Porous-surfaced dental implants (endopores implants) were used for the sol–gel coating of sintered porous surface structures. The porous surface was created by sintering Ti–6Al–4V microspheres of 45 to 150 μm in diameter onto a machined Ti–6Al–4V substrate. The films were prepared using both an inorganic precursor solution (with calcium nitrate tetrahydrate and ammonium dihydrogen phosphate) and an organic precursor solution (with calcium nitrate tetrahydrate and triethyl phosphite). They reported that both approaches resulted in the formation of nanocrystalline carbonated HAp films but with different Ca/P ratios and structures. They commented that while both the inorganic and organic methods resulted in films with nanocrystalline or submicron crystalline carbonated HAp films, the inorganic method resulted in films that differed significantly in structure, displayed a more irregular surface texture, and were less dense. Cross-sectional TEM studies revealed an interfacial reaction product phase when using the inorganic method, and calcium titanium oxide was developed.

In order to improve thermal stability and strength of hydroxyapatite powder during thermal or plasma spraying, fluorine is added to hydroxyapatite to form HAp/fluoroapatite (FA) solid solution.

In 2001, Cheng et al. (2001) developed a sol–gel method to synthesize a (HAp)/(FA) solid solution. Calcium nitrate–4 hydrate, phosphoric pentoxide, and trifluoroacetic acid (TFA) were used as the precursors. Triethanolamine (TEA) was used as a promoter for incorporating fluorine into Ca phosphates. Mixed ethanol solutions of the Ca and P precursors in Ca/P ratio of 1.67 with different amounts of TFA and TEA were prepared; the mixed solutions were dried on a hot plate to convert them to the as-prepared powders. HAp/FA solid solutions were obtained after the powders were calcined at temperatures up to 900°C.

Cheng et al. (2004) utilized a sol–gel method to synthesize a fluoridated hydroxyapatite (FHAp) phase. Calcium nitrate tetrahydrate, phosphoric pentoxide, and ammonium hexafluorophosphate were used as precursors. The Ca, P, and F precursors were mixed under designated proportions to form solutions with a Ca/P ratio of 1.67. In order to obtain an FHA phase with various fluorine contents, different amounts of ammonium hexafluorophosphate were added in the Ca–P mixed solutions.

The synthesis of HAp nanopowders using a sol–gel route with calcium nitrate and ammonium hydrogen phosphate as calcium and phosphorous precursors, respectively, were described by Bose and Saha (2003). Sucrose was used as the template material, and alumina was added as a dopant to study its effects on particle size and surface area. The average particle size of porous HAp samples was between 30 and 50 nm.

Hsieh et al. (2002) successfully developed a simple rapid-heating method for calcium phosphate coatings on Ti–6Al–4V substrates deposited by using a sol–gel derived precursor. The preparation of the precursor was carried out by mixing $Ca(NO_3)_2{\cdot}4H_2O$ and $(C_2H_5O)_3PO$ in 2-methoxy ethanol. Upon aging, the as-prepared solution was closely capped and placed in an oil bath for 16 h. Upon gelation (drying), the solvent was evaporated in the same oil bath so that a viscous precursor was obtained. Adhesive strength tests were conducted and the results indicated that, at the first coating layer using either spin or dip coating, the breakages occur at the glue-coating interface, representing an adhesive strength higher than 90 MPa. Thus, the first layer is firmly adhered to the substrate. Hsieh et al. also found that a porous structure, with a pore size of 10 to 20 μm, was formed on the outermost coating surface. It was reported that this structure is due to the fast decomposition during rapid heating of the precursor deposited on the substrate, and is very suitable for ingrowth of living cells. Although this comment is true for cell penetration it does not allow vascularization, which requires pore sizes of 140 to 500 μm.

Lim et al. (2001) investigated the bioactivities of the coating by analyzing the variation of ion concentrations of Ca and P in simulated body fluid after soaking, using an inductively coupled plasma–atomic emission spectrometer. Ti/HAp coating solutions with variable HAp concentrations were derived from calcium nitrate ($Ca(NO_3)_2{\cdot}4H_2O$) and phosphoric acid (H_3PO_4) that were dissolved in ethylene glycol monomethyl ether ($CH_3OCH_2CH_2OH$). Coating surfaces, after soaking in simulated body fluid, indicated significant morphological changes when investigated by field emission-scanning electron microscopy.

Dicalcium Phosphate Dihydrate

The crystal growth and morphology of the nanosized HAp powders synthesized from dicalcium phosphate dihydrate ($CaHPO_4{\cdot}2H_2O$) and $CaCO_3$ have been investigated by Shin et al. (2004). The nanosized HAp powders were obtained from the hydrolysis of dicalcium phosphate dihydrate and $CaCO_3$ with NaOH. They discovered that the only product synthesized from dicalcium phosphate dihydrate was HAp, and the crystallinity of the HAp was improved with increasing annealing temperature. The crystallite size of the HAp samples with Ca/P equal to 1.0 was about 50 nm thick and 100 nm long. As the Ca/P ratio increased by adding $CaCO_3$, the particle size increased to 200 nm thick and 500 nm long.

Sol–Gel Hydroxyapatite-Nanocoated Coralline Apatite

Coral mineral has had considerable success as a bone graft material in view of its interconnected porous structure, which ranges from 150 to 500 μm (Figure 2.10). In morphology, it is similar to the human cancellous bone and is one of a limited number of materials that will form chemical bonds with bone and soft tissue in vivo. On the other hand, unless it is modified by chemical means, coral as calcium carbonate is unsuitable for bone graft applications due to its high dissolution rate. Conversion to hydroxyapatite and the use of nanocoatings improves a range of properties. Nanocoated coralline hydroxyapatite has been reported to have enhanced bioactivity and strength (Hu et al. 2001; Ben-Nissan et al. 2004).

Natural Skeletons

Using natural skeletons in a direct way as a scaffold for growing cells into tissue emerged for making new bone tissue as a product of hydrothermal processing (Weber et al. 1974; Roy et al. 1974). Transformed coral has been the primary source of natural skeletons for bone tissue engineering because of its chemical, crystallographic, and structural similarity to human bone.

Since then researchers have attempted to make use of the skeletons of hydrozoans, cuttlefish (Rocha et al. 2005), marine sponges (Green et al. 2003), nacre seashell, and echinoderm spines (Martina et al. 2005; Roy et al. 1974) as templates with optimal ranges of pore sizes, channels, and structural networks for organizing and nourishing the growth of human tissues as a prelude to transplantation into the patient.

In a number of studies, various candidate biomatrices were identified in nature with varied chemical homologies and structural analogies to human extracellular matrices and whole tissues (Green 2003; Green and Ben-Nissan 2008). They include nacre marine shell,

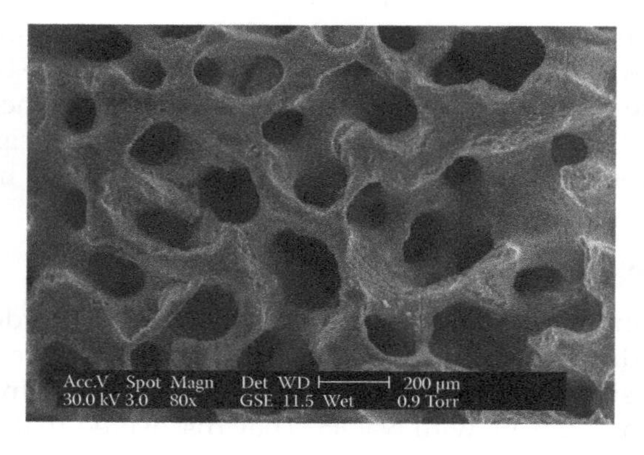

FIGURE 2.10
Natural coral containing interconnected pores.

marine sponge skeletons, echinoderm skeletal elements, and coral skeletons. The utility of selected species of these marine animals has been applied to the regeneration of human bone and cartilage. However, their full utility in these tissues and other tissues has yet to be harnessed and exploited.

Coral and Coralline Apatite

Natural coral exoskeletons have been used widely as a bone replacement in orthopedic, craniofacial, dental, and neurosurgery owing to their combination of good mechanical properties, open porosity, and ability to form chemical bonds with bone and soft tissues in vivo (Ben-Nissan 2004). In fact corals have the best mechanical properties of the porous calcium-based ceramics and resorb at a rate equivalent to host bone formation.

The abundance, conformation, and composition of the organic matrices are responsible for successful biological integration of coral with human host (Dauphin 2003). Use of coral skeletons for general routine orthopedic surgery and tissue engineering has so far been limited to external fixation devices as they are inappropriate for strictly load-bearing applications. Sol–gel coating technologies can be used to enhance the strength of corals and this enables them to be used at more skeletal locations. Corals offer great opportunities to tissue engineering of bone either in their natural form or as hybridized synthetic forms (Petite et al. 2000). Coral skeleton combined with in vitro expanded human bone marrow stromal cells (HBMSC) increased osteogenesis more than that obtained with scaffold alone or scaffold with fresh marrow. In vivo large animal segmental defect studies led to complete recorticalization and formation of a medullary canal with mature lamellar cortical bone giving rise to clinical union in a high number of cases (Petite et al. 2000). Structural and biomineralization studies of coral can be used as a guide for the development of new advanced functional materials because of the unique nanoscale organization of organic tissue and mineral as highlighted by Ehrlich et al. (2006). At a macrostructural level, the deep-sea bamboo coral exhibited bonelike biochemical and mechanical properties. A specialized collagen matrix (acidic fibrillar) serves as a model for future potential tissue engineering applications. The matrix supported both osteoblast and osteoclast growth and the exceptional bioelastomeric properties of the collagen matrix (gorgonin) of this coral make it potentially suitable for blood vessel implants. Quinones cross-link and harden the collagenous gorgonin proteins and closely resemble human keratin. The mechanism by which gorgonin is synthesized and interacts with the process of mineralization may provide lessons for the generation of a synthetic collagen-like material (Ehrlich et al. 2006).

Nanocoated Coralline Apatite

Current commercially available bone graft materials using hydrothermal conversion only achieve partial conversion of coralline calcium carbonate to HAp. Unfortunately, being limited to the outer surface, the inner core remains as unconverted calcium carbonate of the original coral (Shors 1999). This material has the advantage of retaining a favorable pore size and bioactivity, with improved properties, compared to native coral. Unfortunately, this also generates an unknown factor of biodegradation due to the differing solubility rates of hydroxyapatite and unconverted calcium carbonate. As a result, this material is subject to fast dissolution in the physiologic environment, compromising strength, durability, tissue integration, and ultimately the longevity.

It was discovered (Hu et al. 2001; Ben-Nissan et al. 2004) that the application of a hydroxyapatite sol–gel coating onto the monophasic HAp derived from the hydrothermally converted coral increased its mechanical properties. This nanocoating was reported to increase all of the mechanical properties. Coral, in addition to the macropores, also contains meso- and nanopores ranging between 5 and 50 nm within a fibrous structure that constitutes the interpore area between the large macropores.

The method involves a unique patented two-step conversion procedure. In the first stage, corals possessing a suitable macropore structure are converted to pure HAp, with complete replacement of calcium carbonate by phosphatic material throughout the specimen. The HAp can be prepared from coral by a hydrothermal reactor. The reaction can be carried out at 250°C with an ammonium monohydrogen phosphate solution for a predetermined period of time. Additional stage involves the use of sol–gel derived HAp with the converted coralline apatite.

In general, the alkoxide method used involves the formulation of a homogeneous solution containing all of the component metals in the correct stoichiometry. Mixtures of metal alkoxides and/or metal alkanoates in organic solvents that have been stabilized against precipitation by chemical additives (amines, glycols, acetylacetone, etc.) have proven the most successful.

All synthetic procedures for the preparation of sols were carried out in a dry nitrogen atmosphere due to the hygroscopic nature of the starting alkoxide precursors. The calcium alkoxide precursor solution was prepared by dispersing calcium diethoxide ($Ca(OEt)_2$) in absolute ethanol (Et(OH)). Phosphorous precursor solution was then prepared by diluting triethyl phosphite ($P(OEt)_3$) in absolute Et(OH) (Ben-Nissan et al. 2001).

After complete dissolution of the calcium diethoxide, the phosphorous precursor solution can be added to the calcium precursor solution. The clear solutions were aged at ambient temperature before being used. Coatings were formed using these solutions followed by subsequent heat treatment for further densification.

Detailed analyses using SEM revealed that the coating step effectively obliterates the surface meso- and nanopore systems while leaving the macropore system intact (Figure 2.11).

Application of nanocoating had two major effects; first, the improvement of the mechanical properties compared to traditional coral materials, and second, it enhanced the bioactivity of the material. Mechanical testing indicated that all properties have increased including compression, biaxial, flexural strengths, and the elastic modulus (Ben-Nissan

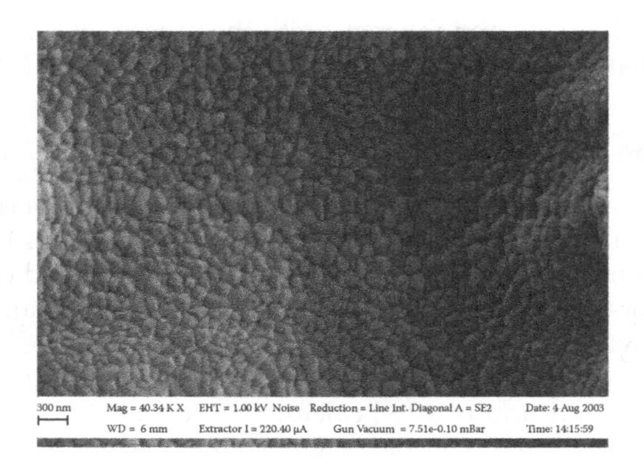

FIGURE 2.11
SEM reveals that the coating step effectively obliterates the surface meso- and nanopore systems, whilst leaving the macropore system intact.

et al. 2004). It is anticipated that this new patented process and material can be applied to bone graft applications where high strength requirements and longevity are pertinent.

Mechanical Properties of Thin Films

Understanding of the long-term mechanical reliability of biomedical thin films is pertinent in clinical applications. Hence, a number of methods capable of quantitatively measuring the mechanical properties are required. Since the 1980s there have been constant improvements and developments in equipment capable of extracting the structure and properties of thin films and also the adhesion of the coating to an underlying substrate (Ben-Nissan and Pezzotti 2002).

A general review of thin film mechanical properties of coatings is given by Nix (2006). According to his work on both thin and thick film coatings, the main factors that can influence mechanical reliability are many; however, the most important ones are the interfacial properties, residual stresses for thick coatings, substrate, and thin film thickness and its geometry.

The evaluation of stress in a nanocoating due to deposition technique and heat treatments applied plays an important role in regards to mechanical stability. The potential for cracking and spalling of the coating due to inbuilt stresses (whether they are tensile or compressive) or from external mechanical loading plays a key part in the successful use of biomaterial implants. The stress in a film is a combination of the following components and is described in Equation 2.4: intrinsic (deposition, mode of growth, structure), thermal expansion mismatch between film and substrate (specifically in thick films) due to changes in temperature and externally applied stresses (Lepienski et al. 2004):

$$\sigma_{\mathrm{f}} = \sigma_{(\mathrm{intrinsic})} + \sigma_{(\mathrm{thermal})} + \sigma_{(\mathrm{external})} \tag{2.4}$$

Stress measurement by substrate curvature is a simple method requiring either (1) a stylus profilometer capable of scans 10 mm in length or more, or (2) using a phase shifting interferometer. The advantages of using an optical method such as interferometry are high accuracy of about 6 nm, substrates with curvature of up to 3 µm are acceptable, and it is a rapid and straightforward technique to use.

In stylus profiometry, the substrate needs to be sufficiently thin for adequate measurement of the curvature. The method requires careful and precise placement of the sample, so that a cross scan in the x and y directions can be made on the surface (preferably both sides) before and after coating.

The stress in the coating (intrinsic + thermal) can be evaluated using the Stoney formula without prior knowledge of the coating properties. The information that is required is coating thickness, substrate thickness, and its Young's modulus. Stoney's equation (Stoney 1909) shows the relationship between the change in the radius of a coated and uncoated substrate and the corresponding stress in the layer (Equation 2.5):

$$\sigma = \frac{1}{6}\left[\frac{1}{R_{\mathrm{f}}} - \frac{1}{R_{\mathrm{i}}}\right]\frac{E_{\mathrm{s}}}{(1-\nu_{\mathrm{s}})}\frac{t_{\mathrm{s}}^2}{t_{\mathrm{f}}} \tag{2.5}$$

where R_i is the radius of curvature before coating, R_f after coating, E_s and v_s the modulus and Poisson's ratio of the substrate, t_s the substrate thickness, and t_f the film thickness. Assuming that the scan length L of the substrate is much greater than the final bow B of the substrate, the radius R can be calculated using Equation 2.6.

$$R = \frac{L^2}{8B} \tag{2.6}$$

Compressive stress in the film leads to a convex deflection, whereas tensile stress results in concave deflection. Measurements can be made in situ during deposition or thermal treatment with optical means by interferometry or deflection method (cantilever beam) using a low-power laser. Similarly, elastic strain in films can be measured by x-ray diffraction from the change in crystal lattice *d*-spacing, from which the stress can be determined given knowledge of Young's modulus and strain-free lattice spacing (which may be unknown in many cases) (Tsui et al. 1998).

The most commonly used methods for characterizing the performance of micro- and nanocoatings on substrates can generally be divided into the measurement of coating properties and adhesion strength. There are a number of excellent methods that can be used in thin film mechanical properties evaluation, and some of the commonly used methods are nanoindentation, tensile testing, scratch testing, adhesion and wear testing, pin-on-disk testing, pull-out test, and bending and bulge testing. Some of these are shown in Figure 2.12a, b, c, and d.

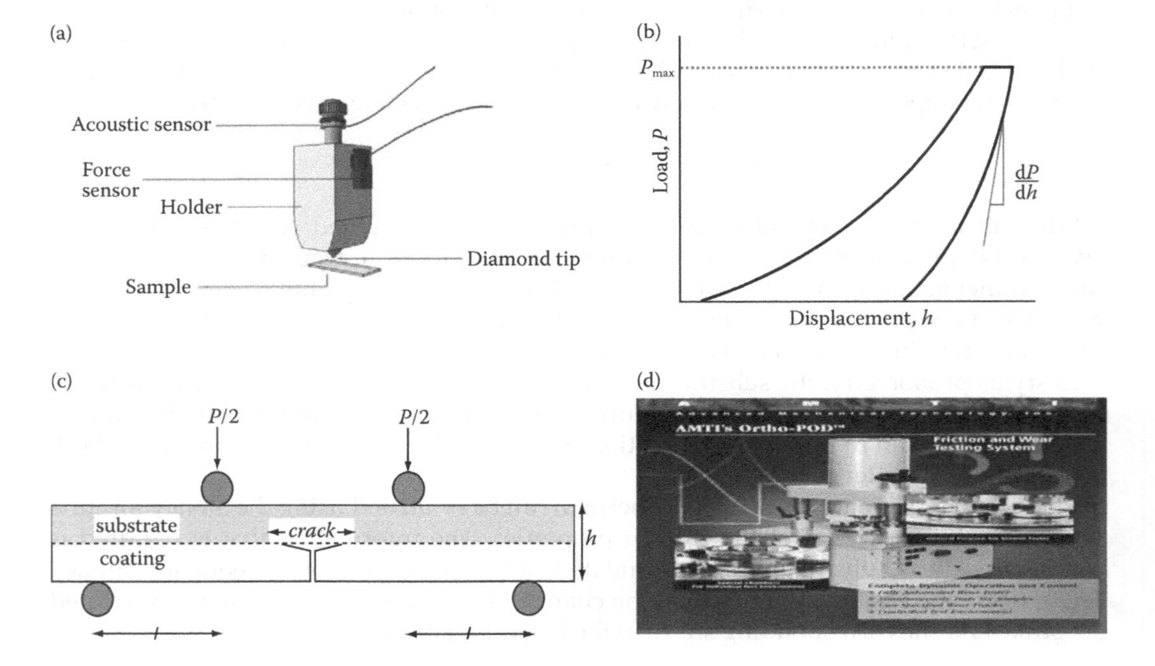

FIGURE 2.12
Some of the thin film testing methods: (a) typical scratch testing device (based on the Quad Group Inc. Romulus III universal test equipment), (b) schematic of a nanoindentation load vs. displacement load and unloading curve from an indentation experiment, (c) schematic of the four-point bend delamination method, and (d) Orthopod® pin on disk wear tester.

Adhesion testing is essential to ensure the coating will adhere properly to the substrate to which it is applied. Many techniques have been used for adhesion measurement of films and coatings as demonstrated by Mittal (1995). The most popular test methods for measuring the bond strength of film on substrate systems include pull-off, cross-cut, indentation scratching at increasing loads, and pin-on-disk. Microtensile testing is also an excellent method to determine the adhesion integrity of nanocoatings.

Pull-off testing is perhaps the most common method for determining the bond strength between a thin film and a thick substrate. Many types of configurations have been proposed (Vallin et al. 2005) using universal testing machines or dedicated tensile testers. The main requirements are that the alignment of grips and sample fixture is precise to ensure uniform loading and that the adhesive used to bond the sample to the fixture is sufficiently strong (stronger than the bond strength of the film–substrate) and does not penetrate the interface of interest. The bond strength is determined from the critical load required to separate the film–substrate contact area. The main advantage of pull-off testing is its applicability and versatility to a wide range of coating/substrate systems. It can be used for both soft flexible coating as well as hard brittle ones. The weakness in typical pull testing is the wide variation in data. One must perform multiple tests on a given sample and statistical analysis to obtain reliable quantitative data. In biomaterials, pull-out is a more common mode of failure of a bone implant than bone fracture. Pull-out may not necessarily occur at the interface between bone and coating, but instead between the metal and the hydroxyapatite coating.

Pin-on-disk tribometers are used to determine the wear resistance and friction coefficient of surfaces. The tester consists of a pin (normally a ruby, tungsten carbide, or metal sphere) under a static load in contact with a rotating sample. Wear coefficients for the pin and disk material are calculated from the volume of material lost during the test. The method facilitates the study of friction and wear behavior of many material combinations with or without lubricant. Pin-on-disk test can be run for an extended period of time either in air or a simulated body environment to provide information on the degradation of the coating with time (sliding distance).

Similar devices that are used in biomaterials research are pin-on-plate type wear testing machines, such as the Ortho-Pod instrument (Advanced Mechanical Testing, Inc., Watertown, MA) (Figure 2.12d). This has six stations for the pins with independent servo-controlled variables that correspond to rotary motion of both the plate and the pins and the normal load applied to each of the six pins. The pin rotation feature gives this machine the ability to generate pin/plate sliding motions that are typically not available on standard pin-on-disk machines. The Ortho-pod is an excellent tool for testing implant materials whose wear characteristics depend upon various sliding directions (crossings) as well as load, in either dry or a fully lubricated environment (serum or other fluids).

Scratch testers (Figure 2.12a) use a small diamond stylus or hard metal (such as tungsten carbide) normally with a 200-μm radius that is drawn across the coated surface at a constant velocity at increasing load. The load on the diamond causes stresses to be increased at the interface between the coating and the substrate, which can result in flaking or chipping of the coating. The load at which the coating first delaminates is called the critical load and is a measure of coating adhesion. Coating failure can be determined from load and the distance at which delamination begins using microscopy, or from the change in friction or using an acoustic emission sensor. In addition to the critical load, the applied normal force, the tangential (friction) force, and the penetration depth are obtained.

Examining scratch test results is difficult due to the complex stress states involved and the broad array of damage processes that can occur depending on film thickness and the mechanical properties of the film and substrate. The test is sensitive to loading rate, stylus shape, environment (humidity), and scratch speed. Thus, it is difficult to relate the critical load to film adhesion.

Three- and four-point bending methods have been used to ascertain the interfacial fracture resistance between dissimilar materials and films on substrates and to provide quantitative measures of the interfacial fracture energy. The thicknesses of these substrates are usually much smaller than their lateral dimensions, so that simple beam bending mechanics can be applied to describe their elastic response (Saha and Nix 2002).

A fracture-mechanics-based method for four-point bending developed by Charalambides et al. (1989) for interfaces between dissimilar materials has been applied in many areas including biomaterials research (Angelelis et al. 1998; Kuper et al. 1997; Dauskardt et al. 1998; Hofinger et al. 1998; Suansuwan and Swain 2003) to measure interface fracture energy. The method requires a bend bar of the coated substrate with a notch machined in the coated layer (Figure 2.12c). As the bending moment increases, a crack initiates from the notch and propagates to the interface. For a sufficiently weak interface bond, the cracks deflect and propagate along the interface. The interfacial fracture energy is given by Equation 2.7:

$$\gamma = \frac{21P_c^2 l^2 \left(1 - v_s^2\right)}{16E_s b^2 h^3} \tag{2.7}$$

where b is the specimen or beam width, h is the total thickness, l is the moment arm (distance between inner and outer loading lines), P_c is the critical load for stable crack propagation, and v_s and E_s are Poisson's ratio and Young's modulus of the substrate, respectively. This method has the advantage that the interface fracture energy is independent of the crack length as long as the crack tip is not too close to the precrack or the loading points.

In bulge and blister testing, the film–substrate system is pressurized with a fluid or gas through a hole in the substrate. The height of the resulting hemispherical bulge in the film is then measured by optical microscopy or an interferometer. The pressure and deflection height can be used to provide in-plane information on elastic, plastic, and time-dependent deformation.

In blister testing the pressure is increased until the film starts to debond from the substrate. The interfacial energy can be determined from the critical pressure for debonding as shown in Equation 2.8 (Bennet et al. 1974):

$$\gamma = \frac{p^2 \left(3 - v_f^2\right) r^4}{16E_f t_f^3} \tag{2.8}$$

where p is the applied pressure, r is the radius of the hole, E_f is Young's modulus of the film, v_f is Poisson's ratio of the film, and t_f is the film thickness.

Two of these commonly used methods, namely, microtensile testing and nanoindentation, are discussed in more detail below given their relevance in biomaterial property evaluations and based on studies by the main author's research group.

Microtensile Testing

The method is suitable for determining properties of both thin and thick coatings on a variety of ductile substrates and provides insights into interfacial delamination susceptibility by the application of controlled external stresses (Filiaggi et al. 1996; Wang et al. 1998; Roest et al. 2004; Latella et al. 2007a, 2007b).

In this adhesion test, the coating is deposited on a tensile coupon, which can then be pulled in a universal testing machine or a specialized device that can be placed under the objective lens of an optical microscope or in a scanning electron microscope. Figure 2.13a shows a schematic of a tensile sample with a thin coating layer that can be uniaxially loaded at defined rates. The cracking, damage evolution, and failure in the coating can be viewed in situ or ex situ after application of specific strains. Brittle coatings on ductile substrates when uniaxially stressed produce parallel cracks in the coating layer perpendicular to the tensile axis and normal to the interface as demonstrated in Figure 2.13b for a sol–gel silica film on stainless steel strained to about 15%. These cracks generally extend through the thickness of the coating and along the width of the sample and increase in number with additional elongation, leading to a decrease in the crack spacing. For some systems, cracks may also be accompanied by localized delamination of the coating from the substrate. Eventually, delamination of the coating signals the end of the lifetime of the coated system.

For softer and more compliant films, cracking can be irregular and film debonding reduced substantially. The drawback with these semibrittle films is that quantitative analysis becomes more difficult.

Tensile testing is advantageous in that the stress field is uniform along the gauge length of the sample and relatively small specimens can be used. Similarly, using optical or scanning electron microscopy to view the damage in situ during loading offers useful insights into material failure mechanisms (Ignat et al. 1999; Latella et al. 2004). The only prerequisite for this type of test is that for analysis of the coating behavior, the residual stress, and Young's modulus of the coating are required by other means, such as from substrate curvature measurements and nanoindentation, respectively.

Microtensile tests provide insights into delamination and fracture processes and for ranking the practical adhesion performance of different coatings. The film debonding behavior is essential to the reliability of film–substrate systems, particularly where mechanical loading and chemical interactions are encountered. For films that crack and debond in a controlled fashion, one can use linear elastic fracture mechanics relations to

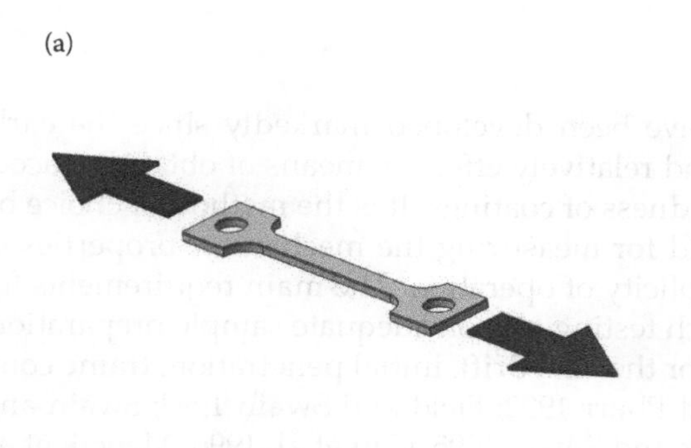

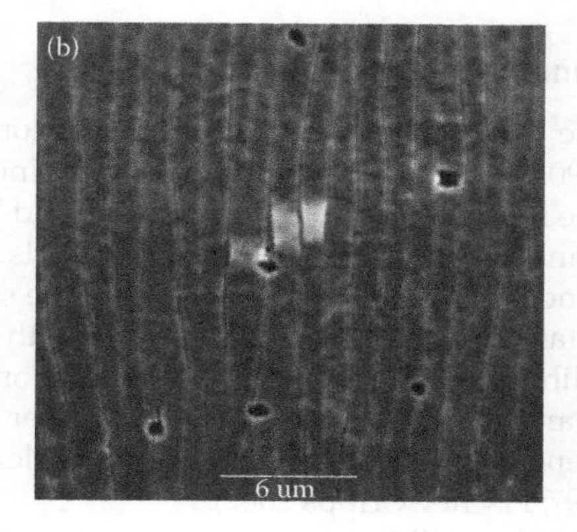

FIGURE 2.13
(a) Shows a schematic of the tensile test specimen, (b) parallel cracks and damage in a sol–gel silica coating on stainless steel strained to about 15% (tensile axis is in the horizontal direction). Small debonded film region between cracks can be seen in the center of the image.

extract intrinsic film properties (strength and fracture toughness) and interfacial adhesion characteristics (Ignat 1996; Harry et al. 1998; Scafidi and Ignat 1998).

On tensile straining, the coating-substrate sample is examined to determine the instant of first cracking in the coating, which corresponds to a strain ε_c. Using Young's modulus of the film (E_f) the critical stress, σ_c, for cracking may be calculated as follows:

$$\sigma_c = \varepsilon_c E_f + \sigma_r \tag{2.9}$$

where σ_r is the residual stress of the coating.

The fracture energy of the coating is obtained from the following equation (Hu and Evans 1989):

$$\gamma_f = \frac{\sigma_c^2 h}{E_f}\left(\pi g(\alpha) + \frac{\sigma_c}{3\tau}\right) \tag{2.10}$$

where γ_f is the fracture energy (J m^{-2}), h is the thickness of the coating, and α is Dundar's parameter $\alpha = (E_f - E_s)/(E_f + E_s)$, where E_s is Young's modulus of the substrate. The $g(\alpha)$ is obtained from Beuth and Klingbeil (1996) and $\tau = \sigma_y/\sqrt{3}$, where σ_y is the yield stress of the substrate.

The toughness of the film is then given by

$$K_{IC} = \sqrt{\gamma_f E_f} \tag{2.11}$$

Adhesion of the film to the substrate is determined by the measurement of the interfacial fracture energy. During tensile straining, the instant of first debonding of the film corresponds to a strain ε_d. The interfacial fracture energy is calculated as follows:

$$\gamma_i = \frac{1}{2} E_f h \varepsilon_d^2 \tag{2.12}$$

Nanoindentation

The methodology and instrumentation have been developed markedly since the early 1990s and it is now considered a routine and relatively effective means of obtaining accurate measures of Young's modulus and hardness of coatings. It is the method of choice by many practitioners in the biomaterials field for measuring the mechanical properties of nanocoatings and implants due to the simplicity of operation. The main requirements for obtaining the best possible results with such testing rely on adequate sample preparation, calibration of equipment, and corrections for thermal drift, initial penetration, frame compliance, and indenter tip shape (Oliver and Pharr 1992; Field and Swain 1993; Swain and Mencik 1994; Field and Swain 1995; Mencik and Swain 1995; Gan et al. 1996; Mencik et al. 1997; Fischer-Cripps 2002).

In the well-known conventional microindentation testing, a load is applied through a diamond tip of known geometry (typically Rockwell, Vickers, or Knoop) into the material surface and then removed and the area of the residual impression is measured by optical means to give the material hardness, an example of which is shown by Kealley et al. (2008)

for HAp ceramics. By contrast, in nanoindentation testing the size of the residual impressions are often only a few microns and this makes it very difficult to obtain a direct measure using optical techniques. In nanoindentation a set load (in the mN range) is applied to the indenter in contact with the specimen. As the load is applied the penetration depth is measured (nm range). At maximum load the area of contact is determined by the depth of the impression and the known angle or radius of the indenter. The result is a continuous measurement of the load and displacement (Figure 2.12b) as a function of time that yields contact pressure or hardness as well as Young's modulus from the shape of the unloading curve using software based on the model and the diamond indenter type (pointed, i.e., Berkovich, Vickers, Knoop, or spherical) (Field and Swain 1995). Likewise different types of loading and unloading methods can be used to extract desired properties as a function of depth of penetration (Fischer-Cripps 2002; Gan and Ben-Nissan 1997a, 1997b; Fischer-Cripps 2006).

In the analysis of nanoindentation the elastic modulus is obtained from the contact stiffness S, which is the slope of the unloading portion of an indentation load–displacement curve at maximum load (Figure 2.12b):

$$S = \frac{\mathrm{d}P}{\mathrm{d}h} = \frac{2}{\sqrt{\pi}} E^* \sqrt{A} \tag{2.13}$$

with A the contact area at maximum load and E^* is the combined elastic modulus of the indenter and specimen expressed as:

$$\frac{1}{E^*} = \frac{\left(1 - v_\mathrm{i}^2\right)}{E_\mathrm{i}} + \frac{\left(1 - v_\mathrm{s}^2\right)}{E_\mathrm{s}} \tag{2.14}$$

where E_i, v_i and E_s, v_s are Young's modulus and Poisson's ratio of the indenter and specimen, respectively. Equation 2.13 is valid for elastic contacts of axis-symmetric indenters (i.e., spherical, conical, and cylindrical punches). The hardness or mean contact pressure for indentation is obtained from the maximum load, P, over the projected contact area, A:

$$H = \frac{P}{A} \tag{2.15}$$

The contact area, A, is determined by the indenter geometry and the contact depth (Fischer-Cripps 2002).

Nanoindentation not only provides a comprehensive assessment of hardness and Young's modulus of the coating but shows the elastic–plastic response from the loading and unloading curves based on the coating–substrate combination (i.e., soft/hard and rigid/compliant coating on soft/hard and rigid/compliant substrate). Furthermore, many tests can be performed in selected regions or in specific areas of interest that may show local variations in properties. Nanoindenters have been used to measure residual stress, coating adhesion from the load at which delamination occurs (taken from the pop-in that corresponds to a plateau or discontinuity in the load–displacement curve) and also function as scratch testers depending on the equipment capability (Fischer-Cripps 2002). Similarly, creep and viscoelastic behavior can be examined (Fischer Cripps 2004; Latella 2008) for softer materials and is particularly relevant in bone, dental composites/resins, and biological tissue studies.

TABLE 2.2

Mechanical Property Data of Sol–Gel Derived HAp Coatings Compared to HAp from Other Deposition Techniques and Other Coatings

Coating on Substrate	Deposition Method	Hardness (GPa)	Young's Modulus (GPa)	Strength (MPa)	Interface Fracture Energy (J/m^2)	Study
HAp on pure titanium	Sol–gel	0.38	25	481 ± 38	0.45 ± 0.1	Roest (2010)
HAp on Ti6Al4V	Sol–gel	-	42.73 ± 4.4	598.22 ± 61.6	-	Zhang et al. (2007)
HAp on stainless steel (316)	Plasma-spray	1.5-5.0	60-100	-	-	Dey et al. (2009)
HAp on Ti6Al4V	Plasma-spray	-	23-33	-	-	Yang and Lui (2008)
ZrO2 on pure titanium	Sol–gel	4.2	138	480 ± 50	4 ± 0.8	Roest (2010)
SiO2 on polyester	Sol–gel	2.5 ± 0.27	13.6 ± 0.4	-	-	Chan et al. (2000)
SiO2 on copper	Sol–gel	2.4 ± 0.29	42.66 ± 2.33	1706	20	Atanacio et al. (2005)
Thermally grown TiO2 on pure titanium	Thermal oxidation	13.9 ± 0.2	259	1340 ± 60	-	Latella et al. (2007a)
Dense HAp (bulk ceramic) ≈ 1% porosity	Sintered	16.1 ± 0.5	137 ± 3	-	-	Kealley et al. (2008)
Porous HAp (bulk ceramic) ≈ 50% porosity	Sintered	0.79 ± 0.02	20.01 ± 0.23	-	-	He et al. (2008)
Compact human bone	-	-	17-18.9 (p)[a] 11.5 (n)	124-174 (p) 49 (n)	-	Suchanek and Yoshimura (1998)
Dry trabeculae		0.52-0.74	19.4 ± 2.3 (p) 15 ± 2.5 (n)	-	-	Rho et al. (1999)
Enamel occlusal section (human tooth)	-	3.23 ± 0.38	94 ± 5	-	-	Xu et al. (1998)

Note: Comparative data is provided for bulk HAp, bone, and dentin.

Tensile strength – testing direction parallel (p) or normal (n) to the axis of the bone.

A selection of micromechanical property data based on nanoindentation and tensile testing of HAp coatings deposited on titanium substrates by the sol–gel method are given in Table 2.2 along with comparisons to other deposition techniques and other coatings on different substrates, from a range of literature sources. Also provided for comparative purposes are data for bulk HAp ceramics (dense and porous), human bone, and dentin. There is a clear difference in the hardness and elastic modulus of bone compared to dentin. The properties of porous HAp (50% porosity) are similar to bone and the range in data for HAp coatings indicates that there is plenty of scope for selecting appropriate properties and film microstructures that can be matched to bone where applicable. It must be emphasized that there is a degree of compromise involved in any implants or restorations with bioactivity and in vivo response being critical along with judicious selection of coating properties and adequate adhesive bonding to the underlying substrate.

Future Perspective

One of the major disadvantages of current synthetic implants is their failure to adapt to the local tissue environment. Recently, tissue engineering has been directed toward taking advantage of the combined use of living cells and three-dimensional ceramic scaffolds to deliver vital cells to damaged sites in the body.

Stem cells have been incorporated into a range of bioceramics. The use of stem cells in regenerative medicine has increased the potential to restore a greater range of tissues in a more sustainable manner and for longer than with conventional tissue-specific differentiated cells. Cultured bone marrow cells derived from adult stem cells can be considered as mesenchymal precursor cell populations and are similar to stem cells in that they can also differentiate into different lineages, which are osteoblasts, chondrocytes, adipocytes, and myocytes. When implanted, these cells can combine with mineralized three-dimensional scaffolds to form highly vascularized bone tissue.

These nanocoated and nanoscale cultured cell/bioceramic composites can be used to treat full-thickness gaps in lone bone shafts with excellent integration of the ceramic scaffold with bone and good functional recovery.

Nanostructured materials are associated with a variety of uses within the medical field, such as nanoparticles in slow drug delivery systems, in diagnostic systems, in devices, and in regenerative medicine.

Tissue engineers are faced with the challenge of developing scaffolds with diverse functions that must be bioresponsive and evolve in real time to a dynamic host environment. Nanoscale coatings and surface modification methods are currently being used to produce body-interactive materials, helping the body to heal, and promoting regeneration of tissues, thus restoring physiological function. This approach is being explored in the development of a new generation of nanobioceramics with a widened range of applications in maxillofacial and orthopedic surgery.

While the impact of nanotechnology is generally considered to be very beneficial, consideration has to be given to the potential risk associated with nanoparticles and nanopowders. Problems can arise from their unsafe use; for example, in the workplace, while their long-term health effects in products used by humans (e.g., sunscreens) are still unknown. A number of research institutions are currently working on the diagnostic methods and to improve the safe work practices.

Conclusion

Both thick and thin nanocoatings offer the opportunity to modify the surface properties of surgical-grade materials to achieve improvements in biocompatibility, reliability, and performance. In recent years, the use of hydroxyapatite as coatings for drug-delivery systems and medical devices has gone through a transformation from being a rarity to being an absolute necessity. Sol–gel derived coatings demonstrate significant promise in clinical applications due to their relative ease of production and the ability to form a chemically and physically uniform and pure coating over complex geometric shapes. Sol–gel derived coatings also have the potential to deliver exceptional mechanical properties owing to their nanocrystalline structure.

Currently used micro- and macrohydroxyapatite coatings on titanium alloys and cobalt chromium alloy implants have had nearly 20 years of clinical use, and their success rate has been controversial and in some instances negative. The equipment used is expensive and control of the production factors is cumbersome. The work on sol–gel derived nanocrystalline hydroxyapatite both in vitro and in vivo studies are very promising and their application at tissue-implant interfaces on knee, hip, and dental implants due to their bioactivity can be advantageous and can help to improve reliability and longevity of the implants.

References

Aksakal, B. and Hanyaloglu, C. 2008. Bioceramic dip-coating on Ti–6Al–4V and 316L SS implant materials. *J. Mater. Sci.: Mater. Med.* 19:2097–2104.

Anast, M., Bell, J., Bell, T., and Ben-Nissan, B. 1992. precision ultra-microhardness measurements of sol–gel derived zirconia thin films. *J. Mater. Sci. Lett.* 11:1483–1485.

Anast, M. 1996. Production and characterization of sol–gel derived thin film ceramic coatings. M.Sc. thesis, University of Technology, Sydney, Australia.

Anderson, P., and Klein, L.C. 1987. Shrinkage of lithium aluminosilicate gels during drying. *J. Noncryst. Solids* 93:415–422.

Andersson, J., Areva, S., Spliethoff, B., and Lindén, M. 2005. Sol–gel synthesis of a multifunctional, hierarchically porous silica/apatite composite. *Biomaterials.* 26:6827–6835.

Angelelis, C., Ducarroir, M., Felder, E., Ignat, M., and Scordo, S. 1998. Mechanical testing by bending, nano- and macro-indentation of micro-wave PACVD sic coatings on steel. *Ann. Chim.-Sci. Mater.* 23:891–898.

Atanacio, A.J., Latella, B.A., Barbe, C.J., and Swain, M.V. 2005. Mechanical properties and adhesion characteristics of hybrid sol–gel thin films. *Surf. Coat. Technol.* 192:354–364.

Balamurugan, A., Michel, J., Fauré, J., Benhayoune, H., Wortham, L., Sockalingum, G., Banchet, V., Bouthors, S., Laurent-Maquin, D., and Balossier, G. 2006. Synthesis and structural analysis of sol gel derived stoichiometric monophasic hydroxyapatite. *Ceramic-Silikáty* 50:27–31.

Bartlett, J.R. and Woolfrey, J.L. 1990. Preparations of multicomponent ceramic powders by sol–gel processing, 191–196. In *Better Ceramics Through Chemistry,* 4th Edition. B.J.J. Zelinski, C.J. Brinker, D.E. Clark, and D.R. Ulrich (eds.). Pittsburgh, PA: Materials Research Society.

Ben-Nissan, B. 2004. Nanoceramics in biomedical applications. *MRS Bull.* 29, 1:28–32.

Ben-Nissan, B., Anast, M., Bell, J.M., Johnston, G.E., West, B.O., Spiccia, L., de Villiers D., and Watkins, I.D. 1994. Production and characterisation of sol–gel derived zirconia thin films. *J. Aust. Ceram. Soc.* 30, 2:68–75.

Ben-Nissan, B. and Chai, C.S. 1995. Sol–gel derived bioactive hydroxyapatite coatings. In *Advances in Materials Science and Implant Orthopedic Surgery,* NATO ASI Series, Series E: Applied Sciences, 294:265–275. R. Kossowsky and N. Kossovsky (eds.). Germany: Kluwer Academic Publishers.

Ben-Nissan, B., Green, D.D., Kannangara, G.S.K., Chai, C.S., and Milev, A. 2001. ^{31}P NMR studies of diethyl phosphite derived nanocrystalline hydroxyapatite. *J. Sol–Gel Sci. Technol.* 21:27–37.

Ben-Nissan, B., Milev, A., Vago, R., Conway, M. and Diwan, A. 2004. Sol–gel derived nano-coated coralline hydroxyapatite for load bearing applications. *Key Eng. Mater.* 254–256:301–304.

Ben-Nissan, B. and Pezzotti, G. 2002. Bioceranics: Processing routes and mechanical evaluation. *J. Ceram. Soc. Jpn.* 110:601–608.

Bennet, S.J., Devries, K.L., and Williams, M.L. 1974. Adhesive fracture mechanics. *Int. J. Fracture* 10:33–43.

Berndt, C.C., Haddad, G.N., Farmer, A.J.D., and Gross, K.A. 1990. Thermal spraying for bioceramic applications. *Mater. Forum* 14:161–173.

Beuth, J.L. and Klingbeil N.W. 1996. Cracking of thin films bonded to elastic–plastic substrates. *J. Mech. Phys. Solids* 44(9):1411–1428.

Bogdanoviciene, I., Beganskiene, A., Tõnsuaadu, K., Glaser, J., Meyer, H.J., and Kareiva, A. 2006. Calcium hydroxyapatite, $Ca_{10}(PO_4)_6(OH)_2$ ceramics prepared by aqueous sol–gel processing. *Mater. Res. Bull.* 41:1754–1762.

Bose, S. and Saha, S.K. 2003. Synthesis of hydroxyapatite nanopowders via sucrose-templated sol–gel method. *J. Am. Ceram. Soc.* 86:1055–1057.

Bradley, D.C., Mehrota, R.C., and Gaur, D.P. 1978. *Metal Alkoxides.* London, UK: Academic Press.

Brinker, C.J., Clark, D.E., and Ulrich, D.R. (eds.). 1988. *Better Ceramics Through Chemistry,* 3rd Edition. Pittsburgh, PA: Materials Research Society.

Brinker, C.J. and Scherer, G.W. 1990. *Sol–Gel Science: The Physics and Chemistry of Sol–Gel Processing.* London: Academic Press.

Cassidy, D. Woolfrey, J.J.L., Bartlett, J.R., and Ben-Nissan, B. 1997. The effect of precursor chemistry on the crystallisation and densification of sol–gel derived mullite gels and powders. *J. Sol–Gel Sci. Technol.* 10(6):19–30.

Chai, C., Ben-Nissan, B., Pyke, S., and Evans, L. 1995. Sol–gel derived hydroxyapatite coatings for biomedical applications. *Mater. Manuf. Process.* 10(2):205–216.

Chai, C.S., Gross, K.A., and Ben-Nissan, B. 1998a. Critical ageing of hydroxyapatite sol–gel solutions. *Biomaterials* 19:2291–2296.

Chai, C.S., Gross, K.A., Hanley, L. and Ben-Nissan, B. 1998b. Critical ageing and chemistry of nano-crystalline hydroxyapatite sol–gel solutions. *J. Aust. Ceram. Soc.* 34:263–268.

Chai, C. and Ben-Nissan, B. 1999. Bioactive nano-crystalline sol–gel hydroxyapatite coatings. *J. Mater. Sci.: Mater Med.* 10:465–469.

Chan, C.M., Cao, G.Z., Fong, H., Sarikaya, M., Robinson, T. and Nelson, L. 2000. Nanoindentation and adhesion of sol–gel-derived hard coatings on polyester. *Mater. Res. Soc.* 15:148–154.

Charalambides, P.G., Lund, J., Evans, A.G., and McMeeking, R.M. 1989. A test specimen for determining the fracture resistance of biomaterial interfaces. *J. Appl. Mech.* 56:77–82.

Chen, T.S. and Lacefield, W.R. 1994. Crystallisation of ion beam deposited calcium phosphate coatings. *J. Mater. Res.* 9:1284–1296.

Cheng, K., Shen, G., Weng, W.J., Han, G.R., Ferreira, J.M.F., and Yang, J. 2001. Synthesis of hydroxyapatite/fluoroapatite solid solution by a sol–gel method. *Mater. Lett.* 51:37–41.

Cheng, K., Weng, W.J., Du, P.Y., Shen, G., Han, G.R., and Ferreira, J.M.F. 2004. Synthesis and characterization of fluoridated hydroxyapatite with a novel fluorine-containing reagent. *Key Eng. Mater.* 254–256:331–334.

Choi, A.H. and Ben-Nissan, B. 2007. Sol–gel production of bioactive nanocoatings for medical applications: Part II. current research and development. *Nanomedicine* 2(1):51–61.

Cihlar, J. and Castkova, K. 1998. Synthesis of calcium phosphates from alkyl phosphates by the sol–gel method. *Ceramics-Silikaty* 42:164–170.

Colby, M.W., Osaka, A., and Mackenzie, J.D. 1988. Temperature dependence of the gelation of silicon alkoxides. *J. Noncryst. Solids* 99:129–139.

Cromme, P., Zollfrank, C., Müller, L., Müller, F. A., and Greil, P. 2007. Biomimetic mineralisation of apatites on Ca^{2+} activated cellulose templates. *Mater. Sci. Eng. C* 27:1–7.

Dauphin, Y. 2003. The organic matrices of corals and biocompatibility. In *NATO ASI Symposium: Learning from Nature How to Design New Implantable Biomaterials.* R. Reis and S. Weiner (ed.). Alvor Portugal, Poster presentation 76, *NATO Science Series*, vol. 171. The Netherlands: Kluwer Academic Publishers.

Dauskardt, R.H., Lane, M., and Ma, Q. 1998. Adhesion debonding of multi-layer thin film structures. *Eng. Fract. Mech.* 61:141–162.

de Kambilly, H. and Klein, L.C. 1989. Effect of methanol concentration on lithium aluminosilicates. *J. Noncryst. Solids* 109:69–78.

Dey, A., Mukhopadhyay, A.K., Gangadharan, S., Sinha, M.K., Basu, D., and Bandyopadhyay, N.R. 2009. Nanoindentation study of microplasma sprayed hydroxyapatite coating. *Ceram. Int.* 35:2295–2304.

Dislich, H. 1988. Thin films from the sol–gel process, 50–77. In *Sol–Gel Technology for Thin Films, Fibers, Preforms, Electronics and Specialty Shapes.* L.C. Klein (ed.). Park Ridge, NJ: Noyes Publishing.

Dorozhkin S.V. 2009. Nanodimensional and nanocrystalline apatites and other calcium orthophosphates in biomedical engineering, biology and medicine. *Materials* 2:1975–2045.

Ducheyne, P., Radin, S., Heughebaert, M., and Heughebaert, J.C. 1990. Effect of calcium phosphate ceramic coatings on porous titanium: Effect of structure and composition on electrophoretic deposition, vacuum sintering and in vitro dissolution. *Biomaterials* 11:244–254.

Ebelmen, J. 1846. Untersuchungen über die Verbindung der Borsaure und Kieselsaure mit Aether. *Ann. Chim. Phys.* Ser. 3, 57:319–355.

Ehrlich, H., Etnoyer, P., Litvinov, S.D., Olennikova, M.M., Domaschke, H., Hanke, T., Born, R.H., Meissner, H., and Worch, H. 2006. Biomaterial structure in deep-sea bamboo coral (Anthozoa: Gorgonacea: Isididae): Perspectives for the development of bone implants and templates for tissue engineering. *Materwiss. Werksttech.* 37(6):552–557.

Eichorst, D.J. and Payne, D.A. 1988. Sol–gel processing of lithium niobates thin layers on silicon, 773–778. In *Better Ceramics Through Chemistry*, Third Edition. Brinker, C.J., Clark, D.E. and Ulrich D.R. (eds). Pittsburgh, PA: Materials Research Society.

Field, J. S. and Swain, M.V. 1993. A simple predictive model for spherical indentation. *J. Mater. Res.* 8:297–306.

Field, J.S. and Swain, M.V. 1995. Determining the mechanical properties of small volumes of material from submicrometer spherical indentations. *J. Mater. Res.* 10:101–112.

Filiaggi, M.J., Pilliar, R.M., and Abdulla, D. 1996. Evaluating sol–gel ceramic thin films for metal implant applications: II. Adhesion and fatigue properties of zirconia films on Ti–6Al–4V. *J. Biomed. Mater. Res.* 33:239–256.

Fischer-Cripps, A.C. 2002. *Introduction to Nanoindentation.* New York: Springer.

Fischer-Cripps, A.C. 2004. A simple phenomenological approach to nanoindentation creep. *Mater. Sci. Eng. A* 385:74–82.

Fischer-Cripps, A.C. 2006. Critical review of analysis and interpretation of nanoindentation test data. *Surf. Coat. Technol.* 200:4153–4165.

Floch, H.G., Belleville, P.F., Priotton, J.J., Pegon, P.M., Dijonneau, C.S., and Guerain, J. 1995. Sol–gel optical coatings for lasers. *I. Am. Ceram. Soc. Bull.* 74:60–63.

Gabriel, A.O. and Riedel, R. 1997. Novel non-oxide sol–gel process to Si–C–N ceramics. *Ceram. Eng. Sci. Proc.* 18:713–720.

Gan, L. and Pilliar, R. 2004. Calcium phosphate sol–gel derived thin films on porous-surfaced implants for enhanced osteoconductivity: Part I. Synthesis and characterization. *Biomaterials* 25:5303–5312.

Gan, L.B., Ben-Nissan, B., and Ben-David, A. 1996. Modelling and finite element analysis of ultra-microhardness indentation of thin films. *Thin Solid Films* 290–291:362–366.

Gan, L.B. and Ben-Nissan, B. 1997a. The effect of mechanical properties of thin films on nano-indentation data: Finite element analysis. *Comput. Mater. Sci.* 8:273–281.

Gan, L.B. and Ben-Nissan, B. 1997b. Finite element analysis and the behaviour of sol–gel derived thin films under ultra-microhardness indentation. *J. Aust. Ceram. Soc.* 32:51–55.

Gao, J., Xiao, H., Li, Z., and Du, H. 1997. Preparation of nanosized silicon nitride powders by ammonic sol–gel process. *Trans. Nonferrous Met. Soc. China* 7:21–24.

Geffcken, W. and Berger, E. 1939. Änderung des Reflexionsvermogens Optischer Gläser. German Patent 736411.

Green, D.D. 2001. Characterisation of hydroxyapatite powders produced by an efficient alkoxide sol–gel process. MSc thesis, University of Technology, Sydney, Australia.

Green, D.W., Howard, D., Yang, X.B., Kelly, M., and Oreffo, R.O.C. 2003. Natural marine sponge fibre skeleton: A biomimetic scaffold for human osteoprogenitor cell attachment, growth and differentiation. *Tissue Eng.* 9, 6:1159–1166.

Green, D.W. and Ben-Nissan, B. 2008. Bio-inspired engineering of human tissue scaffolding in regenerative medicine, 364–388. In *Biomaterials in Asia.* Tateishi, T. (ed). Singapore: World Scientific Publishing Co. Pte. Ltd.

Gross, K.A., Chai, C.S., Kannangara, G.S.K., Ben-Nissan, B. and Hanley, L. 1998. Thin hydroxyapatite coatings via sol–gel synthesis. *J. Mater. Sci.: Mater. Med.* 9(12):839–843.

Gottardi, V., Guglielmi, M., Bertoluzza, A., Fagnano, C., and Morelli, M.A. 1984. Further investigations on Raman spectra of silica gel evolving toward glass. *J. Noncryst. Solids* 63:71–80.

Han, Y.C., Li, S.P., Wang, X.Y., and Chen, X.M. 2004. Synthesis and sintering of nanocrystalline hydroxyapatite powders by citric acid sol–gel combustion method. *Mater. Res. Bull.* 39:25–32.

Harris, M.T., Byers, C.H., and Brunson, R.R. 1988. A study of solvent effects on the synthesis of pure component and composite ceramic powders by metal alkoxide hydrolysis, 287–292. In *Better Ceramics Through Chemistry*, 3rd Edition. Brinker, C.J., Clark, D.E., and Ulrich D.R. (eds.). Pittsburgh, PA: Materials Research Society.

Harris, E.E. and Malyango, A.A. 2005. Evolutionary explanations in medical and health profession courses: Are you answering your students' 'why' questions? *BMC Med. Educ.* 5:16.

Harry, E., Rouzaud, A., Ignat, M., and Juliet, P. 1998. Mechanical properties of W and W(C) thin films: Young's modulus, fracture toughness and adhesion. *Thin Solid Films* 332:195–201.

Hasegawa, I., Nakamura, T., Motojima, S., and Kajiwara, M. 1997. Synthesis of silicon carbide fibers by sol–gel processing. *J. Sol–Gel Sci. Technol.* 8:577–579.

He, L.H., Standard, O.C., Huang, T.T.Y., Latella, B.A., and Swain, M.V. 2008. Mechanical behaviour of porous hydroxyapatite. *Acta Biomater.* 4:577–586.

Heimke, G. and Griss, P. 1980. Ceramic implant materials. *Med. Biol. Eng. Comput.* 18:503–510.

Hench, L.L. 1991. Bioceramics: From concept to clinic. *J. Am. Ceram. Soc.* 74(7):1487–1510.

Hench, L.L. and West, J.K. 1990. The sol–gel process. *Chem. Rev.* 90:33–72.

Hofinger, I., Oechsner, M., Bahr, H.A., and Swain, M.V. 1998. Modified four-point bending specimen for determining the interfacial fracture energy for thin, brittle layers. *Int. J. Fract.* 92:213–220.

Hofmann, I., Mülloer, L., Greil, P., and Müller, F.A. 2006. Calcium phosphate nucleation on cellulose fabrics. *Surf. Coat. Technol.* 201:2392–2398.

Hollister, S.J. 2005. Porous scaffold design for tissue engineering. *Nat. Mater.* 4:518–524.

Hollister, S.J. and Lin, S.Y. 2007. Computational design of tissue engineering scaffolds. *Comput. Methods Appl. Mech. Eng.* 196:2991–2998.

Hsieh, M.F., Perng, L.H., and Chin, T.S. 2002. Hydroxyapatite coating on Ti6Al4V alloy using a sol–gel derived precursor. *Mater. Chem. Phys.* 74(3):245–250.

Hu, M. S. and Evans, A. G. 1989. The cracking and decohesion of thin films on ductile substrates. *Acta Metall.* 37(3):917–925.

Hu, J., Russell, J.J., Ben-Nissan, B., and Vago, R. 2001. Production and analysis of hydroxyapatite from Australian corals via hydrothermal process. *J. Mater. Sci. Lett.* 20:85–87.

Hulbert, S.F., Young, F.A., Mathews, R.S., Klawitter, J.J., Talbert, C.D., and Stelling, F.H. 1970. Potential of ceramic materials as permanently implantable skeletal prostheses. *J. Biomed. Mater. Res.* 4(3):433–456.

Ignat, M. 1996. Mechanical response of multilayers submitted to in-situ experiments. *Key Eng. Mater.* 116–117:279–290.

Ignat, M., Marieb, T., Fukimoto, H., and Flinn, P.A. 1999. Mechanical behaviour of submicron multilayers submitted to microtensile experiments. *Thin Solid Films* 353:201–207.

Jimenez, C. and Langlet, M. 1994. Formation of TiN by nitration of TiO_2 films deposited by ultrasonically assisted sol–gel technique. *Surf. Coat. Technol.* 68–69:249–252.

Kealley, C.S., Latella, B.A., Van Riessen, A., Elcombe, M., and Ben-Nissan, B. 2008. Micro- and nanoindentation of a hydroxyapatite–carbon nanotube composite. *J. Nanosci. Nanotechnol.* 8:3936–3941.

Kim, H.W., Kim, H.E., Salih, V., and Knowles, J.C. 2005. Hydroxyapatite and titania sol–gel composite coatings on titanium for hard tissue implants; mechanical and in vitro biological performance. *J. Biomed. Mater. Res. Part B: Appl. Biomater.* 72B:1–8.

Kim, S.S., Park, M.S., Gwak, S.J., Choi, C.Y., and Kim, B.S. 2006. Accelerated bonelike apatite growth on porous polymer/ceramic composite scaffolds in vitro. *Tissue Eng.* 12:2997–3006.

Kirk, P. and Pilliar, R. 1999. The deformation response of sol–gel-derived thin films on 316L stainless steel using a substrate straining test. *J. Mater. Sci.* 34:3967–3975.

Klein, L.C. (ed.). 1988. *Sol–Gel Technology for Thin Films, Fibers, Preforms, Electronics and Specialty Shapes*. Park Ridge, NJ: Noyes Publishing.

Kokubo, T., Kushitani, H., Ohtsuki, C., Sakka, S., and Yamamuro, T. 1992. Chemical reaction of bioactive glass and glass–ceramics with a simulated body fluid. *J Mater Sci: Mater. Med.* 3(2):79–83.

Kokubo T., Kim, H.M., Kawashita M., and Nakamura T. 2000. Novel ceramics for biomedical applications. *J. Aust. Ceram. Soc.* 36:37–46.

Kokubo, T. and Takadama, H. 2006. How useful is SBF in predicting in vivo bone bioactivity? *Biomaterials* 27:2907–2915.

Kolos, E.C., Ruys, A.J., Rohanizadeh, R., Nuir, M.M., and Roger, G. 2006. Calcium phosphate fibres synthesized from a simulated body fluid. *J. Mater. Sci.: Mater. Med.* 17:1179–1189.

Kraus, G.T., Oldweiler, C.S., and Giannelis, E.P. 1996. Synthesis and oxidation kinetics of sol–gel and sputtered tantalum nitride thin films. 410, 295–300. In *Covalent Ceramics III—Science and Technology of Non-Oxides*. Pittsburgh, PA: Materials Research Society.

Kuper, A., Clissold, R., Martin, P.J., and Swain, M.V. 1997. A comparative assessment of three approaches for ranking the adhesion of TiN coatings onto two steels. *Thin Solid Films* 308–309:329–333.

Latella, B.A., Ignat, M., Barbé, C.J., Cassidy, D.J., and Li, H. 2004. Cracking and decohesion of sol–gel hybrid coatings on metallic substrates. *J. Sol–Gel Sci. Technol.* 31:143–149.

Latella, B.A., Gan, B., and Li, H. 2007a. Fracture toughness and adhesion of thermally grown titanium oxide on medical grade pure titanium. *Surf. Coat. Technol.* 201:6325–6331.

Latella, B.A., Triani, G., and Evans, P. 2007b. Toughness and adhesion of atomic layer deposited alumina films on polycarbonate substrates. *Scr. Materi.* 56:493–496.

Latella, B.A., Gan, B.K., Barbé, C.J., and Cassidy, D.J. 2008. Nanoindentation hardness, Young's modulus, and creep behavior of organic–inorganic silica-based sol–gel thin films on copper. *J. Mater. Res.* 23(9):2357–2365.

Layrolle, P. and Lebugle, A. 1994. Characterization and reactivity of nanosized calcium phosphate prepared in anhydrous ethanol. *Chem. Mater.* 6:1996–2004.

Layrolle, P., Ito, A., and Tateishi, T. 1998. Sol–gel synthesis of amorphous calcium phosphate and sintering into microporous hydroxyapatite bioceramics. *J. Am. Ceram. Soc.* 81:1421–1428.

LeGeros, R.Z. 1991. In *Calcium Phosphates in Oral Biology and Medicine. Monographs in Oral Sciences*, Vol. 15. Myers, H. (ed). Basel: S. Karger.

LeGeros, R.Z. 1993. Biodegradation and bioresorption of calcium phosphate ceramics. *Clin Mater.* 14:65–88.

LeGeros, R.Z., Coelho, P.G., Holmes, D., Dimaano, F., and LeGeros, J.P. 2011. Orthopedic and dental implant surfaces and coatings. 295–328. *In Biological and Biomedical Coatings: Applications*, Zhang, S. (ed). Boca Raton, Florida: CRC Press.

Lee, J.W., Won, C.W., Chun, B.S., and Sohn, H.Y. 1993. Dip-coating of alumina films by the sol–gel method. *J. Mater. Res.* 8:3151–3157.

Lepienski, C.M. Pharr, G.M., Park, Y.J., Watkins, T.R., Misra, A., and Zhang, X. 2004. Factors limiting the measurement of residual stresses in thin films by nanoindentation. *Thin Solid Films* 447–448:251–257.

Lim, Y.M., Hwang, K.S., and Park, Y.J. 2001. Sol–gel derived functionally graded TiO_2/HAp films on Ti–6Al–4V implants. *J. Sol–Gel Sci. Technol.* 21:123–128.

Liu, Y., Hunziker, E.B., Layrolle, P., Van Blitterswijk, C., Calvert, P.D., and de Groot, K. 2003, Remineralization of demineralized albumin–calcium phosphate coatings. *J. Biomed. Mater. Res. Part A* 67(4):1155–1162.

Martina, M., Subramanyam, G., Weaver, J.C., Hutmacher, D.W., Morse, D.E., and Valiyaveettil, S. 2005. Developing macroporous bicontinuous materials as scaffolds for tissue engineering. *Biomaterials* 26:5609–5616.

Masuda, Y., Matubara, K., and Sakka, S. 1990. Synthesis of hydroxyapatite from metal alkoxides through sol–gel technique. *J. Ceram. Soc. Jpn.* 98:84–94.

Mazdiyasni, K.S. 1982. Powder synthesis form metal–organic precursors. *Ceram. Int.* 8:42–56.

Melpolder, S.M. and Coltrain, B.K. 1988. Optimization of sol–gel film properties, 811–816. In *Better Ceramics Through Chemistry,* 3rd Edition. Brinker, C.J., Clark, D.E., and Ulrich D.R. (eds.). Pittsburgh, PA: Materials Research Society.

Mencik, J. and Swain, M.V. 1995. Errors associated with depth-sensing microindentation tests. *J. Mater. Res.* 10:1491–1501.

Mencik, J., Munz, D., Qut, E., Weppelmann, E.R., and Swain, M.V. 1997. Determination of elastic modulus of thin layers using nanoindentation. *J. Mater. Res.* 12:2475–2484.

Milev, A., Kannangara, G.S.K., and Ben-Nissan, B. 2002. Ligand substitution and complex formation in hydroxyapatite sol–gel system. *Key Eng. Mat.* 218–220:79–84.

Milev, A., Kannangara, K., and Ben-Nissan, B. 2003. Morphological stability of plate-like carbonated hydroxyapatite. *Mater. Lett.* 57(13–14):1960–1965.

Mittal, K.L. 1995. Adhesion measurement of films and coatings: A commentary. In *Adhesion Measurements of Films and Coatings.* Mittal, K.L. (ed.) Utrecht: VSP.

Nix, D.W. 2006. Mechanical properties of thin films (class notes for a graduate class at Stanford University), iMechanica, http://imechanica.org/node/530.

Oliver, W.C. and Pharr, G.M. 1992. A new improved technique for determining hardness and elastic modulus using load and sensing indentation experiments. *J. Mater. Res.* 7:1564–1582.

Orcel, G. and Hench, L.L. 1986. Effect of formamide additive on the chemistry of silica sol–gels: Part I. NMR of silica hydrolysis. *J. Noncryst. Solids* 79:177–194.

Oonishi, H., Aoki, H., and Sawai, K. (eds.) 1988. *Bioceramics*, Volume 1. Proceedings of 1st International Symposium on Ceramics in Medicine, Ishiyaku EuroAmerica, Inc. Tokyo.

Parker, A.R. and Townley, H.E. 2007. Biomimetics of photonic nanostructures. *Nat. Nanotechnol.* 2:347–353.

Parker, A.R. and Martini, N. 2006. Structural colour in animals—Simple to complex optics. *Optics Laser Technol.* 38:315–322.

Percy, M.J., Bartlett, J.R., Spiccia, L. West, B.O., and Woolfrey, J.L. 2000. The influence of b–diketones on hydrolysis and particle growth from zirconium (IV) *N*-propoxide in *n*-propanol. *J. Sol–Gel Sci. Technol.* 19:315–319.

Pettit, R.B., Ashley, C.S., Reed, S.T., and Brinker, C.J. 1988. Antireflective films from the sol–gel process, 80–109. In *Sol–Gel Technology for Thin Films, Fibers, Performs, Electronics, and Specialty Shapes.* Klien, L.C. (ed.) Park Ridge, NJ: Noyes Publishing.

Petite, H., Viateau, V., Bensaïd, W., Meunier, A., de Pollak, C., Bourguignon, M., Oudina, K., Sedel, L., and Guillemin, G. 2000. Tissue-engineered bone regeneration. *Nat. Biotechnol.* 18:959–963.

Paterson, M.J., Paterson P.J.K., and Ben-Nissan, B. 1998. The dependence of structural and mechanical properties on film thickness in sol–gel zirconia films. *J. Mater. Res.* 13(2):388.

Raman, V., Bahl, O.P., and Dhawan, U. 1995. Synthesis of silicon carbide through the sol–gel process from different precursors. *J. Mater. Sci.* 30:2686–2693.

Rho, J.Y., Roy, M.E., Tsui, T.Y., and Pharr, G.M. (1999). Properties of microstructural components of human bone tissue as measured by nanoindentation. *J. Biomed. Mater. Res.* 45:48–54.

Rocha, J.H.G., Lemos A.F., Agathopoulos, S., Valero, P., Kannan, S., Oktar, F.N., and Ferriera, J.M.F. 2005. Scaffolds for bone restoration from cuttlefish. *Bone* 850–857.

Roest, R. 2010. Interfacial characterisation of sol–gel derived coatings of hydroxyapatite and zirconia thin films with anodised titanium substrates. Ph.D. thesis, University of Technology, Sydney, Australia.

Roest, R. and Ben-Nissan, B. 2001. Surface modification of anodized titanium for calcium phosphate coatings. *Proceedings of the Engineering Materials 2001*, Pereloma, E. and Raviprasad, K. (eds.), 115–120.

Roest, R., Eberhardt, A.W., Latella, B.A., Wuhrer, R., and Ben-Nissan, B. 2004. Adhesion of sol–gel derived zirconia nano-coatings on surface treated titanium. In *Bioceramics* 16. *Key Eng. Mat.* 254–256:455–458.

Roy, R. 1987. Ceramics by the solution–sol–gel route. *Science* 238(4834):1664–1669.

Roy, D.M. and Roy, R. 1954. An experimental study of the formation and properties of synthetic sepentines and related layer silicates. *Am. Mineral.* 39:957–975.

Saha, R. and Nix, W. D. 2002. Effects of the substrate on the determination of thin film mechanical properties by nanoindentation. *Acta Material.* 50:23–38.

Sakka, S., Kamiya, K, Makita, K., and Tamamoto, Y. 1984. Formation of sheets and coating films from alkoxide solutions. *J. Noncryst. Solids* 63:223–235.

Sarig, S. and Kahana, F. 2002. Rapid formation of nanocrystalline apatite. *J. Cryst. Growth* 237–239:55–59.

Scafidi, P. and Ignat, M. 1998. Cracking and loss of adhesion of Si_3N_4 SiO_2:P films deposited on Al substrates. *J. Adhes. Sci. Technol.* 12:1219–1242.

Schmidt, H., Rinn, G., Nab, R., and Sporn, D. 1988. Film preparation by inorganic–organic sol–gel synthesis. *Mater. Res. Soc. Symp. Proc.* 32:743–754.

Schroder H. 1966. New sun-shielding glasses for architectural purposes. *Vetro Silicati.* 10:10–14.

Schroeder, H. 1965. Water-dispersed industrial and architectural coatings. *Paint Varnish Prod.* 55:31–46.

Schwart, I., Anderson, P., de Lambilly, H., and Klein, L.C. 1986. Stability of lithium silicate gels. *J. Noncryst. Solids* 83:391–399.

Scriven, L.E. 1988. Physics and application of dip coating and spin coating. *Mater. Res. Soc. Symp. Proc.* 121:717–729.

Sengers B.G., Please, C.P., and Oreffo, R.O.C. 2007. Experimental characterization and computational modeling of two-dimensional cell spreading for skeletal regeneration. *J. R. Soc. Interface* 4:1107–1117.

Shih, W.J., Chen, Y.F., Wang, M.C., and Hon, M.H. 2004. Crystal growth and morphology of the nanosized hydroxyapatite powders synthesized from $CaHPO_4{\cdot}2H_2O$ and $CaCO_3$ by hydrolysis method. *J. Cryst. Growth* 270:211–218.

Shors, E.C. 1999. Porous ceramics and bone growth factors for bone grafting: Now and into the millennium. 12th International Symposium on Ceramics in Medicine, Bioceramics 12. Nara, Japan.

Stoch, A., Jastrzebski, W., Dlugon, E., Lejda, W., Trybalska, B., Stoch, G.J., and Adamczyk, A. 2005. Sol–gel derived hydroxyapatite coatings on titanium and its alloy Ti6Al4V. *J. Mol. Struct.* 744–747:633–640.

Stoney, G.G. 1909. The tension of thin metallic films deposited by electrolysis. *Proc. R. Soc. London A* 82:172–173.

Strawbridge, I. and James, P.F. 1986. Thin silica films prepared by dip coating. *J. Noncryst. Solids* 82:366–372.

Suansuwan, N. and Swain, M.V. 2003. Adhesion of porcelain to titanium and a titanium alloy. *J. Dent.* 31:509–518.

Suchanek, W. and Yoshimura, M. 1998. Processing and properties of hydroxyapatite-based biomaterials for use as hard tissue replacement implants. *J. Mater. Res.* 13:94–117.

Swain, M.V. and Mencik, J. 1994. Mechanical property characterization of thin films using spherical tipped indenters. *Thin Solid Films* 253:204–211.

Tas, A.C. and Bhaduri, S.B. 2004. Rapid coating of Ti6A14V at room temperature with a calcium phosphate solution similar to 10× simulated body fluid. *J. Mater. Res.* 19: 2742–2749.

Thomas, I.M. 1988. Multicomponent glasses from the sol–gel process, 2–15. In *Sol–Gel Technology for Thin Films, Fibers, Preforms, Electronics and Specialty Shapes*. Klein, L.C. (ed.). Park Ridge, NJ: Noyes Publishing.

Tkalcec, E., Sauer, M., Menninger, R., and Schmidt, H. 2001. Sol–gel derived hydroxyapatite powders and coatings. *J. Mater. Sci.* 36:5253–5263.

Turner, C.W. 1991. Sol–gel process—Principles and applications. *Ceram. Bull.* 70:1487–1490.

Tsui, Y.C., Doyle, C., and Clyne, T.W. 1998. Plasma sprayed hydroxyapatite coatings on titanium substrates—Part 1: Mechanical properties and residual stress levels. *Biomaterials* 19:2015–2029.

Tjong, T. and Chen, H. 2004. Nanocrystalline materials and coatings. *Mater. Sci. Eng. R* 45:1–88.

Vallin, O., Jonsson, K., and Lindberg, U. 2005. Adhesion quantification methods for wafer bonding. *Mater. Sci. Eng. R.* 50:109–165.

Wallace, S. and Hench, L.L. 1984. Metal organic-derived 20L gel monoliths. *Ceram. Eng. Sci. Proc.* 5:568–573.

Wang, H.S., Wang, G.X., and Pan, Q.X. 2005. Electrochemical study of the interactions of DNA with redox-active molecules based on the immobilization of dsDNA on the sol–gel derived nano porous hydroxyapatite–polyvinyl alcohol hybrid material coating. *Electroanalysis* 17:1854–1860.

Wang, J.S., Sugimura, Y., Evans, A.G., and Tredway, W.K. 1998. The mechanical performance of DLC films on steel substrates. *Thin Solid Films* 325:163–174.

Weng, W.J., Han, G.R., Du, P.Y., and Shen, G. 2002. The effect of citric acid addition on the formation of sol–gel derived hydroxyapatite. *Mater. Chem. Phys.* 74:92–97.

Weber, J.N. and White, E.W. 1973. Carbonate minerals as precursors of new ceramic, metal, and polymer materials for biomedical applications. *Miner. Sci. Eng.* 5(2):312–323.

Williams, G.C. and Nesse, R.M. 1991. The dawn of Darwinian medicine. *Q. Rev. Biol.* 66(1):1–22.

Wu, C., Chang, J., Zhai, W., and Ni, S. 2007. A novel bioactive porous bredigite ($Ca_7MgSi_4O_{16}$) scaffold with biomimetic apatite layer for bone tissue engineering. *J. Mater. Sci.: Mater. Med.* 18:857–864.

Xu, H.H.K., Smith, D.T., Jahanmir, S., Romberg, E., Kelly, J.R., Thompson, V.P., and Rekow, E.D. 1998. Indentation damage and mechanical properties of human enamel and dentin. *J. Dent. Res.* 77:472–480.

Yang, C.W. and Lui, T.S. 2008. Microstructural self-healing effect of hydrothermal crystallization on bonding strength and failure mechanism of hydroxyapatite coatings. *J. Eur. Ceram. Soc.* 28:2151–2159.

Yang, Z., Huang, Y., Chen, S.T., Zhao, Y.Q., and Li, H.L. 2005. Template synthesis of highly ordered hydroxyapatite nanowire arrays. *J. Mater. Sci.* 40:1121–1125.

Yoldas, B.E. 1984. Wide-spectrum anti-reflective coatings for fused silica and other glasses. *Appl. Opt.* 23:1418.

Zhang, S., Wang, Y.S., Zeng, X.T., Cheng, K., Qian, M., Sun, D.E., Weng, W.J., and Chia, W.Y. 2007. Evaluation of interfacial shear strength and residual stress of sol–gel derived fluoridated hydroxyapatite coatings on Ti6Al4V substrates. *Eng. Fract. Mech.* 74:1884–1893.

Zheng, H., Colby, M.W., and Mackenzie, J.D. 1988. The control of precipitation in sol–gel solutions, 537–540. In *Better Ceramics Through Chemistry,* 3rd Edition. Brinker, C.J., Clark, D.E., and Ulrich, D.R. (eds). Pittsburgh, PA: Materials Research Society.

Zreiqat, H., Valenzuela, S.M., Ben-Nissan, B., Roest, R., Knabe, C., Radlanski, R.J., Renz, H., and Evans, P.J. 2005. The effect of surface chemistry modification of titanium alloy on signalling pathways in human osteoblasts. *Biomaterials.* 26:7579–7586.

3

Hydroxyapatite and Other Biomedical Coatings by Electrophoretic Deposition

Charles C. Sorrell, Hariati Taib, Timothy C. Palmer, Fei Peng, Zengmin Xia, and Mei Wei

CONTENTS

Introduction

In his extensive review of bioceramics, Hench [1] indicated that one of two primary clinical applications of porous ceramics was in the form of *hydroxyapatite coatings* for (1) prostheses as alternatives to cement fixation and (2) dental implants for bioactive fixation. Although there are many reports of methods that can be used to fabricate thin (and thick) films of ceramics on the surfaces of substrates and their properties, the most common types of fabrication can be categorized generally according to Figure 3.1 [2–17].

The focus of the present work is *electrophoretic deposition*, particularly of hydroxyapatite ($Ca_{10}[PO_4]_6[OH]_2$), which is one of two well-known analogs of electrodeposition [18,19]:

- Electrolytic deposition: surface coating produced from *dissolved* ions or complexes
- Electrophoretic deposition: surface coating produced from *suspended* particles

Table 3.1 [20,21] summarizes the differences between these two techniques for surface coating application.

Although electrolytic deposition is well known as the process by which metals are plated on other metals, there has been a number of reports of the use of this technique to produce ceramic coatings, including Al_2O_3, TiO_2, and hydroxyapatite [19].

In electrophoretic deposition, what are typically colloidal particles are deposited onto a conductive substrate in the presence of an external electrical field [20,22]. These particles, which are conductive owing to surface electrical charge, migrate to the substrate of opposite charge, and so particle deposition may occur either on the cathode or anode. Generally, any solid that can be suspended, typically in the form of a powder less than ~30 μm in size, can be used for electrophoretic deposition [19,23]. This process is applicable to many types of materials, including oxides, carbides, nitrides, glasses, metals, and polymers.

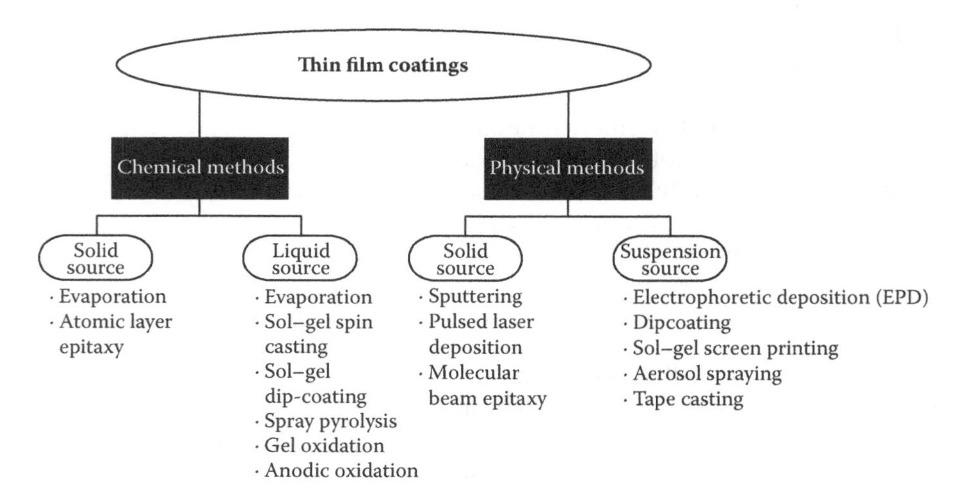

FIGURE 3.1
Summary of fabrication methods for ceramic thin films.

TABLE 3.1

Comparison between Electrophoretic and Electrolytic Deposition Processes

Parameter	Electrophoretic Deposition	Electrolytic Deposition
System	Suspension	Solution
Moving species	Particles	Ions or complexes
Electrode reactions	None	Electrogeneration of OH^- and neutralization of cationic species
System electrical conductivity	Low	High
Deposited material	Ceramics or metal	Metal
Deposition rate	10^0–10^3 μm/min	10^{-3}–10^0 μm/min
Deposit thickness	10^0–10^3 μm	10^{-3}–10^1 μm
Deposit composition control	By powder stoichiometry	By solution composition

Source: Heavens, S.N., *Advanced Ceramic Processing and Technology*, William Andrews Publishing/Noyes, Park Ridge, NJ, 1990; Besra, L., Liu. M., *Prog. Mater. Sci.*, **52**, 1, 1–61, 2007. With permission.

There are two basic components of electrophoretic deposition: electrophoresis and deposition [22]. That is, the process includes movement of charged particles in a suspension toward an electrode under the influence of an electric field followed by deposition on the electrode. Calcination or firing generally follows in order to (1) convert the weak initial physical bond to a stronger chemical bond, (2) pyrolyze any binder (if used), and (3) densify the deposit. A schematic of the process of cathodic electrophoretic deposition is shown in Figure 3.2.

In addition to the fabrication of coatings, electrophoretic deposition can be used to produce the following [20,22,24]:

- Die-formed monolithic shapes
- Free-standing monolithic shapes
- Laminates
- Infiltrated porous bodies
- Infiltrated woven fiber preforms

In the fabrication of coatings, electrophoretic deposition offers a number of advantages over other methods of fabrication:

- Even (matched) profile over irregular surfaces
- Highly precise and reproducible coating thicknesses
- High deposition rates
- Operation in air
- Simplicity of materials and process
- Low cost of infrastructure and operation
- Capacity to produce patterned coatings (using a mask)
- Capacity to produce composite coatings (as above)
- Capacity to operate continuously

For these reasons, electrophoretic deposition is of considerable interest from the technical and commercial perspectives.

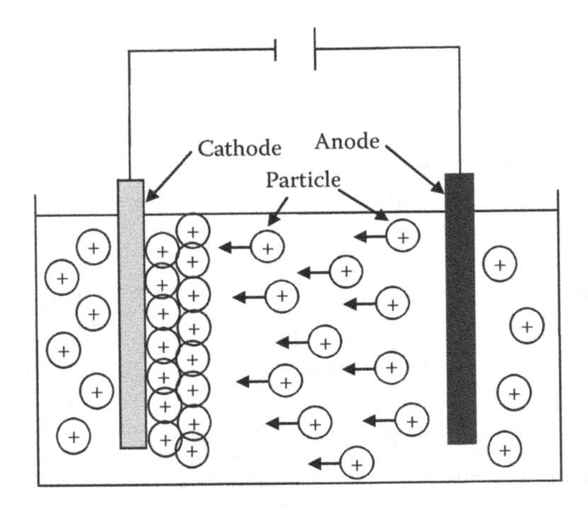

FIGURE 3.2
Schematic of cathodic electrophoretic deposition.

Principles of Electrophoresis

Double Layer

Figure 3.3 illustrates the nature of a particle and the *surface potential* (ψ) associated with the unsaturated chemical bonds that are present at the terminating grain surface [24–26]. A *double layer* forms when a charged particle in suspension is surrounded by ions of opposite charge in concentrations higher than that of the bulk concentration of these ions in the medium. The electrochemical double layer formed around the particle surface consists of an inner *Stern layer* of counterions fixed on the particle surface, which produce the *Stern potential* (ψ_S), and an outer *diffuse layer*. The *Debye length* $\left(\frac{1}{\kappa}\right)$ is determined by the point at which the effects of the electrical forces are countered by random thermal motion. The *zeta potential* (ζ; or *electrokinetic potential*), which is used widely to assess the magnitude of the electrical charge at the double layer, is the electrical potential at the *slipping plane*, which is the interface between the stationary adsorbed liquid layer and the mobile medium beyond it.

The stability of a suspension (its resistance to gravitational settling) is determined by the Debye length, which is defined in Equation 3.1 [19,22,27]

$$\frac{1}{\kappa} = \frac{\varepsilon\varepsilon_o kT}{e^2 \sum n_i z_i} = \frac{k' \varepsilon_o^2 kT}{e^2 \sum n_i z_i} \tag{3.1}$$

where

ε = permittivity of medium

ε_o = permittivity of vacuum

$\frac{1}{\kappa}$ = Debye length

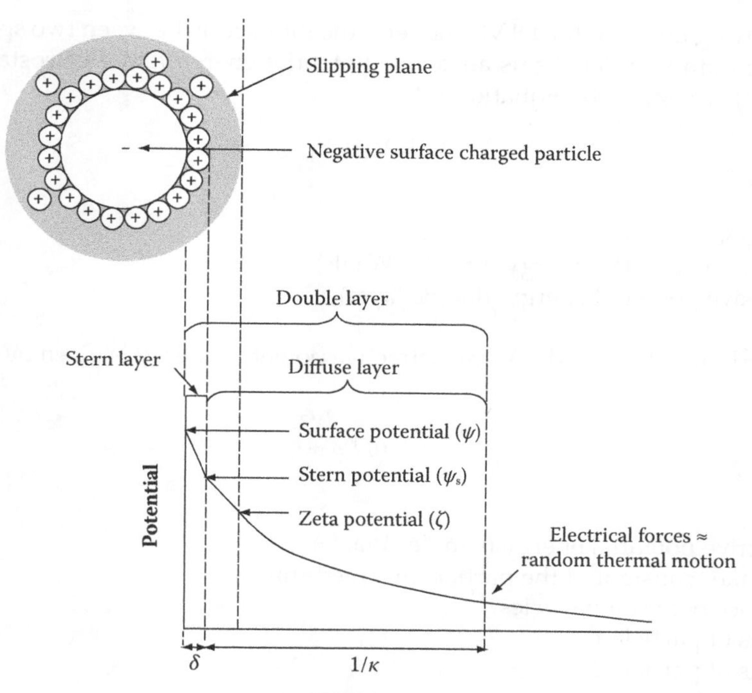

FIGURE 3.3
Schematic of a particle and associated surface charge. (Adapted from Van der Biest, O.O. and Vandeperre, L.J., *Annu. Rev. Mater. Sci.*, 29 [1] 327–52 (1999); Usui, S., Electric Charge and Charge Neutralization in Aqueous Solutions, pp. 432–39 in *Powder Technology Handbook*. Marcel Dekker, New York, 1991; Cazes, J. (ed.)., *Encyclopedia of Chromatography*, 3rd Edition, CRC Press, Boca Raton, FL, 2005.)

k = Boltzmann constant
T = absolute temperature
e = electron charge
n_i = concentration of ions
z_i = valence of ions
k' = dielectric constant of medium ($\varepsilon/\varepsilon_o$ [28])

A high surface charge on a particle, regardless of the charge type, results in the formation of a thick double layer [29]. This condition prevents particles from approaching closely to one another owing to electrostatic repulsion. This condition typically results in suspensions of low viscosities, deflocculation, and high stability. With lower surface charges and thinner double layers, suspensions typically exhibit high viscosities, flocculation, and rapid gravitational settling.

Derjaguin, Landau, Verwey, and Overbeek Theory

The most commonly applied theoretical model describing the force between charged surfaces in a liquid medium is the Derjaguin, Landau, Verwey, and Overbeek (DLVO) theory, which is applicable for dilute suspensions [19,21,22,29,30]. However, the Gouy–Chapman (GC) theory [31] and the Gouy–Chapman–Stern–Grahame (GCSG) theory [26] also are used. The starting point for the DLVO model is the interaction between two spheres, which are subject to both van der Waals attractive potential energy and electrostatic repulsive potential energy, as given by Equation 3.2:

$$V_T = V_A + V_R \tag{3.2}$$

where:
V_T = total potential energy
V_A = attractive potential energy (van der Waals)
V_R = repulsive potential energy (double layer)

In simplified form, the van der Waals attractive potential energy is given by Equation 3.3:

$$V_A = -\frac{A}{6D}\frac{r_1 r_2}{r_1 + r_2} \tag{3.3}$$

where:
V_A = attractive potential energy (van der Waals)
A = Hamaker constant of the particle in a medium
D = distance between particles
r_1 = radius of particle 1
r_2 = radius of particle 2

The double layer repulsive potential energy generally is given in terms of a single particle radius by Equation 3.4:

$$V_R = \frac{\varepsilon \psi r}{2}\ln\left(1 + e^{-\kappa D}\right) \tag{3.4}$$

where:
V_R = Repulsive potential energy (double layer)
ε = Permittivity of medium
ψ = Surface potential
r = Radius of particle
$\frac{1}{\kappa}$ = Debye length
D = Distance between particles

Using these equations, the potential energy of the interaction between particles can be shown schematically, which is done in Figure 3.4. This can be interpreted in terms of the following phenomena [22,29]:

- *Point A.* At $D \approx 0$, the particles are in contact, with maximal attractive potential energy (V_A), which dominates the total potential energy (V_T).
- As the distance between the particles increases, the balance between the attractive potential energy (V_A) and repulsive potential energy (V_R) shifts in favor of the latter.
- *Point B.* At the maximal V_T, an energy barrier (E_B) to particle flocculation is established, so *deflocculation* occurs.

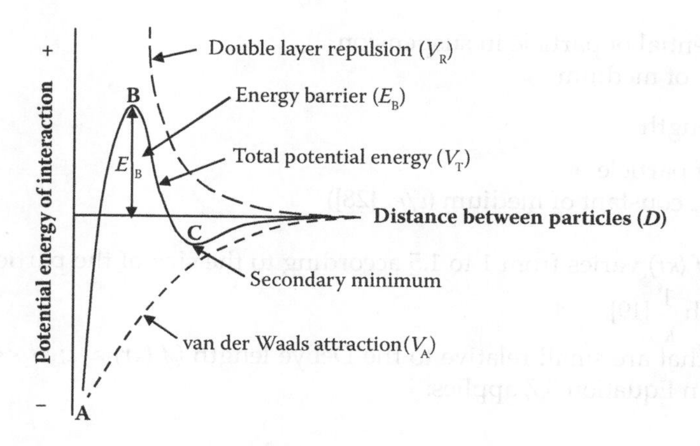

FIGURE 3.4
Schematic of interaction energy between two particles. (Adapted from Sarkar, P. and Nicholson, P.S. *J. Am. Ceram. Soc.*, 79 [8] 1987–2002 (1996).)

- As the distance between the particles increases, the balance between the attractive potential energy (V_A) and repulsive potential energy (V_R) shifts in favor of the former.
- *Point C.* At the secondary minimum (the primary minimum is off-scale, beyond point A), if the concentration of counterions is sufficient, *flocculation* occurs.

Electrophoretic Mobility

Electrophoresis generally occurs when the distance over which the double layer charge falls toward zero is large compared to the particle size [20]. Hence, the effect of an applied electric field is greater on the particle and so it will move under its influence. The velocity at which this occurs is given by Equation 3.5 [19]:

$$v = \mu E \tag{3.5}$$

where:
v = particle velocity
μ = electrophoretic mobility
E = applied electric field

The electrophoretic mobility for a rigid spherical particle is given by Equation 3.6 [20]:

$$\mu = \frac{2\varepsilon\varepsilon_0\zeta}{3\eta} f(\kappa r) = \frac{2k'\varepsilon_o^2\zeta}{3\eta} f(\kappa r) \tag{3.6}$$

where
μ = electrophoretic mobility of particle
ε = permittivity of medium
ε_o = permittivity of vacuum

ζ = zeta potential of particle in suspension
η = viscosity of medium
$\frac{1}{\kappa}$ = Debye length
r = radius of particle
k' = dielectric constant of medium ($\varepsilon/\varepsilon_o$ [28])

The function $f(\kappa r)$ varies from 1 to 1.5 according to the size of the particle compared to the Debye length $\frac{1}{\kappa}$ [19].

For particles that are small relative to the Debye length ($f(\kappa r) \approx 1$; $\kappa r << 1$), the Hückel formula, given in Equation 3.7, applies:

$$\mu = \frac{2\varepsilon\varepsilon_0\zeta}{3\eta} = \frac{2k'\varepsilon_0^2\zeta}{3\eta} \tag{3.7}$$

For particles that are large relative to the Debye length ($f(\kappa r) \approx 1.5$; $\kappa r >> 1$), the Smoluchowski formula, given in Equation 3.8, applies:

$$\mu = \frac{\varepsilon\varepsilon_0\zeta}{\eta} = \frac{k'\varepsilon_0^2\zeta}{\eta} \tag{3.8}$$

where:
μ = electrophoretic mobility of particle
ε = permittivity of medium
ε_o = permittivity of vacuum
ζ = zeta potential of particle in suspension
η = viscosity
k' = dielectric constant of medium ($\varepsilon/\varepsilon_o$ [28])

Zeta Potential

As mentioned, the zeta potential is used widely to assess the magnitude of the electrical charge at the double layer. It also is known as the *electrokinetic potential*. Figure 3.3 illustrates that the zeta potential is the electrical potential at the interface between the stationary adsorbed liquid layer and the mobile medium beyond it.

For effective suspension of particles, which generally is a prerequisite to electrophoretic deposition, a high and uniform surface charge on the particles is desirable [21]. In this regard, the zeta potential is important to this process by determining the following:

- Level of repulsive interaction and consequent suspension stabilization
- Direction and speed of particle migration
- Green (unfired) bulk density of the deposit

It is possible to manipulate the zeta potential through the use of *charging agents*, including acids, bases, and adsorbed ions and polyelectrolytes [19]. This manipulation can extend to complete reversal of the sign of the zeta potential (positive versus negative).

A common method of altering the surface charge is by metal oxide or metal hydroxide surface hydrolysis through particle surface ionization. This may occur either by protonation or deprotonation of acid or base groups by changing the pH. For example, when oxide particles are dispersed in an aqueous medium, the surfaces are coordinated by water molecules to form hydroxylated surfaces. The charge of the particle surface then depends on the pH, as shown in Reactions **1** and **2** [19,30]:

$$\text{pH} < 7: \quad \text{M-OH} + \text{H}^+ \leftrightarrow \text{M-OH}_2^+ \qquad \text{Reaction } \mathbf{1}$$

$$\text{pH} > 7: \quad \text{M-OH} + \text{OH}^- \leftrightarrow \text{M-O}^- + \text{H}_2\text{O} \qquad \text{Reaction } \mathbf{2}$$

There are two terms used to define the state of the solid/medium interface of dispersed particles. The *isoelectric point* corresponds to the condition where the zeta potential of a particle surface is zero ($\zeta = 0$) [32]. This also is considered that point at which the surface charge of the particle only is zero [33]. The pH at which this occurs is the pH_{iep}. The other related parameter is the *point of zero charge*, which corresponds to the condition where positive ([M-OH_2^+]) and negative ([M-O^-]) surface electrolyte concentrations are equal (i.e., $\psi = 0$) [32]. This also is considered the point at which the net total of the external and internal surface charges of the particle is zero [33]. The pH at which this occurs is the pH_{zpc}.

The isoelectric point and point of zero charge often are used interchangeably. However, they are equivalent only if the sorption of ions and dissociation of counterions are ignored [32]. Whether this is the case depends principally on the method of powder fabrication, stoichiometry, crystal structure, degree of surface hydration, leaching, and impurities. Consequently, the differences between these two parameters can be significant. In general, it can be observed that (1) the pH_{zpc} tends to be close to the natural pH of a suspension [22] but (2) the pH_{iep} is strongly influenced and altered by the preceding factors. In this sense, the zero point charge can be considered more of an intrinsic quantity while the isoelectric point can be viewed pragmatically as an extrinsic quantity. In effect, the ease of altering the surface isoelectric point explains why it is used to control the surface charge more frequently than the point of zero charge.

Table 3.2 [25,34] provides a selection of pH values for isoelectric points (pH_{iep}) determined for some oxide ceramic powders.

The Australian authors of the present work recently have described the relation between the pH, zeta potential, and rheology of suspensions in terms of charge saturation at the particle surface [35]. This model differs from the conventional approach in three principal ways:

- Conventionally, particles are considered to have only intrinsic positive *or* negative surface charge. In the present model, they possess both positive *and* negative surface charges, which result from the anisotropic directional bonding in most crystal structures, although only one typically dominates.
- Conventionally, the solid/liquid interface is viewed in terms of homogeneous and complete saturation of the solid by oppositely charged species in the medium, as shown in Figure 3.3. In the present model, while the surface charge is assumed to be homogeneous, it is not assumed to be saturated.
- Conventionally, flocculation is viewed to result from compression of the repulsive double layer with increasing electrolyte concentration [19]. In the present model, anisotropic surface charges contribute to this compression.

TABLE 3.2
Selected pH Values of Isoelectric Points for Oxide Powders

Oxide	pH_{iep}	Reference
MgO	12.4	34
La_2O_3	10.4	34
CuO	9.5	34
Al_2O_3	9.4	25
ZnO	8.8	25
Cr_2O_3	7.0	34
CeO_2	6.7	34
Fe_2O_3	6.7	25
Fe_3O_4	6.5	25
TiO_2	6.0	25
SnO_2	5.4	25
Amorphous SiO_2	2.5	25

Source: Usui, S., *Powder Technology Handbook*, Marcel Dekker, New York, 1991; Lewis, J.A., *J. Am. Ceram. Soc.*, 83, 10, 2341–59, 2000, With permission.

These concepts are illustrated schematically in Figures 3.5 and 3.6. In effect, this model attempts to provide a phenomenological interpretation of the effect of pH and charge anisotropy on the zeta potential. However, Figure 3.6 is an idealized curve that is applicable to any suspended particle, regardless of whether the surface charge is isotropic or anisotropic. The model merely clarifies the change in behavior in terms of physical parameters.

The nominated values of zeta potential (±30 and ±60 mV) are based on well-known observed thresholds for suspension stability. The terms *overly stable* and *appropriately stable* (right side of Figure 3.6) and $E_{\text{particle repulsion}}$ and $E_{\text{external field}}$ (left-hand side of Figure 3.6) are relevant to electrophoresis, where it is possible for the suspension to be too stable because

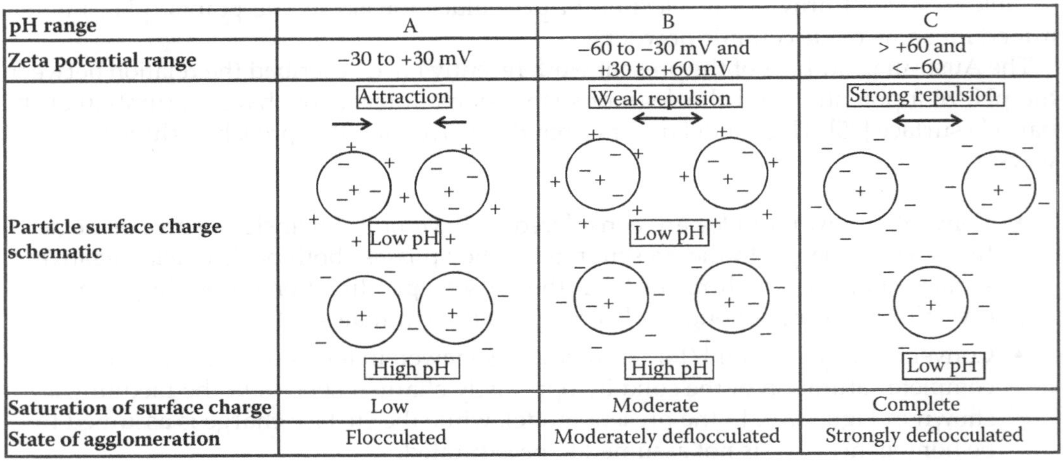

pH range	A	B	C
Zeta potential range	−30 to +30 mV	−60 to −30 mV and +30 to +60 mV	> +60 and < −60
Particle surface charge schematic	Attraction Low pH High pH	Weak repulsion Low pH High pH	Strong repulsion Low pH
Saturation of surface charge	Low	Moderate	Complete
State of agglomeration	Flocculated	Moderately deflocculated	Strongly deflocculated

FIGURE 3.5
Effects of surface charge anisotropy on suspensions. (Reprinted from Taib, H., Synthesis and Electrophoretic Deposition of Tin Oxide (SnO_2). Ph.D. Thesis, University of New South Wales, 2009. With permission.)

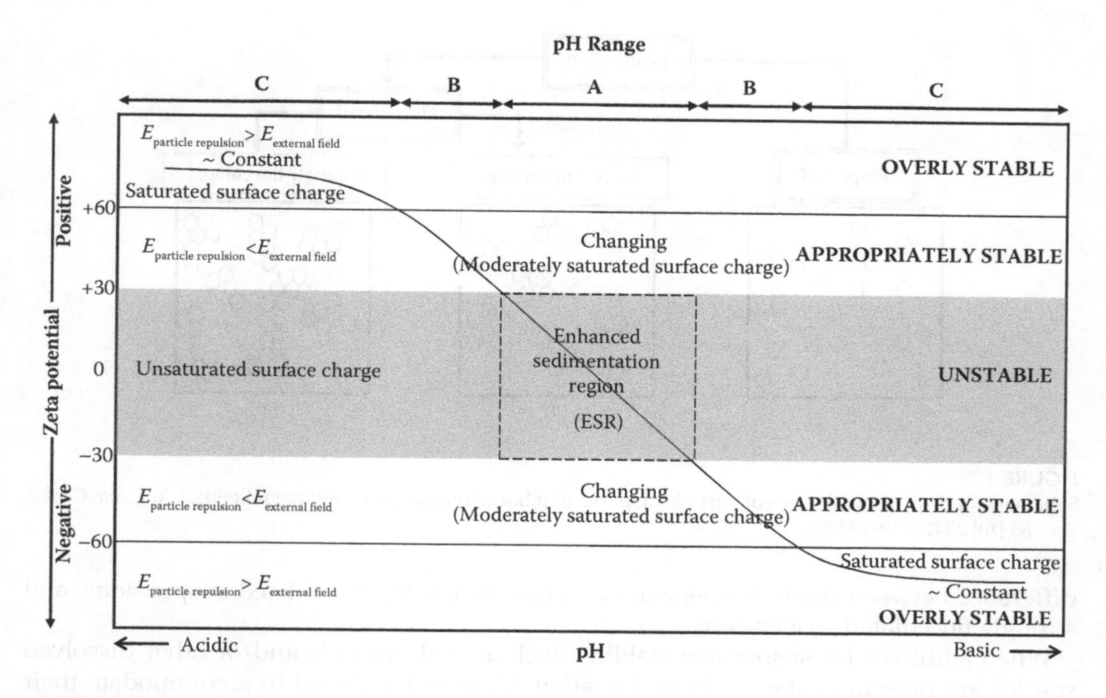

FIGURE 3.6
Effects of surface charge on pH–zeta potential relation during electrophoresis. (Reprinted from Taib, H., Synthesis and Electrophoretic Deposition of Tin Oxide (SnO_2). Ph.D. Thesis, University of New South Wales, 2009. With permission.)

the repulsive forces between particles cannot be overcome by the electric field (E), thereby hindering deposition [19]. Accordingly, it has been commented that a suspension benefits from being unstable near the electrode [22].

Suspension Stability

Suspension Stabilization

As mentioned, the effectiveness of electrophoretic deposition depends significantly on the suspension stability. There are two types of suspension media used for electrophoretic deposition [21]:

1. Aqueous (water-based)
2. Nonaqueous (organic)

Traditionally, suspensions and electrophoresis have been considered in terms of *colloidal* particles, which can remain relatively stable in suspension since Brownian motion is able to overcome gravitational settling of these particles of size ~1 μm or less [21]. Stable suspensions present minimal tendency to flocculate, and upon eventual settling, pack densely owing to the near-absence of irregular agglomerates [20]. Figure 3.7 illustrates the

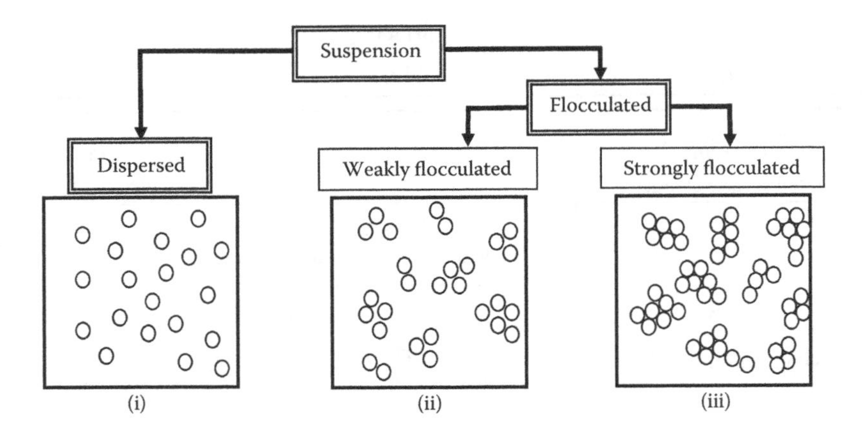

FIGURE 3.7
Schematic of three general states of particle dispersion in liquid media. (Adapted from Lewis, J.A. *J. Am. Ceram. Soc.*, 83 [10] 2341–2359 (2000).)

difference between stable (dispersed) suspensions, weakly flocculated suspensions, and strongly flocculated suspensions.

When additives for suspension stability such as deflocculants and/or other dissolved species are present in the medium, Equation 3.2 must be altered to accommodate their effects. This is shown in Equation 3.9 [34]:

$$V_{\text{total}} = V_{\text{vdw}} + V_{\text{elect}} + V_{\text{steric}} + V_{\text{struct}} \tag{3.9}$$

where:
V_{total} = total potential energy (V_T)
V_{vdw} = attractive potential energy (van der Waals; V_A)
V_{elect} = repulsive potential energy (electrostatic interaction between double layers; V_R)
V_{steric} = repulsive potential energy (steric interactions between particle surfaces)
V_{struct} = attractive or repulsive potential energy (nonadsorbed species in solution)

When additives are used, the energy associated with each of these can play a critical role in the stabilization of the suspension. Figure 3.8 schematically illustrates these mechanisms [29,34]:

- *Electrostatic stabilization.* Repulsive electrostatic double-layer forces at the solid/liquid interface are responsible for the stabilization of the suspension. This approach, which is what has been considered up to this point and shown in Figure 3.3, is more effective with aqueous media owing to the ready generation of $M\text{-}OH_2^+$ and $M\text{-}O^-$ electrolytes, as shown in Reactions **1** and **2** [19].
- *Steric stabilization.* The addition of what usually are long-chain organic species effectively coat the particles with an adlayer sufficiently thick to (1) overcome van der Waals attraction between particles and (2) avoid adsorbing on multiple particles (*bridging flocculation* [36]). Alternatively, short-chain, functionalized, polar polymers also can achieve the same outcome. The polymer adlayer provides effective interparticle steric repulsion. This approach can be used with both aqueous and organic media.

- *Electrosteric stabilization.* The addition of what usually are long-chain polyelectrolytes with at least one type of ionizable group, such as a carboxylic or sulfonic acid group, combine electrostatic and steric stabilization. In this case, the adlayer can be attached more strongly than the preceding case of polar attraction owing to the ionization. This approach can utilize cationic and anionic polyelectroytes and it can be used in both aqueous and organic media.

Concerning the potential energy from V_{struct}, the effect of the nonadsorbed species in solution can increase or decrease stability [34]. This is likely to depend largely upon the type and scale of their charge.

Initial Assessment of Suspension Stabilization

The dispersion of suspensions generally is assessed initially through simple experimentation on the settling behavior as a function of pH and/or deflocculant addition. This is done by placing suspensions with different pH, deflocculant addition, medium, and/or solids loading in test tubes, agitating, and allowing to settle for an extended period, usually up to a

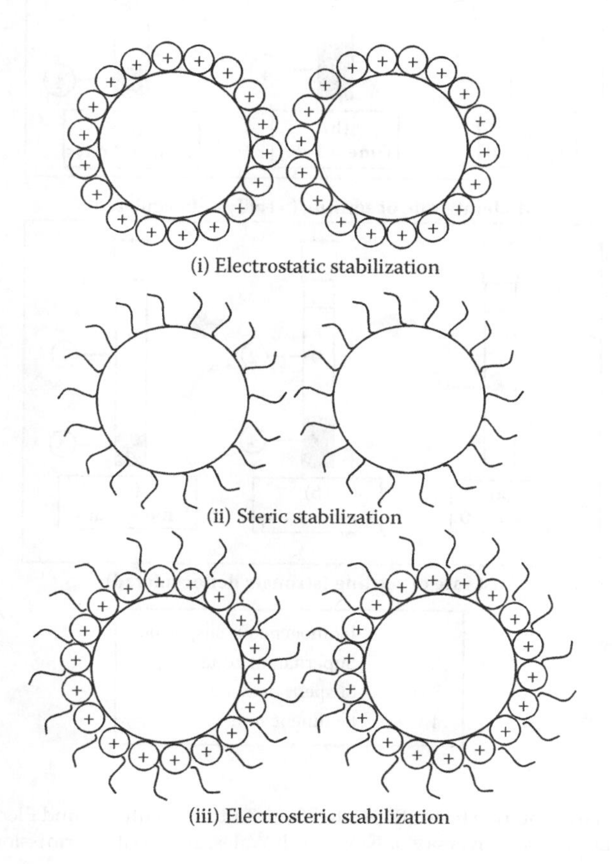

FIGURE 3.8
Principal mechanisms of suspension stabilization. (Adapted from Cao, G., *Nanostructures and Nanomaterials—Synthesis, Properties and Applications.* Imperial College Press, London, 2004; Lewis, J.A. *J. Am. Ceram. Soc.*, 83 [10] 2341–59 (2000).)

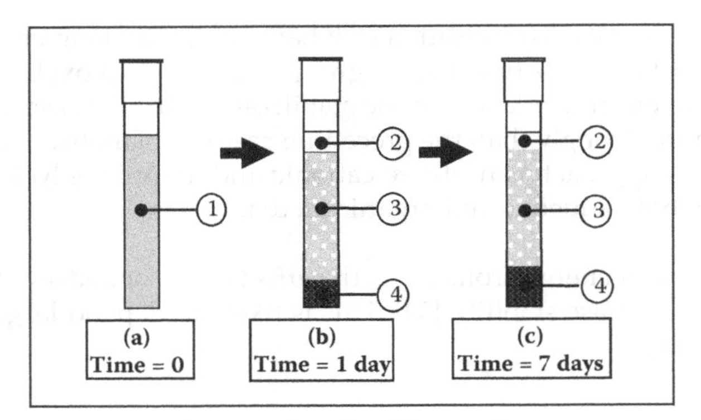

Slow rate of settling (dispersed)

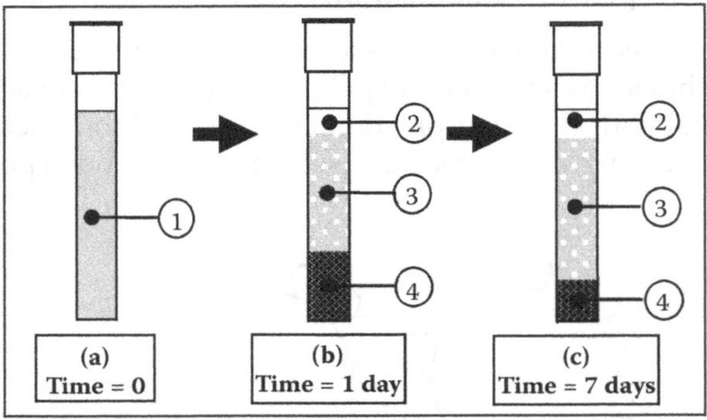

Moderate rate of settling (weakly deflocculated)

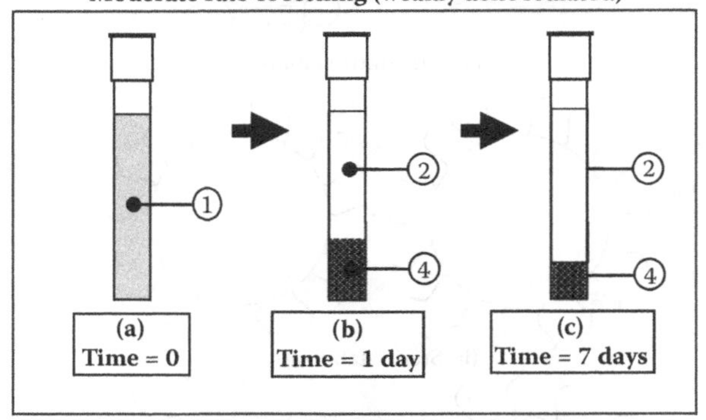

Fast rate of settling (strongly deflocculated)

1	—	Homogeneous suspension
2	—	Supernatant zone
3	—	Suspension zone
4	—	Sediment zone

FIGURE 3.9
Typical results of initial sedimentation tests. (Reprinted from Taib, H., Synthesis and Electrophoretic Deposition of Tin Oxide (SnO_2). Ph.D. Thesis, University of New South Wales, 2009. With permission.)

week. The results are interpreted in terms of the appearance of the resultant layers that can be detected. Figure 3.9 [35] summarizes typical observations for this experimentation.

Aqueous Suspensions

In aqueous media, there are four common ways by which the surface charge of particles can be altered [30]:

- *Dissociation.* Partial dissociation of the particle surface provides ions to the suspension. This can be controlled by pH alteration; addition of a solvent, such as high-valence ions, to the solution; and addition of a polyelectrolyte (cationic or anionic).
- *Nernstian charging.* Adsorption or desorption of lattice ions can be altered through the common ion effect, in which a solution of two solutes with the same ion can have its equilibrium shifted owing to different levels of ionization. This can be controlled through the addition of a solute that increases the solubility of the particle.
- *Metal hydrolysis.* The surface of a metal oxide or metal hydroxide hydrolyzes by protonation or deprotonation of acid or base groups. This principle is indicated in Reactions **1** and **2**. This typically is done by control of the pH.
- *Metal hydrolysis and dissolution.* The surface of a metal oxide or metal hydroxide can dissolve incongruently (particle composition $\neq$ solute composition) into one or more cationic species. This usually is done with complex metal oxides, where ions of different valence are leached and then adsorb in the Stern layer. This is controlled by pH, solute concentration, and solids loading.

It is perceived widely that aqueous suspensions are problematic for electrophoretic deposition. The main reason for this is that there are several shortcomings that create the following risks:

- Electrolysis of the water at low field strengths, which produces gas bubbles that disrupt the process and may introduce porosity in the deposit
- High current densities, which cause Joule heating
- Potential dissolution of the substrate at unsuitable pH values
- Potential dissolution of the deposit at unsuitable pH values

However, the main advantages are:

- Easy manipulation of the surface charge through pH alteration
- Low processing costs
- Low environmental impact

Table 3.3 [37–85] provides a representative example of reports of the aqueous electrophoretic deposition of a range of bioceramics.

TABLE 3.3

Summary of Reported Work on Aqueous and Organic Electrophoretic Deposition of Other Bioceramics

Coating	Particle Size	Medium Type	Substrate	Suspension Medium	Solids Loading	Voltage (V)	Time (min)	Temp. (°C)	Heat Treatment	Deposit Properties	Reference
α-Al_2O_3	0.5 μm	Aqueous	Anode: Pt Cathode: Zn Electrode separation: 2 cm	Medium: H_2O Dispersant: Dolapix CE64	5, 20 wt.%	100+	30	25	1550°C, 2 h	Deposit thickness: 0.5–1.8 mm	37
α-Al_2O_3		Aqueous	Anode: graphite, Zn Cathode: graphite, Zn Electrode separation: 2 cm	Medium: H_2O Dispersant: Dolapix CE64 (0–5 wt.%)	5, 10, 20 wt.%		10–30	25–40	None	Deposit thickness: 2.13–2.23 mm	38
α-Al_2O_3	0.20 μm	Aqueous	For $pH < pH_{iep}$ Anode: stainless steel Cathode: Pd For $pH > pH_{iep}$ Anode: Zn Cathode: Pd	Medium: H_2O Suspension pH: 2 to 11 pH adjustment: HCl, NaOH	3 wt.%	0–160	3	25	None		39
α-Al_2O_3	0.5 μm	Aqueous	Anode: graphite Cathode: Pd Electrode separation: 2 cm	Medium: H_2O Suspension pH: 2 to 11 pH adjustment: HCl, NaOH Dispersant: Dolapix CE64 (0.35 wt.%)	5 wt.%	10–700	2, 5	24, 31, 38	1550°C, 2 h		40
α-Al_2O_3	0.5 μm	Aqueous	Anode: stainless steel Cathode: Pt Electrode separation: 1.8 cm	Medium: H_2O Suspension pH: 10 pH adjustment: HNO_3 Dispersant: Dolapix ET85, PC33 Binder: 2% PVA[a] in water	10, 20, 30 wt.%	30–250	2, 5, 10			Deposit thickness: 10–60 μm	41

α-Al_2O_3		Aqueous	Anode: graphite Cathode: Pt Electrode separation: 2 cm	Medium: H_2O Suspension pH: 10 pH adjustment: HNO_3 Dispersant: ester polyphosphate (C213), Darvan 821-A	5 wt.%	50–700	10	23–33			42
α-Al_2O_3	0.6 μm	Nonaqueous	Anode: stainless steel Cathode: stainless steel Electrode separation: 0.35 cm	Medium: methylamylketone, *n*-butylamine, ethanol, HNO_3 Suspension pH: 0.78	0.05–0.4 wt.%	150, 300	6			Thin deposit	43
α-Al_2O_3	1.4 μm	Nonaqueous	Anode: stainless steel Cathode: stainless steel Electrode separation: 0.5 cm, 3 cm	Medium: ethanol Suspension pH: 3 pH adjustment: glacial acetic acid Dispersant: citric acid	2.6, 15, 20 vol.%	1, 20	0.5, 5				44
α-Al_2O_3	150 nm	Nonaqueous	Electrode separation: 2 cm	Medium: ethanol Suspension pH: 4, 7, 11 pH adjustment: glacial acetic acid, tetramethyl ammonium hydroxide Dispersant: polyethylene imine	20–70 vol.%	80	5	25	1250°C 2 h, air; HIPed[b] 180 MPa, 1250°C, 2 h, Ar	Full density with solids loading of 50 vol.%	45
α-Al_2O_3	0.15 nm	Aqueous	Interposing membrane: cellulose	Medium: H_2O Suspension pH: 7.5–9.0 Dispersant: Darvan C	25 wt.%			25	1200°C, 2 h, air; HIPed[b], 160 MPa, 1250°C, 2 h, Ar		46
α-Al_2O_3	0.15 μm	Aqueous	Cathode: Pd Electrode separation: 2 cm	Medium: H_2O Suspension pH: 4	10 vol.%			25	1600°C, 2 h	Deposit thickness: 150 μm, alternating layers, no cracking,	47

(continued)

TABLE 3.3 (Continued)

Summary of Reported Work on Aqueous and Organic Electrophoretic Deposition of Other Bioceramics

Coating	Particle Size	Medium Type	Substrate	Suspension Medium	Solids Loading	Voltage (V)	Time (min)	Temp. (°C)	Heat Treatment	Deposit Properties	Reference
α-Al_2O_3	0.3-0.5 μm	Nonaqueous	Electrode separation: 3.5 cm	Medium: ethanol + *n*-butylamine Dispersant: Dolapix CE64	100 g/L			25	1550°C, 2 h		48
α-Al_2O_3	0.2–0.4 μm	Nonaqueous	Electrode separation: 0.6 cm	Medium: ethanol Dispersant: polyacrylic acid, polyethylene imine	60 wt.%	50	10	25		Deposit thickness: 4–5 mm	49
α-Al_2O_3	0.7 μm	Aqueous versus nonaqueous	Anode: steel Cathode: Zn Electrode separation: 2 cm	Medium: H_2O, ethanol Dispersant: Dolapix CE64, citric acid	50 wt.%	5–60		25	1550°C, 2 h		50
β-Al_2O_3	1 μm	Nonaqueous	Anode: stainless steel Cathode: graphite	Medium: dichloromethane	40 g/L	100–500	0–5	25	1700°–1750°C, 1–5 h		51
β-Al_2O_3		Nonaqueous	Anode: stainless steel, Ni, Invar Cathode: stainless steel	Medium: *n*–amyl alcohol	40–750 g/L	200–1000		25	1700°–1825°C		52
γ-Al_2O_3	37 nm	Aqueous	Anode: graphite Cathode: Cu Electrode separation: 2 cm	Medium: H_2O Suspension pH: 2 and 11 pH adjustment: HCl, NaOH	0.01–0.16 vol.%	30		25	1050°C, 1 h	Porous deposit, Pore size 18–25 nm	53
γ-Al_2O_3	33 nm	Aqueous	Anode: stainless steel Cathode: Pd Electrode separation: 2 cm	Medium: H_2O Suspension pH: 5–6 pH adjustment: HCl, NaOH	3–5 wt.%						54

α-Al_2O_3		Nonaqueous	Anode: graphite Electrode separation: 1 cm	Medium: ethanol	10 vol.%	0–600	0–5	25	1550°C, 6 h	Al_2O_3 deposit thickness: 60–180 μm	55
Y-ZrO_2 (YSZ[c])										YSZ[c] deposit thickness: 30–110 μm	
α-Al_2O_3	0.6 μm	Nonaqueous	Anode: stainless steel Cathode: stainless steel Electrode separation: 0.35 cm	Medium: ethanol pH adjustment: HCl, NaOH Dispersant: Darvan C + *n*-butylamine	α-Alumina 2.5 vol.%	100, 300	20				56
Ce-ZrO_2 (CeSZ[d])	0.32 μm				Ce-ZrO_2 1.5 vol.%						
α-Al_2O_3 + ZrO_2	0.02 μm 60 nm	Aqueous	Anode: stainless steel Cathode: stainless steel, Ni, Pt, Pd	Medium: H_2O Suspension pH: 4	5 vol.%	5–120 (over time)	30	25	1350°C, 2 h	Al_2O_3 + ZrO_2 laminate	57
α-Al_2O_3 + ZrO_2	220 nm 75 nm	Nonaqueous	Anode: stainless steel Cathode: stainless steel	Medium: ethanol pH adjustment: HCl, NaOH Dispersant: triethylamine + citric acid	5 wt.%	20, 15	3, 5			Deposit thickness: 10 μm, 15 μm	58
α-Al_2O_3 + Y-ZrO_2 (YSZ[c])	470 nm 170 nm	Nonaqueous	Anode: stainless steel Cathode: stainless steel Electrode separation: 2.6 cm	Medium: monochloroacetic acid in isopropanol	15 wt.%	85–105	0–30	25	1500°C, 2 h	Deposit thickness: ≤1250 μm	59, 60

(*continued*)

TABLE 3.3 (Continued)

Summary of Reported Work on Aqueous and Organic Electrophoretic Deposition of Other Bioceramics

Coating	Particle Size	Medium Type	Substrate	Suspension Medium	Solids Loading	Voltage (V)	Time (min)	Temp. (°C)	Heat Treatment	Deposit Properties	Reference
Y-ZrO_2 (YSZ[c])		Nonaqueous	Anode: porous Ni-cermet/Cu Cathode: Cu Electrode separation: 1 cm	Medium: ethanol pH adjustment: glacial acetic acid Dispersant: polyethylene imine	2 vol.%	1–30	1–4			Deposit thickness: 12 μm	61
Y-ZrO_2 (YSZ[c])		Aqueous	Cathode: Pt Electrode separation: 2 cm	Medium: H_2O + acetic acid	40 wt.%	5–30	20–60	25	1450°C, 2 h	Deposit thickness: 2–4 mm, porous, no cracking	62
Y-ZrO_2 (CSZ[e])		Aqueous	Anode: steel Cathode: corrugated steel	Medium: H_2O Suspension pH: 3–7 pH adjustment: 0.1 M HCl	4–8 wt.%				1000°C, 45 min	Deposit thickness: 5 μm in trenches, 2 μm on top of profile	63
Y-ZrO_2 (CSZ[e])	0.26 μm	Nonaqueous	Anode: Fecralloy Cathode: Fecralloy Electrode separation: 1 cm	Medium: acetylacetone Suspension pH: 4.4–8.4 pH adjustment: acetic acid, triethanolamine	25 g/L	60	0.5–2	25	1200°C, 6 h	Deposit thickness: 50 μm, no cracking	64
Y-ZrO_2 (CSZ[e])		Nonaqueous	Anode: NiO–YSZ[c] + graphite Cathode: stainless steel Electrode separation: 1 cm	Medium: acetylacetone, ethanol		0–50	0–15	25	1400°C, 2 h	Deposit thickness: 13–32 μm, no cracking	65

Y-ZrO_2 (CSZ[e])		Nonaqueous	Anode: NiO–YSZ[c] Cathode: stainless steel	Medium: ethanol, isopropanol, acetylacetone, *n*-propanol, ethanol + acetylacetone	0.01 g/mL	50	3	25		Deposit thickness: 5 μm	66
Y-ZrO_2 (YSZ[c]) Y-ZrO_2 (YSZ[c]) + α-Al_2O_3	0.26 μm 0.26 μm		Anode: Cu + plaster Cathode: Pt	Medium: ethanol Dispersant: PVA, diethyl amine, polyethylene-imine, benzoic acid, 4-hydroxybenzoic acid Binder: Butvar B-98	50–60 wt.%	30	10, 15, 20	25	1450°–1500°C, 1 h	Deposit thickness: 600–1200 μm, no cracking	67
Y-ZrO_2 (YSZ[c]) + α-Al_2O_3		Nonaqueous	Anode: stainless steel Cathode: stainless steel Electrode separation: 3.5 cm	Medium: methyl ethyl ketone pH adjustment: glacial acetic acid Dispersant: *n*-butylamine Binder: nitrocellulose	150 g/L	300	5			Thick deposit	68
Y-ZrO_2 (YSZ[c]) + Bioglass		Nonaqueous	Anode: stainless steel Cathode: Ti6Al4V Electrode separation: 4 cm	Medium: ethanol, H_2O Dispersant: PVA	YSZ[c] 0.5 wt.% Bioglass 1 wt.%	50, 200	1	25	900°C, 2 h, Ar	Deposit thickness: 30 μm, no cracking	69
$ZrO_2 + Y_2O_3$ $ZrO_2 + Y_2O_3$ α-Alumina	10 μm 1.73 μm 1.0 μm 0.29 μm 1.27 μm	Aqueous	Anode: stainless steel Cathode: stainless steel Electrode separation: 1 cm	Medium: H_2O Suspension pH: 2 pH adjustment: HCl, tetramethylammonium hydroxide (TMAH) Dispersant: Dolapix CE64	10 wt.%	0.5–5	10		None		70
Y-ZrO_2 (CSZ[e]) + α-Al_2O_3 + Glass	10 μm	Nonaqueous	Anode: Fecralloy Cathode: Fecralloy Electrode separation: 1 cm	Medium: acetylacetone	50 g/L	100–300	0.5–1	25	1100°C, 20 h	Deposit thickness: 50 μm	71

(continued)

TABLE 3.3 (Continued)

Summary of Reported Work on Aqueous and Organic Electrophoretic Deposition of Other Bioceramics

Coating	Particle Size	Medium Type	Substrate	Suspension Medium	Solids Loading	Voltage (V)	Time (min)	Temp. (°C)	Heat Treatment	Deposit Properties	Reference
SiO_2	3.2 µm	Nonaqueous	Anode: Al Cathode: stainless steel Electrode separation: 1 cm	Medium: acetone		10–100	1–5	25			72
SiO_2	12 µm	Nonaqueous	Working electrode: Al Cathode: stainless steel Electrode separation: 0.5 cm	Medium: acetone	3–10 g/L	10–200	1–10	25	Calcined 300°C, 8 h	Deposit thickness: 100 µm	73
TiO_2 (Rutile)	0.48 µm	Aqueous	Anode: stainless steel Cathode: stainless steel Electrode separation: 1 cm	Medium: H_2O pH adjustment: titanium tetraisopropoxide, lactic acid	20 vol.%		15	25	1000°C, 2 h		74
TiO_2 (Rutile)	30 nm	Aqueous	Anode: stainless steel Cathode: Pd Electrode separation: 2 cm	Medium: H_2O pH adjustment: HCl and ammonia solution Dispersant: polyethylenimine	5 vol.%			25			75
TiO_2 (Rutile)	0.4 µm	Aqueous	Anode: alumina coated with 100 nm layer of Au 80%/Pd 20% Cathode: alumina coated with 100 nm layer of Au 80%/Pd 20% Electrode separation: 2 cm	Medium: H_2O Suspension pH: 10 pH adjustment: nitric acid Dispersant: tetraethylammonium hydroxide, sodium salt of polymethacrylic acid, Tiron Cosolvent: ethanol	5–20 vol.%		10	25		Deposit thickness: 0.5 µm – 5 mm	76

TiO_2 (Anatase)		Nonaqueous	Anode: Al Cathode: stainless steel Electrode separation: 1.0 cm	Medium: isopropanol	20 g/L	200	0.5–2	25	500°C, 0.5 h	Deposit thickness: 30–80 μm	77
TiO_2 (Anatase)	7 nm	Nonaqueous	Anode: stainless steel Cathode: stainless steel	Medium: acetone Suspension pH: 3–5	0.3 g/L	10–240	0–10	25	600°–800°C, 1 h	Thick film	78
TiO_2 (Rutile + Anatase)	Nanopowder	Nonaqueous	Cathode: stainless steel, Ti Electrode separation: 1 cm	Medium: acetylacetone Dispersant: iodine	1.05 wt.%	10	2.0	25	700°–900°C, Ar	Deposit thickness 10–20 μm, cracking after heat treatment	79
TiO_2	5 nm	Nonaqueous	Anode: stainless steel Cathode: stainless steel Electrode separation: 1 cm	Medium: isopropanol Dispersant: triethanolamine	250 g/L	5–20	0.1–1	25			80
TiO_2		Nonaqueous	Anode: Al Cathode: stainless steel mesh Electrode separation: 1 cm	Medium: isopropanol	20 g/L	195	0.5	25	500°C, 1 h	Deposit thickness: 8 μm (smooth) 10 μm (thick), no cracking	81
TiO_2 Nanotubes	12 nm Ø, 200–400 nm L	Nonaqueous	Anode: SnO_2-glass Cathode: stainless steel Electrode separation: 1 cm	Medium: ethanol Suspension pH: 4 pH adjustment: nitric acid Dispersant: PVB[f]	50 g/L	10–30	8	25	350°–550°C, 2 h	Thin film	82

(continued)

TABLE 3.3 (Continued)

Summary of Reported Work on Aqueous and Organic Electrophoretic Deposition of Other Bioceramics

Coating	Particle Size	Medium Type	Substrate	Suspension Medium	Solids Loading	Voltage (V)	Time (min)	Temp. (°C)	Heat Treatment	Deposit Properties	Reference
Zeolite (Clinoptilolite)	150 μm	Nonaqueous	Anode: stainless steel Cathode: stainless steel	Medium: ethanol Binder: TEOS[g], NaOH	8 g/L	50–200	5.0	25		No cracking	83
$CaSiO_3$ (Wollastonite)	1.7–3.7 μm	Aqueous versus nonaqueous	Anode: austenitic steel Cathode: austenitic steel Electrode separation: 1 cm	Medium: H_2O, ethanol	7.5 g/L	50	3	25	1100°–1300°C, 1 h	Porous thick film	84
PEEK[h]	20 μm	Nonaqueous	Anode: Nitinol wires on stainless steel Cathode: stainless steel Electrode separation: 2.0 cm	Medium: ethanol pH adjustment: NaOH Dispersants: HCl	1–6 wt.%	3–50	2–20	25	340°C, 0.33 h, Ar	Deposit thickness: 10–15 μm, no cracking	85
PEEK[h] + Bioglass®	20 μm 1–50 μm										

[a] PVA, polyvinyl alcohol.
[b] HIPed, hot isostatically pressed.
[c] YSZ, yttria partially stabilized zirconia.
[d] CeSZ, ceria partially stabilized zirconia.
[e] CSZ, cubic stabilized zirconia.
[f] PVB, polyvinyl butyral.
[g] TEOS, tetraethyl orthosilicate.
[h] PEEK, polyetheretherketone.

Organic Suspensions

Conversely to the case of aqueous suspensions, a general perception is that organic liquids are associated with the following advantages [24]:

- No risk of electrolysis
- Little risk of Joule heating, so high electrical field strengths can be applied
- No risk of chemical attack of the substrate
- No risk of chemical attack of the deposit

However, there also are some disadvantages [24]:

- Low dielectric constants, which limit the amount of surface charge
- High costs of media
- Necessity of proper disposal of waste media

With organic media, it appears that electron transfer between solid and liquid is the means by which the surface charge changes [20,24]. There is evidence that it is possible to use the pH and the zeta potential to assess the suspensions, analogously to the behavior in water. However, in this case, the relevant phenomenon is the *electron donicity*, which is defined as a measure of the tendency of the medium to donate electrons. If the medium has a higher electron donicity than the particle, then the former will donate electrons to the latter, thereby facilitating a particle of negative surface charge. Conversely, if the donicity of the medium is lower than that of the particle, then the latter will donate electrons to the former, thereby forming a positive surface charge.

Alcohols are regarded as neutral amphiprotic media and so they can donate or accept H^+ and OH^- ions [24]. Hence, they are similar to water in their effect on the surface charge and so the preceding comments concerning aqueous media are relevant to alcohols. In the case of proton donation, the mechanism of particle charging in alcohol is [86]:

$$\text{Pure alcohol:}\quad RCH_2OH + RCH_2O\text{-}OH \leftrightarrow RCH_2O^- + RCH_2OH_2^+ \qquad \text{Reaction 3}$$

$$\text{Aqueous alcohol:}\quad RCH_2O\text{-}H + H_2O \leftrightarrow RCH_2O^- + H_3O^+ \qquad \text{Reaction 4}$$

For the pure alcohol, the adsorbed alcohol ionizes into a protonated alcohol ($RCH_2OH_2^+$) and an alkoxide ion (RCH_2O^-), followed by the dissociation of the protonated alcohol [86]. The dissociated alcohol and the alkoxide ion then desorb into the solution, leaving the proton on the particle surface.

On the other hand, ketones and ethers are aprotic media and so they cannot donate or accept a proton (i.e., the hydrogen ion is nondissociable) [20]. They have relatively low dielectric constants and it has been observed that relatively high dielectric constants, in the limited range 12 to 25, are necessary for electrophoresis. Equation 3.1 shows that the Debye length is proportional to the dielectric constant, so low values are equivalent to compression of the repulsive double layer. It is apparent that the ionization of these media is insufficient to donate charge to the particle surface.

Table 3.3 [37–85] provides a representative example of reports of the organic electrophoretic deposition of a range of bioceramics.

Other Factors Affecting Electrophoretic Deposition

Overview

Although the preceding text provides general coverage of a range of features relevant to the success or failure of electrophoretic deposition, there are some other specific parameters that are critical to the process [21]. These are more of a practical nature than those discussed to this point and these points are made only briefly. These features can be separated into two categories, as shown in Table 3.4.

Suspension Parameters

Particle Size

Particle sizes in the range 1 to 20 μm have been suggested to ensure good deposition [20]. Larger particles have a tendency to settle rapidly, so their suspension requires either a stronger surface charge or a thicker double layer [21]. If large particles are subject to rapid settling during the process, then nonuniform and inhomogeneous films result.

Electrical Conductivity of Suspension

It has been shown that the dielectric constant and bulk electrical conductivity for solid-liquid mixtures show a linear proportionality [87]. Hence, the electrical conductivity must be sufficiently high to facilitate ionization and thus charging but sufficiently low so that excessive ionization does not compress the double layer [21]. This is why deposition occurs only over a limited range of dielectric constants (12–25) for aprotic media.

An alternative approach to overcome this limitation is the addition of polyelectrolytes or temperature regulation to control a suspension's electrical conductivity. It is known that the electrical conductivity of a suspension is proportional to the ionic strength of the suspension in acidic or basic conditions [88]. Hence, when the pH is close to the pH_{iep}, the electrical conductivity is low. Conversely, when the electrical conductivity is high, the main current carriers are the free ions in the suspension rather than the particles, so particle motion is reduced.

Dielectric Constant of Medium

As mentioned, the dielectric constant of aprotic organic media should be neither too low nor too high [20]. A range of 12 to 25 has been observed to be advantageous. More generally, for aqueous and amphiprotic media, high dielectric constants are advantageous. The

TABLE 3.4

Summary of Parameters Relevant to Electrophoretic Deposition

Suspension Parameters	Processing Parameters
Particle size	Applied voltage and deposition time
Electrical conductivity of suspension	Solids concentration
Dielectric constant of medium	Electrical conductivity of substrate
Solids loading	Surface area of substrate
Viscosity of medium	Electrode separation

high dielectric constant of water of 80 is one of the reasons for its widespread use as a suspending medium [89].

Solids Loading

The DLVO theory is applicable to dilute suspensions because its starting point is two spheres free of influence from the electric fields of other spheres [19,21,22,29,30]. Thus, in a real suspension, the proximity of other particles affects the probability of agglomeration. With dilute suspensions, this generally is not a concern. However, when the solids loading increases, then the distance between particles decreases, thereby increasing the likelihood of agglomeration and altering the shape of the curve for the total potential energy (V_T) in Figure 3.4 through the effect on Equations 3.3 and 3.4.

Viscosity of Medium

The viscosity of the medium can have a beneficial or deleterious effect. If the particles are large, then a viscous medium causes drag on the particles and assists in resisting sedimentation. However, if the particles are small, then the drag from a viscous medium retards electrophoretic mobility, as shown in Equations 3.7 and 3.8.

Processing Parameters

Applied Voltage and Deposition Time

The rate of deposition depends principally on the following factors:

- Voltage
- Current
- Solids concentration

Most electrophoresis power supplies operate on the principle of a voltage set point, with the current's not being controlled. The solids concentration tends to be sufficiently high so that the amount of deposit is so low that it does not change the remaining solids concentration significantly during the process.

Curves for the measurement of the deposit weight as a function of time vary according to the conditions of constant or variable voltage, current, and solids concentration [22]. Figure 3.10 represents the most common observation for these measurements, which usually show an initial linear rate followed by a logarithmically decreasing rate.

These curves are assigned to the following simplistic phenomenological scenario:

- *Linear segment.* The circuit is overbiased from an excessive voltage setting, resulting in a steady-state drive to satisfy Ohm's law through increasing resistance of the deposit as it thickens.
- *Logarithmic segment.* Once Ohm's law has been satisfied, further resistance increase from the thickening deposit at constant voltage requires a decrease in the current and thus a corresponding decrease in particle movement.

The effect of increasing deposition rate with increasing voltage is simply a response to a greater level of overbias. That is, for the same thickness of deposit at two different voltages,

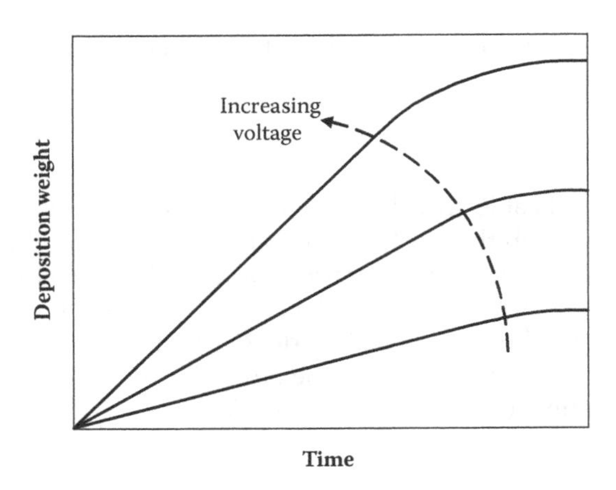

FIGURE 3.10
Effect of voltage on rate of deposition.

since the resistances are the same, then the current associated with the higher voltage must be higher, and so the rate of deposition also must be higher.

Electrical Conductivity of Substrate

Most electrophoresis work is done using conducting substrates, including metals and graphite. It is obvious that a highly conducting substrate is desirable in order to reduce the resistance of the circuit. However, there have been a number of studies of deposition of ZrO_2 on porous insulating substrates backed by an electrically conducting surface. These reports are summarized in Table 3.5 [90–95]. In these studies, it is considered that the porosity is essential as it provides a pathway to complete the circuit to the conducting back surface.

However, doubt has been cast on this requirement by recent work by the Australian authors of the present work [35]. This work revealed that tin oxide (SnO_2) could be deposited on single-crystal sapphire (Al_2O_3) backed by graphite tape. The deposits were very thin but they were coherent, flat, and of even thickness.

Surface Area of Substrate

When the current is reported, it usually is done in terms of the current density, which is the current divided by the surface area of the substrate. It is clear that this will have a significant impact on the rate of deposition because a higher current density deposits more quickly. That is, for the same voltage setting, a small substrate will be coated more rapidly than a large one owing to the greater current.

Electrode Separation

The intensity of the electric field (V/cm) is a direct function of the electrode separation. Since the voltage affects the rate of deposition, as shown in Figure 3.10, then a higher field strength resulting from a smaller electrode separation increases the deposition rate.

TABLE 3.5

Summary of Reported Work on Electrophoretic Deposition on Insulating Substrates

Material and Suspension	Electrodes	Processing Parameters	Remarks	Ref.
Material: Y-ZrO_2 (YSZ^A) Solids loading: 4 g/L Suspension medium: ethanol	Anode: porous NiO–YSZ, reverse-coated with graphite (commercial graphite spray coating, layer thickness 0.6–1 μm) Cathode: stainless steel	Voltage: 400–900 V Time: 0.5 min Electrode separation: 1 cm Stirring during process: yes	• Dense deposits of thickness ~5–10 μm on porous substrates • No deposition on dense substrates • Good coating adherence • Grain growth during firing	90
Material: Y-ZrO_2 (YSZ^A) Solids loading: 4 g/L Suspension medium: ethanol	Anode: porous NiO–YSZ reverse-coated with graphite (commercial graphite spray coating, layer thickness 0.6–1 μm) Cathode: stainless steel	Voltage: 400 V Time: 0.5 min Electrode separation: 1 cm Stirring during process: yes	• Dense and continuous deposits of thickness ~5–10 μm on porous substrates • No deposition on dense substrates	91
Material: Y-ZrO_2 (YSZ^A) Solids loading: 10 g/L Suspension medium: acetyl acetone	Anode: Pt Cathode: porous NiO–YSZ (thickness 300 μm) of different porosities	Voltage: 50–300 V Time: 1–5 min Electrode separation: 1.5 cm Stirring during process: yes	• Deposit weight proportional to applied voltage • Deposit thickness ~6 μm at 50 V • Deposit density increased with substrate porosity • Dense deposits with good adherence to the substrate • Some closed porosity • No deposition on dense substrates	92
Material: Y-ZrO_2 (YSZ^A) Solids loading: 10 g/L Suspension medium: acetyl acetone	Anode: Pt Cathode: porous NiO–YSZ (thickness 300 μm) of different porosities, carbon sheet backing	Voltage: 25–100 V Time: 1–3 min Electrode separation: 1.5 cm Stirring during process: yes	• Deposit density increased with substrate porosity at 25 V and 100 V, reaching a stable value with time • Minimal threshold substrate porosity level for electrophoresis to take place obtained from extrapolation of deposition curve • Threshold substrate porosity level decreased with increasing voltage • Deposits were dense, with good adherence and little closed porosity • Deposit thickness ~40 μm at 100 V	93

(*continued*)

TABLE 3.5 (Continued)

Summary of Reported Work on Electrophoretic Deposition on Insulating Substrates

Material and Suspension	Electrodes	Processing Parameters	Remarks	Ref.
Material: Y-ZrO_2 (YSZ[a]), 0.3 μm Solids loading: 2.5–20 g/L Suspension medium: acetyl acetone, acetone, ethanol, mixture of acetone and ethanol (3:1) Dispersant: iodine	Anode: Pt Cathode: Porous $La_{0.85}Sr_{0.15}MnO_3$ (LSM), LSM–YSZ composite	Voltage: 5–40 V Time: 3–30 min Electrode separation: 1.5 cm Stirring during process: yes	• Dense, pore-free, crack-free deposits on LSM and LSM–YSZ obtained by controlling parameters (sintering temperature, heating rate) • Optimal deposition time 8 min • Deposit thickness ~10 μm • Optimal solids loading 9 g/L (<5g/L gave low deposition rate) • Iodine increased electrical conductivity in 3:1 acetone:ethanol • Best quality suspensions and deposits were from acetone:ethanol	94
Material: wollastonite, 3 μm Solids loading: 0.5 g/mL Suspension medium: acetone Dispersant: iodine	Anode: Au Interposing membrane: porous alumina (10 μm pore size) Cathode: Au	Voltage: 1,000 V Time: 1 min Electrode separation: 30 mm Stirring during process: no	• Wollasonite penetration of pores • Apatite formed after soaking in simulated body fluid	95

[a] YSZ, Yttria partially stabilized zirconia.

Electrophoretic Deposition of Hydroxyapatite

Electrophoretic Deposition

Electrophoretic deposition for the fabrication of hydroxyapatite (HAp) coatings onto metallic substrates was reported first in 1986 [96]. A survey of more recent studies (since 1997) is given in Table 3.6 [86,88,96–150]. Under an applied electric field, the HAp particles exhibit a net positive charge and so they deposit on the cathode. Organic liquids have been used consistently as the media when suspending and depositing HAp. Homogenous HAp coatings can be formed easily on different metallic substrates, such as Ti, Ti6Al4V, and 316L stainless steel.

The effects of coating and associated parameters, including medium, applied voltage, current density, time, deposit weight and thickness, homogeneity, and crack formation have been studied extensively [101,107]. These studies revealed that, as expected, the coating thickness increased with applied voltage and deposition time. However, an important observation was that increasing the applied voltage also led to enhanced coating roughness. Consequently, it was necessary to adjust the applied voltage and current so that the coating morphology could be controlled appropriately [101]. At relatively low deposition voltages, fine and densely packed HAp particles were obtained. In contrast, higher voltages yielded porous coatings containing large HAp particles. Further, it has been reported that, at high applied current densities, porous HAp scaffolds with interconnected pores could be fabricated using electrophoretic deposition [107].

Many studies have indicated that the suspension stability plays an important role in the electrophoretic deposition process [106,123,151]. Using fine, unagglommerated HAp particles favors the formation of a stable suspension and the fabrication of high-quality HAp coatings. When submicron, well-dispersed, HAp particles were deposited under optimal coating conditions, a high-quality, dense, HAp coating was achieved [106]. Figure 3.11 shows cross sections of the HAp coating before and after sintering. The as-deposited coating was homogeneous, with a thickness of ~30 μm; after sintering, the HAp layer became translucent owing to significant densification and the coating thickness reduced to ~20 μm. It also is known that the HAp synthesis method, particle size, and particle shape also play important roles in determining the quality of green deposits [108,117]. Consequently, optimization of the powder fabrication, suspension, and deposition parameters are standard procedures for the fabrication of high-quality electrophoretically deposited coatings.

Ceramic–Metal Interface

One of the main shortcomings of electrophoretic deposition is the low adhesive bonding strength between the deposit and the substrate. In general, a post-heating process is required to densify the coating and improve the bonding but this process imposes conflicting requirements [96]. On the one hand, low densification temperatures result in poorly bonded low-density coatings. On the other hand, high densification temperatures may improve the bulk density and interfacial bonding but these come at the cost of potential degradation of the HAp coating and deterioration of the metal substrate. In general, pure bulk HAp decomposes in the temperature range 1250°C to 1450°C [152]. However, when in contact with an underlying metal substrate, such as Ti, Ti6Al4V, or stainless steel, HAp coatings may decompose at temperatures as low as 800°C to 900°C [101,153,154]. This results

TABLE 3.6

Summary of Recent Studies of Electrophoretic Deposition of Hydroxyapaptite (HAp)

Coating	HAp Type	Substrate	Medium	HAp Concentration	Voltage (V)	Time (min)	Temperature (°C)	Sintering	Quality (Cracks)	Thickness (μm)	Reference
HAp, TCP[a]	Precipitated HAp	Ti	2-Propanol, ethanol, methanol	0.2–8 vol.%	300–600	0.01–10	25	1000°C, 2 h, Ar	Yes/No	50	86
HAp	Submicron HAp powder	Carbon rod	Ethanol–HNO_3	~20 g/L	<150	>1.5	25	1150°–1300°C, 2 h	No	50–200	88
HAp	Precipitated HAp, HAp powder	Ti6Al4V	Isopropanol		75–300	0.2–2	25	900°C, 1 h, Ar, vacuum		>15	96
HAp	Nanomonetite	Ti	Ethanol–HCl	10 g/L	10–50	1–30	25				97
HAp		Gold surface on quartz crystal microbalance			10, 50, 100	5				0.01–0.02	98
HAp	Calcined HAp powder	Ti6Al4V	Ethanol		10, 20, 50, 200	1	40	1000°C, 1 h, Ar	No	30	99
HAp	HAp powder	Pyrolytic carbon-coated carbon–carbon composite rod	Ethanol–glycol	5 g/L	300	0.2–3	20–80	1000°C, 1 h, vacuum	Yes		100
HAp		316L stainless steel	Isopropanol		30, 60, 90	1–5, 3		800°C, 1 h, 10^{-4-5} Torr	No	20–120	101
HAp	Nano-HAp	Ti	Ethanol	15 g/L	150	1		950°C, 1 h			102
HAp	Nano-HAp	Ti	Acetic anhydride		10	1	25	800°C, 1 h	No		103
HAp	HAp powder	Fecralloy, 22 wt.% Cr, 4.8 wt.% Al	Ethanol	30 g/L	80	0.5		1000°–1150°C, 2 h			104
HAp	Nano-HAp, polystyrene spheres for pores	Ti	Ethanol		100	1		450°–1000°C, 1 h, air			105

HAp	Nano-HAp	Ti6Al4V, femoral shaft of hip prosthesis	Ethanol	58 wt.%	10–30	5–11		500°C, 1 h		20–30	106
HAp	Nano-HAp	Ti	Ethanol-PVA[b]-*N,N*-dimethyl-formamide	0.10 wt.%	20, 200 (dynamic)			800°C, 2 h, Ar	No		107
HAp	HAp powder	Ti, Ti6Al4V, 316L stainless steel	Ethanol	5 g/L	50			875°, 900°, 950°, 975°, 1000°, 1050°C, 1 h, Ar			108
HAp		Stainless steel cortical screws			50–200	2		950°C, 1 h, Ar			109
HAp	HAp powder	316L stainless steel	Isopropanol	2.50 wt.%	60	2–5		800°C, 1 h, 10^{-5} Torr			110
HAp	Submicron HAp	316L stainless steel	Ethanol		200, 400, 800	0.05		800°C, 2 h	No		111
HAp	Nano-HAp, polystyrene spheres for pores	Ti	Ethanol		100			900°C, 1 h			112
HAp	Hap powder 0.3 μm		Ethanol–HNO_3	30 g/L		1		1200°C, 2 h	No	50	113
HAp		316L stainless steel	Isopropanol		30–90	3		800°C, 1 h, 10^{-5} Torr			114
HAp	Stoichiometric and calcium-deficient Hap powder	Ti	Ethanol–HCl	5 g/L	12	2–5		800°C, 2 h	Yes	5–15	115
HAp	HAp powder	Ti6Al4V	H_2O–ethylenediol	3 g/L	400	10	25–75				116

(continued)

TABLE 3.6 (Continued)

Summary of Recent Studies of Electrophoretic Deposition of Hydroxyapaptite (HAp)

Coating	HAp Type	Substrate	Medium	HAp Concentration	Voltage (V)	Time (min)	Temperature (°C)	Sintering	Quality (Cracks)	Thickness (μm)	Reference
HAp	Uncalcined HAp	Ti, Ti6Al4V, 316L stainless steel	Ethanol	5 g/L	50	5		875°, 900°, 950°, 975°, 1000°, 1050°C, 1 h, Ar	Yes		117
HAp	Raw uncalcined HAp	Ti6Al4V	Ethanol	15 g/L	200	0.3			Yes		118
HAp	Precipitated HAp	Ti	Ethanol	5 g/L	12	2–5	25	800°C, 2 h partial Ar	Yes/No	5–15	119
HAp	Precipitated HAp	Ti6Al4V	Isopropanol	30 g/L	10–200	0.1–300	25	930°C, 2 h vacuum			120
HAp	Natural HAp (from bovine cortical bone)	316L stainless steel	Isopropanol, polyethylenimine	40 g/L	30, 60, 90	1–5	25		Yes/No	30–140	121
HAp	HAp powder	Ti	Ethanol–PVA[b]	0.05–0.5 wt.%	10–200	3–10	25	800°C, 0.25 h, vacuum	Yes/No		122
HAp	Precipitated HAp	Ti	*n*–Butanol, *n*–propanol, ethanol, methanol, triethanolamine dispersant	100 g/L	30	1	25	850°C, 2 h			123
HAp	Synthetic HAp	Ti dental implant	Ethanol–HCl		24	3	25		Yes	4–8	124
HAp	Precipitated HAp	Ti	Ethanol–HCl	2–40 g/L	50–300	1–10	25	930°C, 2 h, O_2	No		125
HAp	HAp powder	Ti	Ethanol				25	700°–800°C, 2 h, Ar			126
HAp	Precipitated HAp	Carbon fiber (Tenax), carbon felt (Lydall)	Isopropanol	30 g/L	10, 50	0.2–5	25	900°C pyrolysis, 1200°C	No	200	127
HAp	HAp powder	Ti6Al4V	Ethylenediol	3 g/L	400–450	5–10	25-75			15–30	128

HAp	Precipitated HAp	Carbon fiber (Tenax), carbon felt (Lydall)	Isopropanol	30–100 g/L	50–200	0.2–10	25		No		129
Si-HAp	Si-substituted HAp	Ti	*n*–Butanol–chloroform–triethanolamine	20 g/L	30	1.5		700°C, 2 h			130
Si-HAp	Precipitated Si-substituted HAp	Ti	*n*–Butanol, triethanolamine	12.5 g/L	40	2–10	25	820°C	No	6–30	131
HAp HAp + YSZ[c]	Precipitated HAp		Acetic acid, ethanol, isopropanol	0.25–10 g/L	100		25				132
HAp Al_2O_3	Precipitated HAp	Carbon-coated alumina	Ethanol, acetylacetone		30, 60, 90	0.5–6	25	1400°C			133
HAp + CNT[d]	Submicron HAp	Ti6Al4V	Ethanol	2.5 wt.%	200	30	25	800°C, 1 h, 5 Torr vacuum	No	10	134
HAp + CNT[d]	Nano-HAp	Ti6Al4V	HCl solution–Darvan C	5 wt.%	20	4		600°C, 2 h, N_2	No	25	135
HAp + CNT[d]	Nano-HAp	Ti	Ethanol (pH 4–5)	5 g/L	30	1	25	700°C, 2 h, Ar	No	10–20	136
HAp + CNT[d]	Nano-HAp	Ti wire	Ethanol (pH 3.5)		20	1–3			Yes	10	137
HAp + CNT[d]	Precipitated HAp	Ti6Al4V	H_2O–triethanolamine	5 wt.%	20		25	600°C, 2 h, N_2		10–15	138
HAp + CNT[d]	Precipitated HAp	Graphite, NiTi shape memory alloy	Ethanol–H_2O	4 g/L	10–50		20	≤800°C		0.5–10	139
HAp + TCP[a] + Ca_2SiO_4	Precipitated HAp	Ni foil, carbon felt, graphite	Isopropanol–PVB[e]	30–200 g/L	50–200	≤1	25	25			140
HAp + $CaSiO_3$ (Wollastonite)	Precipitated HAp	Ti	Ethanol	2 g/L		1	25			10	141
HAp + glass	Nano-HAp	Ti6Al4V	Ethanol–H_2O–PVB[e]	8 wt.%	20	3		600°C pyrolysis, 950°C, N_2	No		142
HAp + glass	Nano-HAp	Ti6Al4V		8 wt.%	20	7–8	25	950°C, N_2	No		143

(continued)

TABLE 3.6 (Continued)

Summary of Recent Studies of Electrophoretic Deposition of Hydroxyapaptite (HAp)

Coating	HAp Type	Substrate	Medium	HAp Concentration	Voltage (V)	Time (min)	Temperature (°C)	Sintering	Quality (Cracks)	Thickness (μm)	Reference
HAp + chitosan	Nano-HAp	316L stainless steel (foil, wire)	Ethanol–H_2O					1000°C		~60	144
HAp + chitosan	Precipitated HAp	Pt, stainless steel (plate, wire), graphite	Ethanol–H_2O–chitosan	8 g/L			25	≤1200°C	No	50	145
HAp + SiO_2 + chitosan	HAp	Ti (foil), graphite, 316L stainless steel (foil, wire)	Ethanol–H_2O	2.5 g/L	10–30	1–10	25		No	~100	146
HAp + $CaSiO_3$ + chitosan	Nanoneedle HAp	316L stainless steel	Ethanol–H_2O	0.5–1.0 g/L	20			1000°C		0.1–20 (single layer)	147
HAp + bioglass + chitosan HAp + bioglass + alginate	Nanoneedle HAp	Pt (foil), Ti (wire), platinized Si wafer	H_2O–chitosan–sodium alginate	0–1 g/L	10–30		25	≤1000°C	No		148
HAp + chitosan + heparin	Nanoneedle HAp	304 stainless steel, Pt (foil), graphite	H_2O–acetic acid	0.5–1.0 g/L	10–30					2–100 (Multilayered)	149
HAp + bioglass + chitosan + heparin	Nano-HAp	NiTi shape memory alloy	Ethanol–H_2O	0.5 g/L chitosan	10–30		25			1–30	150

[a] TCP, tricalcium phosphate.
[b] PVA, polyvinyl alcohol.
[c] YSZ, yttria partially stabilized zirconia.
[d] CNT, carbon nanotubes.
[e] PVB, polyvinyl butyral.

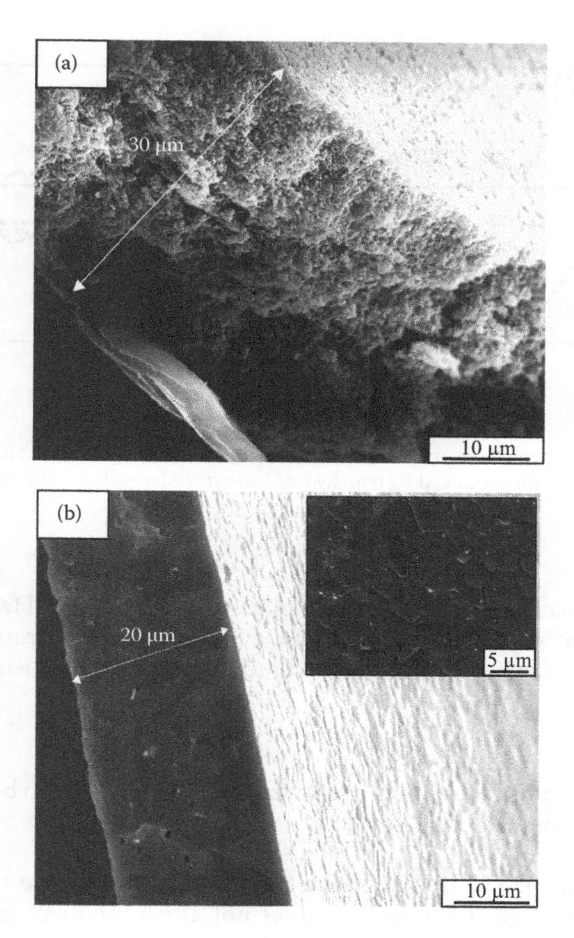

FIGURE 3.11
SEM images of a deposited HAp layer (a) cross-section of the fracture surface before sintering and (b) cross-section of coating after sintering at 1300°C (inset: higher magnification of the surface). (Reproduced by courtesy of *Journal of Materials Science Materials*.)

from diffusion of the metallic ions into the HAp structure, resulting in decomposition and associated decrease in the HAp decomposition temperature [154].

At the HAp–Ti interface, a large-scale graded microstructure was observed following heat treatment [155–157]. It was found that these implants displayed a graded structure of different compounds at the microscopic and macroscopic levels. Under reducing or non-oxidizing atmospheres, a layer of Ti–P phase was formed and HAp decomposed into tetracalcium phosphate [157]. Under oxidizing atmospheres, $CaTiO_3$ was formed at the interface and HAp decomposed into tricalcium phosphate.

Energy dispersive spectroscopy (EDS) scans of the principal elements of the HAp coating (Ca, P, and O) and the Ti substrate (Ti) at the interface between the two supported the preceding observation, as shown in Figure 3.12 [154]. These elemental scans revealed that Ca ions diffused into the Ti substrate at the interface while Ti ions diffused into the HAp coating. X-ray diffraction (XRD) results confirmed that substantial chemical reaction occurred at the interface. In addition to HAp decomposition, a significant amount of $CaTiO_3$ formed.

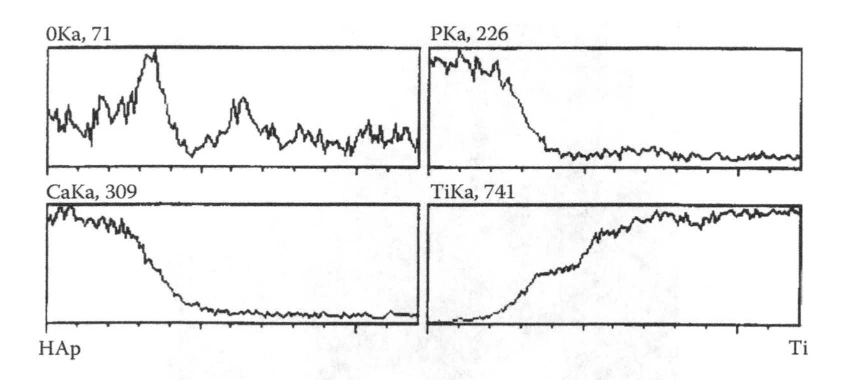

FIGURE 3.12
Energy dispersive spectroscopy line scans across a HAp–Ti (left to right) interface (12 μm length; 1 μm divisions), heat-treated at 950°C for 1 h. (Reproduced by courtesy of *Journal of Materials Science Materials in Medicine.*)

Previous studies revealed that many other oxides in contact with HAp also cause decomposition [158,159]. These phases included Al_2O_3, SiO_2, ZrO_2, SiC, graphite, and 316L stainless steel, all of which reacted with HAp and reduced the decomposition temperature.

Metallic Substrates

Concerning titanium substrates, there are several problems that can be expected from heat treatment at high temperatures, which are:

- *Phase transformation.* The $\alpha \rightarrow \beta$ phase transformation in pure titanium occurs at 882°C [160]. Although this normally does not affect the mechanical properties, it could disrupt the HAp microstructure. The use of alloying elements to stabilize the α or β phase is well known [161]. Aluminum additions stabilize the α phase by increasing the transformation temperature while vanadium additions stabilize the β phase by decreasing it. As a result, the phase transition temperature of Ti6Al4V is 1000°C.
- *Grain growth.* In general, grain coarsening in metals degrades the mechanical properties. This has been demonstrated in titanium alloys [162].
- *Oxidation.* Both Ti and Ti6Al4V are very reactive and so they are susceptible to oxygen dissolution and rapid oxidation reaction at high temperatures, which are well known to cause embrittlement [154].

In light of these risks, it is desirable to minimize the heat treatment temperatures of HAp-coated Ti and Ti6Al4V, which typically are in the range 600°C to 1050°C, depending on the HAp powder, particle size, and substrate [154]. In general, for uncalcined and other fine particles, densification can be done at relatively low temperatures; coarser calcined powders require higher temperatures.

In comparison, 316L stainless steel (16–18 wt.% Cr, 10–14 wt.% Ni, 2–3 wt.% Mo, 0.03 wt.% C, and 0.1 wt.% N) and Fecralloy (22 wt.% Cr and 4.8 wt.% Al) are less susceptible to high-temperature oxidation and elevated temperature strength degradation than are Ti and Ti6Al4V [104,160]. In particular, Fecralloy has good high-temperature stability, which allows it to be heated to high temperatures without sacrificing its mechanical properties.

Interfacial Stresses and Adhesion

Despite the achievement of chemical bonding formed at the HAp/metal interface, the adhesion of the HAp layer to the substrate tends to be extremely weak [163]. This outcome is largely a result of stresses at the HAp/metal interface [164]:

- *Drying shrinkage (HAp).* When the HAp is removed from the suspension, it dries and undergoes shrinkage while the Ti does not.
- *Heating expansion (Ti).* When the coated substrate is heated initially, the Ti expands significantly while the deposit, which expands to a lower degree, is unfired and very weak.
- *Thermal expansion mismatch.* Upon cooling, the brittle ceramic, which is bonded to the metal, is subjected to tensile stress owing to the different coefficients of thermal expansion (α) [165]:

$$\alpha_{HAp} = 11\text{–}14 \times 10^{-6}\,°C^{-1}$$

$$\alpha_{Ti} = 8.7\text{–}10.1 \times 10^{-6}\,°C^{-1}$$

$$\alpha_{Ti6Al4V} = 8.7\text{–}9.8 \times 10^{-6}\,°C^{-1}$$

Owing to the stresses arising from these mismatches, slow heating and cooling rates are required.

Metals with coefficients of thermal expansion similar to that of HAp have attracted considerable attention. Fecralloy, with a coefficient of thermal expansion of $11.1 \times 10^{-6}\,°C^{-1}$, has been used as a substrate for HAp coatings, resulting in dense and crack-free HAp coatings [104]. Another advantage of using Fecralloy is that a dense, alumina, passivating layer forms in situ on the metal surface during the sintering process and this can protect the metal from corrosion in the body environment. Metals with much higher coefficients of thermal expansion than that of HAp also have been used. The coefficient of thermal expansion of 316L stainless steel is 16.0 to $19.0 \times 10^{-6}\,°C^{-1}$, which is advantageous because it places the HAp in compression during and after cooling [117,166]. It is well known that ceramics are brittle and hence weak in tension but they are very strong in compression.

There have been considerable efforts made to improve the interfacial strength between the HAp coating and the substrate. One method involved the fabrication of a dual-layer electrophoretic deposit strategy, which required applying a HAp coating and heat treating twice [117]. The purpose of this was to use the bottom layer as a diffusion barrier for metallic ions, thereby reducing the decomposition of the HAp coating in the top layer. Since the top coating layer was applied seamlessly to the bottom coating layer, it filled the cracks created in the bottom layer, thus improving the adhesive strength of the coating to the substrate. Shear strengths up to 23 MPa were achieved.

Another method is to obtain densified HAp coatings without significantly increasing the heat treatment temperature. This has been approached by electrophoretically depositing a well-packed green ceramic coating. The two main methods of doing this are careful adjustment of the coating parameters [167] or use of fine HAp particles, especially nanoHAp

[168]. Fine uncalcined HAp powders were electrophoretically deposited as high-density coatings and heat treated at 1050°C [169]. Another study confirmed that submicron-scale HAp particles can be densified at relatively low heating temperatures [119].

In general, HAp approaches full density at temperatures in the range 1100°C to 1400°C but fine HAp particles can achieve relatively high densities at lower heat treatment temperatures. It has been demonstrated that well-dispersed HAp particles are crucial for producing densely packed deposits [123]. Citric acid (2 wt.% relative to the weight of HAp powder) was used as a dispersant [106]. Citric acid was found to be effective in preventing the reagglomeration of the HAp particles after ball milling, suspension, and coating. The well-dispersed HAp particles contributed to the formation of an even and dense HAp coating.

The efforts to obtain high-quality materials also have extended to optimization of the media in order to stabilize suspensions. A mixture of *n*-butanol, chloroform, and triethanolamine was found to give results superior to those for *n*-butanol alone in the suspension of nanorod-like Si-substituted HAp (Si-HAp) [167]. The particles were found to exhibit superior bonding within the deposit across the Si-HAp/metal interface. After heating at only 700°C for 2 h, a shear strength of ~20 MPa was achieved.

Good results also were achieved with a medium of acetic anhydride [168]. After heat treatment at 800°C to 900°C, the HAp particles were densified and adhered to the substrate, giving a uniform and crack-free coating.

The effects of different substrates coated with HAp also have received attention [114]. HAp was electrophoretically deposited on 316L stainless steel and heated in air and vacuum at 900°C for 1 h. Heating in air resulted in severe oxidation of the metallic substrate and the decomposition of HAp into tricalcium phosphate. In comparison, heating in vacuum at the same temperature for the same time led to the formation of adherent stoichiometric HAp. In order to reduce the decomposition of HAp and minimize oxidation of the metallic substrates, besides vacuum, protective atmospheres such as argon [115] and nitrogen [170] also have been used during heat treatment.

Calcium-deficient HAp was electrophoretically deposited on Ti sheets and heated at 800°C for 2 h in a partial argon atmosphere [115]. This coating resembled biological apatite and remained stable during the heating process. HAp reinforced with carbon nanotube (CNT) was electrophoretically deposited Ti6Al4V and heated at 600°C for 2 h in flowing nitrogen [170]. Crack-free and well-bonded composite coatings were obtained.

In an attempt to minimize the damage to the metallic substrate but densify the HAp coating, laser surface treatment was used and resulted in a seamless bond between HAp and Ti [171]. The composition of the laser-treated surface was comprised mainly of HAp, Ti, and $CaTiO_3$. This treatment substantially improved the bond strength as well as the microhardness of the coating. The three-point flexural strength of the HAp coating reached as high as 87.5 ± 15 MPa and the Vickers microhardness was relatively high at 582 ± 98 H_V in the Ti–HAp composite region.

An intermediate layer with coefficient of thermal expansion between those of HAp and the metal substrate has been used to reduce the thermal stresses created during the heating and cooling. A titanium dioxide layer (coefficient of thermal expansion = $9.19 \times 10^{-6}\,°C^{-1}$) has been used as an intermediate layer with HAp coatings on Ti6Al4V and Ti substrates [99,103]. Improved bonding strengths relative to controls without the intermediate layer were reported. The use of a titania layer yielded shear strengths in the range 12 to 21 MPa, depending on the applied voltage used during electrophoretic deposition. At lower voltages, less cracking occurred during the drying process [99]. When nano-HAp particles were used in combination with the titania intermediate layer, an average shear strength

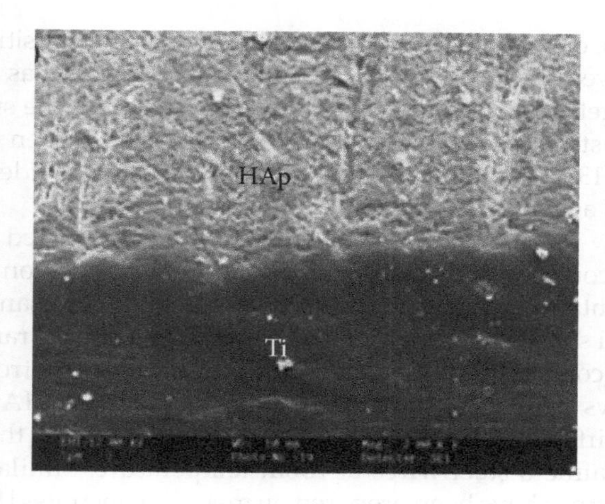

FIGURE 3.13
SEM image of the cross-section of a dense nano-HAp coating on a Ti substrate. (Reproduced by courtesy of *Journal of Biomedical Materials Research B: Applied Biomaterials*.)

of 18 MPa was obtained, with a maximum of 47 MPa [103]. Figure 3.13 shows the dense nano-HAp coating that was formed on the surface of a Ti substrate using electrophoretic deposition.

In order to reduce the thermal expansion mismatch between the HAp coating and the underlying metallic substrate, glass has been codeposited with HAp for improved bonding strength [133,142]. Homogenous and crack-free HAp–glass composite coatings on acetabular cup implants were fabricated by electrophoretic deposition [142]. A composite coating of calcium phosphate glass and HAp powder was used as an adhesive layer adjacent to the substrate for improvement in the bonding strength of a multilayered apatite composite coatings [133].

Recently, multiwalled carbon nanotubes (MWNTs) have been added to the suspension and codeposited with HAp onto the substrate to form composite coatings [135]. The addition of carbon nanotubes not only substantially improved the microhardness and elastic modulus of the coating but it also significantly increased the shear strength of deposited layers. The MWNTs provided reinforcement to the deposit and helped prevent its peeling.

Crack-free coatings as thick as 25 μm were produced using codeposited nano-HAp (20 nm) and MWNTs on Ti6Al4V substrates [170]. The samples were heated for 2 h at the unusually low heat treatment temperature of 600°C, which probably explains the relatively low bond strength of 2.9 MPa. In a similar study, MWNT-reinforced nano-HAp (30–50 nm) was electrophoretically deposited on Ti sheet at thicknesses of 10 to 20 μm and heated at 700°C for 2 h in a flowing argon [136]. A shear strength as high as 35 MPa was obtained. The corrosion resistance of the coated metal also was said to be superior to that of the bare metal. Coatings of CNT-reinforced HAp showed increased microhardness while retaining adequate corrosion resistance and adhesive strength [134].

Hydroxyapatite–Polymer Composite Coatings

In 2005, the organic phase *chitosan* was introduced to HAp for the first time to produce HAp/polymer composites at room temperature [172]. In this method, the chitosan was applied by electrolytic deposition followed by electrophoretic deposition of the HAp coating. The polymer served the two important functions of (1) acting as an adhesive to bind the HAp particles together and (2) adhering the HAp coating to the substrate. More complex composites consisting of HAp, chitosan, and MWNTs have been used to improve the corrosion resistance [139]. This coating also was observed to provide protection for NiTi shape-memory alloys against Ringer's solution.

Recent studies show that HAp-chitosan coatings with a laminated microstructure or a graded composition could be achieved by electrophoretic deposition [146,149,150]. For an instance, coatings containing multiple alternating layers of chitosan and HAp-chitosan were attained on NiTi shape-memory alloy with thicknesses in the range 1 to 30 μm [150]. HAp-chitosan–silica coatings also have been produced using electrophoretic deposition [146]. Figure 3.14 shows cross sections of these microstructures for HAp–chitosan composites prepared using different solids loadings. Crack-free coatings as thick as ~100 μm were deposited on 316L stainless steel wires at room temperature. Similarly, HAp–chitosan–silicate composite coatings have been prepared on metallic substrates [147]. HAp–chitosan–$CaSiO_3$ composite coatings with the composition's being controlled by adjusting the HAp and $CaSiO_3$ concentrations were prepared by adding the solids to a chitosan suspension. The results from potentiodynamic polarization and electrochemical impedance spectros-

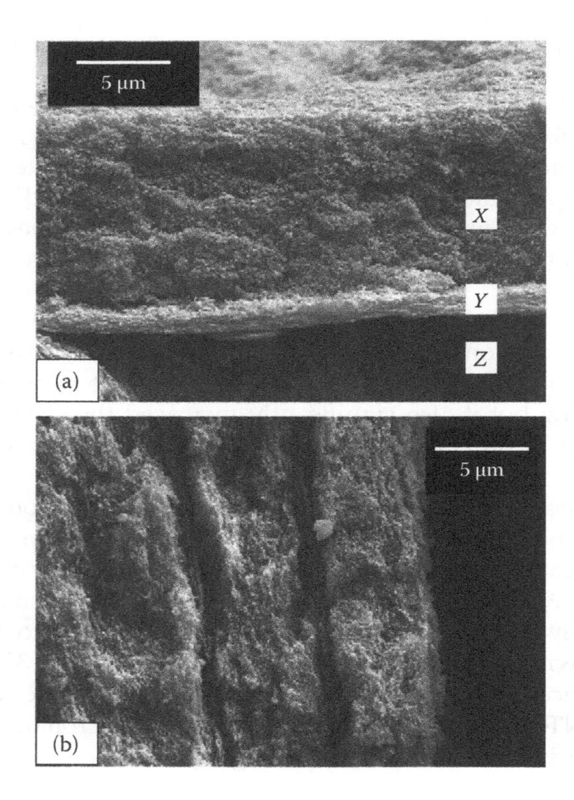

FIGURE 3.14
(a) Graded microstructure: cross-section of thick-layer high-solids-loading HAp–chitosan [X]; cross-section of thin-layer low-solids-loading HAp–chitosan [Y]; graphite substrate [Z]. (b) Laminated HAp–chitosan microstructure: cross-section of two types of layers with different solids loadings. (Reproduced by courtesy of *Materials Characterization*.)

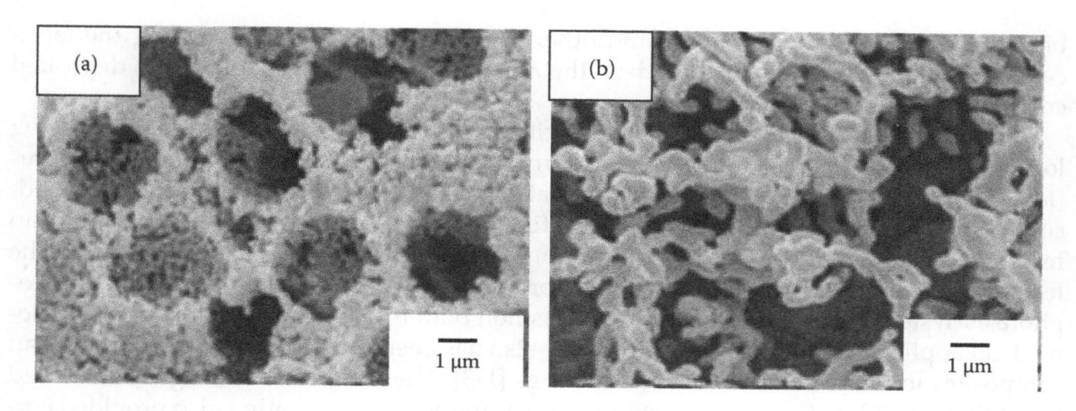

FIGURE 3.15
SEM images of porous HAp coatings electrophoretically deposited on Ti substrates and sintered at (a) 900°C and (b) 1000°C for 1 h in air. (Reproduced by courtesy of *Journal of the Ceramic Society of Japan*.)

copy studies indicated that the composite coating provided corrosion protection to the substrates in simulated physiological solution.

HAp–chitosan–bioactive glass and HAp–alginate–bioactive glass composite coatings were fabricated using electrophoretic deposition on a range of substrates, including 316L stainless steel, Pt foil, Ti wire, and platinized silicon wafers [148]. The use of chitosan and alginate enabled electrosteric stabilization and effective deposition of both HAp and bioactive glass. Both the composition and the microstructure of the ceramic–polymer composite coatings could be adjusted by controlling the HAp and glass concentrations in the suspensions.

Silicon-substituted HAp (Si-HAp) and poly(ε-caprolactone) (PCL) were used to fabricate composite coatings on Ti substrates using electrophoretic deposition [130]. It was discovered that the PCL significantly improved the bonding strength of the green coating but it also reduced the deposition rate of the Si–HAp coating.

Finally, macroporous HAp coatings were produced using electrophoretic deposition by codeposition of polymer microspheres and hydroxyapatite nanoparticles, followed by heat treatment [105,112]. By carefully choosing the processing parameters, a highly ordered porous structure was created by three-dimensional assembly using a polymer microsphere template and a ceramic outer layer. The microstructure of the coating was dependent largely on the coating parameters and heat treatment conditions. At a sintering temperature of 900°C, a porous HAp coating with good adhesive strength was achieved, as shown in Figure 3.15. However, when the sintering temperature was increased to 1000°C, the ordered porous structure of the HAp coating was destroyed owing to grain growth of the HAp particles.

Biomedical Considerations

Perhaps the most exciting development in these materials and techniques is that the HAp–chitosan composite coatings hold out the potential to resolve the long-standing problems associated with high-temperature heat treatment required following electrophoretic deposition. HAp coatings produced at room temperature will allow the fabrication of bioactive organic–inorganic composite coatings suitable for many different types of biomedical applications. More importantly, this new approach allows the incorporation of drugs and bioagents, such as growth factors and other proteins into the coating during the fabrication process, which further broadens the applications of electrophoretically deposited coatings.

Heparin has already been codeposited with HAp–chitosan composite coatings, being located in the top layer of multilayered or functionally graded composite microstructures [149]. Heparin is an anticoagulant drug that has been used to modify different blood-contacting materials surfaces. By incorporating it into the top layer of the coating, it can improve the blood biocompatibility of the implant. This discovery has demonstrated the feasibility of adding other drugs, such as proteins and growth factors, into the electrophoresis system, thereby facilitating codeposition onto implant surfaces for different biomedical applications. Besides heparin, silver also has been codeposited with HA–chitosan composites to fabricate antimicrobial coatings [173]. The composite coating was attained by adding $AgNO_3$ to the coating medium. It was found that the coating also provided corrosion protection to the underlying 316L stainless steel substrate.

More broadly, the biocompatibilities of HAp coatings and HAp–polymer composite coatings produced by electrophoretic deposition have been evaluated in vitro and in vivo. Both silicon-substituted HAp coatings and silicon-substituted HAp–poly(ε-caprolactone) composite coatings have the ability to induce bonelike apatite formation after immersion in simulated body fluid for ~1 week, indicating the good bioactivity of these coatings [130,167]. Moreover, these coatings support the attachment, proliferation, and mineralization of osteoblast cells and stem cells [103,104,171]. In vitro studies have shown that HAp coatings support the attachment and growth of human primary osteoblast cells (HOBs) and they exhibit greater mineralization than uncoated substrates [104]. Laser-treated HAp coatings have shown superior biocompatibility than Ti controls. After 11 days of culture with the osteoblast precursor cell line (OPC1), coated surfaces indicated good cell spreading and coverage [171]. Figure 3.16 shows the morphology of rabbit mesenchymal stem cells (MSC) growing on nano-HAp coatings after 2 and 10 days of culture [103]. After 10 days, the cells were well spread on the substrate and formed a confluent monolayer.

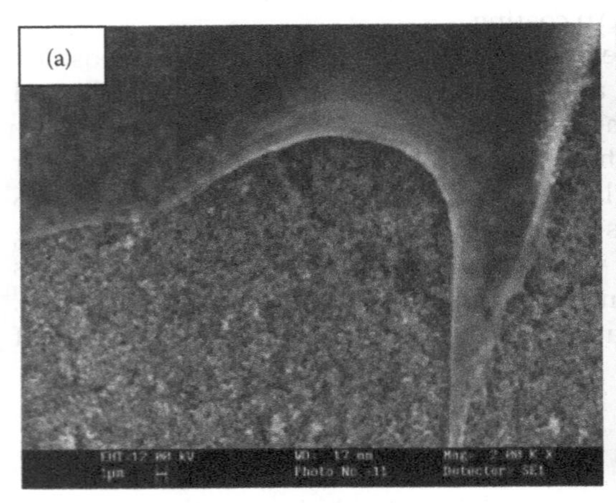

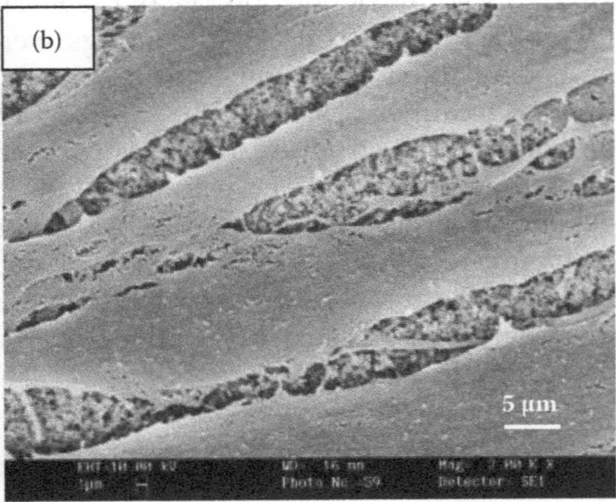

FIGURE 3.16
Scanning electron microscope (SEM) images of human primary osteoblast cells (HOBs) growing on the surface of a nano-HAp coating produced by electrophoretic deposition. (a) After 2 days, the pseudopod of cells can be seen clearly. (b) After 10 days, the surface is extensively covered by cells, which are flattened and form a confluent monolayer. (Reproduced by courtesy of *Journal of Biomedical Materials Research B: Applied Biomaterials*.)

The surface bioactivity of CNT- or MWNT-reinforced HAp coatings also has been studied in vitro. The addition of CNTs increased the hardness of the HAp coating without compromising the biocompatibility. Apatite could grow on CNT-HAp coatings after immersion in Hanks' solution for 4 weeks, indicating superior bioactivity of the coating [134]. In vitro cell culture studies also were conducted on MWNT–HAp composite coatings using osteoblast-like MG63 cells. This work demonstrated that MG63 cells attach and grow well on the composite coating surface [136]. The cells exhibited high affinity for the coating. A porous HAp coating with a uniform and interconnected pore structure was fabricated using electrophoresis by repeated deposition [113]. It was reported that the coating scaffold provided good support for human fibrosarcoma (HT1080) cell seeding and anchoring, maintaining cell viability.

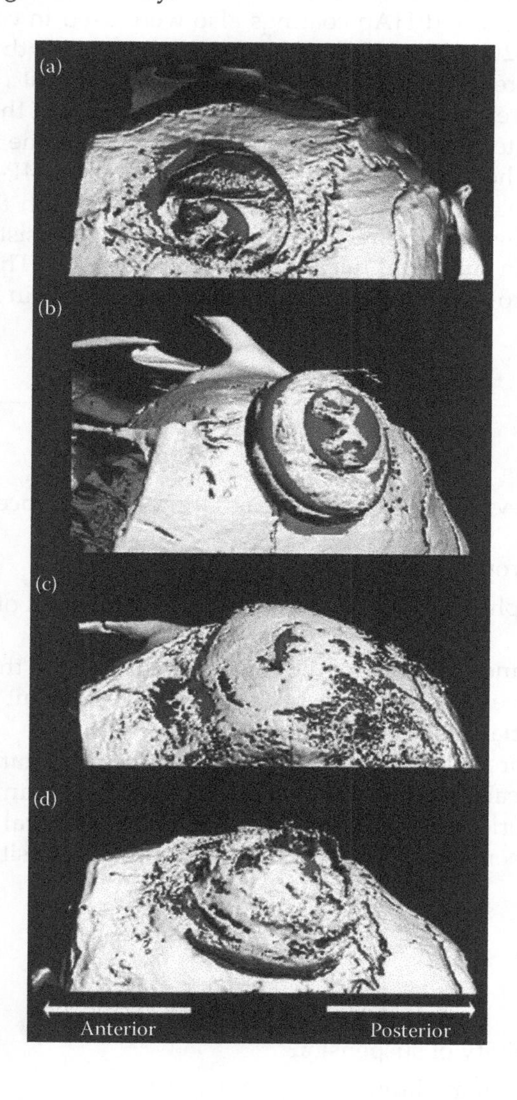

FIGURE 3.17
Three-dimensional micro-CT reconstructions of mouse calvariae and implants (solid grey shading) retrieved 21 days after implantation: (a) control Ti (no new bone formation), (b) HAp (no new bone formation), (c) ng/rhBMP-2 (new bone stimulated), (d) HAp + ng/rhBMP-2 (nearly complete coverage). (Reproduced by courtesy of *Bone*.)

In vivo tests also demonstrated that HAp coatings produced by electrophoretic deposition on the surface of cortical screws have excellent biocompatibility and osteoconductivity [109]. Three groups of samples were prepared, these being uncoated, HAp-coated, and coated with HAp + a xonotlite ($6CaO{\cdot}6SiO_2{\cdot}H_2O$) interlayer. As with Al_2O_3 and TiO_2, xonotlite has a coefficient of thermal expansion between that of HAp and Ti. The samples were heated at 950°C for 1 h in argon. They then were implanted into sheep femurs for 2 months. After sacrifice, it was found that the bond at the bone/screw interface was much stronger in the testing groups than that in the uncoated control. Extensive bone ingrowth was observed for both test groups. The torques required to extract the test groups were much greater than that for the control. Consequently, the screws with the electrophoretically deposited HAp coating had significantly improved bone-to-implant integration.

Electrophoretically deposited HAp coatings also were used in combination with bone morphogenetic protein-2 (ng/rhBMP-2) to guide new bone growth in a murine calvarial model [174]. Following retrieval after 3 weeks, it was found that the untreated implant, which was a Ti dental screw, moved when touched. In comparison, the HAp-coated implant demonstrated much better stability, even though no apparent bone formation occurred in either case after such a short implantation period. When ng/rhBMP-2 was added, substantially more supracalvarial bone formation was observed in both the implants with and without the HAp coating. It appeared that the HAp coating assisted in retention of the ng/rhBMP-2, resulting in sustained release of the growth factor. Three-dimensional computer tomography (micro-CT) images of the implants are shown in Figure 3.17.

Summary

The present work has reviewed two main areas, citing 174 references:

- Principles of electrophoretic deposition
- Reports of electrophoretic deposition of hydroxyapatite and other biomaterials

The importance of the underpinning of the concepts of the DLVO theory, and in particular the double layer, has been emphasized. Likewise, the assessment of the double layer in terms of the zeta potential has been highlighted.

Complementing the preceding has been coverage of the importance of producing stable suspensions and the means of doing so in both aqueous and organic media. These means include electrostatic, steric, and electrosteric stabilization. Practical issues associated with the achievement of suspension stability and electrophoretic deposition that have been discussed briefly include:

Suspension parameters

- Particle size
- Electrical conductivity of suspension
- Dielectric constant of medium
- Solids loading
- Viscosity of medium

Processing parameters

- Applied voltage and deposition time
- Electrical conductivity of substrate
- Surface area of substrate
- Electrode separation

The DLVO and other theories assume that the surface charge of particles is isotropic. While this is the case in cubic and amorphous materials, this is not so with other crystalline materials. Hence, the present work introduces a new consideration in the form of the (1) effect of anisotropic surface charge on the suspension and electrophoretic deposition of powders and (2) effect of surface charge saturation. These considerations were explained briefly in the text but they were clarified more fully in graphical form.

A large range of published studies of the electrophoretic deposition of hydroxyapatite has been presented. This coverage was categorized according to the following topics:

- Electrophoretic deposition
- Ceramic–metal interfaces
- Metallic substrates
- Interfacial stresses and adhesion
- Hydroxyapatite–polymer composite coatings
- Biomedical considerations

Probably the most encouraging information is embodied in the recent work on hydroxyapatite–chitosan composites, where the polymer phase provides both bonding between the ceramic particles and to the metallic substrate, thereby obviating the need for high-temperature densification and fixation to the substrate, which often is associated with intractable shortcomings in the resultant materials.

The present work has been complemented by extensive tabulated data that summarize the materials, processing parameters, and outcomes of published work in the following areas:

- Electrophoretic deposition of alumina, zirconia, and other oxides in aqueous and organic media
- Electrophoretic deposition of zirconia on insulating substrates
- Electrophoretic deposition of hydroxyapatite in organic media

References

1. L. Hench, Bioceramics, *J. Am. Ceram. Soc.*, **81** [7] 1705–28 (1998).
2. D. Manno, G. Micocci, R. Rella, A. Serra, A. Taurino, and A. Tepore, Titanium Oxide Thin Films for NH_3 Monitoring: Structural and Physical Characterizations, *J. Appl. Phys.*, **82** [1] 54–59 (1997).

3. M.H. Park, Y.J. Jang, H.M. Sung-Suh, and M.M. Sung, Selective Atomic Layer Deposition of Titanium Oxide on Patterned Self-Assembled Monolayers Formed by Microcontact Printing, *Langmuir*, **20** [6] 2257–60 (2004).
4. P.S. Shinde and C.H. Bhosale, Properties of Chemical Vapour Deposited Nanocrystalline TiO_2 Thin Films and their Use in Dye-Sensitized Solar Cells, *J. Anal. Appl. Pyrolysis*, **82** [1] 83–88 (2008).
5. J.Y. Kim, S.H. Kim, H.H Lee, K. Lee, W. Ma, X. Gong, and A.J. Heeger, New Architecture for High-Efficiency Polymer Photovoltaic Cells Using Solution-Based Titanium Oxide as an Optical Spacer, *Adv. Mater.*, **18** [5] 572–76 (2006).
6. M. Hemissi, H. Amardjia-Adnani, and J.C. Plenet, Titanium Oxide Thin Layers Deposited by Dip-Coating Method: Their Optical and Structural Properties, *Curr. Appl. Phys.*, **9** [4] 717–21 (2009).
7. H.P. Deshmukh, P.S. Shinde, and P.S. Patil, Structural, Optical and Electrical Characterization of Spray-Deposited TiO_2 Thin Films, *Mater. Sci. Eng. B*, **130B** [1–3] 220–27 (2006).
8. H.Z. Abdullah and C.C. Sorrell, Preparation and Characterisation of TiO_2 Thick Films by Gel Oxidation, *Mater. Sci. Forum*, **561–565**, 2167–70 (2007).
9. H.Z. Abdullah and C.C. Sorrell, Preparation and Characterisation of TiO_2 Thick Films Fabricated by Anodic Oxidation, *Mater. Sci. Forum*, **561–565**, 2159–62 (2007).
10. G.K. Mor, O.K. Varghese, M. Paulose, K.G. Ong, and C.A. Grimes, Fabrication of Hydrogen Sensors with Transparent Titanium Oxide Nanotube-Array Thin Films as Sensing Elements, *Thin Solid Films*, **496** [1] 42–48 (2006).
11. M. Walczak, E.L. Papadopoulou, M. Sanz, A. Manousaki, J.F. Marco, and M. Castillejo, Structural and Morphological Characterization of TiO_2 Nanostructured Films Grown by Nanosecond Pulsed Laser Deposition, *Appl. Surf. Sci.*, **255** [10] 5267–70 (2009).
12. X. Weng, P. Fisher, M. Skowronski, P.A. Salvador, and O. Maksimov, Structural Characterization of TiO_2 Films Grown on $LaAlO_3$ and $SrTiO_3$ Substrates Using Reactive Molecular Beam Epitaxy, *J. Cryst. Growth*, **310** [3] 545–50 (2008).
13. H.Z. Abdullah and C.C. Sorrell, Preparation and Characterisation of TiO_2 Thick Films Fabricated by Electrophoretic Deposition, *Mater. Sci. Forum*, **561–565**, 2163–66 (2007).
14. R. Rohanizadeh, M. Al-Sadeq, and R.Z. LeGeros, Preparation of Different Forms of Titanium Oxide on Titanium Surface: Effects on Apatite Deposition, *J. Biomed. Mater. Res. A*, **71A** [2] 343–52 (2004).
15. I. Seigo, P. Chen, P. Comte, M.K. Nazeeruddin, P. Liska, P. Péchy, and M. Grätzel, Fabrication of Screen-Printing Pastes from TiO_2 Powders for Dye-Sensitised Solar Cells, *Prog. Photovoltaics Res. Appl.*, **15** [7] 603–12 (2007).
16. R. Vaßen, Z. Yi, H. Kaßner, and D. Stöver, Suspension Plasma Spraying of TiO_2 for the Manufacture of Photovoltaic Cells, *Surf. Coat. Technol.* **203** [15] 2146–49 (2009).
17. K.H. Zuo, D.L. Jiang, J.X. Zhang, and Q.L. Lin, Forming Nanometer TiO_2 Sheets by Nonaqueous Tape Casting, *Ceram. Int.*, **33** [3] 477–81 (2007).
18. R. Gould, Thin Films, pp. 659–716 in *Springer Handbook of Electronic and Photonic Materials*. Springer US, New York, 2006.
19. I. Zhitomirsky, Cathodic Electrodeposition of Ceramic and Organoceramic Materials. Fundamental Aspects, *Adv. Coll. Interface Sci.*, **97** [1–3] 277–315 (2002).
20. S.N. Heavens, Electrophoretic Deposition as a Processing Route for Ceramics, pp. 255–279 in *Advanced Ceramic Processing and Technology*. William Andrews Publishing/Noyes, Park Ridge, NJ, 1990.
21. L. Besra and M. Liu, A Review on Fundamentals and Applications of Electrophoretic Deposition (EPD), *Prog. Mater. Sci.*, **52** [1] 1–61 (2007).
22. P. Sarkar and P.S. Nicholson, Electrophoretic Deposition (EPD): Mechanisms, Kinetics, and Application to Ceramics, *J. Am. Ceram. Soc.*, **79** [8] 1987–2002 (1996).
23. A.R. Boccaccini and I. Zhitomirsky, Application of Electrophoretic and Electrolytic Deposition Techniques in Ceramics Processing, *Curr. Opin. Solid State Mater. Sci.*, **6** [3] 251–60 (2002).

24. O.O. Van der Biest and L.J. Vandeperre, Electrophoretic Deposition of Materials, *Ann. Rev. Mater. Sci.*, **29** [1] 327–352 (1999).
25. S. Usui, Electric Charge and Charge Neutralization in Aqueous Solutions, pp. 432–39 in *Powder Technology Handbook*. Marcel Dekker, New York, 1991.
26. J. Cazes, Editor, *Encyclopedia of Chromatography*, 3rd Edition. CRC Press, Boca Raton, FL, 2005.
27. L. Bergström, Colloidal Processing of Ceramics, pp. 201–18 in *Handbook of Applied Surface and Colloid Chemistry*. John Wiley & Sons Ltd., West Sussex, UK, 2001.
28. J. Speight, *Lange's Handbook of Chemistry*, 16th Edition. McGraw Hill, New York, 2005.
29. G. Cao, *Nanostructures & Nanomaterials–Synthesis, Properties & Applications*. Imperial College Press, London, 2004.
30. J.H. Adair, E. Suvaci, and J. Sindel, Surface and Colloid Chemistry, pp. 8996–9006 in *Encyclopedia of Materials Science and Technology*. Edited by K.H.J. Buschow, R.W. Cahn, M.C. Flemings, B. Ilschner, E.J. Kramer, and S. Mahajan. Elsevier Science Ltd., Oxford, 2001.
31. D.J. Shaw, *Introduction to Colloid and Surface Chemistry*, 2nd Edition. Butterworths, London, 1970.
32. J.J. Gulicovski, L.S. Čerović, and S.K. Milonjić, Point of Zero Charge and Isoelectric Point of Alumina, *Mater. Manuf. Proc.*, **23** [6] 615–19 (2008).
33. J.A. Menéndez, M.J. Illán-Gómez, C.A. León y León, and L.R. Radovic, On the Difference between the Isoelectric Point and the Point of Zero Charge of Carbons, *Carbon*, **33** [11] 1655–59 (1995).
34. J.A. Lewis, Colloidal Processing of Ceramics, *J. Am. Ceram. Soc.*, **83** [10] 2341–59 (2000).
35. H. Taib, Synthesis and Electrophoretic Deposition of Tin Oxide (SnO_2). Ph.D. Thesis, University of New South Wales, 2009.
36. M. Fellows and W.O.S. Doherty, Insights into Bridging Flocculation, *Macromol. Symp.*, **231** [1] 1–10 (2006).
37. B. Ferrari, J.C. Fariñas, and R. Moreno, Determination and Control of Metallic Impurities in Alumina Deposits Obtained by Aqueous Electrophoretic Deposition, *J. Am. Ceram. Soc.*, **84** [4] 733–39 (2001).
38. R. Moreno and B. Ferrari, Effect of the Slurry Properties on the Homogeneity of Alumina Deposits Obtained by Aqueous Electrophoretic Deposition, *Mater. Res. Bull.*, **35** [6] 887–97 (2000).
39. T. Uchikoshi and Y. Sakka, Electrophoretic Deposition Characteristics of Alumina Particles in Aqueous Media, *J. Ceram. Soc. Japan*, **112** [1] S63–S66 (2004).
40. B. Ferrari and R. Moreno, Electrophoretic Deposition of Aqueous Alumina Slips, *J. Eur. Ceram. Soc.*, **17** [4] 549–56 (1997).
41. K. Simović, V.B. Mišković-Stanković, D. Kićević, and P. Jovanić, Electrophoretic Deposition of Thin Alumina Films from Water Suspension, *Colloids Surf. A Physicochem. Eng. Aspects*, **209A** [1] 47–55 (2002).
42. B. Ferrari and R. Moreno, The Conductivity of Aqueous Al_2O_3 Slips for Electrophoretic Deposition, *Mater. Lett.*, **28** [4–6] 353–55 (1996).
43. G. Anné, K. Vanmeensel, J. Vleugels, and O. Van der Biest, A Mathematical Description of the Kinetics of the Electrophoretic Deposition Process for Al_2O_3-Based Suspensions, *J. Am. Ceram. Soc.*, **88** [8] 2036–39 (2005).
44. M. Menon, S. Decourcelle, N. Attia, S. Ramousse, and P.H. Larsen, Stabilization of Ethanol Based Ceramic Suspensions for Electrophoretic Deposition, *Ceram. Eng. Sci. Proc.*, **26** [3] 239–46 (2005).
45. M. Shan, X. Mao, J. Zhang, and S. Wang, Electrophoretic Shaping of Sub-Micron Alumina in Ethanol, *Ceram. Int.*, **35** [5] 1855–61 (2009).
46. A. Braun, G. Falk, and R. Clasen, Transparent Polycrystalline Alumina Ceramic with Sub-Micrometre Microstructure by Means of Electrophoretic Deposition, *Materialwiss. Werkst.*, **37** [4] 293–97 (2006).
47. T. Uchikoshi, T.S. Suzuki, H. Okuyama, Y. Sakka, and P.S. Nicholson, Electrophoretic Deposition of Alumina Suspension in a Strong Magnetic Field, *J. Eur. Ceram. Soc.*, **24** [2] 225–29 (2004).

48. L. Zhang, A.K. Kanjarla, J. Vleugels, and O. Van der Biest, Textured α–Alumina through Electrophoretic Deposition and Templated Grain Growth, *Key Eng. Mater.*, **412**, 261–66 (2009).
49. K. Moritz and E. Müller, Investigation of the Electrophoretic Deposition Behaviour of Non-Aqueous Ceramic Suspensions, *J. Mater. Sci.*, **41** [24] 8047–58 (2006).
50. S. Novak and K. König, Fabrication of Alumina Parts by Electrophoretic Deposition from Ethanol and Aqueous Suspensions, *Ceram. Int.*, **35** [7] 2823–29 (2009).
51. J.H. Kennedy and A. Foissy, Fabrication of Beta-Alumina Tubes by Electrophoretic Deposition from Suspensions in Dichloromethane, *J. Electrochem. Soc.*, **122** [4] 482–86 (1975).
52. R.W. Powers, The Electrophoretic Forming of Beta-Alumina Ceramic, *J. Electrochem. Soc.*, **122** [4] 490–500 (1975).
53. W.J. Seng and C.H. Wu, Aggregation, Rheology and Electrophoretic Packing Structure of Aqueous Al_2O_3 Nanoparticle Suspensions, *Acta Mater.*, **50** [12] 3757–66 (2002).
54. F. Tang, T. Uchikoshi, K. Ozawa, and Y. Sakka, Electrophoretic Deposition of Aqueous Nano-γ-Al_2O_3 Suspensions, *Mater. Res. Bull.*, **37** [4] 653–60 (2002).
55. P.S. Nicholson, P. Sarkar, and X. Haung, Electrophoretic Deposition and its Use to Synthesise ZrO_2/Al_2O_3 Micro-Laminate Ceramic/Ceramic Composites, *J. Mater. Sci.*, **28** [23] 6274–78 (1993).
56. A.M. Popa, J. Vleugels, J. Vermant, and O. Van der Biest, Influence of Ammonium Salt of Poly-Methacrylic Acid and Butyl Amine Addition on the Viscosity and Electrophoretic Deposition Behaviour of Ethanol-Based Powder Suspensions, *Colloids Surf. A Physicochem. Eng. Aspects*, **267A** [1–3] 74–78 (2005).
57. T. Uchikoshi, K. Ozawa, B.D. Hatton, and Y. Sakka, Dense, Bubble-Free Ceramic Deposits from Aqueous Suspensions by Electrophoretic Deposition, *J. Mater. Res.*, **16** [2] 321–24 (2001).
58. M.F.D. Riccardis, D. Carbone, and A. Rizzo, A Novel Method for Preparing and Characterizing Alcoholic EPD Suspensions, *J. Colloid Interface Sci.*, **307** [1] 109–15 (2007).
59. H. Hadraba, K. Maca, and Z. Chlup, Alumina and Zirconia Based Composites: Part 1 Preparation, *Key Eng. Mater.*, **412**, 221–26 (2009).
60. Z. Chlup and H. Hadraba, Alumina and Zirconia Based Composites: Part 2 Fracture Response, *Key Eng. Mater.*, **412**, 227–32 (2009).
61. J. Will, M.K.M. Hruschka, L. Gubler, and L.J. Gauckler, Electrophoretic Deposition of Zirconia on Porous Anodic Substrate, *J. Am. Ceram. Soc.*, **84** [2] 328–32 (2001).
62. K. Moritz and T. Moritz, Electrophoretically Deposited Porous Ceramics and their Characterisation by X-ray Computer Tomography, *Key Eng. Mater.*, **412**, 255–60 (2009).
63. A. Pfrengle, H. von Both, R. Knitter, and J. Haußelt, Electrophoretic Deposition and Sintering of Zirconia Layers on Microstructured Steel Substrates, *J. Eur. Ceram. Soc.*, **26** [13] 2633–38 (2006).
64. H. Xu, I.P. Shapiro, and P. Xiao, pH Effect on Electrophoretic Deposition in Non-Aqueous Suspensions and Sintering of YSZ Coatings, *Key Eng. Mater.*, **412**, 165–70 (2009).
65. T. Talebi, B. Raissi, and A. Maghsoudipour, Electrophoretic Deposition of YSZ Electrolyte on Porous NiO-YSZ Substrate for Solid Oxide Fuel Cells, *Key Eng. Mater.*, **412**, 215–20 (2009).
66. I.A. Borojeni, B. Raissi, A. Maghsoudipour, M. Kazemzad, and E. Marzbanrad, Aging Behavior of Yttria Stabilized Zirconia (YSZ), *Key Eng. Mater.*, **412**, 279–86 (2009).
67. T. Moritz, W. Eiselt, and K. Moritz, Electrophoretic Deposition Applied to Ceramic Dental Crowns and Bridges, *J. Mater. Sci.*, **41** [24] 8123–29 (2006).
68. G. Anne, K. Vanmeensel, B. Neirinck, O. Van der Biest, and J. Vleugels, Ketone-Amine Based Suspensions for Electrophoretic Deposition of Al_2O_3 and ZrO_2, *J. Eur. Ceram. Soc.*, **26** [16] 3531–37 (2006).
69. S. Radice, P. Kern, G. Bürki, J. Michler, and M. Textor, Electrophoretic Deposition of Zirconia-Bioglass® Composite Coatings for Biomedical Implants, *J. Biomed. Mater. Res. A*, **82A** [2] 436–44 (2007).
70. S. Bonas, J. Tabellion, and J. Hauβelt, Effect of Particle Size Distribution and Sedimentation Behaviour on Electrophoretic Deposition of Ceramic Suspensions, *Key Eng. Mater.*, **314**, 69–74 (2006).

71. I.P. Shapiro, X. Zhao, H. Xu, and P. Xiao, Monitoring Constrained Sintering of YSZ Coatings Using Fluorescence Spectroscopy and Micro-Hardness, *Key Eng. Mater.*, **412**, 177–82 (2009).
72. A. Miyamoto, H. Negishi, A. Endo, B. Lu, K. Sakaki, T. Ohmori, H. Yanagishita, and K. Watanabe, Electrophoretic Deposition Mechanism of Mesoporous Silica Powder in Acetone, *Key Eng. Mater.*, **412**, 131–36 (2009).
73. H. Negishi, A. Endo, A. Miyamoto, K. Sakaki, and T. Ohmori, Influence of Water on the Preparation of Thick Mesoporous Silica Coatings by the Electrophoretic Deposition Method, *Key Eng. Mater.*, **412**, 171–76 (2009).
74. O. Sakurada, M. Komaba, S. Obata, M. Hashiba, and Y. Takahashi, Electrophoretic Deposition on Anodes from Aqueous Titania Suspensions with Titanate Solution, *Key Eng. Mater.*, **412**, 313–16 (2009).
75. F. Tang, T. Uchikoshi, K. Ozawa, and Y. Sakka, Effect of Polyethylenimine on the Dispersion and Electrophoretic Deposition of Nano-Sized Titania Aqueous Suspensions, *J. Eur. Ceram. Soc.*, **26** [9] 1555–60 (2006).
76. S. Lebrette, C. Pagnoux, and P. Abélard, Fabrication of Titania Dense Layers by Electrophoretic Deposition in Aqueous Media, *J. Eur. Ceram. Soc.*, **26** [13] 2727–34 (2006).
77. S. Yanagida, A. Nakajima, Y. Kameshima, N. Yoshida, T. Watanabe, and K. Okada, Preparation of a Crack-Free Rough Titania Coating on Stainless Steel Mesh by Electrophoretic Deposition, *Mater. Res. Bull.*, **40** [8] 1335–44 (2005).
78. C.K. Lin, T.J. Yang, Y.C. Feng, T.T. Tsung, and C.Y. Su, Characterisation of Elecrophoretically Deposited Nanocrystalline Titanium Dioxide Films, *Surf. Coat. Tech.*, **200** [10] 3184–89 (2006).
79. M.J. Santillán, N. Quaranta, F. Membrives, J.A. Roether, and A.R. Boccaccini, Processing and Characterization of Biocompatible Titania Coatings by Electrophoretic Deposition, *Key Eng. Mater.*, **412**, 189–94 (2009).
80. M. Ghorbani and M. Roushanafshar, Electrophoretic Deposition of Titania Nanopowders, *Key Eng. Mater.*, **412**, 77–82 (2009).
81. S. Yanagida, A. Nakajima, Y. Kameshima, and K. Okada, Photocatalytic Destruction of 1,4-Dioxane in Aqueous System by Surface-Roughened TiO_2 Coating on Stainless Mesh, *Key Eng. Mater.*, **412**, 137–41 (2009).
82. N. Wang, H. Lin, J. Li, X. Yang, and B. Chi, Electrophoretic Deposition and Optical Property of Titania Nanotubes Films, *Thin Solid Films*, **496** [2] 649–52 (2006).
83. S. Hayashi, J. Onoe, K. Ebina, and N. Kodama, Electrophoretic Deposition/Infiltration of Natural Zeolite Particles on/into Various Substrates, *Key Eng. Mater.*, **412**, 119–23 (2009).
84. S. Hayashi, Z. Nakagawa, A. Yasumori, and K. Okada, Effects of H_2O in EtOH–H_2O Disperse Medium on the Electrophoretic Deposition of $CaSiO_3$ Fine Powder, *J. Eur. Ceram. Soc.*, **19** [1] 75–79 (1999).
85. A.R. Boccaccini, C. Peters, J.A. Roether, D. Eifler, S.K. Misra, and E.J. Minay, Electrophoretic Deposition of Polyetheretherketone (PEEK) and PEEK/Bioglass® Coatings on NiTi Shape Memory Alloy Wires, *J. Mater. Sci.*, **41** [24] 8152–59 (2006).
86. R. Damodaran and B.M. Moudgil, Electrophoretic Deposition of Calcium Phosphates from Non-Aqueous Media, *Colloids Surf. A Physicochem. Eng. Aspects*, **80A** [2–3] 191–95 (1993).
87. M. Persson, Evaluating the Linear Dielectric Constant-Electrical Conductivity Model Using Time-Domain Reflectometry, *Hydrol. Sci. J.*, **47** [2] 269–77 (2002).
88. C. Wang, J. Ma, W. Cheng, and R. Zhang, Thick Hydroxyapatite Coatings by Electrophoretic Deposition, *Mater. Lett.* **57** [1] 99–105 (2002).
89. D.R. Lide, Editor, *CRC Handbook of Chemistry and Physics*, 76th Edition. CRC Press, Boca Raton, FL, 1995.
90. M. Matsuda, T. Hosomi, K. Murata, T. Fukui, and M. Miyake, Direct EPD of YSZ Electrolyte Film onto Porous NiO–YSZ Composite Substrate for Reduced-Temperature Operating Anode-Supported SOFC, *Electrochem. Solid-State Lett.*, **8** [1] A8–A11 (2005).
91. T. Hosomi, M. Matsuda, and M. Miyake, Electrophoretic Deposition for Fabrication of YSZ Electrolyte Film on Non-Conducting Porous NiO–YSZ Composite Substrate for Intermediate Temperature SOFC, *J. Eur. Ceram. Soc.*, **27** [1] 173–78 (2007).

92. L. Besra, C. Compson, and M. Liu, Electrophoretic Deposition of YSZ Particles on Non-Conducting Porous NiO/YSZ Substrates for Solid Oxide Fuel Cell Applications, *J. Am. Ceram. Soc.*, **89** [10] 3003–3009 (2006).
93. L. Besra, C. Compson, and M. Liu, Electrophoretic Deposition on Non-Conducting Substrates: The Case of YSZ Film on NiO–YSZ Composite Substrates for Solid Oxide Fuel Cell Application, *J. Power Sources*, **173** [1] 130–36 (2007).
94. F. Chen and M. Liu, Preparation of Yttria-Stabilized Zirconia (YSZ) Films on $La_{0.85}Sr_{0.15}MnO_3$ (LSM) and LSM-YSZ Substrates Using an Electrophoretic Deposition (EPD) Process, *J. Eur. Ceram. Soc.*, **21** [2] 127–34 (2001).
95. S. Yamaguchi and T. Yao, Development of Bioactive Alumina–Wollastonite Composite by Electrophoretic Deposition, *Key Eng. Mater.*, **284–286**, 863–68 (2005).
96. P. Ducheyne, W.V. Raemdonck, J.C. Heughebaert, and M. Heughebaert, Structural Analysis of Hydroxyapatite Coatings on Titanium, *Biomaterials*, **7** [2] 97–103 (1986).
97. M.S. Djošić, V.B. Mišković-Stanković, Z.M. Kačarević-Popović, B.M. Jokić, B.M.N. Bibić, M. Mitrić, S.K. Milonjić, R. Jančić-Heinemann, and J. Stojanović, Electrochemical Synthesis of Nanosized Monetite Powder and its Electrophoretic Deposition on Titanium, *Colloids Surf. A Physicochem. Eng. Asp.*, **341A** [1–3] 110–17 (2009).
98. T. Ikoma, M. Tagaya, N. Hanagata, T. Yoshioka, D. Chakarov, B. Kasemo, and J. Tanaka, Protein Adsorption on Hydroxyapatite Nanosensors with Different Crystal Sizes Studied in situ by a Quartz Crystal Microbalance with the Dissipation Method, *J. Am. Ceram. Soc.*, **92** [5] 1125–28 (2009).
99. O. Albayrak, O. El-Atwani, and S. Altintas, Hydroxyapatite Coating on Titanium Substrate by Electrophoretic Deposition Method: Effects of Titanium Dioxide Inner Layer on Adhesion Strength and Hydroxyapatite Decomposition, *Surf. Coat. Tech.*, **202** [11] 2482–87 (2008).
100. L. Gao and J. Lin, Electrophoretic Coating of Hydroxyapatite on Pyrolytic Carbon Using Glycol as Dispersion Medium, *J. Wuhan Univ. Tech. Mater. Sci. Ed.*, **23** [3] 293–97 (2008).
101. M. Javidi, S. Javadpour, M.E. Bahrololoom, and J. Ma, Electrophoretic Deposition of Natural Hydroxyapatite on Medical Grade 316L Stainless Steel, *Mater. Sci. Eng. C*, **28C** [8] 1509–15 (2008).
102. M. Roy, A. Bandyopadhyay, and S. Bose, Laser Surface Modification of Electrophoretically Deposited Hydroxyapatite Coating on Titanium, *J. Am. Ceram. Soc.*, **91** [11] 3517–21 (2008).
103. F. Chen, W.M. Lam, C.J. Lin, G.X. Qiu, X.H. Wu, K.D.K. Luk, and W.W. Lu, Biocompatibility of Electrophoretical Deposition of Nanostructured Hydroxyapatite Coating on Roughened Titanium Surface: In Vitro Evaluation Using Mesenchymal Stem Cells, *J. Biomed. Mater. Res. B*, **82B** [1] 183–91 (2007).
104. X. Guo, J. Gough, and P. Xiao, Electrophoretic Deposition of Hydroxyapatite Coating on Fecralloy and Analysis of Human Osteoblastic Cellular Response, *J. Biomed. Mater. Res. A*, **80A** [1] 24–33 (2007).
105. J. Hamagami, Y. Ato, and K. Kanamura, Macroporous Hydroxyapatite Ceramic Coating by Using Electrophoretic Deposition and then Heat Treatment, *J. Ceram. Soc. Jap.*, **114** [1] 51–54 (2006).
106. H. Mayr, M. Ordung, and G. Ziegler, Development of Thin Electrophoretically Deposited Hydroxyapatite Layers on Ti6Al4V Hip Prosthesis, *J. Mater. Sci.*, **41** [24] 8138–43 (2006).
107. X. Meng, T.-Y. Kwon, Y. Yang, J.L. Ong, and K.-H. Kim, Effects of Applied Voltages on Hydroxyapatite Coating of Titanium by Electrophoretic Deposition, *J. Mater. Res. B*, **78B** [2] 373–77 (2006).
108. M. Wei, A.J. Ruys, B.K. Milthorpe, and C.C. Sorrell, Precipitation of Hydroxyapatite Nanoparticles: Effects of Precipitation Method on Electrophoretic Deposition, *J. Mater. Sci. Mater. Med.*, **16** [4] 319–24 (2005).
109. O.S. Yildirim, B. Aksakalb, H. Celik, Y. Vangolu, and A. Okur, An Investigation of the Effects of Hydroxyapatite Coatings on the Fixation Strength of Cortical Screws, *Med. Eng. Phys.*, **27** [3] 221–28 (2005).
110. N. Eliaz, T.M. Sridhar, U. Kamachi Mudali, and Baldev Raj, Electrochemical and Electrophoretic Deposition of Hydroxyapatite for Orthopaedic Applications, *Surf. Eng.*, **21** [3] 238–42 (2005).

111. P. Mondragón-Cortez and G. Vargas-Gutiérez, Electrophoretic Deposition of Hydroxyapatite Submicron Particles at High Voltages, *Mater. Lett.*, **58** [7–8] 1336–39 (2004).
112. J. Hamagami, Y. Ato, and K. Kanamura, Fabrication of Highly Ordered Macroporous Apatite Coating onto Titanium by Electrophoretic Deposition Method, *Solid State Ionics*, **172** [1–4] 331–34 (2004).
113. J. Ma, C. Wang, and K.W. Peng, Electrophoretic Deposition of Porous Hydroxyapatite Scaffold, *Biomater.*, **24** [20] 3505–10 (2003).
114. T.M. Sridhar, U.K. Mudali, and M. Subbaiyan, Sintering Atmosphere and Temperature Effects on Hydroxyapatite Coated Type 316L Stainless Steel, *Corr. Sci.*, **45** [10] 2337–59 (2003).
115. L.A. de Sena, M.C. de Andrade, A.M. Rossi, and G. de Almeida Soares, Hydroxyapatite Deposition by Electrophoresis on Titanium Sheets with Different Surface Finishing, *J. Biomed. Mater. Res. A*, **60A** [1] 1–7 (2002).
116. X. Nie, A. Leyland, A. Matthews, J.C. Jiang, and E.I. Meletis, Effects of Solution pH and Electrical Parameters on Hydroxyapatite Coatings Deposited by a Plasma-Assisted Electrophoresis Technique, *J. Biomed. Mater. Res. A*, **57A** [4] 612–18 (2001).
117. M. Wei, A.J. Ruys, B.K. Milthorpe, C.C. Sorrell, and J.H. Evans, Electrophoretic Deposition of Hydroxyapatite Coatings on Metal Substrates: A Nanoparticulate Dual-Coating Approach, *J. Sol–Gel Sci. Tech.*, **21** [1–2] 39–48 (2001).
118. M. Wei, A.J. Ruys, B.K. Milthorpe, and C.C. Sorrell, Solution Ripening of Hydroxyapatite Nanoparticles: Effects on Electrophoretic Deposition, *J. Biomed. Mater. Res. A*, **45A** [1] 11–19 (1999).
119 L. Ágata de Sena, M. Calixto de Andrade, A.M. Rossi, and G. de Almeida Soares, Hydroxyapatite Deposition by Electrophoresis on Titanium Sheets with Different Surface Finishing, *J. Biomed. Mater. Res. A*, **60A** [1] 1–7 (2002).
120. I. Zhitomirsky and L. Gal-Or, Electrophoretic Deposition of Hydroxyapatite, *J. Mater. Sci. Mater. Med.*, **8** [4] 213–19 (1997).
121. M. Javidi, S. Javadpour, M.E. Bahrololoom, and J. Ma, Electrophoretic Deposition of Natural Hydroxyapatite, *Key Eng. Mater.*, **412**, 183–88 (2009).
122. X. Meng, T.-Y. Kwon, and K.-H. Kim, Different Morphology of Hydroxyapatite Coatings on Titanium by Electrophoretic Deposition, *Key Eng. Mater.*, **309–311**, 639–42 (2006).
123. X.F. Xiao and R.F. Liu, Effect of Suspension Stability on Electrophoretic Deposition of Hydroxyapatite Coatings, *Mater. Lett.*, **60** [21–22] 2627–32 (2006).
124. C.C. Almeida, L.A. Sena, A.M. Rossi, M. Pinto, C.A. Muller, and G.A. Soares, Effect of Electrophoretic Apatite Coating on Osseointegration of Titanium Dental Implants, *Key Eng. Mater.*, **254–256**, 729–32 (2004).
125. Z. Feng, Q. Su, and Z. Li, Electrophoretic Deposition of Hydroxyapatite Coating, *J. Mater. Sci. Tech.*, **19** [1] 30–32 (2003).
126. A. Stoch, A. Brożek, G. Kmita, J. Stoch, W. Jastrzębski, and A. Rakowska, Electrophoretic Coating of Hydroxyapatite on Titanium Implants, *J. Mol. Struct.*, **596** [1–3] 191–200 (2001).
127. I. Zhitomirsky, Electrophoretic Hydroxyapatite Coatings and Fibres, *Mater. Lett.*, **42** [4] 262–71 (2000).
128. X. Nie, A. Leyland, and A. Matthews, Deposition of Layered Bioceramic Hydroxyapatite/TiO_2 Coatings on Titanium Alloys Using a Hybrid Technique of Micro-Arc Oxidation and Electrophoresis, *Surf. Coat. Tech.*, **125** [1–3] 407–14 (2000).
129. I. Zhitomirsky, Electrophoretic and Electrolytic Deposition of Ceramic Coatings on Carbon Fibers, *J. Eur. Ceram. Soc.*, **18** [7] 849–56 (1998).
130. X. Xiao, R. Liu, and X. Tang, Electrophoretic Deposition of Silicon-Substituted Hydroxyapatite/Poly(ε-Caprolactone) Composite Coatings, *J. Mater. Sci. Mater. Med.*, **20** [3] 691–97 (2009).
131. F.J. Xiao, Y. Zhang, and L.J. Yun, Electrophoretic Deposition of Titanium/Silicon-Substituted Hydroxyapatite Composite Coating and its Interaction with Bovine Serum Albumin, *Trans. Nonferrous Met. Soc. China*, **19** [1] 125–30 (2009).
132. K. Yamashita, M. Nagai, and T. Umegaki, Fabrication of Green Films of Single- and Multicomponent Ceramic Composites by Electrophoretic Deposition Technique, *J. Mater. Sci.*, **32** [24] 6661–64 (1997).

133. K. Yamashita, E. Yonehara, X. Ding, M. Nagai, T. Umegaki, and M. Matsuda, Electrophoretic Coating of Multilayered Apatite Composite on Alumina Ceramics, *J. Biomed. Mater. Res. B*, **43B** [1] 46–53 (1998).
134. C.T. Kwok, P.K. Wong, F.T. Cheng, and H.C. Man, Characterization and Corrosion Behavior of Hydroxyapatite Coatings on Ti6Al4V Fabricated by Electrophoretic Deposition, *Appl. Surf. Sci.*, **255** [13–14] 6736–44 (2009).
135. C. Kaya, Electrophoretic Deposition of Carbon Nanotube-Reinforced Hydroxyapatite Bioactive Layers on Ti–6Al–4V Alloys for Biomedical Applications, *Ceram. Inter.*, **34** [8] 1843–47 (2008).
136. C. Lin, H. Han, F. Zhang, and A. Li, Electrophoretic Deposition of HA/MWNTs Composite Coating for Biomaterial Applications, *J. Mater. Sci. Mater. Med.*, **19** [7] 2569–74 (2008).
137. I. Singh, C. Kaya, M.S.P. Shaffer, B.C. Thomas, and A.R. Boccaccini, Bioactive Ceramic Coatings Containing Carbon Nanotubes on Metallic Substrates by Electrophoretic Deposition, *J. Mater. Sci.*, **41** [24] 8144–51 (2006).
138. C. Kaya, F. Kaya, J. Cho, J.A. Roether, and A.R. Boccaccini, Carbon Nanotube-Reinforced Hydroxyapatite Coatings on Metallic Implants Using Electrophoretic Deposition, *Key Eng. Mater.*, **412**, 93–97 (2009).
139. K. Grandfield, F. Sun, M. FitzPatrick, M. Cheong, and I. Zhitomirsky, Electrophoretic Deposition of Polymer–Carbon Nanotube–Hydroxyapatite Composites, *Surf. Coat. Tech.*, **203** [10–11] 1481–87 (2009).
140. I. Zhitomirsky, Electrophoretic Deposition of Chemically Bonded Ceramics in the System CaO–SiO_2–P_2O_5, *J. Mater. Sci. Lett.*, **17** [24] 2101–2104 (1998).
141. S. Sharma, V.P. Soni, and J.P. Bellare, Chitosan Reinforced Apatite–Wollastonite Coating by Electrophoretic Deposition on Titanium Implants, *J. Mater. Sci. Mater. Med.*, **20** [7] 1427–36 (2009).
142. H. Zhang, J. Krajewski, Z. Zhang, T.D. Xiao, and D. Reisner, Nano-Hydroxyapatite Coated Acetabular Cup Implant by Electrophoretic Deposition, *NSTI-Nanotech*, **2**, 99–102 (2006).
143. H. Zhang, J. Krajewski, Z. Zhang, M. Masopust, and D.T. Xiao, Nano-Hydroxyapatite Coated Femoral Stem Implant by Electrophoretic Deposition, *Mater. Res. Soc. Symp. Proc.*, **975E**, Symposium DD, Paper 0975–DD06–05 (2007).
144. X. Pang and I. Zhitomirsky, Electrophoretic Deposition of Composite Hydroxyapatite-Chitosan Coatings, *Mater. Character.*, **58** [4] 339–48 (2007).
145. X. Pang and I. Zhitomirsky, Electrodeposition of Composite Hydroxyapatite-Chitosan Films, *Mater. Chem. Phys.*, **94** [2–3] 245–51 (2005).
146. K. Grandfield and I. Zhitomirsky, Electrophoretic Deposition of Composite Hydroxyapatite-Silica-Chitosan Coatings, *Mater. Character.*, **59** [1] 61–67 (2008).
147. X. Pang, T. Casagrande, and I. Zhitomirsky, Electrophoretic Deposition of Hydroxyapatite–$CaSiO_3$–Chitosan Composite Coatings, *J. Colloid Interface Sci.*, **330** [2] 323–29 (2009).
148. D. Zhitomirsky, J.A. Roether, A.R. Boccaccini, and I. Zhitomirsky, Electrophoretic Deposition of Bioactive Glass/Polymer Composite Coatings with and without HA Nanoparticle Inclusions for Biomedical Applications, *J. Mater. Proc. Tech.*, **209** [4] 1853–60 (2009).
149. F. Sun, X. Pang, and I. Zhitomirsky, Electrophoretic Deposition of Composite Hydroxyapatite–Chitosan–Heparin Coatings, *J. Mater. Proc. Tech.*, **209** [3] 1597–1606 (2009).
150. F. Sun, K. Sask, J. Brash, and I. Zhitomirsky Surface Modifications of Nitinol for Biomedical Applications, *Colloids Surf. B Biointerfaces*, **67B** [1] 132–39 (2008).
151. M. Javidi, M.E. Bahrololoom, S. Javadpour, and J. Ma, Studying Surface Charge and Suspension Stability of Hydroxyapatite Powder in Isopropyl Alcohol to Prepare Stable Suspension for Electrophoretic Deposition, *Adv. Appl. Ceram.*, **108** [4] 241–48 (2009).
152. A.J. Ruys, M. Wei, C.C. Sorrell, M.R. Dickson, A. Brandwood, and B.K. Milthorpe, Sintering Effects on the Strength of Hydroxypatite, *Biomater.*, **16** [5] 409–15 (1995).
153. J. Weng, X. Liu, X. Zhang, and K. de Groot, Integrity and Thermal Decomposition of Apatite in Coatings Influenced by Underlying Titanium during Plasma Spraying and Post-Heat-Treatment, *J. Biomed. Mater. Res. A*, **30A** [1] 5–11 (1996).

154. M. Wei, A.J. Ruys, M.V. Swain, B.K. Milthorpe, and C.C. Sorrell, Hydroxyapatite-Coated Metals: Interfacial Reactions during Sintering, *J. Mater. Sci. Mater. Med.*, **16** [2] 101–106 (2005).
155. H. Ji and P.M. Marquis, Effect of Heat Treatment on the Microstructure of Plasma-Sprayed Hydroxyapatite Coating, *Biomater.*, **14** [1] 64–68 (1993).
156. P. Ducheyne and K.E. Healy, The Effect of Plasma-Sprayed Calcium Phosphate Ceramic Coatings on the Metal Ion Release from Porous Titanium and Cobalt–Chromium Alloys, *J. Biomed. Mater. Res.*, **22** [12] 1137–63 (1988).
157. P. Ducheyne, P.D. Bianco, and C. Kim, Bone Tissue Growth Enhancement by Calcium Phosphate Coatings on Porous Titanium Alloys: The Effect of Shielding Metal Dissolution Product, *Biomater.*, **13** [9] 617–24 (1992).
158. A.J. Ruys, M. Wei, B.K. Milthorpe, A. Brandwood, and C.C. Sorrell, Hydrothermal Sintering of ZrO_2 and Al_2O_3 Fibre-Reinforced Hydroxyapatite, *J. Aust. Ceram. Soc.*, **29** [1/2] 51–56 (1993).
159. A.J. Ruys, K.A. Zeigler, B.K. Milthorpe, and C.C. Sorrell, Hydroxyapatite-Ceramic/Metal Composites: Quantification of Additive-Induced Dehydration, pp. 591–97 in *Ceramics: Adding the Value*. Edited by M.J. Bannister. CSIRO, Melbourne, 1992.
160. J.B. Park and R.S. Lakes, *Biomaterials: An Introduction*, 2nd Edition. Plenum Press, New York, NY, 1992.
161. Hugh Baker, Editor, *ASM Handbook, Volume 3: Alloy Phase Diagrams*. ASM International, Materials Park, OH, 1992.
162. L.S. Moroz and I.N. Razuvaeva, Effect of β Stabilizers on the Mechanical Properties of Titanium Alloys with an α Structure, *Metall. Termich. Obrab. Metall.*, [3] 34–39 (1971).
163. L.M. Boulton, P.J. Gregson, M. Tuke, and T. Baldwin, Adhesively Bonded Hydroxyapatite Coating, *Mater. Lett.*, **12** [1–2] 1–6 (1991).
164. C.S. Kim and P. Ducheyne, Compositional Variations in the Surface and Interface of Calcium Phosphate Ceramic Coatings on Ti and Ti–6Al–4V due to Sintering and Immersion, *Biomater.*, **12** [5] 461–69 (1991).
165. A. Ravaglioli and A. Krajewski, *Bioceramics: Materials, Properties, Applications*. Chapman & Hall, London, 1992.
166. J. Breme, Y. Zhou, and L. Groh, Development of a Titanium Alloy Suitable for an Optimised Coating with Hydroxyapatite, *Biomater.*, **16** [3] 239–44 (1995).
167. X.F. Xiao, R.F. Liu, and X.L. Tang, Electrophoretic Deposition of Silicon Substituted Hydroxyapatite Coatings from *n*-Butanol–Chloroform Mixture *J. Mater. Sci. Mater. Med.*, **19** [1] 175–82 (2008).
168. Z.C. Wang, F. Chen, L.M. Huang, and C.J. Lin, Electrophoretic Deposition and Characterization of Nano-Sized Hydroxyapatite Particles, *J. Mater. Sci.*, **40** [18] 4955–57 (2005).
169. M. Wei, A.J. Ruys, M.V. Swain, S.H. Kim, B.K. Milthorpe, and C.C. Sorrell, Interfacial Bond Strength of Electrophoretically Deposited Hydroxyapatite Coatings on Metals, *J. Mater. Sci. Mater. Med.*, **10** [7] 401–409 (1999).
170. C. Kaya, I. Singh, and A.R. Boccaccini, Multi-Walled Carbon Nanotube-Reinforced Hydroxyapatite Layers on Ti6Al4V Medical Implants by Electrophoretic Deposition (EPD), *Adv. Eng. Mater.*, **10** [1] 131–38 (2008).
171. M. Roy, A. Bandyopadhyay, and S. Bose, Laser Surface Modification of Electrophoretically Deposited Hydroxyapatite Coating on Titanium, *J. Am. Ceram. Soc.*, **91** [11] 3517–21 (2008).
172. I. Zhitomirsky and X. Pang, Electrodeposition of Composite Hydroxyapatite–Chitosan Films, *Mater. Chem. Phys.*, **94** [2–3] 245–51 (2005).
173. X. Pang and L. Zhitomirsky, Fabrication of Chitosan–Hydroxyapatite Coatings for Biomedical Applications, *ECS Trans.*, **3** [26] 15–22 (2007).
174. M. Freilich, C.M. Patel, M. Wei, D. Shafer, P. Schleier, P. Hortschansky, R. Kompali, and L. Kuhn, Growth of New Bone Guided by Implants in a Murine Calvarial Model, *Bone*, **43** [4] 781–88 (2008).

4

Thermal Sprayed Bioceramic Coatings: Nanostructured Hydroxyapatite (HA) and HA-Based Composites

Hua Li

CONTENTS

The predominant purpose of biomedical materials is to produce a part or facilitate a function of the human body in a safe, reliable, economical, and physiologically acceptable manner. A prerequisite for any synthetic material implanted in the body is that it should be biocompatible in the sense of not producing an inflammatory tissue reaction. In addition, the implanted material is expected to withstand applied physiological forces without substantial dimensional changes, catastrophic brittle fracture, or fracture in the long term from creep, fatigue, or stress corrosion. Accordingly, thermal sprayed bioceramic coatings, which have been extensively proposed as implants for bone and joint replacements, must possess acceptable biocompatibility and sufficient mechanical performances. This chapter addresses the fundamentals of coating deposition of the bioceramics, typically hydroxyapatite (HA) and HA-based composites, apart from other related issues, such as fabrication of nanostructured feedstock, characterization of the nanostructures inside the coatings and their influence on coating properties, effect of the nanostructures and phase compositions on behaviors of the osteoblast cells cultured on the biomedical coatings, co-/postspray treatment of the coatings, and so forth. The biomaterials–cells interactions control dynamic behaviors of the cells, such as adhesion, proliferation, and differentiation, on biomaterial surface. This chapter also discusses the problems encountered during the coating deposition and elucidates the overall fabrication procedure and applications of the thermal sprayed biomedical coatings.

Background and Current Problems

Since a biomaterial is a material in contact with fluids, cells, and tissues of the living body to repair or replace any tissue or organ of the body, prerequisites of the biomaterial include its favorable biocompatibility and sufficient mechanical properties that accomplish its quick fixation after surgery and long-term functional service. According to all the prerequisites, attempts have been made to find suitable materials to repair or replace any deficient tissue or body organ throughout the history of mankind. In orthopedic surgery, biomaterials provide an alternative approach in the treatment of bone defects, with initial emphasis placed on the replacement of the missing tissue with biomaterials designed to induce minimal or no immune response. Among the materials for orthopedic surgery, ceramics play important roles owing to their significant advantages, such as promising mechanical properties, compared to other materials. There are two major classes of ceramics used as biomaterials: structural (or technical) and resorbable (or soluble), the latter includes the so-called bioceramics. In recent decades, several kinds of bioceramics have been used in orthopedic surgery, which can be clinically classified into (1) bioinert, and (2) bioactive ceramics from the point of view of the reactions they elicit in the adjacent tissues (Park 1984). Bioactive implants normally act as a scaffold for cells, enabling them to anchor, attach, and differentiate. Among all the bioceramics explored, hydroxyapatite (HA) ceramics are particularly suitable as bone graft substitutes owing to a chemical composition that is similar to the mineral nature of bone. HA, which is regarded as synthetic bone and the most common calcium phosphate ceramic, is well established as a biocompatible ceramic capable of forming a good bond with natural bone (Jarcho 1981). The first application of calcium phosphate materials as bone substitute or bone graft may be traced to Albee, who reported that a "triple calcium phosphate" compound used in a bony defect promoted osteogenesis or new bone formation (Albee 1920). Application of HA-based bioceramics include dental implants, percutaneous devices, and use in periodontal treatment, alveolar ridge augmentation, orthopedics, maxillofacial surgery, and spinal surgery (Luo et al. 1995).

However, the principal limitation in the clinical use of HA as a load-bearing implant material is its brittleness (tensile strength = ~200 MPa, fracture toughness = 0.5–1.2 MPa $m^{1/2}$). At the same time, ceramics are difficult to shape due to their high melting points as well as limited ductility. Metal alloys such as Ti–6Al–4V have a long clinical history of implantation (Williams 1981). Although metal implants have superior mechanical properties, concern over the toxic responses continues to increase. For example, studies showed that during implantation, metal alloys, in particular titanium, released corrosion products into surrounding tissues and fluids (Healy et al. 1992). Advances in coating technology have brought about a new dimension in the processing of biomaterials. Therefore, there has been a significant interest in the use of HA-coated metal implants (Hardy et al. 1999; Yoshikawa et al. 1996). Figure 4.1 shows the formation of trabecular bone between unsorbed HA coating and bony tissue after 3 years of implantation. Due to the high impact

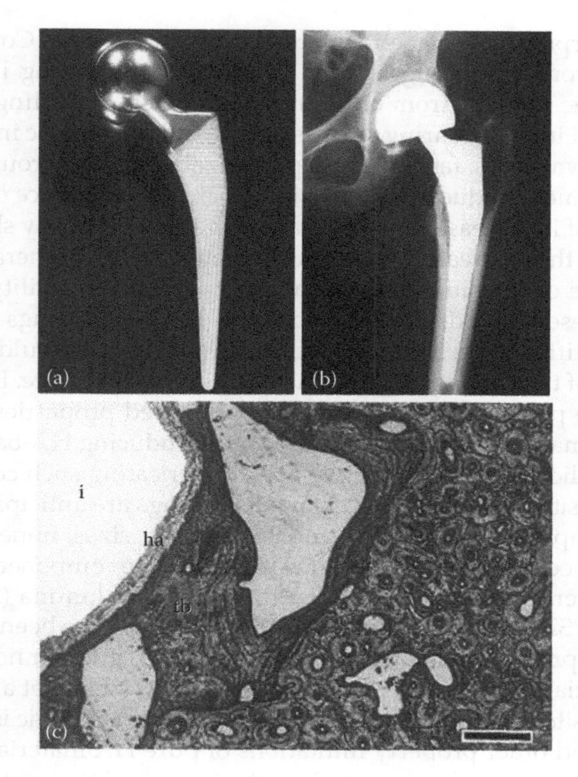

FIGURE 4.1
HA-coated Ti6Al4V femoral implant. (a) Morphology before implantation, and (b) radiograph of the implant 3 years after implantation. Formation of trabecular bone (tb) in the periprosthetic gap and in continuity with the host bone. HA coating appears unabsorbed. (i): metallic implant. Scale bar: 500 μm. (From Hardy, et al., *Eur. J. Orthop. Surg. Traumatol.*, 9, 75–81, 1999. With permission.)

that HA has in biomedical applications, it is very important to investigate the production methods and the properties/processing parameters. Many methods have been used for the production of HA powders and coatings on different substrates, among which thermal spray is the most promising technique for depositing HA coatings with controllable microstructure and properties. To date, the potential medical applications of the HA-coated prosthesis have been investigated. However, in order to achieve those goals, it is essential to optimize production methods for and clarify property/process relationships of the HA coatings. To achieve the properties required by the service circumstance, many manufacturing methods for HA coating preparation have been attempted. In recent years, research on nanobiomaterials has been booming and improved performances have been widely reported, even though synthesis/fabrication of nanobiomaterials in an economic and reliable manner remains challenging. Nevertheless, it seemed clear that surface modification of biomaterials (e.g., nanostructuring) gives rise to enhanced biocompatibility of the biomaterials. The presence of nanostructures within the coatings and at the coating/substrate interface might also enhance the properties of the coatings. Thermal sprayed HA coatings might, through optimized experiment design, be able to provide favorable surface patterns apart from the phases that favor cell attachment and proliferation.

A good prosthetic design should accommodate eventualities such as coating failure without jeopardizing the function of the implant. This perception is important to ensure that the role and purpose of the coatings are not misunderstood. Coatings have specific functions ranging from improving fixation by establishing strong interfacial bonds, to shielding the metallic implant from environmental attack or leading effects (Cheang et al. 1996a). When used in load-bearing such as dental and orthopedic implants, HA coating has the following advantages: fast bony adaptation, absence of fibrous tissue seams, firm implant–bone attachment, reduced healing time, increased tolerance of surgical inaccuracies, and inhibition of ion release. These advantages are of relatively short-term effect, but may provide factors that increase long-term implant stability. Generally, the mechanical properties and phase composition, as well as the operation feasibility, are the most considered factors as these methods are to be adopted. The HA coatings attained from these various techniques differ in chemistry and crystallinity, which would in return affect the biological response of the coatings and ultimately their performance. In addition, composite coatings have the potential of combining the advanced properties of its components. Therefore, there are many attempts in recent years of producing HA-based composite coatings for medical applications. One effective way of fabricating such composite coatings is to deposit precomposite powder so that favorable coatings are anticipated. The criteria for fabricating such composites include controllable particle sizes, none or minor chemical reaction between the components, and unique mixing of the components. Pure HA is quite brittle; therefore, several types of bioinert ceramic, such as alumina (Al_2O_3) and partially stabilized zirconia (PSZ), as well as titanium dioxide (TiO_2), have been chosen as additives in HA coatings to improve the implantation duration based on their nonbiochemical influence on cell differentiation and proliferation (Li et al. 1996; Chang et al. 1997; Champion et al. 1996). The composite coating made from HA and bioinert ceramic is capable of alleviating the brittleness and other property limitations of pure HA material, as well as solving the bioinert instinct of the reinforcements. In order to expand the exploration of the potential use of composite bioceramic coatings, the behavior of the additives in the composites and the strengthening mechanism are important factors that need to be clarified.

There have been attempts in recent years toward the development of processing methods to deposit HA onto metallic substrates while minimizing its inherent mechanical property limitations. A proliferation of studies has taken place in which various processing techniques have been utilized to fabricate HA coatings. Yankee et al. (1990) divided the various methods into categories of "thick coatings" and "thin films" techniques. Most of the processing techniques are listed below.

1. *Sintering method* (Lange et al. 1987; Silva et al. 2001). Thick HA coating (>500 μm) can be rapidly produced with dense microstructure economically by this method. However, there are a number of disadvantages that need to be considered; that is, the elevated temperatures required to sinter dried HA layer tend to degrade the metallic substrate properties and cause the decomposition of HA.
2. *Electrophoresis method* (Wei et al. 1999; Wei et al. 2001). This method is suitable for uniform coating formation with complex shapes such as porous-surfaced implant devices. The process of coating deposition is also relatively rapid. The main shortcomings of this process are porous structure and poor bonding to the substrate because of the low energy with which particles are deposited on the substrate.
3. *Electrochemical route* (Shirkhanzadeh et al. 1995; Vijayaraghavan et al. 1994). An important aspect of this process for fabricating bioactive coatings is that the chemical composition of the electrolyte can be easily altered, and thus coatings with a desired chemical composition may be tailored for specific applications.

Additionally, the operation temperature is low, and process variables can be easily monitored and controlled. However, the resorbability of the coating is a big consideration since the coating is very thin.

4. *Physical vapor deposition (PVD).* Radio frequency sputtering methods have been reported (Yamashita et al. 1994; van Dijk et al. 1998). The main advantage of this method is that a thin coating (~3 μm) with a "clean" interface and dense microstructure as well as good adhesion to substrate can be obtained. However, the potential decomposition of complex target molecules may occur, thus the materials arriving at the substrate may be composed of individual atoms, simple molecules, or ions, rather than stoichiometric HA molecules. The resultant coating may not possess the chemical and structural integrity of initial HA target. Furthermore, the PVD technique cannot produce a thick coating, which is very important for bony tissue fixation with the total implant.
5. *Plasma spraying* (Reis et al. 1996; Gross et al. 1998a; Wang et al. 1993). Plasma spraying is by far the most widely used and the main industrial process to deposit thick HA coatings. The attraction lies in the easy operation and high efficiency to produce HA coatings, as well as relatively low substrate temperature, available technology and equipment, acceptable production costs, and its ability to apply tailored coatings rapidly and reproducibly on complex shapes. However, it is more or less limited by low cohesion and adhesion strength, as well as significant phase transformation of HA that is induced by the extremely high temperature of the plasma torch.
6. *Suspension plasma spraying* (Kozerski et al. 2010). There have been successful efforts in recent years in applying suspension plasma spraying in depositing HA coatings. The major advancement of this technology is its capability of easily producing nanostructured HA coatings. While the challenges for this approach are the potential overheating of the fine HA suspension particles during the spraying, which might trigger unfavorable HA phase transformation.
7. *HVOF spraying* (Cheang et al. 1995; Lugscheider et al. 1996; Sturgeon et al. 1995; Lewis et al. 1998). So far, only preliminary experimental results have been collected on HVOF-sprayed HA coatings. Due to its attractive performances (i.e., high flame velocity and moderate flame temperature), HVOF has received increased attention since its first inception in the early 1980s. Studies showed that the HVOF flame temperature was relatively low, less than 3400°C, which is believed to be an advantage concerning the phase transformation of HA material at elevated temperatures. This process was believed to be one potentially interesting method for HA coating fabrication.
8. *Blast coating* (Ishikawa et al. 1997). The advantage of this method is that the processing can be pursued at room temperature, but adhesion is poor. The low operating temperature leads to little phase transformation, but the mechanical properties of the obtained coatings are rather poor.
9. *Ion beam dynamic mixing (IBDM) method* (Yoshinari et al. 1994; Luo et al. 1999). This method is a combination of ion implantation and physical vapor deposition. The adhesive bonding strength of HA on Ti alloy substrate was reported to be up to 65 MPa (Yoshinari et al. 1994). Thus, the IBDM method was suggested to be useful for creating adherent films. However, the layer is too thin, which is less than 2 μm. Moreover, phase transformation from crystalline HA to amorphous calcium phosphate has been detected.

10. *Pulsed laser deposition* (Cottel et al. 1992). This approach is potentially very interesting because of conservation of the stoichiometry of HA.
11. *Others.* Preparation of HA films by surface-induced mineralization (Campbell et al. 1996), sol–gel technique (Piveteau et al. 1999; Hwang et al. 1999; Weng et al. 1998), and others, has also been reported.

Generally, the mechanical properties and phase composition, as well as operation feasibility, are the main factors used to evaluate processing techniques. HA coatings that are deposited by these techniques possess differences in chemistry and crystallinity, which can affect the biological response to HA and ultimately the coating performance. Among all the surface coating techniques, thermal spraying has shown wide application in depositing HA coatings due to its identified characteristics: low substrate temperature, large coating thickness that can be up to several centimeters, good coating mechanical performance, low cost, and so forth.

Principle of Thermal Spray

Thermal spray is a generic term for a group of coating processes used to apply metallic or nonmetallic coatings (Davis 2004). These processes are grouped into four major categories: flame spray, electric arc spray, cold gas spray, and plasma arc spray. The coating material (in powder, wire, or rod form) is heated by the energy sources and then projected at a high velocity onto a component surface as molten or semimolten or even slightly heated (cold spray) particle that flattens, undergo rapid solidification or solid deformation, and form a deposit through successive impingement. Figure 4.2 shows a schematic diagram of particles impinging onto a substrate in the process. The coatings are generated through continuous overlapping of splats. Intensive cooling at spraying is of primary importance because the temperature gradients within the coating and the substrate, together with the quenching stresses within the individual lamellae (group of splats sprayed per layer), will control the residual stresses of the coatings as well as the formation amorphous phases (Sampath et al. 1996). Thus, a thermal sprayed coating consists of layers of splats (solidified droplets; Pawlowski 2008, Figure 4.2b), which have a lamellar cross section. In fact, virtually all materials can be sprayed. However, special care has to be made when handling the materials that decompose before melting as hydroxyapatite or sublimate as graphite. The effort concerns the powder preparation and choice of spray parameters.

The strength of as-sprayed coatings depends substantially on the features such as porosity and interlamellar strength, originated from the building-up process of solidified droplets, or splats (Pawlowski 1995). These features result from the splat process on the substrate, and thus the properties of coatings are correlated closely to the temperature and velocity of the particles upon impact.

Thermal spraying covers a range of spraying processes that can be employed depending on the materials and desired coating performance. Table 4.1 compares the main thermal spraying techniques being used in the biomedical field for the production of bioactive coatings (Espanol Pons 2003). For comparison purposes, the values on the particles velocity have been given for an alumina powder with an average medium size of 30 μm. It must be noted that thermal spray is an active research area and there has always been

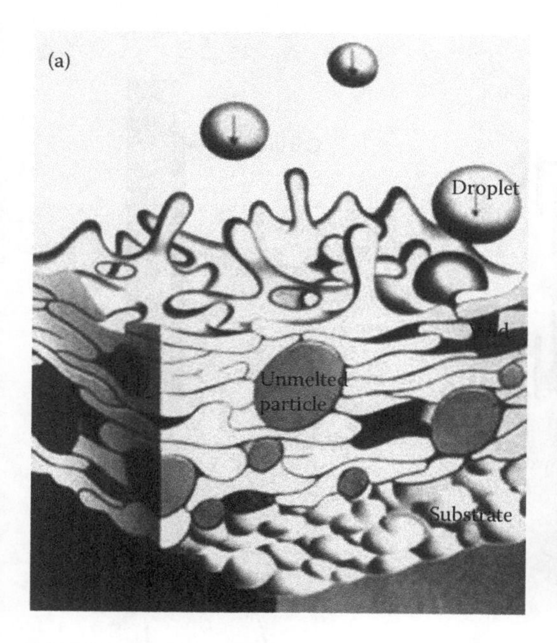

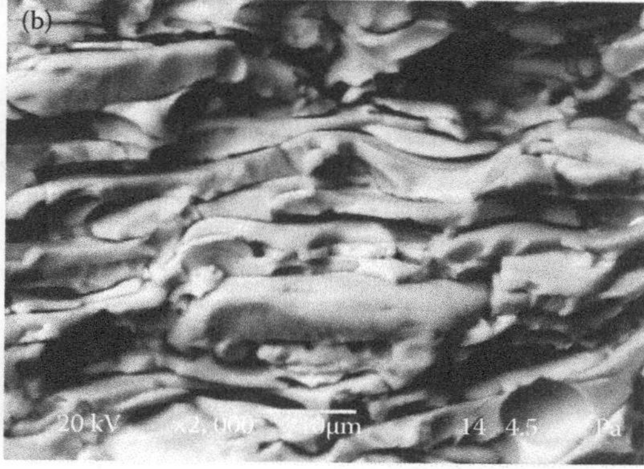

FIGURE 4.2
Buildup process of a coating by accumulation of individual splats (a) and a typical cross-sectional view of plasma sprayed zircon coating showing the layered structure. (From Gordon England, http://www.gordonengland.co.uk/tsc.htm 2010; Li, H., unpublished data, 2004. With permission.)

significant advancement in spray technique development, and hence further improved particle variables (i.e., temperature and velocity) have been achieved.

Among the thermal spray processes, plasma spray and HVOF are the two most widely used processes for HA coating deposition (Figure 4.3). In plasma spraying, the torch operates with a central thoriated tungsten cathode and a water-cooled annular copper anode.

TABLE 4.1
Comparison between Different Thermal Spray Techniques Used to Produce Ha-Based Coatings

	Flame	HVOF	APS	IPS	VPS	RF
Gas temp. (°C)						
P = 100 kPa	2700	3,000	14,000	14,000	–	–
P = 25 kPa	–	–	–	–	10,000	8,000
P = 7 kPa	–	–	–	–	5,000	–
Particle vel. (m/s)						
Al_2O_3, 30 μm						
P = 100 kPa	70	350	230	250	–	–
P = 25 kPa	–	–	–	–	380	30
P = 7 kPa	–	–	–	–	300	–
Flame length (cm)						
P = 100 kPa	<10	<20	<7	<10	–	–
P = 25 kPa	–	–	–	–	<15	<15
P = 7 kPa	–	–	–	–	<50	–
Part. Injection mode	Axial	Axial	Perpendicular to the plasma jet and downstream of the arc			Axial

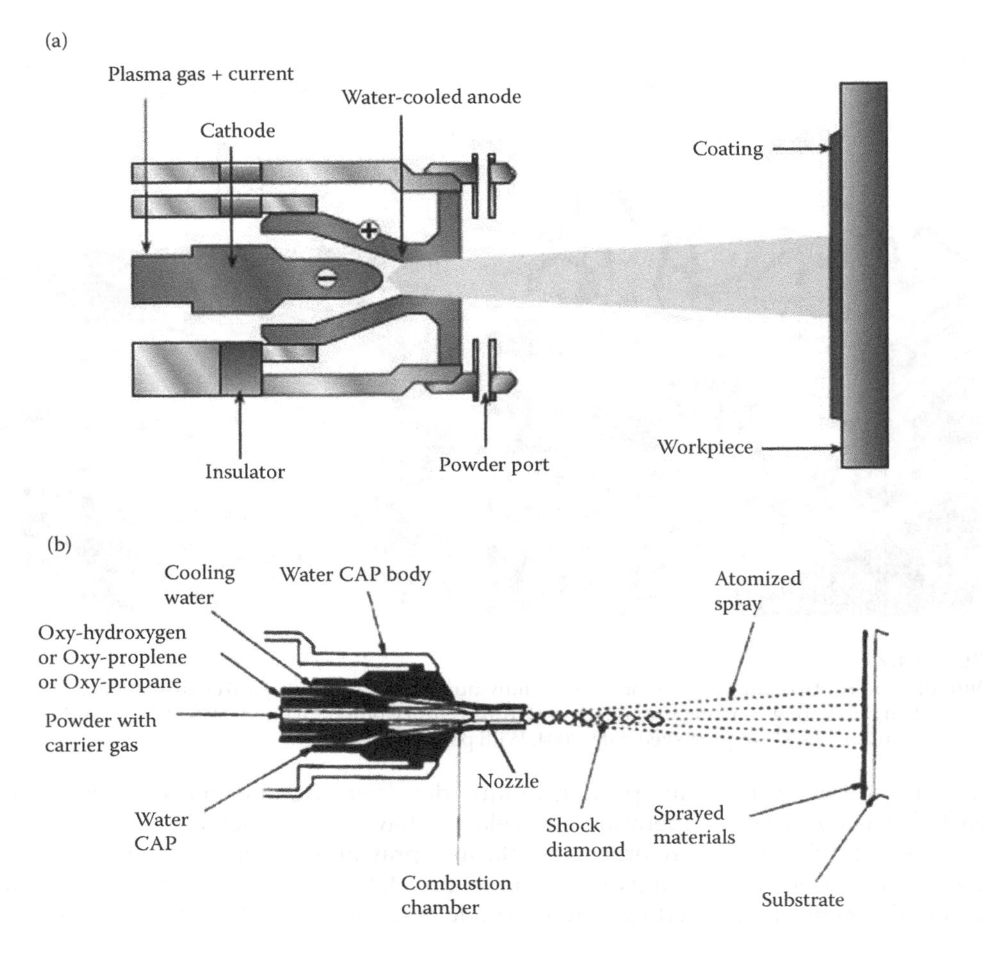

FIGURE 4.3
(a) Sketch of the plasma spraying being used in the biomedical field for the production of HA coatings (http://www.sulzermetco.com). (b) Schematic diagram of HVOF spray (http://www.nationalthermospray.com).

The plasma gas is injected into the gap between the two electrodes. As the gases pass around the arc created between the electrodes, they are heated and partially ionized, emerging from the anode nozzle at high velocity and high temperature. All materials with melting point can be plasma-sprayed because of its high gas temperature.

The HVOF technique was developed in the early 1980s. The principle lies mainly in the use of combustion of fuel gas such as hydrogen, propane, propylene, or acetylene, in oxygen. Supersonic flame can be generated through the combustion of fuel gas in oxygen under high pressure. As shown in Figure 4.3b, the characteristic of the supersonic flame is the appearance of shock diamonds in the flame. Sprayed powders are axially fed into the gun by means of inert carrier gas, then are accelerated and heated in the flame, which is of a high velocity of more than 1000 m/s and a moderate temperature of up to 3400°C depending on fuel gas and oxygen/fuel ratio. Impingement of the heated particles on substrate or precoating could result in a satisfactory coating in terms of dense microstructure and competitive mechanical properties. The unique heated efficiency of the particles can be obtained because of low turbulent degree of the flame. The most notable features of HVOF technique are summarized below (Ahmed et al. 1997; Schroeder et al. 1997; Liao et al. 2000; Thorpe et al. 2000). HVOF processes typically have the highest particle velocities, which result in denser and more uniform coating structures compared to conventional flame spray coatings.

- High density: coatings produced through HVOF develop very high densities because of the high kinetic energy associated with this process
- High adhesive bonding strengths
- Low porosity: less than 1% (with nearly no interconnecting porosity)
- Metalworking capabilities
- Essentially stress-free
- Great thickness (up to several centimeters)
- Low thermal input

Originally, the HVOF process was explored to produce cermet coatings such as WC–Co coating to achieve excellent wear-resistance. High adhesive strength of higher than 100 MPa can also be achieved (Kreye et al. 1986). Due to its high flame velocity and moderate flame temperature, the HVOF technique was extensively employed to deposit alternative materials in recent years.

Synthesis of HA Powder for Coating Deposition

Properties of HA

Natural bone is mainly composed of mineral nanocrystals, water, and collagen fibers. A typical wet cortical bone is composed of 22 wt.% organic matrix, 69 wt.% mineral, and 9 wt.% water (Luo et al. 1995). Because of its chemical similarity to bone, HA can form strong biological bonds with bony tissue without the presence of soft fibrous tissues. Its excellent biointegration makes it an ideal choice for use in orthopedic and dental applications. The stoichiometric Ca/P ratio of HA is 1.67. Its density is 3.21 g/cm^3 (Aoki 1994).

Synthesis and Fabrication of HA Powder

It is a primary knowledge that the properties of the feedstock play an important role among all the considered factors that influence the performances of the coatings and ceramics (Guipont et al. 2002). It is also essential to have complete control of the powder properties, such as particle size, surface area, morphology, and crystallinity, which can be tailored for each specific application in order to maximize the properties of the final biomedical implant. More importantly, it would be exciting to synthesize nanostrucured HA powders so as to make it possible to study the changes of the nanostructural features during the high temperature processing. For the time being, several manufacturing methods for the synthesis of HA powders have been explored, which include liquid reaction, solid phases reaction, hydrothermal reaction, alkoxide method, and flux method (Aoki 1994). The main characteristics of the HA feedstock, including the size, shape, composition, and structure of the powders, have been systematically investigated (Tong et al. 1996; Cheang et al. 1996b; Liu et al. 1994).

The most widely used and well-established method for HA powder synthesis is wet chemical route, which employs the reaction of calcium hydroxide with orthophosphoric acid according to the reaction:

$$10Ca(OH)_2 + 6H_3PO_4 \rightarrow Ca_{10}(PO4)_6(OH)_2 + 18H_2O \quad (4.1)$$

Detailed description of the procedure for the production of the powder was reported (Kweh 2000). Parameters such as temperature, pH, rate of mixing reactants, and maturation time have been carefully controlled to ensure production of an apatite as close as possible to the stoichiometric HA. In addition, special care must be taken to ensure a slow drip rate of the acid onto the alkaline solution to favor the formation of PO_4^{3-} ion and the introduction of OH^- in the lattice. An overview of the synthesis procedure is given schematically in Figure 4.4. It consists primarily of three steps: (1) preparation of the solution, (2) precursor synthesis, and (3) high temperature treatment to consolidate powders.

In order to prepare specific powders, two steps have to be mastered: the slurry stability and the spray drying operating conditions. During spray drying, the solution is extracted from a feed tank and passed through the spray atomizer. It is a result of many interwoven complex mechanisms. The feed materials are either water-based suspensions with air as drying gas or organic solvent-based suspensions (usually ethanol) with nitrogen as drying gas. Compressed air with a selected pressure is used during spraying. The atomized liquid is rapidly dried by a coaxial flow of air that has been previously preheated to a specific temperature. The dried powder is cyclone separated from the flowing airstream.

An important study that has to be carried out especially when nonstoichiometric apatite powder is synthesized is its thermal stability. Only pure HA powder remains stable up to its melting temperature but nonstoichiometric apatite would undergo irreversible decomposition reactions through a wide range of temperatures that can go up to 1000°C. Above this temperature, the reversible decomposition of stoichiometric HA takes place. Rey and

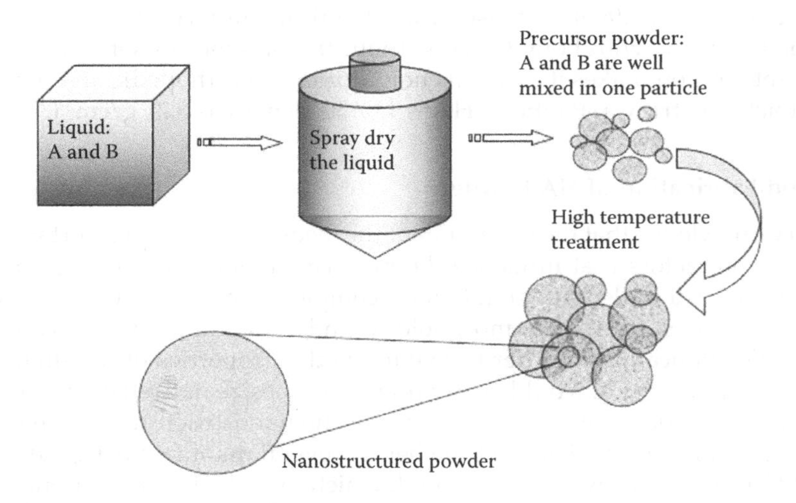

FIGURE 4.4
Schematic illustration of the wet chemical reaction approach. (Li, H., unpublished data, 2004.)

collaborators have summarized, according to the Ca/P ratio of a synthesized apatite, the different phases that are obtained upon heat treatment at 1000°C (Rey et al. 1991):

1.33 > Ca/P > 1.5	α-TCP and/or β-TCP and beta-calcium pyrophosphate
Ca/P = 1.5	β-TCP
1.5 > Ca/P > 1.67	β-TCP and stoichiometric HA
Ca/P = 1.67	stoichiometric HA
Ca/P > 1.67	CaO and stoichiometric HA

Generally, heat treatment at 1000°C was carried out for 4 h on the SDHA powder in order to ascertain the thermal stability of the powder (Espanol Pons 2003).

The spherical HA particles with nanostructures can be synthesized by the wet chemical approach (Li et al. 2007c). Figure 4.5 shows the typical nanostructure of the particles (Li et al. 2007c). The agglomerated nature for the spray-dried HA (SDHA) powder shows rather interconnected porosity between the different grains or crystals in each powder particle (Figure 4.5). The powder must be heat-treated not only to increase crystallinity but

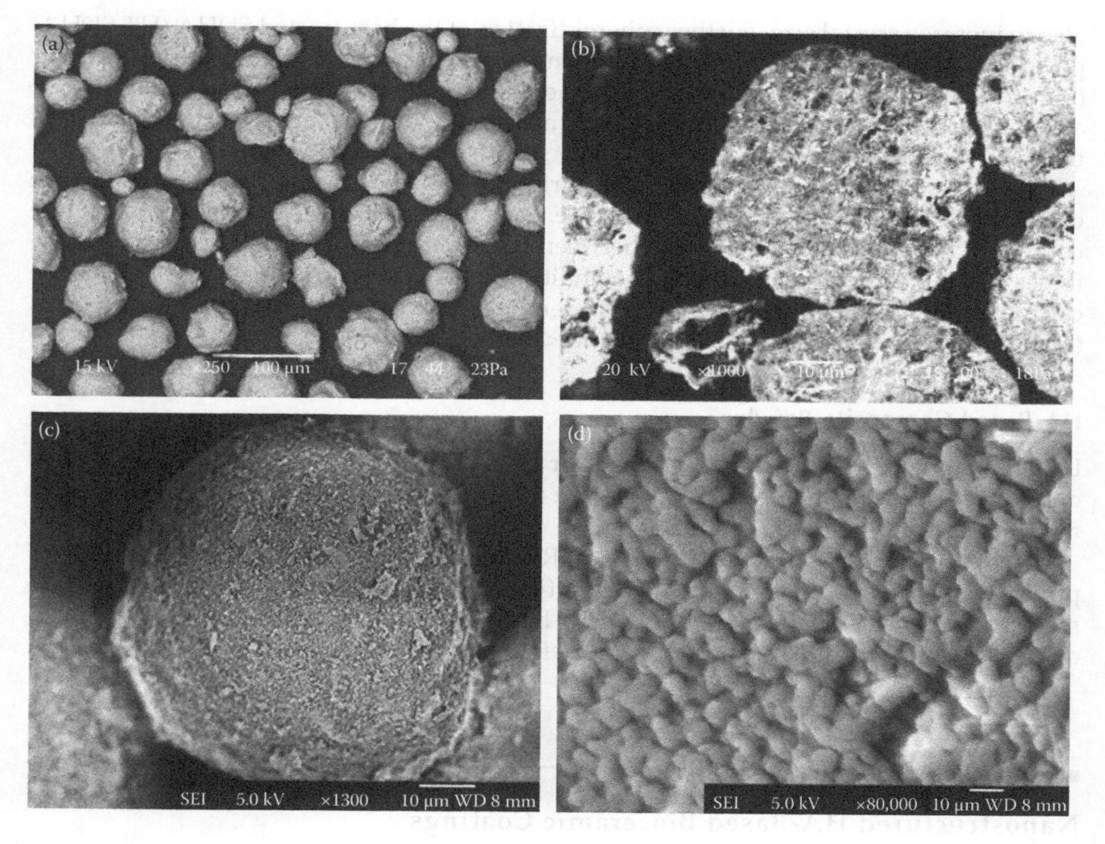

FIGURE 4.5
Nanostructured HA powder. (From Li et al., *Acta Mater.*, 52, 445–453, 2004c; Li et al., *J. Biomed. Mater. Res.*, 82A, 296–303, 2007c; Li et al. *Biomaterials*, 25, 3463–3471, 2004a. With permission.) (a, c, d) Topographical views of the particles and (b) cut-open view of one HA particle.

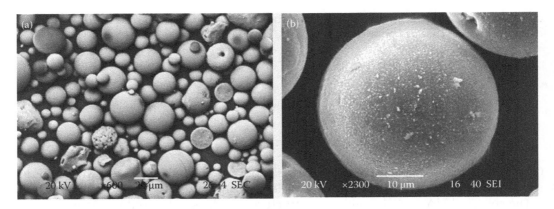

FIGURE 4.6
Spherical HA particles SEM micrographs of the etched cross section of HT–SHA powder (a) dense particles showing columnar and fine equiaxed grains, (b) detail of the columnar grains in the outer layer and equiaxed grains in the core of a newly formed solid particle, (c) detail of the columnar grains in the wall of a hollow sphere, and (d) solid sphere retaining SDHA structure in its core. (From Espanol Pons, M., PhD thesis, Nanyang Technological University, Singapore, 2003. With permission.)

also to increase crystal size. Further spheroidization of the heat-treated SDHA (HT-SDHA) powder can be made using a plasma gun and quenching the product in distilled water (Figure 4.6) (Espanol Pons 2003). The HT-spheroidized HA (HT-SHA) powder was denser and had smoother surfaces than HT–SDHA and that markedly improved the flowability of the HT-SHA powder (Espanol Pons 2003).

The cross-sectional view in Figure 4.5b further demonstrates the highly porous nature of the particle and its agglomerated structure. Each powder consists of an assembly of fine equiaxed crystals. The bond strength between the different crystals will depend on those forces that bind them together and the ability to form interparticle necking during the calcination process. The agglomerated powder particles were composed of nanostructures (with rodlike grains: <230 nm in length and <70 nm in diameter).

HA-Based Composite Powder

Different approaches have been reported for synthesis of the HA-based composite powder (Xu et al. 2005; Kumar et al. 2003). Figure 4.7 shows the HA/titania composite powder made by a slurry-spray-dry approach.

The synthesis of HA/nanozirconia by an RF-plasma spray route provides a method of producing nanozirconia-enwrapped HA particles for thermal spray deposition of the biomedical coatings. Fabrication of the particles has been successful (Figure 4.8) and detailed description of the synthesis approach can be found in the paper (Kumar et al. 2003).

Nanostructured HA-Based Bioceramic Coatings Deposited by Thermal Spray

Hydroxyapatite (HA) coatings deposited using thermal spray techniques on titanium alloy substrates showed capability of avoiding the inherent mechanical property limitations of

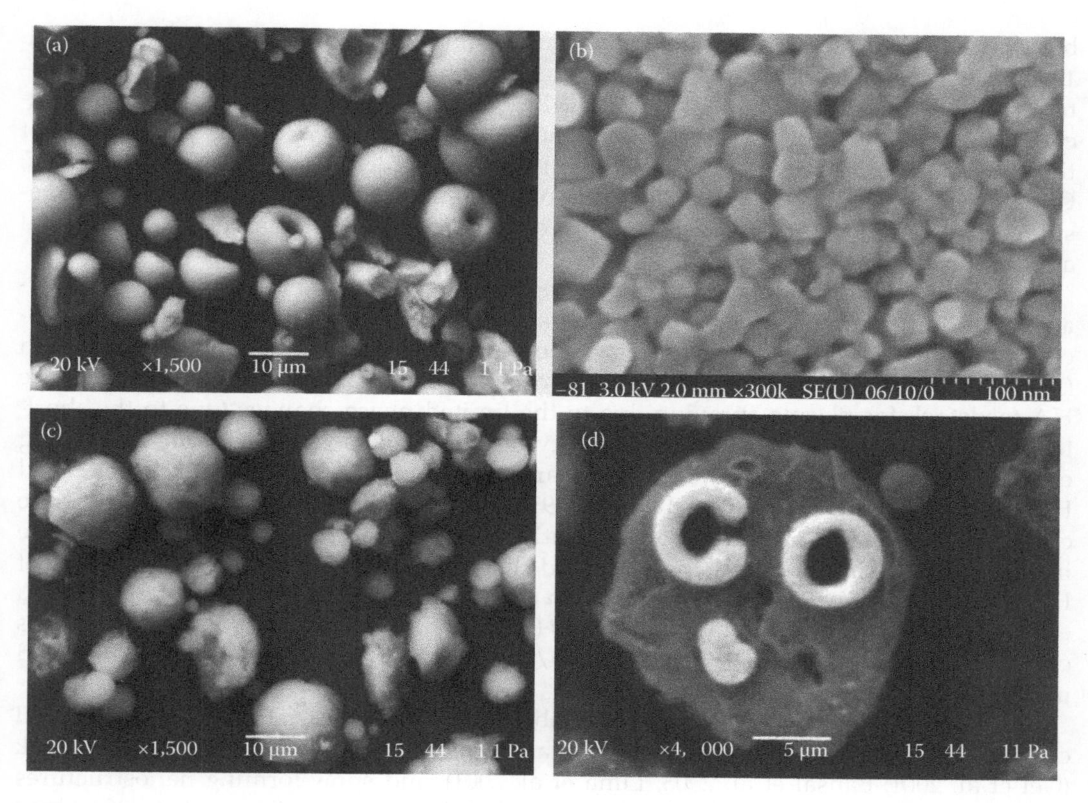

FIGURE 4.7
Slurry-spray-dry approach for fabrication of HA/titania composite powder. (a) Topographical morphology of the nanostructured titania particles showing particle size range of 1–15 µm. (b) Typical cross-sectional view of the titania particles showing the nanostructural feature with the grain sizes of 20–30 nm, (c) surface view, and (d) cross-sectional view of the HA/titania composite powder. (From Li et al., *Therm. Spray Technol.*, 15, 610–616, 2006. With permission.)

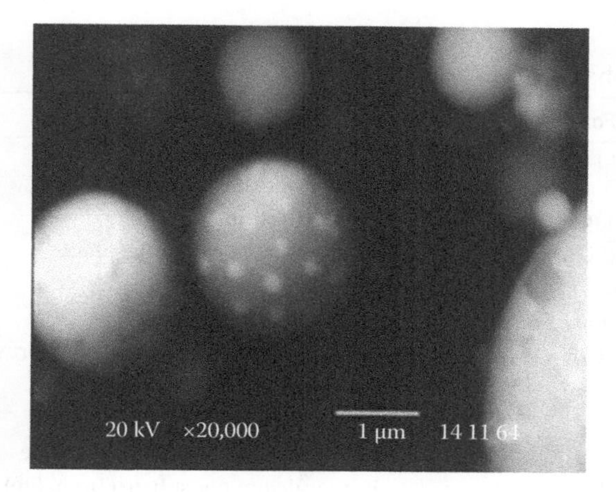

FIGURE 4.8
SEM micrographs of ultrafine ZrO_2/HA composite powders (40 wt.% ZrO_2/HA) showing general morphology of HA with embedded ZrO_2 nanoparticles (spherical). (From Kumar et al., *Biomaterials*, 24, 2611–2621, 2003. With permission.)

bulk HA without remarkable loss in biocompatibility (Oonishi et al. 1989; Hardy et al. 1999). It was found that the macro- and microstructure of HA was particularly important for the apposition of bone (Hing et al. 1999). The biological performance of the calcium phosphate coatings was essentially phase-dependent, and biological behavior of the phases in the calcium phosphate family has been largely elucidated (Yang et al. 1997; Cleries et al. 2000). It is therefore clear that optimization of the phase composition of as-sprayed calcium phosphate coatings is a prerequisite toward their competitive biomedical applications.

Due to the obvious influence of the starting powder on coating performances, a favorable method for HA powder preparation was actively sought. The spheroidization process by using plasma spray was found as one sound method for HA powder preparation (Liu et al. 1994). This process has proven to be the most favorable method to prepare HA feedstock for plasma spraying due to the limited phase changes (due to the short-term stay in the torch) and good flowability of the powders (Cheang et al. 1994; Wang et al. 1999; Oonishi et al. 1987). Different starting HA powder, calcined HA, spray-dried HA, and spheroidized HA (Cheang et al. 1996b) resulted in remarkably different phase composition and microstructure of the coatings. Nearly all the studies involved in the influence of starting HA feedstock revealed that the shape, geometry, and structure of HA powders exhibited significant effects on coating characteristics (Wang et al. 1999; Vu et al. 1996) apart from the spray parameters (Yang et al. 1995; Wang et al. 1993a). Various calcium phosphates with their respective Ca/P ratios in the HA material system are listed in Table 4.2.

Basically, there are two approaches for fabricating nanostructures in thermal sprayed coatings, retaining nanostructures from starting nanophase/nanostructured feedstock (Gel et al. 2001; Bansal et al. 2003; Lima et al. 2001), and spray-forming nanostructures owing to the rapid cooling of the droplets upon their impingement (Tjong et al. 2004; Gang et al. 2003). The use of nanostructured feedstock is a promising way for deposition of nanostructured coatings (Li et al. SCT, 2006). Generally, the spray powder can be fabricated through agglomerating nanosized particles to form big ones (Tjong et al. 2004; Gel

TABLE 4.2

Various Calcium Phosphates with Their Respective Ca/P Atomic Ratios

Ca/P	Formula	Name	Abbreviation
2.0	$Ca_4O(PO_4)_2$	Tetracalcium phosphate (Hilgenstockite)	TCPM (TTCP)
1.67	$Ca_{10}(PO_4)_6(OH)_2$	Hydroxyapatite	HA
	$Ca_{10-x}H_{2x}(PO_4)_6(OH)_2$	Amorphous calcium phosphate	ACP
1.50	$Ca_3(PO_4)_2$	Tricalcium phosphate (α, β, γ)	TCP
1.33	$Ca_8H_2(PO_4)_6 \times 5H_2O$	Octacalcium phosphate	OCP
1.0	$CaHPO_4 \times 2H_2O$	Dicalcium phosphate dihydrate (Brushite)	DCPD
1.0	$CaHPO_4$	Dicalcium phosphate (Monetite)	DCP
1.0	$Ca_2P_2O_7$	Calcium pyrophosphate (α, β, γ)	CPP
1.0	$Ca_2P_2O_7 \times 2H_2O$	Calcium pyrophosphate dehydrate	CPPD
0.7	$Ca_7(P_5O_{16})_2$	Heptacalcium phosphate (Tromelite)	HCP
0.67	$Ca_4H_2P_6O_{20}$	Tetracalcium dihydrogen phosphate	TDHP
0.5	$Ca(H_2PO_4)_2 \times H_2O$	Monocalcium phosphate monohydrate	MCPM
0.5	$Ca(PO_3)_2$	Calcium metaphosphate (α, β, γ)	CMP

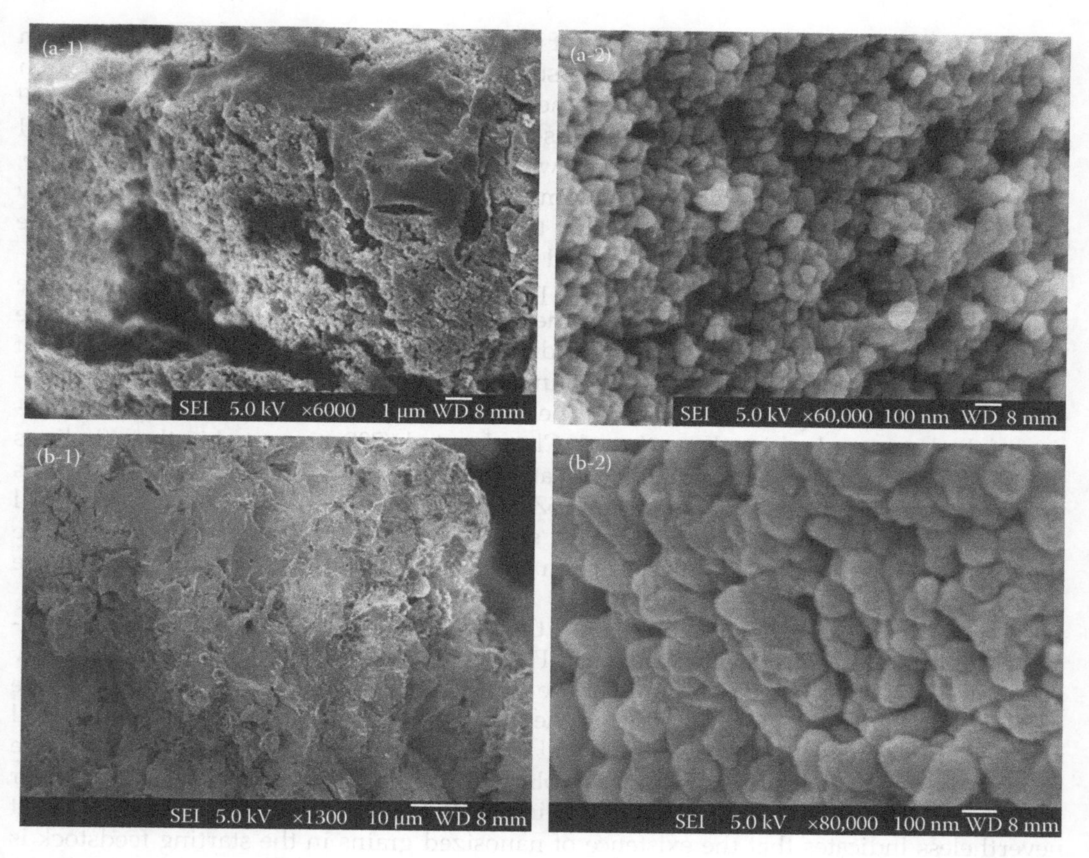

FIGURE 4.9
Typical field-emission SEM (FESEM) pictures of the HVOF coatings (made from 40 ± 10 μm powder) showing nanostructures at (a) their surface and (b) fractured cross sections ((a-2) and (b-2) refer to closer observation on (a-1) and (b-1), respectively). (From Li, H., Khor, K.A., *Surf. Coat. Technol.*, 201, 2147–2154, 2006. With permission.)

et al. 2001). It should be noted that the extent of thermal decomposition of HA to tricalcium phosphate (TCP), tetracalcium phosphate (TTCP), or amorphous calcium phosphate (ACP) is closely related to the heat input, and hence the melt state of HA particles during coating deposition (Gross et al. 1998b, 1998c; Ogiso et al. 1998a; Dyshlovenko et al. 2004; Dyshlovenko et al. 2006).

The HVOF HA coatings show clearly the evidence of the presence of nanostructures at both their surface and cross sections (Figure 4.9) (Li et al. 2006). Similar grain sizes can be seen at both the coating surface and cross sections. In addition, the plasma sprayed HA coatings also show predominate presence of the nanostructures. However, the sizes of the grains (40–90 nm) are slightly smaller than those of the grains in the HVOF coatings (50–110 nm). FESEM observation from the bottom side of the coating (the area with intimate contact with the substrate) showed interesting microstructures (Figure 4.10) (Li et al. SCT 2006). That is, the HVOF sprayed coatings made from the smallest powder (30 ± 10 μm) exhibit typical individual grains with hexagonal prismatic morphology (Figure 4.10a). Most of the grains exhibit a size of <250 nm in height and <50 nm in side length (Figure

4.10a-1). Very few have the enlarged size of 0.4 to 1.2 μm in height and 80 to 120 nm in width. While other coatings do not have such features (Figure 4.10b and c). Research showed evidence of different melt state of the sprayed powder particles during the HVOF spraying (Khor et al. 2004), which will be discussed in a later part. It is further confirmed that during the HVOF spraying, bigger powder particles experienced partial melt state, while the smallest particles were entirely molten. Plasma-sprayed HA particles usually get entirely molten. There is no doubt that the melting of the particles accounts for the reorganization of the rod-shaped nanosized grains in the starting feedstock. The formation of the nanosized grains with hexagonal prismatic morphology indicates the influence of both the melt state and temperature of the HA particles upon their impingement. The partial melt state during HVOF spraying and overheating state during plasma spraying of the HA particles could result in a faster cooling rate of the molten part upon their impingement on the room-temperature substrate. The high cooling rate would influence the formation of the hexagonal grains. Even though Chraska et al. (2001) reported in their findings that the top surface of the first solidified splat causes epitaxial growth of columnar grains in subsequent splats for plasma-sprayed YSZ splats, the study on HA revealed spherical nanosized grains within the second folded splat and there is no experimental evidence showing the presence of columnar grains in other parts in the coatings other than in the first layer splats.

It is noted that the nanostructures in all the coatings showed markedly different features from those in the starting feedstock (Figure 4.5). After the high-temperature spray processing, the rod-shaped nanograins have turned to be nanosized spheres (with a size of 30–120 nm). This suggests that during the melting/resolidification process, individual nanorods were mostly fractured into several individual parts, and with the aid of surface tension, the nanosized spheres were accomplished. Therefore, it can be expected that finer nanostructures in starting feedstock would induce finer nanostructures in the coatings. It nevertheless indicates that the existence of nanosized grains in the starting feedstock is essential for formation of nanostructures in the coatings.

TEM and FESEM observation of the HA splats further reveals the presence of the nanostructures (Figure 4.11) (Li et al. SCT 2006). It is clear that at the areas near to splats' fringes, the structure is actually nanostructures composed of ~30-nm grains (Figure 4.11a and b). The HA particles may have different thermal history during HVOF and plasma spraying. This may influence both the microstructure and phases in the resultant splats/coatings. The unmelted part of the HVOF-sprayed HA splat was also characterized using TEM. The sample was prepared through further ion milling the individual HA splats. As shown in Figure 4.11c, the unmelted part of the splat shows enlarged rod-shaped grains with the dimension of <400 nm in diameter and <550 nm in length. The HVOF coating made from partially melted powder, hence, must have a mixed nano- and microstructure. Enhanced cooling of substrate during coating deposition could effectively increase the content of the nanosized grains in the HA coatings. The nanostructures exhibited within the molten part of the HA splats are consistent with the nanosized grains revealed in the coatings. This, on the other hand, further suggests that during the accumulation of individual HA splats to form bulk coating, there is no obvious grain growth for the nanosized grains. Studies showed the structural features are actually associated closely with melt state of the HA particles experienced during the coating deposition.

The distinguishing structural features could be related to melt state of the sprayed HA powder particles (Khor et al. 2004). The term "melt-state" refers arbitrarily to the extent of melting that took place in the particles prior to impact, and subsequent solidification on the substrate. It would be possible that the phase composition and properties of resultant

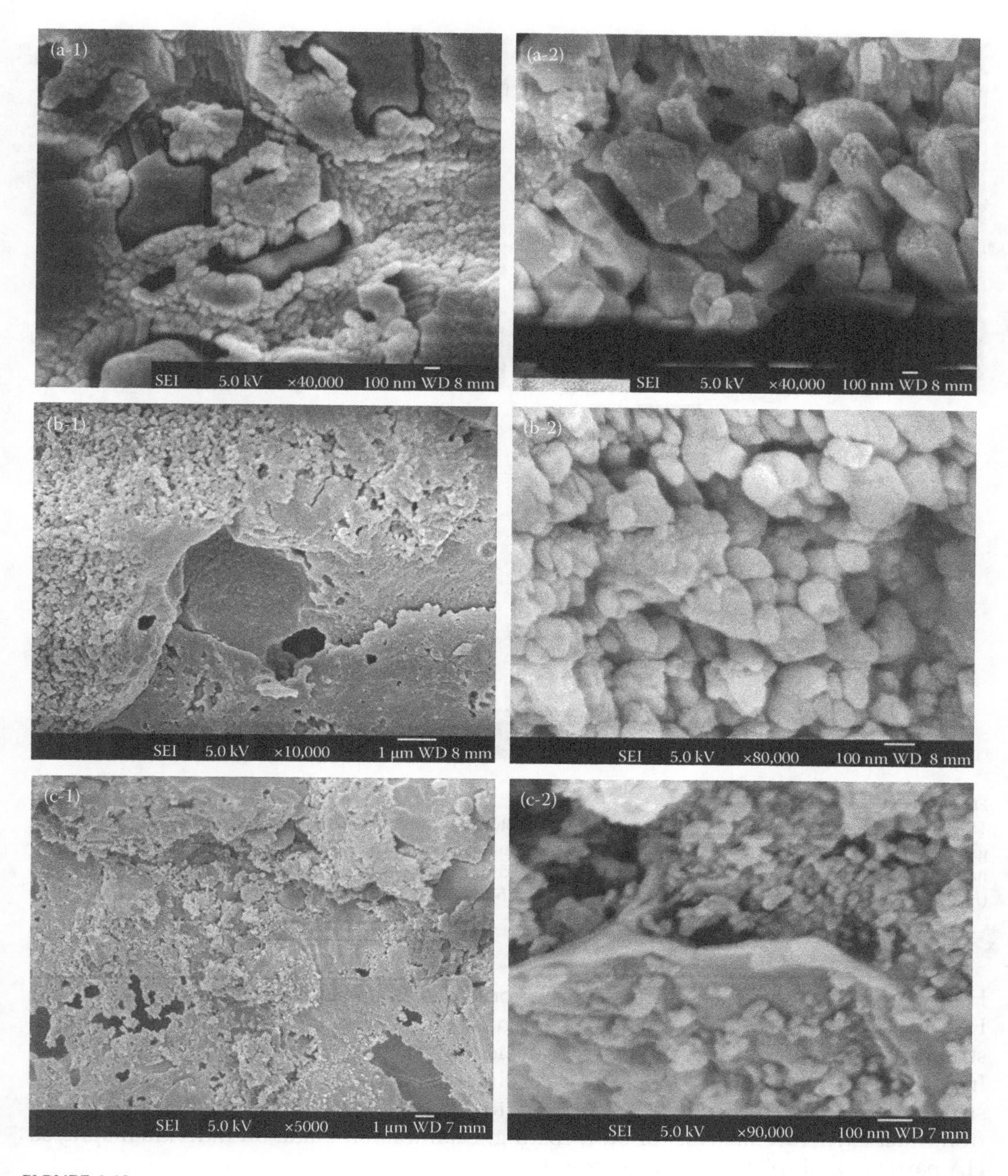

FIGURE 4.10
Typical FESEM photos taken at the coating bottom (with intimate contact with the substrate), (a-1,2) HVOF coating made from 30 ± 10 μm powder showing rectangular nanosized grains with different sizes, (b-1,2) HVOF coating made from 40 ± 10 μm powder showing spherical nanosized grains, (c-1,2) plasma coating showing fine spherical nanosized grains. (From Li, H., Khor, K.A., *Surf. Coat. Technol.*, 201, 2147–2154, 2006. With permission.)

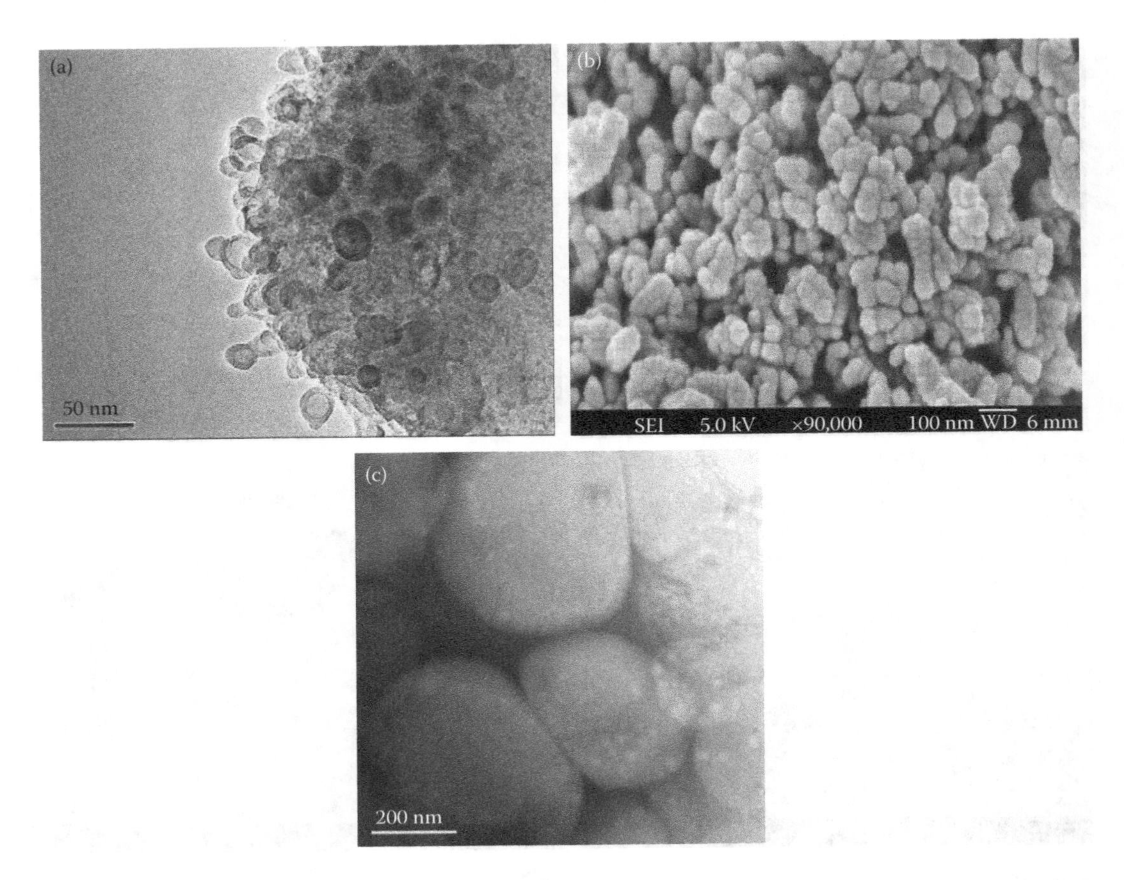

FIGURE 4.11
TEM and FESEM pictures of the HA splats. (a) TEM photo showing the predominant presence of the nanosized grains (~30 nm) at fringes of the splat, (b) FESEM picture taken from the surface of the splat showing consistent nanosized grains, (c) TEM photo showing the enlarged grains at the unmelted part within the HVOF splat. (From Li, H., Khor, K.A., *Surf. Coat. Technol.*, 201, 2147–2154, 2006.)

HA coatings can be achieved through the control of the melt state of HA particle in the HVOF flame. It was evidenced that the molten part of the HA contributed to refined nanostructures, while the unmelted part accounts for enlarged mcrosized grains (Li et al. 2006). Investigation on melt-state of the particles is important toward understanding the microstructure of HA coatings. Since it is difficult to accurately determine the melt state of HA from microstructure analysis of bulk coating, examination made on individual sprayed HA particles and splats has been successful.

Thermal-sprayed coating is composed of liquid droplets that rapidly solidified upon impact. It is likely that some droplets will contain entrapped gases attained during their in-flight stage. Furthermore, it is well known that thermal sprayed coating shows a layered structure, which is a splat-accumulated structure. Apart from the influence of residual stresses, which is generated during coating formation, properties of the bulk coating are essentially derived from the characteristics of the solidified splats (Tadnno et al. 1997; Brown et al. 1994; Brown and Turner 1998). Therefore, the study on the properties of sprayed particles and splats are essentially important.

The molten/unmolten ratio of HVOF-sprayed HA powders was experimentally determined through image analysis. It was found that during the present HVOF spraying, most HA powders were only partially melted, which is schematically shown in Figure 4.12 (Khor et al. 2004). After appropriate grinding and polishing, from the figure, the melt fraction in particle (MFP) of HA powders was defined as the ratio of melted volume to the whole particle's volume (Khor et al. 2004)

$$\text{MFP} = \frac{V_{\text{melted}}}{V_{\text{total}}} = \frac{R^3 - r^3}{R^3} \times 100\% \tag{4.2}$$

where R and r are the radius of HA particle and the unmelted core, respectively. Determination of MFP was performed through deriving the area ratio obtained using the ImagePro image analysis software to volume ratio. From the image analysis, the area ratio of molten part (A) and area of unmelted part (B) can be determined

$$a = \frac{A}{B} = \frac{R^2 - r^2}{r^2} \tag{4.3}$$

Combined with the above definition, the melt fraction of alternative HA particles can be calculated according to the following formula:

$$\text{MFP} = 1 - \left(\frac{1}{1+a}\right)^{\frac{3}{2}} \tag{4.4}$$

The SEM cross-sectional morphology obviously demonstrates the miscellaneous powders' melt state (Figure 4.13) (Khor et al. 2004). It reveals that with the increase in particle size, the melt fraction of the particles decreases. The statistical analysis on the melt fraction of the powders (MFP) is shown in Figure 4.14 (Khor et al. 2004). Under the same spray conditions, fine powders (C-7, 30 ± 10 µm) contained MFP values in excess of 90%, while the large powder (C-4; 50 ± 10 µm) have MFP values that stretches down to ~20%. It also shows that apart from the influence of starting powder size, the increase in flow rate of oxygen and hydrogen, which contributes to an increased flame temperature, also results in increased melt fraction values (cf. C-2 and C-5 in Figure 4.14). Furthermore, the melt-resolidification phenomenon induces a densified structure that compared favorably to the

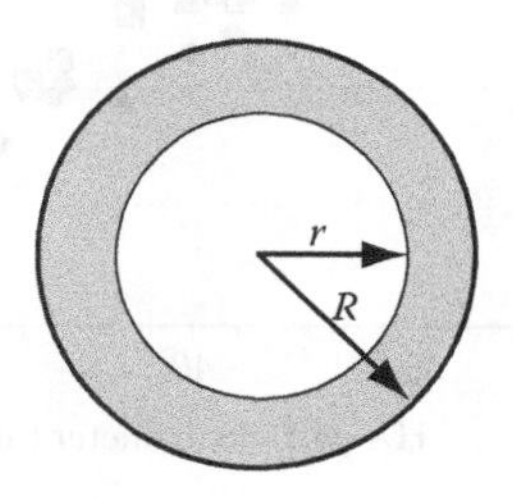

FIGURE 4.12
Sketch of HA particle during HVOF spraying showing partially melted state. R, radius of HA particle; r, radius of unmelted core. (From Khor et al., *Biomaterials*, 25, 1177–1186, 2004. With permission.)

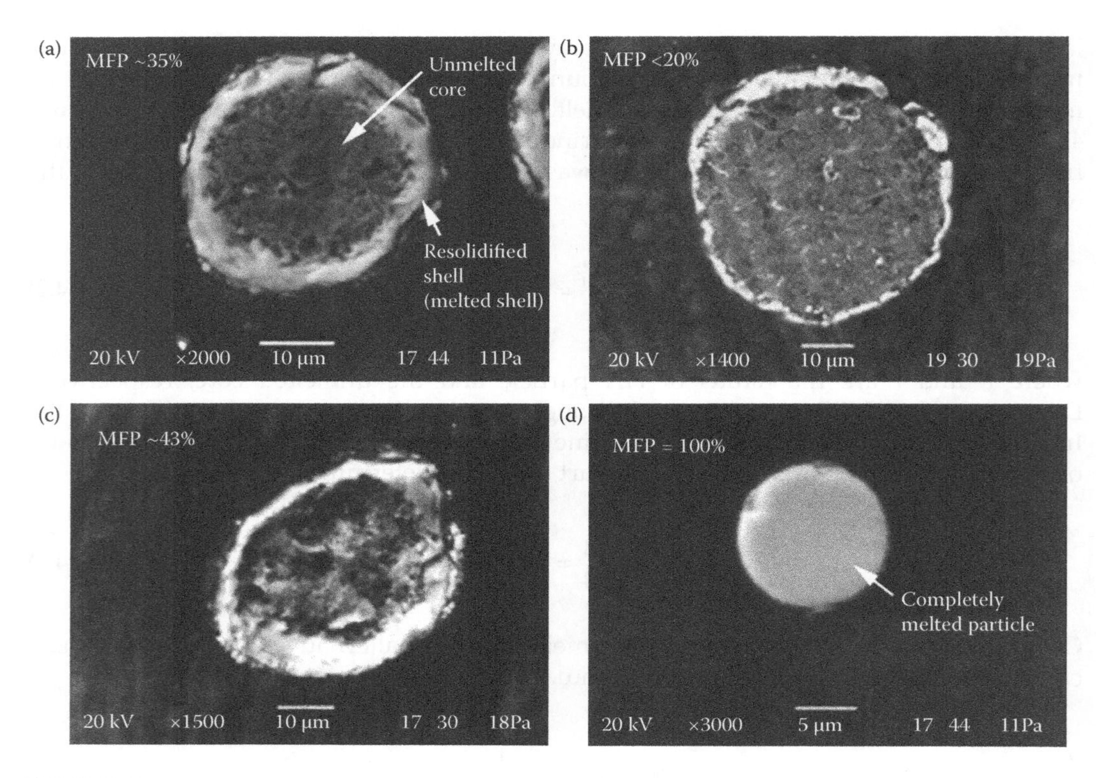

FIGURE 4.13
Cross-sectional morphology of HVOF-sprayed HA particles showing their different melting fraction depending on the altered particle size. (From Khor et al., *Biomaterials*, 25, 1177–1186, 2004. With permission.)

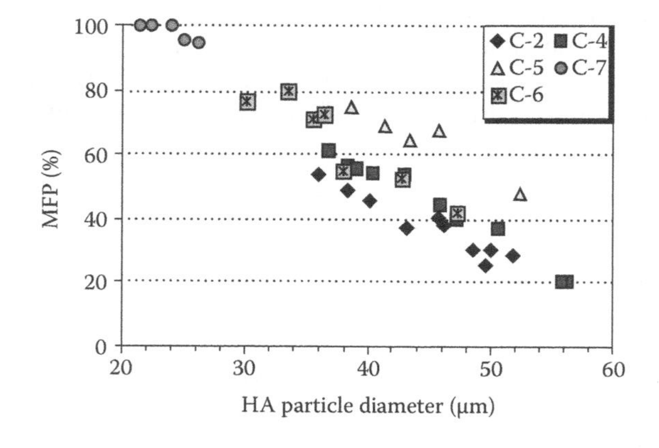

FIGURE 4.14
Melting fraction of HA powders during HVOF spraying, the value was obtained from image analysis on collected HA particles. (From Khor et al., *Biomaterials*, 25, 1177–1186, 2004. With permission.)

starting powders, which exhibit a porous structure. From this point of view, different melt fractions of HA powders correspond to different coating structures. In order to reveal the influence of different melt state of the powders on phase composition of resultant coatings, the coatings, C-4, C-6, and C-7 were analyzed. Figure 4.15 shows the XRD patterns of the three types of coatings. It is found that decrease in powder size results in an increase in ACP phase and extent of thermal transformation of HA. The following formula was widely suggested to describe the decomposition of HA (Ogiso et al. 1998b; Wang et al. 1998; McPherson et al. 1995):

$$Ca_{10}(PO_4)_6(OH)_2 \rightarrow 3Ca_3(PO_4)_2 + CaO + H_2O \tag{4.5}$$

The decomposition of HA during coating deposition can result in some CaO simultaneously, but because of the low content (<1 wt.%), it could not be detected by XRD analysis. The formation of the ACP was apparently associated with partial dehydroxylation of HA (Radin et al. 1992) during melting and subsequent rapid solidification of the powders (Cao et al. 1996). The melted portion of the powder is in direct response to the formation of ACP. Moreover, crystalline HA phase is generally attributed to the retention of original HA phase in the sprayed powders. For near crystalline coatings (crystallinity >90%, determined arbitrarily from XRD technique; Girardin et al. 2000), content of α–TCP was also determined using the Rietveld method, which is shown in Figure 4.16 (Khor et al. 2004). Content of TCP directly reflects the extent of the transformation that occurred following solidification of the droplets on the substrate. Liao et al. (1999) reported that transformation to TTCP occurred at about 1360°C through some transient phases. It has been found that no transformation to α-TCP from a stoichiometric HA (with a Ca/P ratio of 1.67) could be detected up to 1200°C with prolonged heating (Zhou et al. 1993). The appearance of β-TCP in the HA coatings is possibly attributed to the phase transformation from α-TCP at about 1100°C (Reser 1983). Studies already showed that once HA powders had been

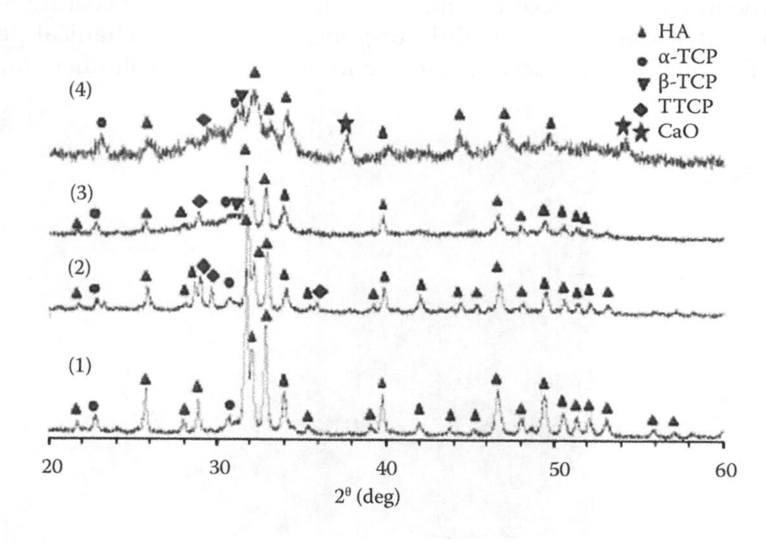

FIGURE 4.15
XRD patterns of the HA coatings (a) and the starting HA powder (b). (1) HVOF HA coating (50 ± 10 μm powder), (2) HVOF HA coating (40 ± 10 μm powder), (3) HVOF HA coating (30 ± 10 μm powder), and (4) plasma HA coating (50 ± 10 μm powder). (From Li, H., Khor, K.A., *Surf. Coat. Technol.*, 201, 2147–2154, 2006. With permission.)

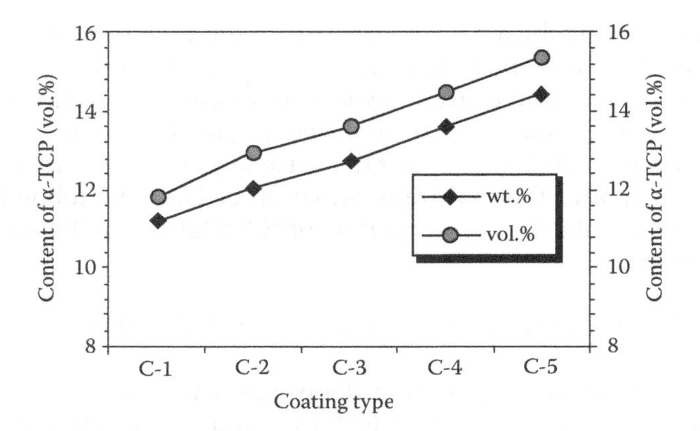

FIGURE 4.16
Content of α-TCP in as-sprayed crystalline coatings that shows the influence of spray parameters on phase composition of the resultant coatings. (From Khor et al., *Biomaterials*, 25, 1177–1186, 2004. With permission.)

totally melted, the phases α-TCP, TTCP, and β-TCP are all exhibited in the resultant coating (Wang et al. 1993a). The difference in the content of α-TCP in the coatings demonstrated in Figure 4.16 further indicates that the extent of HA phase decomposition is significantly related to the MFP during coating formation. From this point of view, the melt fraction of powder is practically meaningful. It is clear that augmentation of starting particle size results in decrease in melt fraction and hence contributes to decreased phase decomposition of HA.

Interestingly, TEM observation evidenced that the melted part shows a smaller grain size than the unmelted part (Figure 4.17) (Khor et al. 2004). It is noted that the HA grains located in the unmelted part are of a far larger size than those in the melted part, which underscores the influence of rapid cooling on grain growth during coating deposition. It should be noted that grain size is mainly responsible for the mechanical performances of materials. The relatively reduced grain size located in the resolidified zone, which is

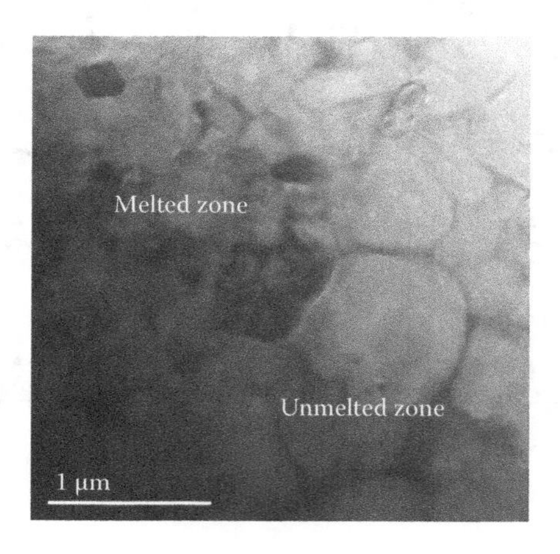

FIGURE 4.17
TEM image of as-sprayed HA coating showing different grain size and the interface between melted and unmelted parts of HA splat. (From Khor et al., *Biomaterials*, 25, 1177–1186, 2004. With permission.)

around the splats' interface, could act as an important factor contributing to improved mechanical properties.

It is evident that partially melted state of HA powders (low MFP values) is beneficial toward obtaining a nanostructured high crystalline HA coating. Furthermore, phase composition analyses indicate that the melted portion of the particles contained predominantly ACP and TCP. Therefore, in order to effectively inhibit HA decomposition, limited melting of the HA powders must be ensured. It was believed that the high levels in crystallinity of HA coatings were beneficial for long-term survivability, and proper functional life in service with regard to the resolvability of different phases in bony tissues; that is, ACP has a far higher resolvability in the bony tissues than crystalline HA (Ducheyne et al. 1993). However, the high resolvability of the amorphous phase is beneficial for accelerated fixation of the implant, and it was also believed that ACP was good for facilitating mechanical mismatch, improving fatigue behavior, and promoting faster bone remodeling and hard tissue attachment (Gross et al. 1998b). In consideration of the above points, HA coatings with a small amorphous content (<15%) would hence be preferred. It should be noted that, during the present HVOF spray study, the particles that have a large diameter (i.e., >30 μm) are only partially melted. Since the thermal transformation of HA generally occurred at the temperatures beyond 1000°C (Aoki 1994), the melted part of HA particle should contribute strongly to the transformation (relatively low temperature transformation by loss of water is also involved to a lesser extent). The present study indicates that during the HVOF spray, the heating of HA powders is rather limited, which further suggests the suitability of HVOF technique for HA coating deposition.

It is well known that a thermal-sprayed coating shows a layered structure, which has an accumulated character composed of individual splats. In order to better understand the coatings, researchers have extensively concentrated on the study of thermal sprayed splats (Bianchi et al. 1997; Montavon et al. 1995; Gougeon et al. 2001). Generally, in most cases, as the substrate temperature is low (e.g., <500°C), splat formation is an isolated procedure, which means minor influence of the subsequent splat on the phases of the former one. Therefore, the overall structure/phases and in vitro behavior of a bulk HA coating can arguably be intimately related to that of individual HA splats. A good understanding of a single HA splat would significantly contribute to the knowledge on structure and dissolution/precipitation mechanism of HA coatings. Therefore, a study on splats is essentially crucial toward establishing an understanding of individual splats' contribution to the phase composition of the thermal-sprayed coating and satisfactory control of phase composition of the coating through elucidation of phases' response within a splat.

In order to characterize the CP phases, which only differentiate slightly in structures, within a splat, a structure-sensitive and localized technique is required. Raman spectroscopy technique could provide information on the short- and intermediate-range ordering in the solids. It allows a direct and nondestructive detection from the sample surface with spatial resolution (micrometric) 100 times higher than the infrared resolution. Since the biological performances of the CP deposits, both in vitro and in vivo, are significantly dependent on their phases (Yang et al. 1997; Cleries et al. 2000), and the local phases play an extremely important role in determining their behaviors (Suominen et al. 1996), the study on the detailed structure information using the Raman spectroscopy technique could be essentially important. It indeed has been successful in using the technique for studying individual HA splats within minor zones (<50 μm) (Li et al. 2004c).

During the in vitro testing, the splats samples were incubated in the SBF solution for various durations to reveal their dissolution behavior. The Kokubo SBF (pH = 7.40) (Kokubo et al. 1990) was used for the in vitro incubation. The solution is composed of 142.0 mM Na^+,

5.0 mM K^+, 1.5 mM Mg^{2+}, 2.5 mM Ca^{2+}, 147.8 mM Cl^-, 4.2 mM HCO_3^-, 1.0 mM HPO_4^{2-}, and 0.5 mM SO_4^{2-}. The in vitro test was conducted in a continuously stirred bath containing distilled water with a stable temperature of 37°C.

As already reported (Li et al. 2004c), the Raman spectra at 200 to 900 cm^{-1} region of the thermal-sprayed HA splats (as-sprayed and heat-treated) with the comparison to those of reference materials are shown in Figure 4.18. While the Raman spectra of the plasma-sprayed HA splats (as-sprayed and heat-treated) at 900 to 2000 cm^{-1} region are typically shown in Figure 4.18d. It is noted that for the plasma-sprayed HA splats, there is a lack of obvious Raman shifts at the miscellaneous locations, as shown in Figure 4.18a(d,e,f) and Figure 4.18d(d,e,f). The broadening and featureless bands at vibration modes u_1 (~950 cm^{-1}), u_2 (~430 cm^{-1}), u_4 (~596 cm^{-1}), and the almost unobservable peaks of u_3 (~1032–1081 cm^{-1}) are typical features of ACP structure (Wen et al. 2000). These indicate the presence of uniform ACP phase within the splat; a result of fully melted HA powders during the plasma-spray process. Upon heat treatment, the bands of the respective vibration modes were narrowed, with an increased intensity and splitting of peaks (u_2: 428 and 447 cm^{-1}; u_3: 1029, 1044, and

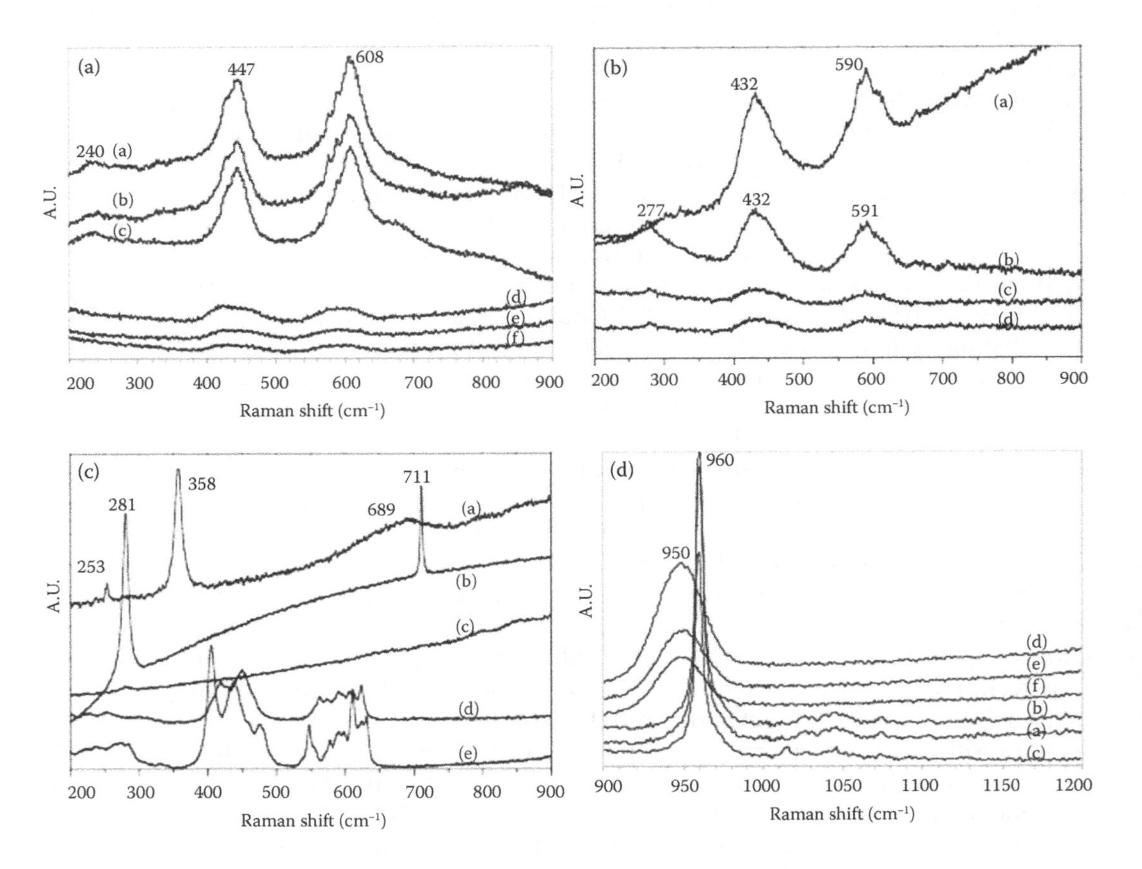

FIGURE 4.18
[a] Raman shifts of heat-treated HA splat (plasma-sprayed) at (a) middle, (b) edge, and (c) center, and as-plasma-sprayed HA splat at (d) edge, (e) middle, and (f) center of splat. [b] Raman shifts of a big HVOF splat at (a) center, (b) edge, and a small HVOF splat at (c) center and (d) edge. [c] Raman shifts of the reference materials (a) $Ca(OH)_2$, (b) $CaCO_3$, (c) CaO, (d) α-TCP and (e) β-TCP. [d] Raman shifts of a typical heat-treated HA splat (plasma-sprayed) at (a) middle, (b) edge, and (c) center, and as-plasma-sprayed HA splat at (d) edge, (e) middle, and (f) center. (From Li et al., *Acta Mater.*, 52, 445–453, 2004c. With permission.)

1075 cm^{-1}; and u_4: 575, 589, and 608 cm^{-1}). The main u_1 peak is also observed to have narrowed and shifted from center of ~950 to ~960 cm^{-1}, which is assigned to a typical feature of crystalline HA (Wen et al. 2000; Cuscó et al. 1998; Silva et al. 2002; Penel et al. 1997). The results from the Raman technique tallies with the postspray heat-treatment studies (Li et al. 2002a), as it was found that the heat treatment bought about full crystallization from ACP to HA. Likewise, it is proposed that for small HVOF splats, HA powders were near fully melted and decomposed during deposition. There is a uniform distribution of ACP, α-TCP, β-TCP, $CaCO_3$, and very small amount of unmelted HA. Overall, the Raman spectra of HVOF splats suggested that the HA powders are only partially decomposed, which must be attributed to their partially melted state during deposition. The highest degree of crystallinity exists at the center of the big splat, with HA and α-TCP being the two main phases. A small HVOF HA splat has a uniform spread of phases, with higher content of α-TCP and $CaCO_3$ and overall lower crystallinity, and TEM analysis has confirmed the presence of α- and β-TCP at the fringes of the splat (Figure 4.19) (Li et al. 2004c). The present Raman results correspond very well with the other findings on the influence of HA particle size on phase composition of resultant HVOF coating (Li et al. 2000).

The in vitro dissolution rates (Figure 4.20) together with the microstructural changes of the splats (Figure 4.21) confirm the possible phases within different locations revealed by the Raman detection (Li et al. 2004c). It was revealed that surrounding parts of the splats preferably dissolved into the SBF. It has been determined that the dissolution rate of different CP phases in the SBF is in the order HA $<$ CDHA $<$ OHA $<$ β-TCP $<$ α-TCP $<$ TTCP $<$ ACP (Ducheyne et al. 1993). The dissolution results of the splats fit very well with their Raman spectra at different zones. It is noted that even under full melt state of the sprayed HA powders, plasma spray (45–75 μm) and HVOF (20–45 μm) showed different effects on the dissolution behaviors of the splats (Li et al. 2004c). The results revealed that under the same full melt state, the dissolution rates of the resultant splats are different depending on the phases present within the splats. On the other hand, the obvious dissolution of the splats has indicated their remarkable biocompatibility. For the plasma-sprayed HA splats, 2 h resulted in full dissolution of the phases, while for HVOF-sprayed HA splats (fully melted), 4 h resulted in full dissolution of the phases (Li et al. 2004c). For the partially melted HVOF splats, a precipitation appeared after 24 h of incubation, and the dissolution reached a proximately stable state after 14 h, which indicates extremely low dissolvability

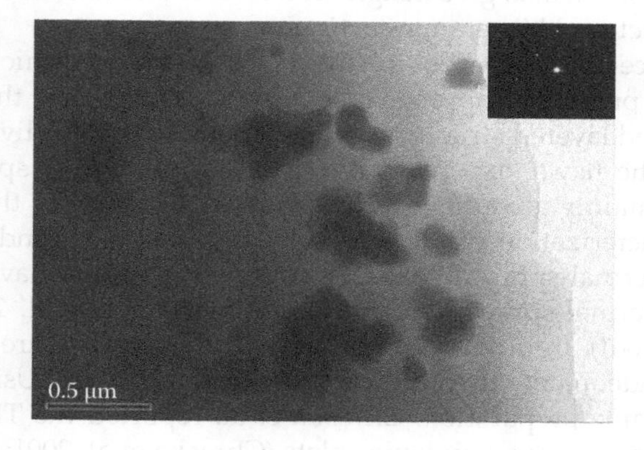

FIGURE 4.19
TEM microstructure of a single HA splat at its fringe showing presence of (a) α-TCP indicated by the selected diffraction pattern from its (001) zone axis, and (b) β-TCP indicated by the selected diffraction pattern from its $(\bar{1}11)$ zone axis. (From Li, H., et al. *Biomaterials*, 25, 3463–3471, 2004a. With permission.)

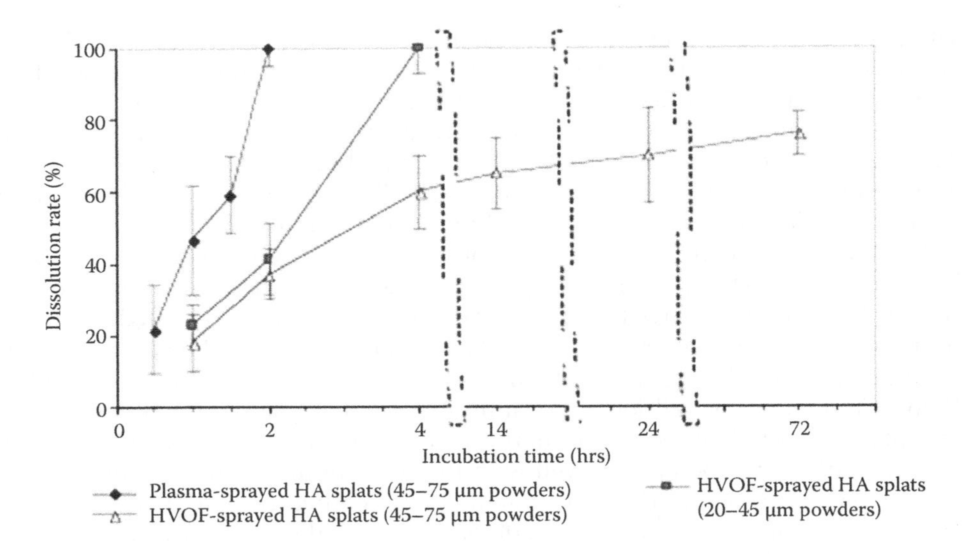

FIGURE 4.20
In vitro dissolution rates of the HA splats prepared by plasma and HVOF spraying. (Li et al. *Acta Mater.*, 52, 445–453, 2004c. With permission.)

of crystalline HA. According to the studies on phase transformations of HA at elevated temperatures (Liao et al. 1999; Zhou et al. 1993), the dissolution results further confirmed that HA decomposition mainly occurred within the melted part of the sprayed particles. In other words, there could be a relationship between melt states of HA particles during the spraying and phase composition of the resultant splat. A previous study (Khor et al. 2003b) and other ancillary results on dissolution behaviors of various CP phases (Cleries et al. 1998) have pointed out that, compared to crystalline HA, TCP, and TTCP, ACP preferably dissolved within SBF. It has also been found that for a structure with a complex phase composition, preferable dissolution still occurred, TCP preferably dissolved and it resulted in remarkable voids within a CP coating (Cleries et al. 1998).

Apart from the capability of elucidating the phase information of individual splats, the in vitro dissolution test can also give insight into formation mechanisms of the nanosized pores in the nanostructured bioceramic coatings.

In order to enhance the properties of the HA-based bioceramic coatings, structure improvement is the preferable approach. It is well known that the coatings actually exhibit an accumulated layered structure, which is composed of individual splats. Besides the contribution of the flaws (e.g., pores and cracks) and among splats, microstructure of individual splats mainly accounts for the apparent structure of the bulk coating. The microstructure characterization of a single splat is essentially fundamental for a good understanding of thermal-sprayed coatings. Interesting results have been reported on microstructure of thermal-sprayed splats (Pasandideh-Fard et al. 2002; Delplanque et al. 1997; Jiang et al. 2001). In order to reveal detailed microstructure features in a single splat, TEM must be adequately involved for the characterization. Using a special polishing tool for their sample preparation, Chraska et al. reported the TEM observations on cross sections of plasma-sprayed zirconia splats (Chraska et al. 2001; Chraska et al. 2002), which revealed columnar grain growth within the splats. Among the structure variables, which are responsible mainly for the mechanical properties, micropores play an important role (Sevostianov et al. 2000; Leigh et al. 1997; Li et al. 1997). The micropores within

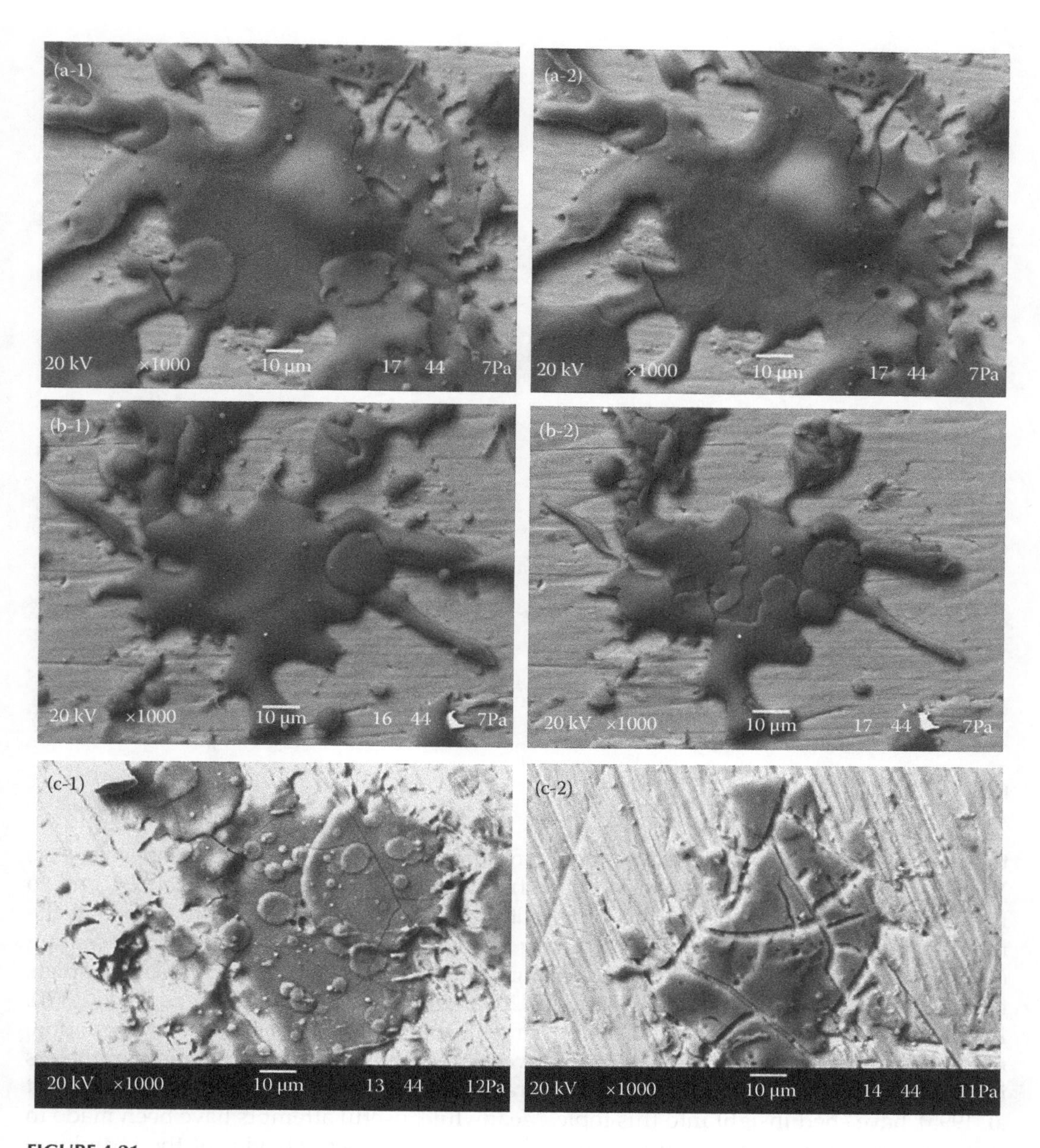

FIGURE 4.21
Typical histological changes of plasma-sprayed HA splats after 30 min (a-1 before, a-2 after) and 1 h (b-1 before, b-2 after) incubation showing obvious dissolution. The substrate temperature is lower than 100°C. Typical histological changes of HVOF-sprayed HA splats after (c) 2 h and (d, e) 3 days in vitro incubation showing remarkable influence of incubation time and particle's melt state on the obvious dissolution (-1 before incubation, -2 after incubation). The micrographs (d, e) have the same magnification as the micrographs (c). The substrate temperature is lower than 100°C. (From Li et al., *Acta Mater.*, 52, 445–453, 2004c. With permission.)

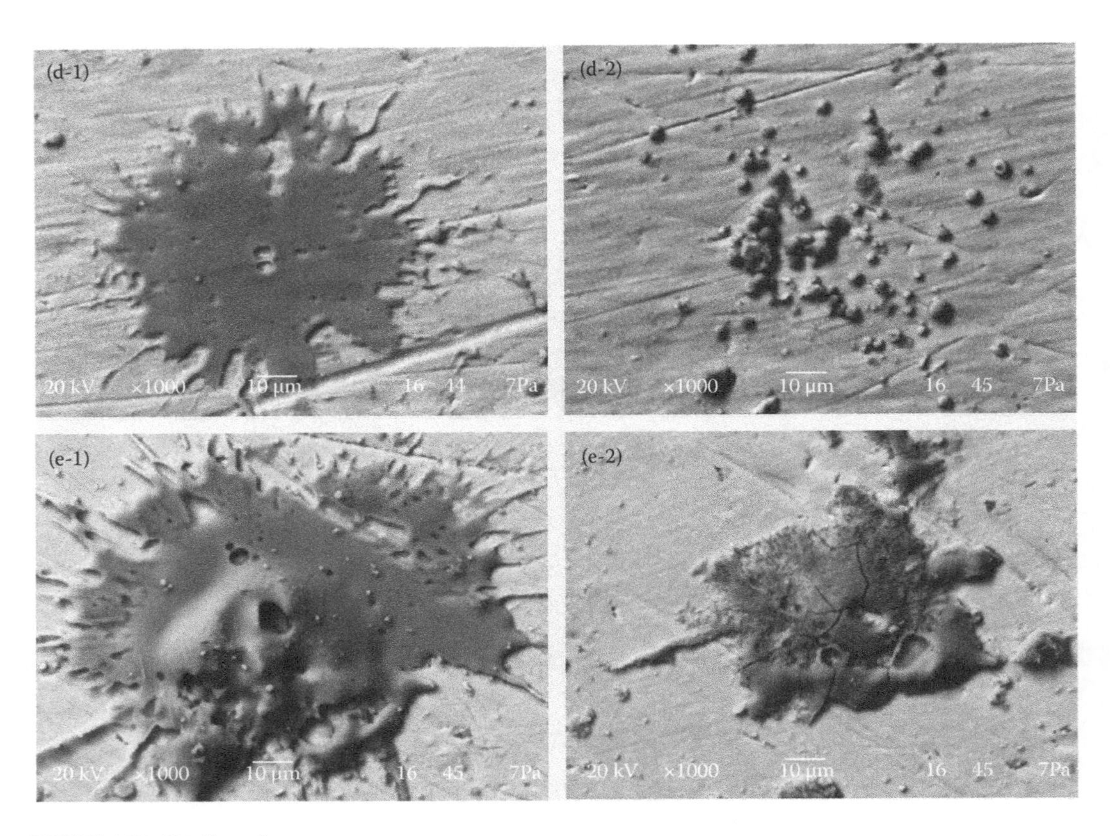

FIGURE 4.21 (Continued)

the thermal-sprayed coatings have significant effect on their mechanical properties (e.g., Young's modulus) (Sevostianov et al. 2000), fracture toughness (Callus et al. 1999), and so forth. The random existence of the pores within a coating was believed to be one of the main factors responsible for the anisotropy in mechanical performances of the coating (Sevostianov et al. 2000). To date, increasing studies on formation mechanism of splats have been conducted (Pasandideh-Fard et al. 2002; Sampath et al. 2001; Gougeon et al. 2001). Additionally, numerous constructive experimental investigations on the splat formation, mainly on clarification of relationships between splat morphology and spray parameters including substrate state (roughness, temperature, etc.) (Sampath et al. 2001; Montavon et al. 1995), have shed insight into this topic. Meanwhile, useful attempts have been made in recent years toward theoretical understanding of the impact behavior of the individual splats during thermal spray (Pasandideh-Fard et al. 2002; Gougeon et al. 2001; Bertagnolli et al. 1997) even though the assumptions for the simulations more or less restricted their valid applications.

Due to the phase transformation of HA during coating formation to tricalcium phosphate (TCP), tetracalcium phosphate (TTCP), CaO, or even amorphous calcium phosphate (ACP) (Gross et al. 1998c; McPherson et al. 1995; Li et al. 2000), full dissolution of the subsequent splat is possible through controlling the dissolution/precipitation procedures during the test (Li et al. 2004c).

Small pores are observed from the surface of the splats prepared by both HVOF and plasma-spray techniques. Typical views under SEM suggest the size of the pores to be 1 to

10 μm (Li et al. 2004a). Furthermore, three categories of the pores exist in the splat: open pores, through-thickness pores, and sealed pores (Figure 4.22) (Li et al. 2004a).

It is noted that for the starting HA particles, a porous structure was demonstrated (Figure 4.5b). During plasma spraying of the HA powders, the particles were assumed to be fully melted, which can be deduced from the complete flattening of the splats. The formation of sealed pores was likely to be the result of a rate balance between gas bubble escaping and particle solidification. Under the same spray conditions, formation of either open pores or through-thickness pores could be attributed to the locations of the original gas bubbles. Partial-melt state of the HA particles during HVOF spraying could be responsible in part for the difference in pore morphology within a splat from that deposited by plasma spray. An earlier study on assessing the significance of the melt state of HVOF-sprayed HA revealed that typically, the melt fraction in the particles ranged from 20% to over 90% depending on the starting particle size. Particles around 20 μm would likely to be over 80% melted. Therefore, apart from porosity of starting powders, the melt state of the particles during spraying is an important factor influencing the final pore structure of bulk coating.

The subsequent droplet (or partially melted particle) could have remarkable influence on the open pores as exhibited by the former splat due to the considerably high velocity of the droplet. Typical morphology changes of the folded splats induced by the in vitro incubation for 1.5 h are shown in Figure 4.23 (Li et al. 2004a). Surprisingly, a trace of liquid filling

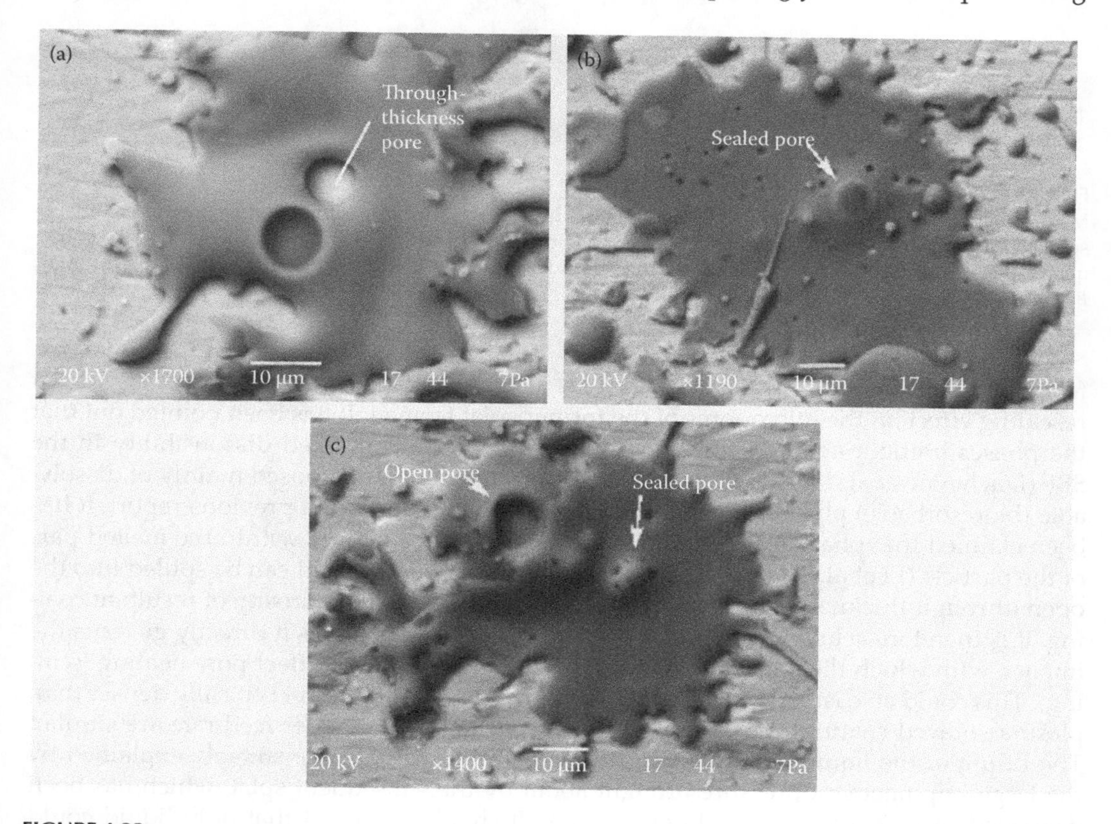

FIGURE 4.22
Typical plasma sprayed HA splats showing three types of pores: open pore, through-thickness pore, and sealed pore. (From Li et al., *Biomaterials*, 25, 3463–3471, 2004a. With permission.)

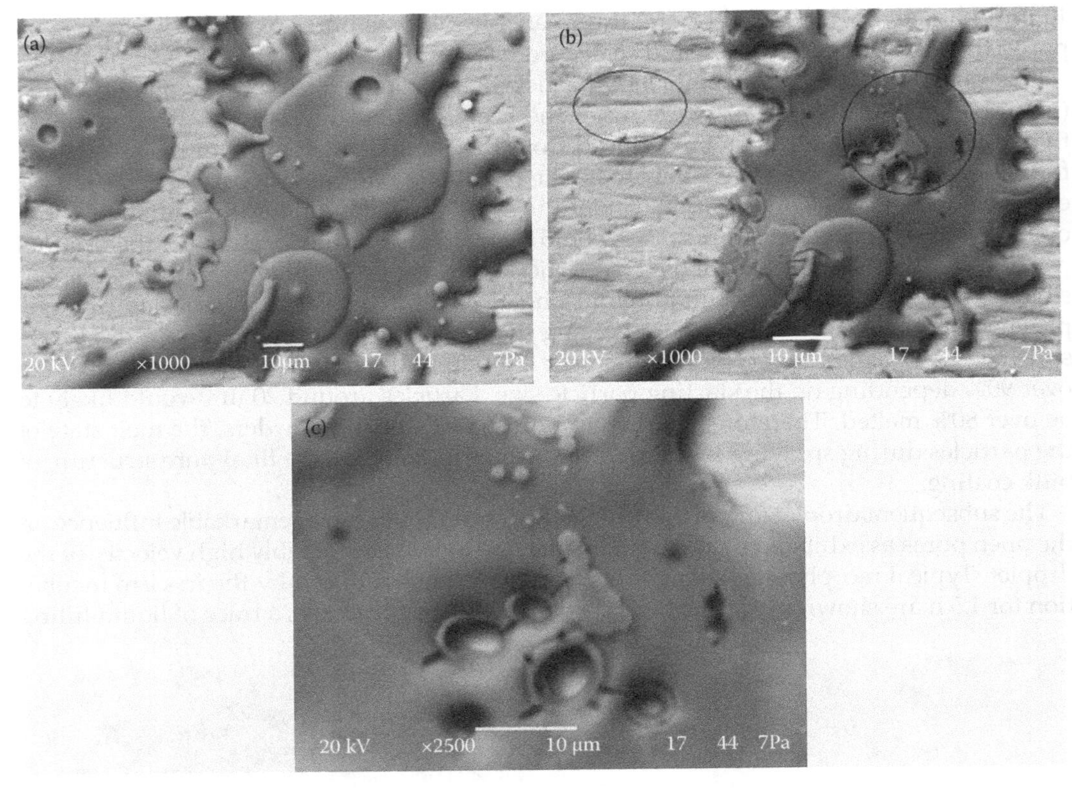

FIGURE 4.23
Microstructure changes of folded HA splats after 1.5-h incubation in vitro showing a healing effect of subsequent splat on the open pores of former splat, (a) before the incubation, (b) after the incubation, the subsequent splat dissolved into the SBF entirely, and (c) under higher magnification of image (b). (From Li et al., *Biomaterials*, 25, 3463–3471, 2004a. With permission.)

from the subsequent droplet is revealed (Li et al. 2004a). The folded splat shows significant resealing effect on the micropores of the former splat formed. It has been pointed out that the phases brought about by the HA transformation have marked dissolvability in the SBF (Ducheyne et al. 1993). It is clear that the injected part is composed mainly of dissolvable (bioresorbable) phases, such as TTCP, TCP, and ACP, and in a previous report, it has been claimed that phase transformation of HA took place mainly within the melted part of the particle (Li et al. 2000). Liquid with high impingement speed can be spilled into the open (through-thickness) pores easily, and hence, decreases the porosity of resultant coating. It is therefore acknowledged that particle velocity is crucial as it directly governs the impact, with which the particle impinges on the former splat to affect pore healing (sealing). This could at least be the partial reason why HVOF coatings are typically denser than plasma-sprayed coatings, given that powder feedstock and powder feed-rate are similar. The filling of the liquid materials into the micropores can also be suitably explained by the large impingement pressure brought about by the subsequent splat, which has been described in an earlier report (Li et al. 2003). It should be noted that only liquid could achieve such improvement. With regard to the healing effect, it can be concluded that only the sealed pores and the unbonded areas among splats contribute predominately to the overall porosity of a bulk coating. Melt state and velocity of the sprayed particles during spray may play the most important role in determining the overall porosity through their influence on pore structure.

Mechanical Properties and Relationship between Nanostructure and Properties

Due to the anomalous inhomogeneous-layered structure, the coatings show a significant dependence of their mechanical performances on the microstructure. Influence of the nanostructures on the mechanical properties such as adhesive strength and Young's modulus is always an important issue that required significant research efforts prior to the applications of the coatings. It was found that for the nanostructured HA coatings the nanostructures contribute to increased Young's modulus values (Li et al. 2006). With the increase of the melted area in the spayed particles (hence the relative content of the nanostructures, HVOF3 vs. HVOF1 in Figure 4.24), the Young's modulus of the corresponding

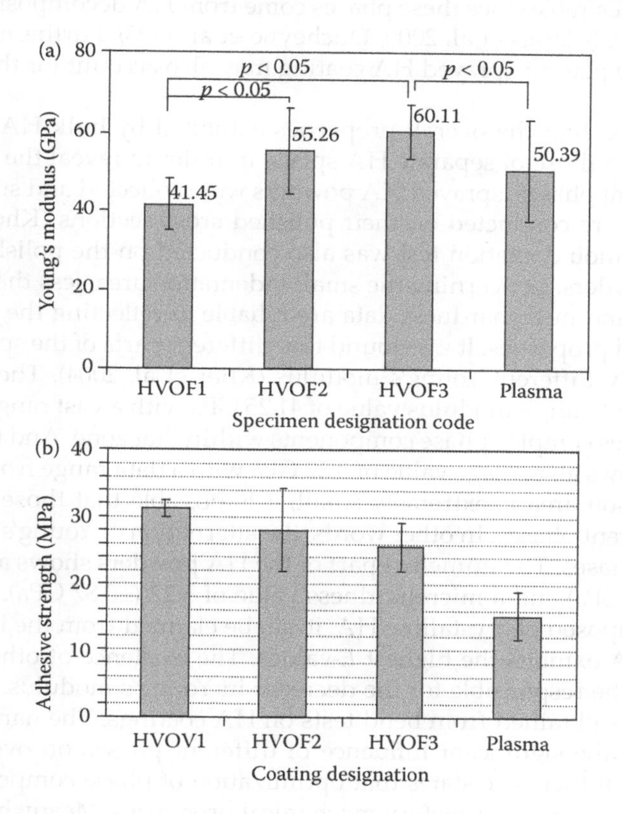

FIGURE 4.24
(a) Young's modulus of the coatings, and (b) adhesive strength of the coatings (HVOF1, HVOF HA coating [50 ± 10 μm powder]; HVOF2, HVOF HA coating [40 ± 10 μm powder]; HVOF3, HVOF HA coating [30 ± 10 μm powder]; Plasma, plasma HA coating (50 ± 10 μm powder). (From Li, H., Khor, K.A., *Surf. Coat. Technol.*, 201, 2147–2154, 2006. With permission.)

coatings increases. However, they showed detrimental effect on adhesive strength (Figure 4.24b). Tensile failure analysis has suggested an entire adhesive failure mode. This in turn indicates that the coating/substrate interface plays a key role in determining the adhesion. The difference of the mechanical properties can be correlated to the nanostructural features (Li et al. SCT 2006). The perpendicular-to-substrate grains might have changed the residual stresses at the coating/substrate interface, or they weakened the mechanical interlocking of the coating with the rough substrate. For a high adhesive strength, formation of the grains with hexagonal prismatic morphology near to the coating/substrate interface must be avoided. The mechanism why the nanostructures benefit high Young's modulus is not clear yet. The presence of nanosized pores among the nanosized grains might be responsible for the increased value, as it has been discussed that irregular pores and large pores can result in decreased modulus (Sevostianov et al. 2000; Shen et al. 1995). Furthermore, high packing density of constituent atom exhibit high values of elastic modulus (Soga 1982). Even though the plasma-sprayed HA coating comprises compatible content of nanostructures, both the low Young's modulus and adhesive strength might be related to the phases present in the coating and the low velocity of in-flight particles (this brought about high porosity). It must be noted that within the nanostructures in the HA splats, there are a lot of phases apart from HA (e.g., ACP, α-TCP, β-TCP) being revealed. These may not be desirable since these phases come from HA decomposition and have less bioactivity than HA (Cleries et al. 2000; Ducheyne et al. 1993). Furthermore, the presence of the phases in the plasma-sprayed HA coating may also account for the low modulus of the coating.

It should be noted that the overall properties exhibited by bulk HA coating could be mainly attributed to those of separate HA splats. In order to reveal the approximate contribution of different phases, sprayed HA powders were collected and subsequently nanoindentation tests were conducted on their polished cross sections (Khor et al. 2004). For comparison, the nanoindentation test was also conducted on the polished cross sections of starting HA powders. Concerning the small indentation area, less than 9×10^4 nm^2, the Young's modulus and microhardness data are reliable in reflecting the relations between microstructure and properties. It was found that different parts of the sprayed HA particle exhibits remarkably different Young's modulus (Khor et al. 2004). The resolidified zone exhibits an average Young's modulus value of 41.25 GPa with a vast range from 23.1 to 65.3 GPa, which indicates complex phase components within that zone. And the corresponding microhardness shows an average value of 3.37 GPa with a data range from 1.72 to 5.93 GPa. Since the indentation area is extremely small, it is possible that those values reflect the properties of different phases. In other words, the alternation of Young's modulus is attributed to different phases. The unmelted part of the HA powders shows a Young's modulus value of 83.9 (±9.4 GPa) and a microhardness value of 5.22 (±0.87 GPa). Since the starting powders were composed of crystalline HA, it can be claimed from the indentation results that crystalline HA exhibits the highest E-values. The existence of other phases, such as α-TCP, ACP, could be responsible for the decrease in Young's modulus. The results correspond well to those obtained from bend tests on HA coatings. The nanoindentation tests further confirmed the significant influence of different phases on overall properties of resultant coatings. It therefore states that optimization of phase components in HA coating is a useful way toward satisfactory mechanical properties. Meanwhile, it is noted that compared to the nanoindentation result on bulk HA coating, which exhibited a Young's modulus of 118 (±5.21 GPa), the sprayed HA particles showed low Young's modulus. The residual stress formed during coating formation could be responsible for the increased E values exhibited by HA coatings.

The major problems pertaining to the HA-coated implants are their poor long-term functional service due to the failure of the coatings. Extensive studies revealed that the long-term functional performance of the CP coated implants was influenced significantly by the microstructure of the coatings (Suominen et al. 1996; Szivek et al. 1996). In addition, HA coating has a potential problem of introducing an additional interface into the implant system. The interface between HA coating and metallic alloy is critical in determining the reliability of the implant (Shaw et al. 1998; Piveteau et al. 1999; Gross et al. 1998c; Bonfield 1987; Krauser et al. 1991). Studies have reported that fracture often occurred at the HA/substrate interface rather than at the bone/HA interface from a direct shear loading (Wang et al. 1993b; Inadome et al. 1995; Hayashi et al. 1993). The analysis of malfunctional dental implants evidenced the failure to be primarily located at HA/metal interface (Krauser et al. 1991). Consequently, estimation of the interface properties is essential for evaluating the HA-coated implants. When used as dental and orthopedic implants, due to identified clinical environment, HA coatings experience compound stresses, which can include shear, bending, tensile, and compressive forces. Among all the mechanical performances required, adhesion and fracture toughness are the most critical variables. Besides the adhesive strength, strain energy release rate is also capable of evaluating the interface (Chung et al. 1997). The strain energy density theory has been extended to study the growth characteristics of three-dimensional cracks within coatings (Sih 1991). Four-point bend test was usually used to determine the strain energy release rate of the coatings at the coating/substrate interface upon the considerations that the interface between the two different materials is usually the weakest part and failure initiated from an interfacial defect was often observed (Howard et al. 1991, 1993, 1994). The four-point bend test to evaluate the bonding between coating and substrate has the advantages of providing stresses more like those experienced in vivo of HA coatings (Haman et al. 1997). As discussed, the strain energy release rate is an appropriate variable for evaluating the energy of the inception of cleavage and dislocation emission along the interface. It is essential to relate the resistance of the material to crack propagation to a parameter that can characterize the fracture toughness of the material. With regard to the complex stresses at the coating/substrate interface, it is not easy to get the fracture toughness to represent interface property. Generally used variable as an alternative of the fracture toughness is based on the determination of strain energy release rate, G. For thermal-sprayed coatings, the four-point bend test was believed to be an effective technique for the determination of critical strain energy release rate (G_{ss}) at the coating/substrate interface (Howard et al. 1994; Clyne et al. 1996). The specimen loaded by four-point bend for the G_{ss} determination is schematically depicted in Figure 4.25. G can be

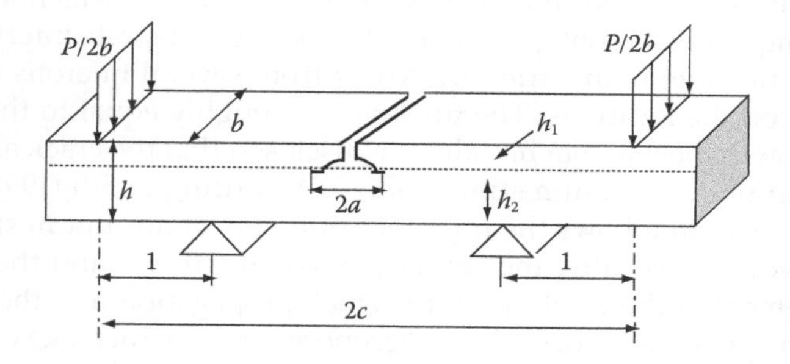

FIGURE 4.25
Schematic depiction of the coating/substrate bimaterial specimen for 4-point bend test (h1, coating thickness; h2, substrate thickness). (From Li et al., *Eng. Fract. Mech.*, 74, 1894–1903, 2007a. With permission.)

obtained from the strain energy, U, per unit cross section according to beam theory under plane strain conditions:

$$G = \frac{\partial U}{\partial a} \tag{4.6}$$

where a is the propagated crack length. G_{ss} during crack propagation can be expressed in the nondimensional form (Charalambides et al. 1989; Murakami 1992):

$$G_{ss} = \frac{M^2\left(1 - v_2^2\right)}{2E_2}\left(\frac{1}{I_2} - \frac{\lambda}{I_c}\right) \tag{4.7}$$

where E is Young's modulus, I is the inertia moment, v is Poisson's ratio, and

$$M = Pl/2b \tag{4.8}$$

$$\lambda = E_2(1 - v_1^2)/E_1(1 - v_2^2) \tag{4.9}$$

$$I_c = h_1^3/12 + \lambda h_2^3/12 + \lambda h_1 h_2 (h_1 + h_2)^2/4(h_1 + \lambda h_2) \tag{4.10}$$

$$I_2 = h_2^3/12 \tag{4.11}$$

In order to determine G_{ss}, both the applied load and the displacement of the loading points were continuously monitored and recorded. The specimen was loaded until both cracks had propagated out to the internal loading points. Stable crack advance should ideally occur at a constant load, whereas a crack burst causes a sharp drop in load between two values having a mean of P_c (Howard et al. 1993).

Critical strain energy release rate value of ~1.1 kJ m^{-2} was revealed for the nanostructured coatings and no significant difference was revealed among the coatings with different nanostructural features (Figure 4.26) (Li et al. 2007a). While the different G_{ss} values can be well explained by the nanostructures of the coatings, in order to reveal the effect of coating microstructure on the G_{ss}, failure mechanism was discussed through observing the worn morphology after bending by SEM (Li et al. 2007a). It was noted that the crack induced by bending stress did not grow along the coating/substrate interface. HA coatings remained on the substrate with varied thickness from several microns to approximately 25 μm depending on the locations. The thickness is roughly equal to that of one splat or two. The crack growth mechanism has already disclosed that the crack always propagates along the direction with minimum strain energy. According to Sih (1991), once a crack is initiated the fracture path follows the trajectory of points of minimum strain energy density remarkably well. Concerning the complex residual stresses and the applied stresses from bending moment at the crack front, the crack propagation into the coating side can be explained by the possible flaws such as micropores and microcracks within the coating. Observation of the microstructure from the cross sections of the coatings gives insight into the flaws inside the coating. There is clear evidence of micro-/nanosized pores and unbonded area between the HA splats. The sizes of the pores in the nanostructured HA

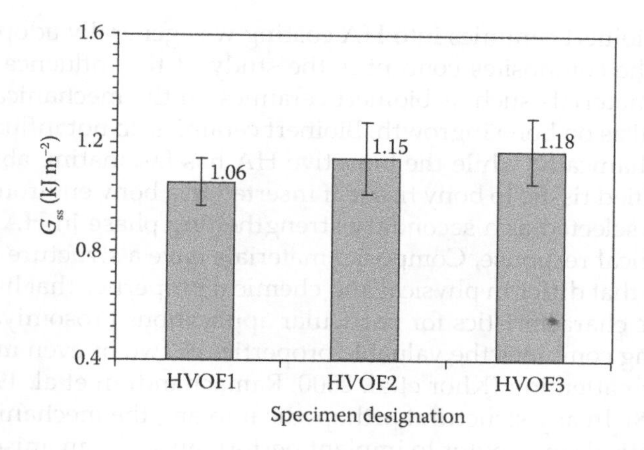

FIGURE 4.26
Critical strain energy release rate (G_{ss}) of the HA coatings obtained from 4-point bend test. (HVOF1, HA coating made from 50 ± 10 μm powder; HVOF2, HA coating made from 40 ± 10 μm powder; HVOF3, HA coating made from 30 ± 10 μm powder.) (From Li et al., *Eng. Fract. Mech.*, 74, 1894–1903, 2007a. With permission.)

coatings are in the range of ~20 to 110 nm (Li et al. 2007a). These should act as the crack path and accelerate the crack propagation as well during the bending. Typical failure morphology reveals that there is no evidence of cracking parallel to the surface of lamellae. The trace of the brittle fracture suggests that the existed defects at the splats' interface might have been connected together as the propagation path of the crack. Furthermore, the size and distribution of pores also play an important role in influencing both the crack initiation and propagation processes (Ishihara et al. 2000); thus failure would occur when sufficient micropores have been connected by an unbonded area between splats and translamella microcracks to separate that region from the remainder of the coating. The effect of micropores located along the crack propagation path on the fracture toughness has been discussed by Leguillon (1997). It was believed that the crack growth was made of successive sudden jumps at each void along the crack path. Thus, the existence of micropores at the crack propagation path (splats' interface in this case) is detrimental to the fracture property. Furthermore, it has been found that the thickness of the retained coating is very much consistent with that of one splat or two. Nevertheless, the cohesion inside individual splats is much better than that between individual HA splats, which also accounts for the bending crack propagation along the splats' interface. Since the fracture occurred within the coating, the existence of the hexagonal nanosized grains did not show obvious influence on the crack growth.

Nanostructured HA-Based Composite Coatings

HA materials are poor in the property, which can lead to the instability of surface crystals in the presence of body fluids and local loading. In addition, HA cannot withstand applied loading force (de Putter et al. 1987). Especially in a body environment, the mechanical strength of HA is further reduced considerably by fatigue (Heimke et al. 1987). Therefore, HA needs to be strengthened. A bond-coat made from bioinert ceramic and the incorporation of bioinert ceramics into HA coating was generally adopted. An important aspect based on the composites concept is the study of the influence of the addition of other osteogenic materials such as bioinert ceramics on the mechanical performances of HA coating as well as on bone ingrowth. Bioinert ceramics do not influence the surrounding tissue biomechanically, while the bioactive HA has fascinating ability to stimulate a deposition of calcified tissue to bony tissue if inserted in a bony environment. The bioinert ceramic is always selected as a secondary strengthening phase in HA coatings owing to its inherent biological response. Composite materials have a structure comprising two or more components that differ in physical and chemical properties that have been combined to provide specific characteristics for particular applications (Yosomiya et al. 1990). Since a composite coating combines the valuable properties of two or even more components, it has attracted much attention (Khor et al. 2000; Ramachandran et al. 1998; Gui et al. 2001; Sordelet et al. 1998). In any structural orthopedic implant, the mechanical behavior of the composites is a critical contributor to implant performance. As an anisotropic, inhomogeneous material, the mechanical behavior of the composite coating is very complex and is a function of the synergistic properties of the second phase, matrix, second phase/matrix interfacial bond, and of geometric properties such as particle size distribution and content in the matrix. Generally, the strengthening mechanism in the composite coating was believed as (Steinhauser et al. 1997):

- The second phase influences coating structure during coating formation.
- The changes of coating property through the mere existence of the second phase.

The distribution, content, shape, and size of the additives can all affect the eventual performances of composite coatings.

Because of the pronounced brittleness of monolithic HA ceramic, there have been many efforts toward improving the strength and the toughness of load-bearing biomedical parts made of HA by adding a second phase. Many ceramic materials have been used in prostheses, especially in load-bearing hip prostheses and dental implants owing to the combination of excellent corrosion resistance, good biocompatibility, high wear resistance, and reasonable strength. They do not influence the surrounding tissue biomechanically and they have a significant level of biocompatibility (Gualtieri et al. 1987). Among the materials used, bioinert ceramics are good at the properties of biocompatibility, biostability, corrosion resistance, compressive strength, impact resistance, fatigue resistance, hardness, scratch resistance, surface polishing, wettability by fluids, sterilization, and tribology. The diverse use of bioinert ceramics in clinical application is mainly due to the following valuable aspects (Heimke et al. 1987):

- Dense, high-purity ceramic does not influence adjacent tissue biochemically.
- Bioinert ceramic does not stimulate immune reactions.
- No material-induced sarcomas could be detected.
- The remodeling processes of body tissue adjacent to the ceramic implant are the same as in fracture healing if the same precautions of relative rest along the interface are observed.
- The direct contact of well-proliferating bony tissue can be maintained during functional loading at all those interfaces along which relative movements can be excluded. A sufficiently dense arrangement of surface undulations can prevent relative movements even along tangentially loaded interfaces by interlocking.

Even though it was found that a bioinert ceramic such as pure alumina prosthesis (Heimann et al. 1998) could not reach an intimate contact with bone owing to its bioinert surface, it is capable of impeding possible diffusion of metal alloy implant to the tissue. Due to the attractive properties of the bioinert ceramics, the clinical-purposed application of these materials has attracted many investigations (Murakami et al. 1996; Patel et al. 1995; Toni et al. 1987; Trentani et al. 1987; Drouin et al. 1997; Labat et al. 1995). They have been widely employed as the skeleton component for maintaining external and internal load in a composite implant.

Many types of bioinert ceramics have been explored as implant materials. Alumina was first used as an implant material in 1964 (Heimke et al. 1987), and some of its modifications were studied experimentally in the late 1960s. Since then, more and more ceramics were attempted for clinical applications. Partially stabilized zirconia has high mechanical strength, low radioactivity, low crystal phase transformation, and high toughness. However, phase transformation among its multiphases—cubic, monoclinic, and tetragonal—can cause the degradation of mechanical strength, thus decreasing its reliability as an implant. Many factors could influence the transformation, even though the tensile stress does not affect it (Fujisawa et al. 1996).

Generally, bioceramics are used as bond coat (Kurzweg et al. 1998; Lamy et al. 1996) or additives to form a composite structure with HA. Bond coat was capable of effectively improving the adhesion properties of HA coatings (Cheang et al. 1996b; Heimann et al. 1998; Tsui et al. 1998). An increase in an order of 20%, up to 15.49 MPa with a bond coat of Ca_2SiO_4 has been reported (Lamy et al. 1996). The adhesion was even further increased by the introduction of Ti bond coat with a thickness of 100 μm (Tsui et al. 1998). In addition to its contribution to the adhesion improvement, which is mostly considered in clinical applications of the ceramic coatings, bond coat could also (Hench 1987; Kurzweg et al. 1998; Lamy et al. 1996):

1. Prevent direct contact between Ti and HA since this is believed to catalyze thermal transformation of HA toward tri- or tetracalcium phosphate or even nonbiotolerant CaO
2. Reduce the release of metal ions from the substrate to surrounding living tissue that has been shown to induce massive hepatic degeneration in mice and impaired development of human osteoblasts
3. Reduce the thermal gradient at the substrate/coating interface caused by the rapid quenching of molten particle splats that leads to deposition of ACP with a concurrent decrease in resorption resistance and hence to reduced in vivo performance
4. Prevent a steep gradient in the coefficients of thermal expansion between substrate and coating that promotes the formation of strong tensile forces in the coating giving rise to crack generation, chipping, and/or delamination
5. Cushion damage by cracking and delamination of the coating initiated by cyclic micromotions of the implant during movement of patient in the initial phase of the healing process

Therefore, it is highly desirable to engineer the substrate/HA coating interface in such a way that by application of a suitable thin biocompatible bond coat layer the advantages addressed above can be realized (Oonishi et al. 1987).

Accompanying with the positive effect brought about by the bond coat, such as the improvement of peeling strength by 20% to 100% (Heimann et al. 1998; Lamy et al. 1996;

Suchanek et al. 1997), there are still some limitations. During the implant's service, the through-thickness direction of HA coating is important for the apposition of bony tissue and the contact zone should be of sufficient wear-resistance property that appears to be necessary for the implant (Gualtieri et al. 1987). Also the incorporation of the bond coat brings about complex operation and extra expense. Even if the functionally graded coating (FGC) that comes from the extension of bond coat can fulfill the biological requirements, there still exist problems of cost and production complexity. Unique incorporation of reinforcements could be more effective.

The tribological property of some bioinert ceramics used as prosthesis has been experimentally investigated (Murakami et al. 1996; Fruh et al. 1997; Patel et al. 1997). Many materials selected to strengthen sintered HA and optimum selections were determined according to phase composition, biocompatibility and phase transformation (Suchanek et al. 1997). It was reported that the incorporation of some glass into HA exhibited a major effect on HA structure (Lopes et al. 1998). Some useful results were also obtained on the reliability of alumina implantation in vivo (Gualtieri et al. 1987; Toni et al. 1987; Trentani et al. 1987).

For pure titanium alloy implant, it was usually found that corrosion was a considerable factor in influencing the duration of the implant in bony tissue. Therefore, in many cases, surface oxidization of the Ti alloy was utilized to promote corrosion resistance (Lausmaa et al. 1986; Lausmaa et al. 1989). Many methods such as thermal oxidization have been employed to produce the oxide layer on the metallic surface. It was found that biocompatibility of the eventual implant seemed to associate with the highly stable protecting surface oxide (Lausmaa et al. 1986). However, all these processes were limited by the thin layer thickness and as a result, the implant may lose its surface protective layer in the long term.

Studies showed that titania ceramics were potentially useful as porous cell carrier material whose properties, such as good permeability, serve to enhance cell vitality (Blum et al. 1996). The potential advantage offered by a porous ceramic implant is its inertness combined with the mechanical stability of the highly convoluted interface developed when bone grows into the pores of the ceramic. In porous materials, the exchange area is high (depending on porosity), which requires a high chemical resistance in biological media. This condition can be met by titania. Study on sintered HA/titania composites revealed effect of sintering temperature on the phases of the composites (Figure 4.27) (Aoki 1994). The effect of different titania materials on cell growth and distribution has also been reported (Blum et al. 1996; Kanagaraja et al. 2001). Results indicate that the porosity of the ceramics should be optimized to levels where release of wear particles does not occur during service. The porous structure needs very coarse powder with a narrow size distribution, coarse grain

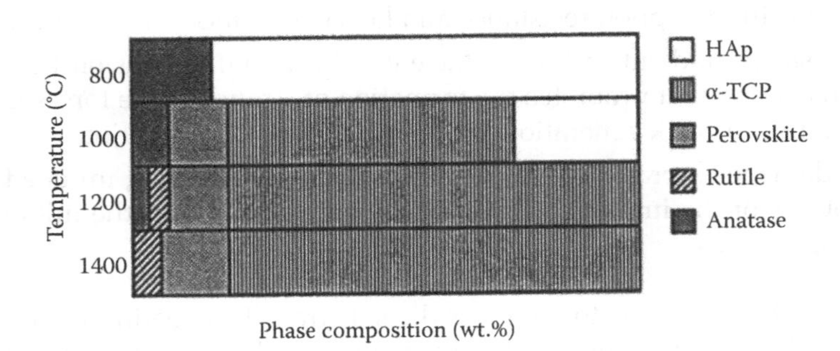

FIGURE 4.27
Influence of TiO_2 on the phase composition of sintered HA. (From Aoki, H., Ishiyaku EuroAmerica, Inc., Tokyo, St. Louis, 1994. With permission.)

sizes lead to low sintering rates, thus the development of pores can be controlled (Eckert et al. 1995). However, commercial titania powder is very fine, around 1 μm. Therefore, certain methods such as thermal and mechanical processing are required to produce the sintered porous TiO_2 materials. The mechanical requirements of the prostheses, however, severely restrict the use of low-strength porous ceramics to nonload-bearing applications. The environmental sensitivity of the ceramics and the loss of strength of porous ceramics with aging are negative aspects (Hench et al. 1982). In vitro investigation of nanoalumina and nanotitania powders has shown the presence of a critical grain size for osteoblast adhesion for the powder (Webster et al. 1999). The study provides evidence of the ability of nanophase alumina and titania to simulate material characteristics of physiological bone that enhance protein interactions and subsequent osteoblast adhesion. Therefore, the composite coating made from titania and HA has attracted attention owing to its ability of combining advantages of the both materials (Weng et al. 1994; Vu et al. 1997). It was believed that titania could work as a skeleton in the composite system. Additionally, according to the formula utilized for coating fracture toughness determination (Beshish et al. 1993), the high Young's modulus of titania material could be useful for the improvement of the fracture toughness of HA, which is very critical for the reliability of the implant for long-term use. Influence of an addition of titanium dioxide on thermal properties of sintered HA has attracted significant attention (Weng et al. 1994; Vu et al. 1997) because titania ceramics are potentially useful as porous cell carrier material whose properties, such as good permeability and high biocompatability, serve to enhance cell vitality. The efficacy of different titanium dioxide materials on cell growth and distribution has been studied (Blum et al. 1996). Study showed that the as-sprayed pure HA coating is mainly composed of crystalline HA and α-TCP (Li et al. 2002b). The crystalline HA, anatase TiO_2, α-TCP, amorphous calcium phosphate, as well as some rutile TiO_2, $CaTiO_3$, and CaO are detected simultaneously in both the composite coatings (Figure 4.28) (Li et al. 2003). The chemical reaction between HA and titania during the thermal spraying was revealed by a high-temperature DSC analysis to be ~1400°C (Li et al. 2002b). And indeed a reaction layer between the HA and titania was distinguished by TEM (Figure 4.29) (Li et al. 2003).

Despite the advantages introduced by TiO_2 addition, a certain negative effect was revealed in the HA/titania composites (Weng et al. 1994; Vu et al. 1997). The main problem is that the existence of TiO_2 can result in the decomposition of HA at a relatively low temperature, such as the considerable decrease in the decomposition temperature from 1300°C to 1400°C for pure HA to 750°C to 1150°C for HA containing oxide additives (Vu et al. 1997). Figure 4.30 shows the influence of the addition of titania powder on phase composition of sintered HA under high sintering temperatures. It shows that the higher the temperature, the more easily the decomposition of HA and chemical reaction between the two components can occur. Although the negative effect of the ceramic additives must be considered, the influence can be neglected if the processing temperature is far lower than the decomposition temperature. HVOF could achieve this due to its relatively low flame temperature. Fortunately, the addition of titania did not trigger obvious deterioration of biocompatibility of the coatings (Li 2002), while the mechanical properties were significantly enhanced (Li et al. 2002b).

Based on the observations, an impact formation model has been proposed (biomat-impact), which correlates the parameters of the in-flight titania particles with the impact formation on preflattened HA splat by elasmic/plasmic deformation (Li et al. 2003). According to the research on HA/titania composite coating (Li et al. 2002b; Li et al. 2003), the addition of TiO_2 is found to improve Young's modulus, fracture toughness, and shear strength of HVOF-sprayed HA-based coatings. This consequence is attributed to the weak chemical

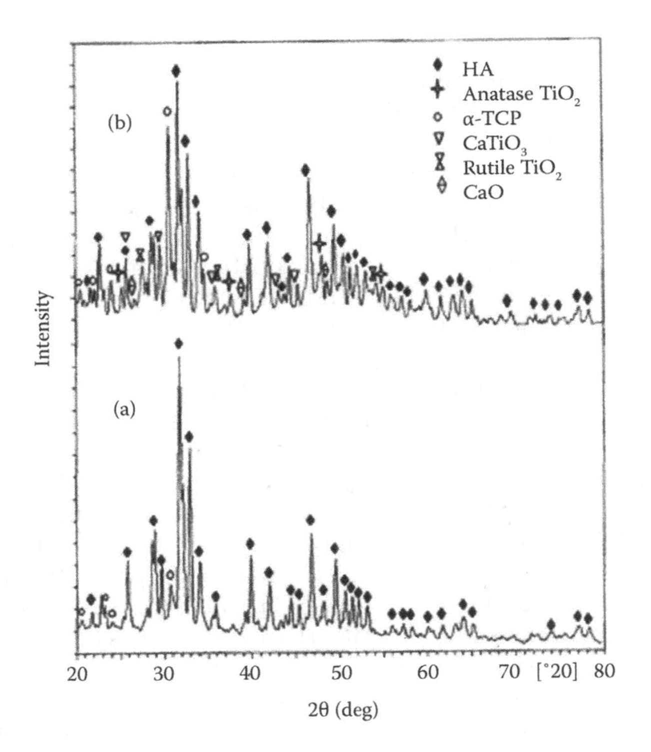

FIGURE 4.28
XRD patterns of the HVOF sprayed (a) pure HA coating and (b) HA + 20 vol.% TiO_2 composite coating. (From Li et al., *Biomaterials*, 24, 949–957, 2003. With permission.)

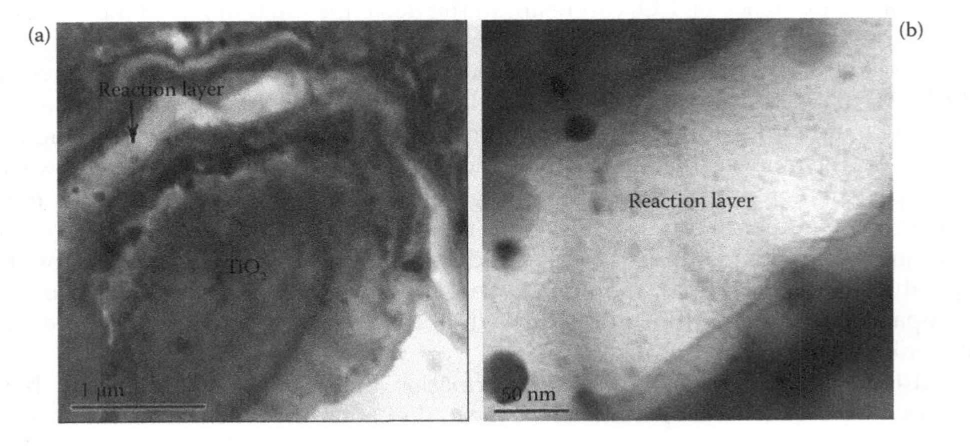

FIGURE 4.29
Morphology of the HA/titania composite structure showing (a) titania is surrounded by a chemical reaction layer, and the enlarged bright interface zone (b) showing that the reaction layer has a thickness of around 140 nm. (From Li et al., *Biomaterials*, 24, 949–957, 2003. With permission.)

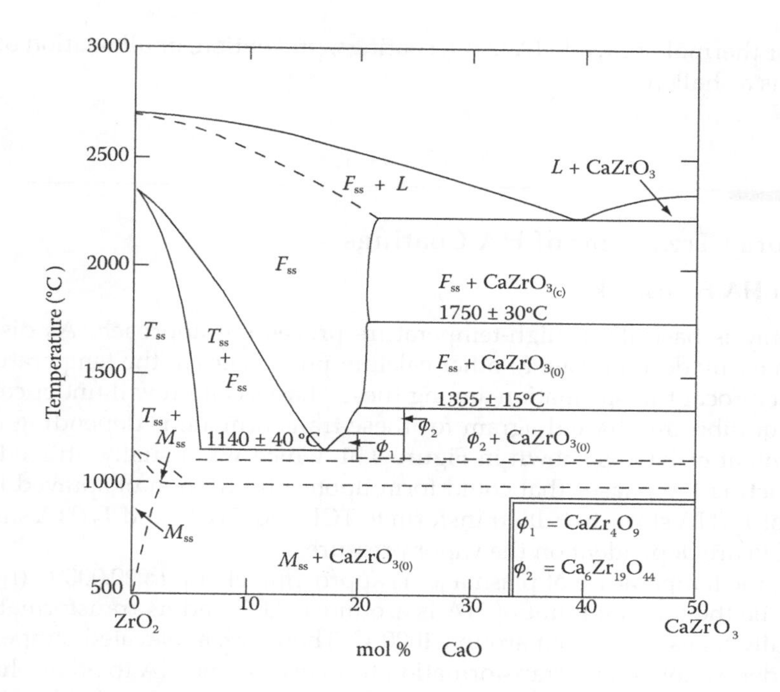

FIGURE 4.30
ZrO_2–CaO phase diagram. (From Stubican, V.S., in *Advances in Ceramics, Volume 24A, Science and Technology of Zirconia III*, American Ceramic Society, Inc., Ohio, pp. 71–82, 1988. With permission.) T_{ss}, tetragonal solid solution; M_{ss}, monoclinic solid solution; F_{ss}, cubic solid solution; *L*, liquid.

bonding and brittle phases that exist at the splats' interface. The increase of titania content from 10 to 20 vol.% induces a small decrease in Young's modulus. Chemical reaction between HA and TiO2 is found to occur during coating deposition. The relatively high fracture toughness exhibited by the composite coating compared to pure HA coating indicates the improved bonding area of splats' interface (Li et al. 2002b).

It deems that the mutual chemical reaction between the two components provides higher density, which was believed as one beneficial factor influencing fracture toughness (Callus et al. 1999).

While reaction between HA and zirconia is also inevitable, since studies on HA/ZrO_2 coatings showed $CaZrO_3$, apart from crystalline HA, α-TCP, and t-ZrO_2 (Li et al. 2004b). The equilibrium ZrO_2–CaO phase diagram (Stubican 1988) depicted in Figure 4.30 illustrates possible reactions between ZrO_2 and CaO in detail. It shows that, under the equilibrium conditions, heating of the zirconia particles up to 1140 ± 40°C caused transformation to a mixture of t-ZrO_2 and c-ZrO_2.

It has been found that when HA decomposition to other phases (e.g., CaO) takes place beyond 1000°C, the gradually increased content of CaO in the present zirconai/HA system makes the reactions between zirconia and CaO more complicated (Li et al. 2004b). The small content change exhibited by α-TCP (increased from 6.7 to 7.5 wt.%) has indicated the low content of CaO. It was pointed out that CaO in preference reacts with t-ZrO_2 to form $CaZrO_3$ (Rao et al. 2002), which can be described as follows:

$$CaO + t\text{-}ZrO_2 \rightarrow CaZrO_3 \quad (4.12)$$

Therefore for thermal-sprayed HA/ZrO_2 coatings, prevention, or alleviation of the chemical reaction is a challenge.

Co-/Postspray Treatment of HA Coatings

Influence of HA Feedstock

Thermal spray is basically a high-temperature processing approach. As discussed earlier, HA can easily decomposite to other calcium phosphates at the temperatures beyond ~1000°C. Reciprocal transformation among these phases can prevail under certain conditions. The equilibrium phase diagram for these transformations depending on temperature and content of P_2O_5 is shown in Figure 4.31, which was usually utilized as a useful tool in predicting the phases that could form upon solidification of sprayed HA powder. The values of T_1 (HA starts to fully transform to TCP and TTCP) and T_2 (HA starts to transform to TTCP) are dependent on the vapor pressure.

Generally, the temperature of plasma jet is approximately up to 20,000°C (Bertagnolli et al. 1995), while the melting point of HA is around 1470°C and its transformation to other phases usually takes place from around 1000°C. Therefore, at elevated temperatures during plasma deposition, phase transformation from crystalline HA to other phases such as TCP or CaO (Aoki 1994; Weng et al. 1994; Vu et al. 1997) seems inevitable. The following decomposition reactions represent the usual chemical decomposition of crystalline HA powders as they are heated and accelerated in the plasma jet or during splat formation:

$$Ca_{10}(PO_4)_6(OH)_2 \rightarrow 2Ca_3(PO_4)_2 + Ca_4P_2O_9 + H_2O\uparrow \tag{4.13}$$

(Liu et al. 1994; Gross et al. 1998a; Ogiso et al. 1998b)

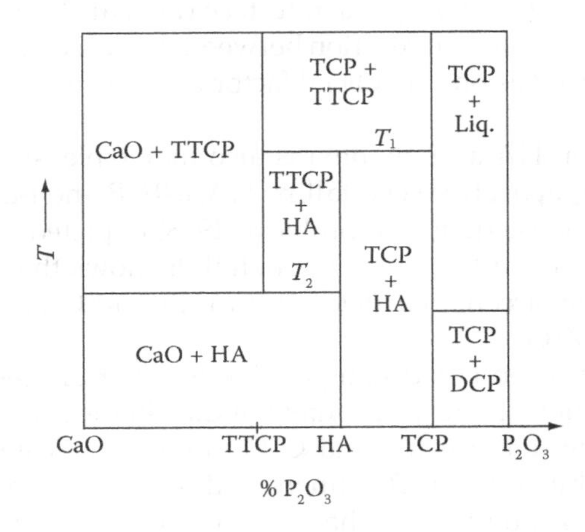

FIGURE 4.31
Schematic representation of CaO–P_2O_5–H_2O system at fixed P_{H2O}. (From Harris, D.H., in *Thermal Spray Research and Applications, Proceedings of the Third NTSC*, Long Beach, CA, May 1990, pp. 419–423. With permission.)

$$Ca_{10}(PO_4)_6(OH)_2 \rightarrow 3Ca_3(PO_4)_2 + CaO + H_2O\uparrow \tag{4.14}$$

(Liu et al. 1994; Gross et al. 1998a).

Due to decomposition, HA coatings can be accompanied by phases such as oxyapatite, tetracalcium phosphate, tricalcium phosphate, calcium oxide, and so forth. The dehydroxylated HA (OHA), TTCP, and TCP obtained from high-temperature processing undergo dissolution and degradation more rapidly than HA in an aqueous environment, which decreases chemical stability and enhances degradation of the implants in vivo (Lin et al. 2000). Like other amorphous phases, the ACP in the as-sprayed coating is thermodynamically metastable. It enhances adhesion to the substrate but dissolves quickly in body fluids, and thus adversely affects bone formation (Guipont et al. 2002). Since HA coatings with lower crystallinity would result in an increased dissolution, a high crystallinity level is desirable in order for the materials to have good bioactive properties (Feng et al. 2000) and/or good biointegration by minimizing the soluble phases. Furthermore, the existence of too much amorphous phases at the interface between the HA deposit and metal alloy implant could be detrimental to the long-term survivability of the implant based on that after some time of implantation, the interface may directly contact with bony tissue (Khor and Cheang 1994a). An appropriate thermal treatment could induce crystallization to occur. That is why the as-sprayed coatings are usually subjected to a postheat-treating cycle. Therefore, it is important to control the relative content of the different phases in as-sprayed coatings. Generally, the appearance of CaO in as-sprayed coatings suggests the loss of P_2O_5 from the starting powders during spraying. Loss of water gives a hydroxyapatite-oxyapatite solid solution in which chains of OH^- are replaced by chains of OH^-, O^{2-}, and vacancies, and the range of composition in equilibrium is given by $Ca_{10}(PO_4)_6(OH)_{2-2x}O_x\otimes_x$, where $x > 0.75$, $\otimes$ = vacancy (McPherson et al. 1995; Antolottin et al. 1998).

Besides decomposition, another problem pertinent to the thermal-sprayed HA coating is the formation of an amorphous phase (Reis et al. 1996; Gross et al. 1998b; Yang et al. 1995), along with the generation of other nonbioactive calcium phosphate phases. Generally, the reason for the formation of amorphous phase in HA coating was believed to be related to the entire melting of the powders and subsequent rapid solidification (Cao et al. 1996). Radin et al. (1992) found that the formation of the amorphous phase was apparently associated with partial dehydroxylation of HA during plasma spray process.

The presence of ACP phase is theoretically undesirable because natural HA in bone is crystalline (Cheang et al. 1996a). Furthermore, a highly crystalline coating is more stable over time in vivo, while a less crystalline coating is subject to slow degradation in the long term but facilitates its substitution by newly formed bone (Tranquilli et al. 1994) because the dissolvability of ACP is far better than that of crystalline one (Ducheyne et al. 1993). Therefore, controlling the amount and location of ACP is very important for proper function of the coated appliance. However, Gross et al. (1988a) stated that ACP was good for absorbing the mechanical mismatch, improve fatigue behavior, and promote fast bone remodeling and attachment. Thus it seemed that HA coatings with limited amorphous phase are preferred in clinical applications (Bioceramics Workshop 1999).

The prevention of phase transformation to ACP could be achieved through the minimal removal of hydroxide and phosphate from HA during processing (Gross et al. 1998a). Especially during plasma spraying, the extreme heating and cooling conditions can produce metastable phases as a result of rapid cooling from high temperatures. Gross and Berndt proposed a visualized model (Gross et al. 1998b), shown in Figure 4.32, to illustrate the equilibrium phase diagram of HA materials during plasma spraying. It is found that phase transformations are produced by (1) preferential removal of hydroxyl and phosphate

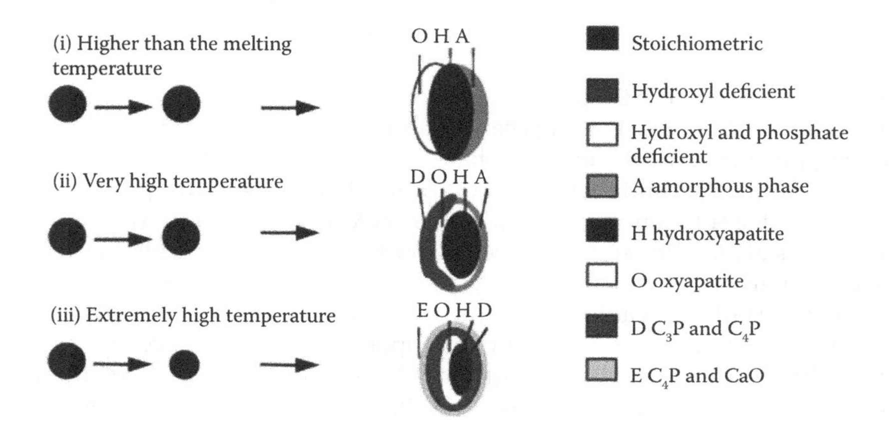

FIGURE 4.32
Proposed model for phase formation of plasma-sprayed HA particles. (From Gross et al., in *Thermal Spray: Meeting the Challenges of the 21st Century, Proceedings of the 15th International Thermal Spray Conference,* Nice, France, 1998a, pp. 1133–1138. With permission.)

leading to a change in melt composition, and (2) the high cooling rate due to the thermal process. Hydroxyl group removal promotes the amorphous phase and oxyapatite. Further heating produces a less viscous melt facilitating decomposition of HA to TCP and TTCP. Phosphate removal during flight produces a more calcium-rich melt preferring TTCP and CaO formation.

The extremely high temperatures easily result in an increased amount of ACP in as-sprayed coatings. It was believed that the cooling rate had significant influence on the resultant phases that transformed from HA (Ruan et al. 1996). Furthermore, partial water vapor pressure acts as an important factor in the phase determination after spraying process. The HA stability as a function of temperature and P_{H2O} is shown in Figure 4.33. It reveals that the decomposition of HA is easier under lower water vapor pressure and higher temperature. (Accordingly, 75% of the water may be lost while retaining the HA crystal

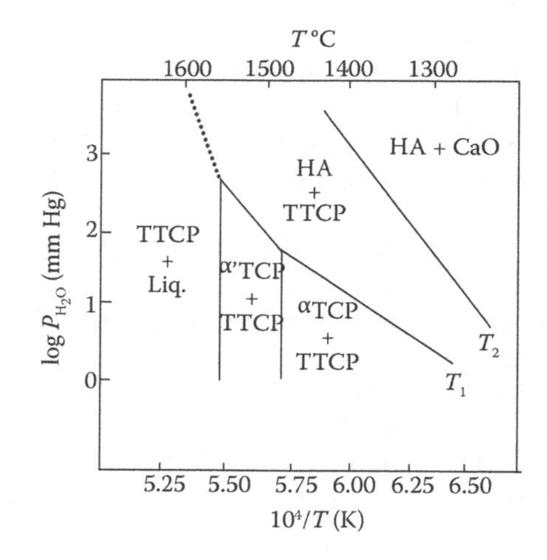

FIGURE 4.33
HA stability as a function of temperature and P_{H_2O}. (From Harris, D.H., in *Thermal Spray Research and Applications, Proceedings of the Third NTSC,* Long Beach, CA, May 1990, pp. 419–423. With permission.)

structure.) The difference in lattice parameter between HA and oxyapatite is reported to be so small that structural changes arising from loss of water are not obvious from XRD patterns. OH^--depleted HA has been shown to be very reactive, absorbing H_2O at ~600°C even in a vacuum of 1.33×10^{-2} Pa (MacPherson et al. 1995).

Generally, the phase transformation may induce the following problems (Ogiso et al. 1998b): (1) stress accumulation in the crystal phase due to volume differences, (2) formation of CaO and TTCP, (3) higher solubility, (4) easier diffusion migration of atoms due to irregular distribution of Ca, and (5) diffusion migration of OH^- group into TCP in vivo. Therefore, the decomposition of HA during coating deposition should be avoided.

The extent of HA decomposition could be examined through determining the Ca/P ratio of the coatings (Gross et al. 1998b). The amount of ACP in most plasma-sprayed HA coating was detected in a range up to 70%. The ACP phase has considerable dissolution ability, which makes the phase dissolve into the tissues quickly and consequently reduces the reliability of the implants. Therefore, the existence of amorphous phase at the coating/substrate interface could weaken the adhesive strength of the coating (Gross et al. 1998a). Furthermore, it is believed that the content of amorphous phase near the coating-substrate interface is more than that within the coating due to the low thermal diffusivity of HA. This phenomenon has been revealed through morphological analysis (Gross et al. JBMR 1998; Ashroff et al. 1996).

The rapid cooling of a splat on substrate surface is the fundamental phenomenon of thermal spray process. Gross et al. (1998b) summarized the factors that mainly influenced the formation of ACP. Dehydroxylation of the molten particle during flight, rapid cooling as the particle impinges onto the metal substrate, and the low substrate temperature are the main variables. They suggested the viscosity of the melted particle as an important variable that influenced the amorphicity. Overheating of the molten particle decreased its viscosity, hence a larger flattened splat would be obtained, which resulted in better cooling and this was beneficial to the formation of the amorphous phase. This was confirmed by experiments through alternative spray angles and spray parameters (Gross et al. 1998b). The effect of dehydroxylation is believed to have a great influence on ACP formation in comparison to the increase in cooling rate.

The presence of water vapor, hydrostatic pressure, or a combination of these could promote the crystallization of hydroxyapatite, which is composition-dependent (Gross et al. 1998c; Yamashita et al. 1994). Furthermore, heat treatment in vacuum at a very high temperature such as 950°C can induce the chemical reaction at the HA/Ti–6Al–4V interface with a titanium phosphide as the resultant compound detected by transmission electron microscope analysis (Ji et al. 1993). This phenomenon can be the proof of the diffusion of Ti or P elements at the coating/substrate interface. Meanwhile Filiaggi et al. (1993) believed that increases in mechanical properties after heat treatment on the as-sprayed coatings can be attributed to diffusion at the interface. Furthermore, the crystallization temperature of the as-sprayed HA coatings differs to some extent depending on the characteristics of the raw HA powder and the spray system employed. Even though the transformation point from amorphous phase to crystalline HA is generally determined, there are still reports that suggest that the crystallization can occur at low temperatures if very long isothermal treatment condition is satisfied (Vogel et al. 1996).

The postspray annealing treatment at 750°C has achieved a complete crystallization of the ACP in the thermal sprayed HA coating (Figure 4.34) (Li et al. 2002a). It is clear that the amorphous phase transformed only to crystalline HA. Through the investigation of the crystallization of amorphous calcium phosphate by Vogel et al. (1996), it was postulated that the thermal decomposition of HA during plasma spraying is reversible when annealed

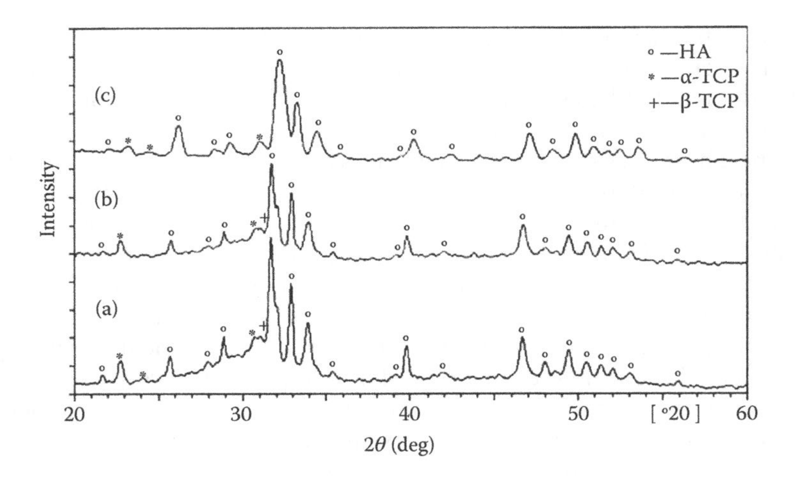

FIGURE 4.34
XRD patterns of heat-treated HA coatings under (b) 500°C and (c) 750°C annealing with the comparison to (a) the as-sprayed coating. (From Li et al., *Biomaterials*, 23, 2015–2112, 2002a. With permission.)

at more than 600°C for 3 h in the presence of water vapor. It was already detected by DSC test that the crystallization temperature of the ACP is about 720°C (Li et al. 2002a).

Postspray heat treatment would further promote the interfaces bonding between the coating and substrates, and is deemed to be a necessary step to transform the amorphous calcium phosphate into HA structure (Yang et al. 1997). As well, the cracks generated by heat treatment should be considered (Cheang et al. 1996a). As discussed earlier, besides the improved phases in the HA coatings, enhanced coating mechanical properties were also reported (Li et al. 2002a; Yang 2007). For example, for HVOF-sprayed HA coatings (Li et al. 2002a), the adhesive strength is significantly improved by the heat treatment at 750°C, increasing from 26 ± 2MPa for the as-sprayed coating to 34 ± 3 MPa. The shear strength is also increased from 11.2 ± 0.9 to 14.1 ± 0.8 MPa.

Generally, according to the mechanism of HA decomposition (Aoki 1994), loss of water is the key reason accounting for the undesirable phase changes of HA during the plasma spraying. It was found that HA gradually releases its OH^- ions and transforms into oxy-apatite (OHAP) in the temperature range of 1000°C to 1360°C. Above 1360°C, OHAP would decompose into TTCP and α-TCP (Liao et al. 1999). It was proposed that the dehydration of HA gives a solid HA-OHAP solution in which chains of OH^- might be replaced by chains of OH^-, O^{2-}, and vacancies (MacPherson et al. 1995). The leave of OH^- groups in terms of water at high temperatures attained by the HA particles leads to lattice changes associated with structure changes (Aoki 1994). Consequently, the plasma-sprayed HA coatings are composed of several CPs with different amounts depending on the extent of the dehydration of HA. Therefore, the possible approaches used for reversing CPs to crystalline HA must involve providing extra water, and hence OH^-. Some researchers have reported their findings that postspray steam treatment on the plasma-sprayed HA coatings from their surface showed evidence of significant reversing effect (Shirkhanzadeh 1994; Yamashita et al. 1994; Cao et al. 1996; Tong et al. 1998; Li et al. 2006). It was believed that oxyapatite remains stable under dry conditions and would readily transform to HA in the presence of moisture (Gross et al. 1998c; Yamashita et al. 1994). It was reported that water vapor treatment pursued under a low temperature, 125°C, was effective in achieving good crystallization (Shirkhanzadeh et al. 1994; Tong et al. 1998).

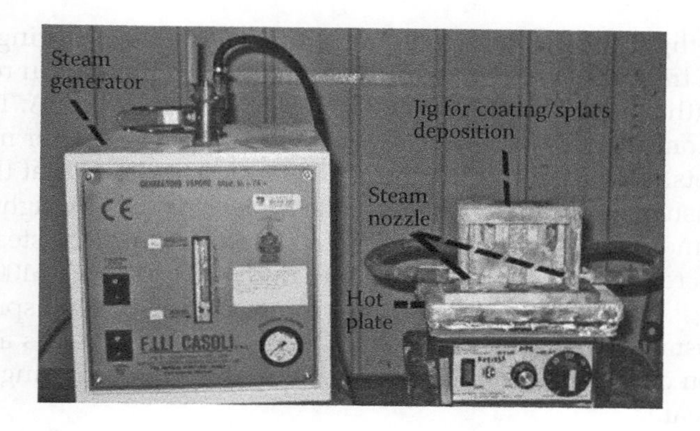

FIGURE 4.35
Facility setup for the HA coating/splat deposition with water steam treatment. (From Li et al., *J. Therm. Spray Technol.*, 15, 610–616, 2006. With permission.)

Another attempt to avoid/reverse the decomposition of HA is to use steam treatment during the spraying process (Li et al. JTST 2006). A steam generator was employed for the steam generation using distilled water. A stable steam with 2 bar (~120°C) was provided through two separate pipes into the jig (Figure 4.35) for the treatment during the spraying. It is interesting to note that the improvement on the crystallinity by the steam treatment is significant for these coatings (Figure 4.36) (Li et al. 2006). Water steam was provided

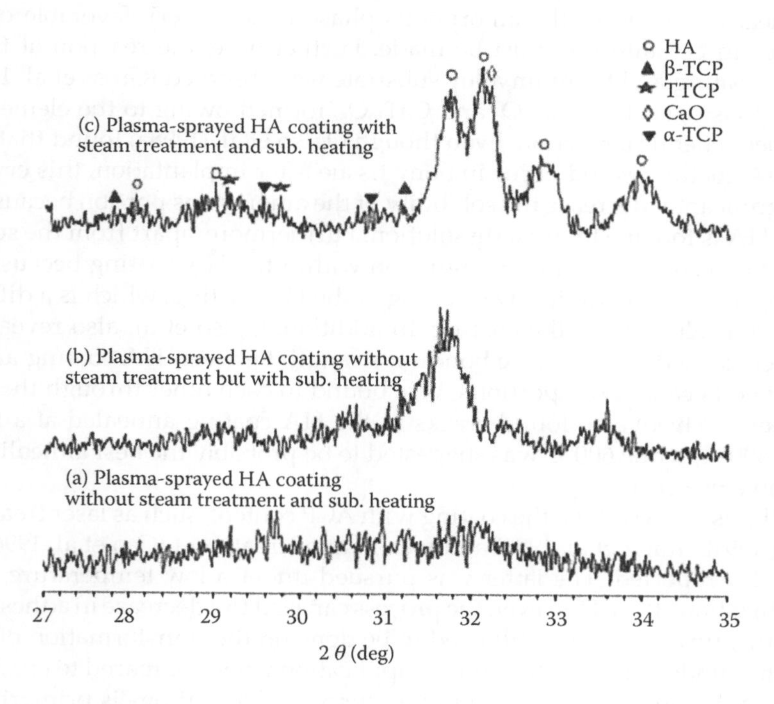

FIGURE 4.36
XRD patterns of the coatings made with the powders with a particle size of less than 25 μm showing a significant effect of the steam treatment. (From Li et al., *J. Therm. Spray Technol.*, 15, 610–616, 2006. With permission.)

accompanying in-flight HA droplets and splats/coating formation during plasma spraying of HA. The steam treatment during the plasma spraying is effective in reversing undesirable phases, ACP (the major effect), TCP, and so forth, to crystalline HA. The mechanism of reversing HA decomposition involves mainly the entrapping of water molecules by individual HA droplets upon their impingement. The results indicate that the phase changes of HA during plasma spraying has already taken place during in-flight stage of the HA particles. Furthermore, apart from reversing HA decomposition, the steam is also capable of significantly increasing the adhesion strength of the coating with >100% (Li et al. 2006). To provide steam is an easy and economical process during plasma spraying. The major problem with plasma spraying of HA seems to be easily solved. It is also expected that phase composition of the HA coatings can be altered through changing the pressure and flow rate of the steam.

Vogel et al. (1996) also reported the crystallization of as-sprayed HA coatings at temperatures around 500°C or above. It was perceived that the decomposition of apatite during plasma spraying was reversible and could be described by a temperature- and time-dependent equilibrium reaction. Furthermore, Tong et al. (1998) found a more stable phase, nanocrystals of HA, after the heat treatment. However, in addition to the recrystallization and element diffusion, one considerable phenomenon appears while the postheat treatment is conducted; that is, new cracks appear as a result of thermal contraction (Gross et al. 1998c; Kijk et al. 1996). HA is 3% denser than oxyapatite, thus the transformation to HA will produce an additional 0.6% contraction (Gross et al. 1998c). The apparent contraction when crystallization occurs can correspond to ~1% in a direction parallel to the lamellae within the coating. Additionally, the contraction is approximately proportional to the amount of amorphous phase (Gross et al. 1998c). The appearance of cracking signifies that heat treatment of the amorphous phase is not a very favorable option when large changes in crystallinity must be made. Furthermore, the reaction at the interface between HA coating and titanium alloy substrate was observed (Gross et al. 1998c). Many unfavorable phases, such as $CaTiO_3$ and $CaTi_2O_5$, formed owing to the element diffusion and subsequent chemical reaction. Even though Ogiso et al. (1998a) found that the crystallization of HA coating would occur in bony tissue after implantation, this crystallization could not significantly decrease the solubility of the amorphous portion because the newly crystallized HA is too fine to resist dissolution. Furthermore, apart from the solubility, the recrystallization causes a stress accumulation within the HA coating because of volume difference, resulting in a physical weakening of the HA coating, which is a different problem besides the solubility of the coating. In addition, Ogiso et al. also revealed that the crystallization caused the adhesive bonding strength between HA coating and substrate to be weakened because both portions were bound to each other through the amorphous phase. Kijk et al. (1996) also found cracks in the HA coating annealed at a temperature higher than 400°C, while 600°C was suggested to be probably the best annealing temperature to obtain a better coating.

Other methods to crystallize the coating with ACP content, such as laser treatment (Khor and Cheang 1994b; Ranz et al. 1998) and water vapor treatment (Cao et al. 1996; Tong et al. 1998), were also reported. The latter was pursued under a low temperature, 125°C, with good crystallization effect. However, the process can lead to a decrease in adhesive strength. In other words, further studies still need to be done on the transformation of amorphous phase, which is undesirable for the clinical application when compared to crystallized HA. After all, the reduction of ACP content in as-sprayed HA coatings is primarily necessary for the solution mentioned above. New deposition methods are required for the HA coating deposition with a low amorphous phase content to avoid the postspray treatment.

Biocompatibility Evaluation of the Nanostructured Bioceramic Coatings by In Vitro Cell Culture

A material must be in contact with living tissues when used as implant during clinical service, thus its biological performance, defined as the interaction between materials and living systems, is important for a favorite functional life. Two aspects of the biological performance, host response and material response, are responsible for overall bioactivity of the implants. Host response (the reaction of a living system to the presence of a material) controls the performance of the patient who received the placement of the implant. It is, however, controlled by the characteristics of the material and especially its chemical stability in the body. These two characteristics—the susceptibility of the material to degradation and the effect such degradation has on the tissue—are the central features of biocompatibility. The mechanism of tissue attachment is directly related to the type of tissue response at the implant interface. So far it seems clear that one of the original goals of implantation, that is, to produce minimal host response, is an outmoded view that may limit further development of implant materials and devices.

Generally, implant materials such as HA coatings must fulfill the following requirements (Wise et al. 2000):

- The elemental chemistry of primarily calcium and phosphate ion substances in Ca/P ratio of 1.67, which is similar to natural bone.
- The controllability of crystalline and physical structures to provide a wide range of in vivo interactions.
- The extensive availability of existing literature on biocompatibility.
- The opportunity for bonding to bone.
- The opportunity to enhance mechanical force transfer allowing for use in load-bearing implants.
- A wide range of crystalline and structural forms can be constituted from reactions between calcium oxide and phosphorous pentoxide, which allows for material properties formulation that better matches requirement.
- The opportunity to introduce other elements or structural defects.
- Microstructures and densities can be varied to provide properties from relatively stable to completely biodegradable.

Biocompatibility was defined as the ability of a biomaterial to demonstrate host and material response appropriate to its intended application (Wise et al. 2000). To be biocompatible, a bioceramic coating must not induce an activation of the immune system or be toxic and carcinogenic, and finally should not disturb the blood flow, intrinsically or via waste products, after being in contact with blood. The simplest form of interaction between implant materials and the biological environment is the transfer of material across the material–tissue interface in the absence of reaction (Black 1999). It was revealed that once the implant was put into the body, complicated behavior took place as a local host response.

In vitro tests have come to be seen as screening tests, serving as precursors for more involved, more costly and time-consuming animal implantation. In vitro testing is a necessary method to evaluate the changes of HA prosthesis in simulated body fluid (SBF) and/or cell culture medium before its direct use in patients' body. Generally used SBF solution is differed according to aimed application circumstances of the implants, and many types of SBF have been reported, such as 0.05 mol Tris(hydroxy)methylaminomethane-HCl (pH = 7.3) (Ducheyne et al. 1993), Hank's balanced salt solution (HBSS) (Reis et al. 1996), isotonic saline solution (0.15M NaCl) (Reis et al. 1996), 37°C sterile Hank's physiologic (pH = 7.2) balanced salt solution (Maxian et al. 1993a), Ringer's solution (Gross et al. 1994), Gomori's buffer (Klein et al. 1994). Nevertheless, the most direct and effect way of validating the biocompatibility of the thermal-sprayed HA coatings is to conduct cell culture experiment. The SBF study is able to give helpful information about the coatings for further investigation.

Different phases in the HA family exhibit different structures and could thus lead to different biological responses in vitro. It was reported that the rate of cell proliferation was highly dependent on the composition of HA powders and sintering characteristics (Best et al. 1997). Because the coating phase composition is significantly dependent on the starting powders, this indicates the effect of final coating composition. Generally, the in vitro behavior of HA coatings mostly involves dissolution/precipitation processes. The variation of the crystal structure and stoichiometry of calcium phosphate ceramics produces dissolution behavior that varies over a wide range. The dissolution rate of monophasic calcium phosphates increases in the following order: HA < CDHA < OHA < β-TCP < α-TCP < TTCP (Ducheyne et al. 1993), even though Maxian et al. reported that crystalline coatings showed significantly greater Ca dissolution than amorphous coatings under some conditions (Maxian et al. 1993a). It was also found that the dissolution of α-TCP phase in TCP coating could favor the precipitation of the nonwell-crystallized apatite phase on the coating surface while for the HA coating the absence of dissolution would delay this precipitation (Cleries et al. 2000). Results indicate the possible mutual effect among different phases in vitro. It was revealed that the precipitation rate of bonelike apatite on their surface was in the order of: β-, α-TCP (β-TCP contains some α-TCP) > HA > Ti > ACP (Cleries et al. 2000). Another study also showed that poorly crystallized coatings resorbed faster and showed greater surface film precipitation and greater chemical changes than amorphous coatings (Maxian et al. 1993b). It suggests that the crystalline structure is indeed important in dictating the differences in the rate of nucleation.

HA coating surface usually plays the most important role in overall dissolution/precipitation behavior. The underlying surface was not a significant factor in Ca dissolution, but was significant for surface chemistry and morphological changes (Maxian et al. 1993). Results already showed that that the precipitation rate was directly influenced by local Ca^{2+} concentration near to the coating surface and dissolution of certain phases accelerated the precipitation of the bonelike apatite (Khor et al. 2003a).

It was revealed that the in vivo behavior of the prosthesis was significantly dependent on its composition (Suominen et al. 1996) regarding degradability and bioactivity of different phases. Despite the content of ACP in HA coatings, it was revealed that once early osteointegration was achieved, biodegradation of a bioactive coating should not be detrimental to the bone/coating/implant fixation (Maxian et al. 1993b). As well, the remodeling process is fundamental for implant fixation and stability for a long term (Pazzaglia et al. 1998). Investigations of the dissolution–reprecipitation phenomena involved in the formation of HA bone bond have identified two joining modes (Mattioli Belmonte et al. 1998): (1) bone tissue components bonded to HA through a recrystallization zone similar in structure to the reprecipitation layer, and (2) bone tissue components bonded directly to HA crystals with no morphologically discernible signs of dissolution. And the reabsorption–reconstruction cycles do not reduce the mechanical fixation of the prosthesis, and do not attain the threshold of loosening (Hardy et al. 1999). Concerning the bonding of bone with

HA, it is interesting to note that the precipitated apatite microcrystals appeared by secondary nucleation and were aggregated around ceramic crystals in bone sites (Rohanizadeh et al. 1999). Available TEM results showed that both HA crystals and precipitated microcrystals had the same D-spacing and the same apatite structure (Rohanizadeh et al. 1999).

Previous study revealed that bioactivity of as-sprayed coatings, especially coating surface bioproperty (Kido et al. 1997), and mechanical properties significantly influenced their functional service in the long run. HA coatings have a favorable effect on bone apposition on the implant and give evidence that this is due to early adhesion of osteoblasts and direct deposition of bone matrix on the HA substrate (Pazzaglia et al. 1998). This proves the importance of early dissolving of HA coating. However, previous studies have raised some concerns regarding the resorption, fracture, fatigue, or macrobiological susceptibility for HA coatings. It should be emphasized that the characteristics of all HA coatings are not always the same, and this may affect the chemical, physical, and mechanical properties of the implants.

Natural HA formed in-bone is initially deposited in the collagen matrix of the bone in a relatively amorphous form that appears to mature into a more crystalline form (Szivek et al. 1996). Perhaps the lower level of crystallinity encourages bone attachment at a faster rate initially because they mimic the naturally occurring newly formed HA surface or because they undergo some resorption that provides an uncontaminated surface for bonding. The relatively amorphous coatings provided better bonding (Szivek et al. 1996). Generally, adhesion of cells to a biomedical coating is believed to involve several steps: adsorption of proteins onto coating surface, attachment of cells by recognizing the adsorbed proteins, spreading of cells, growth/proliferation/differentiation of cells (Silver et al. 2000; Meyer et al. 2006). Adhesive interactions between cells or cells and the extracellular matrix are thought to play an essential role in several biological processes, including cellular recognition, specification and signaling, provision of positional cues during vertebrate development, cell proliferation and differentiation during wound healing, and leukocyte adherence and emigration.

There has been no doubt that HA and HA-based composites are capable of enhancing attachment and proliferation of viable cells (Deligianni et al. 2001; Rose et al. 2004; Carey et al. 2005; Hossain et al. 2005; Knabe et al. 2004; Xie et al. 2004). Fast attachment and proliferation of osteoblast cells on thermal-sprayed HA coatings have been evidenced (Figure 4.37) (Li et al. SCT, 2006).

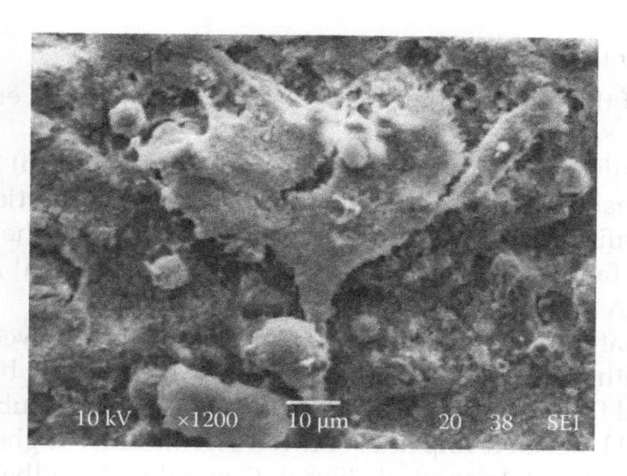

FIGURE 4.37
Typical SEM picture showing the osteoblast cell attached on the HA coating. (From Li et al., *J. Therm. Spray Technol.*, 15, 610–616, 2006. With permission.)

Clear evidence was shown of significantly different cell proliferation rates on the surface of the nanostructured HA coatings and the coatings with more crystalline HA exhibit higher cell proliferation rate (Li et al. 2006). Surprisingly, it was found that since increased surface area undoubtedly furthers cell proliferation, it can be claimed that the nanostructures play a less important role than the phases on the attachment/proliferation of the cells (Li et al. 2006), even though some researchers found that dissolution of the Ca-rich phases was accompanied by good cell attachment (Wang et al. 2004) and high proliferation rate (Kim et al. 2004). Although it was reported that there was increased adhesion with nanophase materials due to the increased surface boundaries (Webster et al. 2004), the bioactivity of the coatings is more dependent on phases than on the nanostructures (Li et al. 2006). Nevertheless, the HA coatings with high content of both crystalline HA and nanostructures are favorably preferred for their biomedical applications.

It has been reviewed that a number of proteins played important roles in mediating the proliferation/differentiation of the osteoblasts and their content changed with the proliferation/differentiation process (Stein et al. 1993). It was revealed that the shape of the nanosized grains at the HA coating surface affects the attachment and proliferation of osteoblast cells and nanosized pores at coating surface promote cell attachment (Li et al. 2007b). Therefore, the nanosized pores instead of the nanosized grains might play the key roles in enhancing the attachment/proliferation of the osteoblast cells.

Even though the resorption, fracture, fatigue, or nanostructure/microstructure of HA coatings have been extensively studied, it should be emphasized that the characteristics of all HA-based coatings are not always the same, and this may affect the chemical, physical, and mechanical properties of the coating. Therefore, a study on the general factors that can influence HA coating properties needs to be conducted. Furthermore, other variables for evaluating the mechanical properties and the intrinsic factors that influence the performance of HA coatings need to be proposed. Generally, HA coatings do not experience pure tensile stress in vivo, while compound stresses are experienced (Haman et al. 1997). In clinical applications, the failure of implantation is usually attributed to many factors. The success or failure of an implant is directly influenced by (Williams et al. 1987):

- The thickness and nature of the implant
- The presence or absence of infection, inflammatory, or foreign body giant cell reactions
- The reactivity of the implant (bioactive, bioresorbable, etc.)
- The structure of the implant (hardness, porosity, crystallinity, etc.)

The major cause of failure of the implantation (apart from infection) is implant loosening (Bonfield 1987). Extensive work has been conducted on the properties of HA coatings in vivo that mostly clarified the effect of implantation duration on the mechanical properties of the implants. Table 4.3 shows previous results on interfacial mechanical strength between bone and HA coating after some time of implantation.

It demonstrated that after long-term implantation, such as 24 weeks, the HA coating would be bonded with bone together firmly, which was indicated by the relatively high bonding strength and the corresponding failure location, coating/substrate interface. And it was revealed that HA-coated implants showed significantly higher push-out strength with bone than dense HA (Ogiso et al. 1998a). Generally, the adhesion of the implants with bony tissue is realized through either mere close (molecular-scale) approximation of tissue and implant or a chemical alteration of the implant surface, a true bonding process

TABLE 4.3
In Vivo Mechanical Properties of Ha Coatings after Implantation Duration

Weeks	Implant	Mechanical Strength MPa (SD)	Type of Test	Comment	Reference
2	HA-coated Ti6Al4V	1.35	Push-out	Goat tibia	Oonishi et al. (1989)
	Uncoated	0.53			
3	HA-coated Ti6Al4V	6.05 (1.94)	Push-out		Thomas et al. (1987)
	Uncoated	4.43 (1.32)			
4	HA-coated Ti6Al4V	3.484 (0.616)	Push-out	Rabbit femoral	Maxian et al. (1993b)
4	HA-coated Ti6Al4V	4.43	Push-out	Goat tibia	Cook et al. (1992)
	Uncoated	1.49			
5	HA-coated Ti6Al4V	9.56 (3.55)	Push-out	Dog femur	Cook et al. (1991)
	Uncoated	4.88 (1.01)			
6	HA-coated Ti6Al4V	14.15	Push-out	Goat tibia	Oonishi et al. (1989)
	Uncoated	7.5			
10	HA-coated Ti6Al4V	14.17 (4.87)	Push-out	Goat tibia	Thomas et al. (1987)
	Uncoated	10.53 (3.29)			
12	HA-coated Ti6Al4V	6.244 (0.282)	Push-out	Rabbit femoral	Maxian et al. (1993b)
12	HA-coated Ti6Al4V	14.71 (2.84)	Push-out	Dog femora	Yang et al. (1997)
12	HA-coated Ti6Al4V	25.41	Push-out	Goat tibia	Oonishi et al. (1989)
	Uncoated	22.5	Push-out	Dog femora	Wang et al. (1996)
	HA-coated Ti6Al4V	11.7 (1.7)			
24	HA-coated Ti6Al4V	14.64 (2.14)	Push-out	Dog femora	Yang et al. (1997)
24	HA-coated Ti6Al4V	12.4 (2.0)	Push-out	Dog femora (failure-c/sub)	Wang et al. (1996)
32	HA-coated Ti6Al4V	12.12 (2.43)	Push-out	Dog femur	Thomas et al. (1987)
	Uncoated	none			

with a continuous gradation of structure and composition across the tissue–implant interface (Black 1999). In either case of integration or bonding, the implant becomes mechanically coupled to the adjacent tissue. For the latter, biomaterials should be in recognition of the necessity of chemical reaction with local host environment prior to bond formation. The satisfactory implantation, which is indicated by high bonding strength, implies adaptive remodeling. It was pointed out that cell adhesion, proliferation, and detachment strength were surface roughness sensitive and increased as the roughness of HA increased (Deligianni et al. 2001). An ideal coating surface might incorporate mechanical interlocks as well as chemical attachment. Generally, it was believed that bonding mechanism of bone with HA seemed to involve dissolution/reprecipitation phenomena (Bagambisa et al. 1993). However, Munting (1996) pointed out that implant fixation must depend on a mechanical interlock with bone and was not related to the duration of implantation.

The strength of interfacial bond that is formed by bioactive materials and adjacent tissue is time-dependent (Laurent et al. 1999). Formation of the bone/HA bond seems to involve dissolution/reprecipitation phenomena. Furthermore, reabsorption of HA is mainly a cell-mediated phenomenon (Kwong et al. 1989). The degree of HA degradation determines the ultramorphological appearance and ultrastructure of the bone/HA bond (Bagambisa et al. 1993). In vivo study of HA-coated cylinders by plasma spraying implanted in femoral diaphyses of sheep showed that the failure during shear test was within the bone, indicating a strong link between bone and implant and between HA coating and titanium substrate (Lopez-Sastre et al. 1998). As the final approach, clinical testing is the only technique by which the true biological performance of implantable biomaterials can be determined. Nevertheless, the only valid subject for study is the human being. Although the information device function (and biological performance of the materials involved) in patients is insufficient yet, there are opportunities for examination of these issues during device retrieval, either subsequent to clinical failure or at autopsy. HA-coated implants have shown their capability of fast bone ingrowth. However, the strongest argument against the routine use of HA-coated implants is the general lack of long-term documentation on HA-coated implant survival, as well as the lack of well-characterized coatings prior to use. In addition, large degrees of variability between studies, involving the definition and length of implant survival/success, implant case and the site selection, surgeon experience, surgical protocols, postoperative regimens, and prosthetic restoration, make direct interstudy comparisons problematic. Future research might cover the issues addressing the problems experienced by the current coated implants. Chemistry and properties are the major concerns for material scientists for biomaterials research. It is anticipated that the well-established theory among processing, micro-/nanostructures, and properties of the HA-based bioceramic coatings for medical applications would give significant insight into the research in thermal sprayed HA-based bioceramic coatings, and in turn would facilitate the final purpose of the research (i.e., medical application for human beings).

References

Ahmed, R. and Hadfield, M. 1997. Wear of high-velocity oxy-fuel (HVOF)-coated cones in rolling contact. *Wear.* 203–204: 98–106.

Albee, F.H. 1920. Studies in bone growth: Triple calcium phosphate as a stimulus to osteogenesis. *Ann. Surg.* 71: 32–39.

Antolottin, N., Bertini, S., and Fanara, C. 1998. Interface characterization of different apatite coatings. In *Thermal Spray: Meeting the Challenges of the 21th Century, Proceedings of the 15th International Thermal Spray Conference*, Nice, France, May 1998, pp. 1121–1126.

Aoki, H. 1994. *Medical Applications of Hydroxyapatite.* Ishiyaku EuroAmerica, Inc., Tokyo, St. Louis.

Ashroff, S., Napper, S.A., Hale, P.N., Siriwardane, U., and Mukherjee, D.P. 1996. Stability of hydroxyapatite coating of different crystallinities on a titanium alloy implant material after cyclic fatigue. *Proc. of 15th Southern Biomedical Engineering Conf.*, pp. 14–17.

Bagambisa, F.B., Joos, U., and Schilli, W. 1993. Mechanisms and structure of the bond between bone and hydroxyapatite ceramics. *J. Biomed. Mater. Res.* 27: 1047–1055.

Bansal, P., Padture, N.P., and Vasiliev, A. 2003. Improved interfacial mechanical properties of Al_2O_3-13wt%TiO_2 plasma-sprayed coatings derived from nanocrystalline powders. *Acta Mater.* 51: 2959–2970.

Belmonte, M.M., de Benedittis, A., Muzzarelli, R.A.A., Mengucci, P., Biagini, G., Gandolfi, M.G., Zucchini, C., Krajewski, A., Ravaglioli, A., Roncari, E., Fini, M., and Giardino, R. 1998. Bioactivity modulation of bioactive materials in view of their application in osteoporotic patients. *J. Mater. Sci.: Mater. Med.* 9: 485–492.

Bertagnolli, M., Marchese, M., and Jacucci, G. 1995. Modeling of particles impacting on a rigid substrate under plasma spraying conditions. *J. Therm. Spray Technol.* 4: 41–49.

Bertagnolli, M., Marchese, M., Jacucci, G., St. Doltsinis, I., and Noelting, S. 1997. Thermomechanical simulation of the splashing of ceramic droplets on a rigid substrate. *J. Comput. Phys.* 133: 205–221.

Beshish, G.K., Florey, C.W., Worzala, F.J., and Lenling, W.J. 1993. Fracture toughness fo thermal spray ceramic coatings determined by the indentation technique. *J. Therm. Spray Technol.* 2: 35–38.

Best, S., Sim, B., Kayser, M., and Downes, S. 1997. The dependence of osteoblstic response on variations in the chemical composition and physical properties of hydroxyapatite. *J. Mater. Sci.: Mater. Med.* 8: 97–103.
Bianchi, L., Leger, A.C., Vardelle, M., Vardelle, A., and Fauchais, P. 1997. *Thin Solid Films* 305: 35.
Bioceramics Workshop. 1999. Public discussion. October, 1999, Singapore.
Black, J. 1999. *Biological Performance of Materials, Fundamentals of Biocompatibility*. Third Edition, Revised and Expanded. Marcel Dekker, Inc.
Blum, J., Eckert, K.-L., Schroeder, A., Petitmermet, M., Ha, S.-W., and Wintermantel, E. 1996. In vitro testing of porous titanium dioxide ceramics. In: Kokubo, T., Nakamura, T., and Miyaji, F. (eds.), *Bioceramics*, Volume 9, *Proceedings of the 9th International Symposium on Ceramics in Medicine*, Utsu, Japan, November 1996, pp. 89–92.
Bonfield, W. 1987. New trends in implant materials. In: Pizzoferrato, A., Marchetti, P.G., Ravaglioli, A., and Lee, A.J.C. (eds.), *Biomaterials and Clinical Applications, Proceedings of the Sixth Conference for Biomaterials*, Bologna, Italy, pp. 13–21.
Brown, S.R. and Turner, I.G. 1998. Acoustic emission analysis of thermal sprayed hydroxyapatite coatings examined under four point bend loading. *Surf. Eng.* 14: 309–313.
Brown, S.R., Turner, I.G., and Reiter, H. 1994. Residual stress measurement in thermal sprayed hydroxyapatite coatings. *J. Mater. Sci. Mater. Med.* 5: 756–759.
Callus, P.J. and Berndt, C.C. 1999. Relationships between the mode II fracture toughness and microstructure of thermal spray coatings. *Surf. Coat. Technol.* 114: 114–128.
Campbell, A.A., Fryxell, G.E., Linehau, J.C., and Graff, G.L. 1996. Surface-induced mineralization: A new method for producing calcium phosphate coatings. *J. Biomed. Mater. Res.* 32: 111–118.
Cao, Y., Weng, J., Chen, J., Feng, J., Yang, Z., and Zhang, X. 1996. Water vapour-treated hydroxyapatite coatings after plasma spraying and their characteristics. *Biomaterials* 17: 419–424.
Carey, L.E., Xu, H.H.K., Simon, C.G., Takagi, S., and Chow, L.C. 2005. Premixed rapid-setting calcium phosphate composites for bone repair. *Biomaterials* 26: 5002–5014.
Champion, E., Gautier, S., and Bernache-Assollant, D. 1996. Characterization of hot pressed Al_2O_3-platelet reinforced hydroxyapatite composites. *J. Mater. Sci.: Mater. Med.* 7: 125–130.
Chang, E., Chang, W.J., Wang, B.C., and Yang, C.Y. 1997. Plasma spraying of zirconia-reinforced hydroxyapatite composite coatings on titanium: Part II. Dissolution behavior in simulated body fluid and bonding degradation. *J. Mater. Sci.: Mater. Med.* 8: 201–211.
Charalambides, P.G., Lund, J., Evans, A.G., and McMeeking, R.M. 1989. A test specimen for determining the fracture resistance of biomaterial interfaces. *J. Appl. Mech.* 56: 77–82.
Cheang, P. and Khor, K.A. 1995. Bioceramic powders and coatings by thermal spray techniques. Proc. of ITSC '95, Kobe, May 1995, pp. 181–186.
Cheang, P. and Khor, K.A. 1996a. Addressing processing problems associated with plasma spraying of hydroxyapatite coatings. *Biomaterials* 17: 537–544.
Cheang, P. and Khor, K.A. 1996b. Properties and microstructure of plasma sprayed hydroxyapatite coatings produced with different powder feedstocks. In: Sudarsan, T.S., Khor, K.A., and Jeandin, M. (eds). *Proceedings of the Tenth International Conference on Surface Modification Technologies*, Singapore, pp. 747–758.
Chraska, T. and King, A.H. 2001. Transmission electron microscopy study of rapid solidification of plasma sprayed zirconia—Part I. First splat solidification. *Thin Solid Films* 397: 30–39.
Chraska, T. and King, A.H. 2002. Effect of different substrate conditions upon interface with plasma sprayed zirconia—A TEM study. *Surf. Coat. Technol.* 157: 238–246.
Chung, H.G.P., Swain, M.V., and Mori, T. 1997. Evaluation of the strain energy release rate for the fracture of titanium–porcelain interfacial bonding. *Biomaterials* 18: 1553–1557.
Cleries, L., Fernandez-Pradas, J.M., Sardin, G., and Morenza, J.L. 1998. Dissolution behaviour of calcium phosphate coatings obtained by laser ablation. *Biomaterials* 19: 1483–1489.
Cleries, L., Fernandez-Pradas, J.M., and Morenza, J.L. 2000. Behavior in simulated body fluid of calcium phosphate coatings obtained by laser ablation. *Biomaterials* 21: 1861–1865.
Clyne, T.W. and Gill, S.C. 1996. Residual stresses in thermal spray coatings and their effect on interfacial adhesion: A review of recent work. *J. Therm. Spray Technol.* 5: 401–418.

Cook, S.D., Thomas, K.A., Dalton, J.E., Volkman, T.K., Whitecloud, T.S., and Kay, J.F. 1992. Hydroxylapatite coating of porous implants improves bone ingrowth and interface attachment strength. *J. Biomed. Mater. Res.* 26: 989–1001.

Cook, S.D., Thomas, K.V., and Kay, J.F. 1991. Experimental coating defects in hydroxylapatite-coated implants. *Clin. Orthop.* 265: 280–290.

Cottel, C.M., Chrisey, D.B., and Grabowski, K.S. 1992. Pulsed laser deposition of hydroxyapatite thin films on Ti–6Al–4V. *J. Appl. Biomater.* 3: 87–93.

Cuscó, R., Guitián, F., de Aza, S., and Artús, L. 1998. Differentiation between hydroxyapatite and β-tricalcium phosphate by means of μ-Raman spectroscopy. *J. Eur. Ceram. Soc.* 18: 1301–1305.

da Silva, A.G., Bavaresco, V.P., Zavaglia, C.A.C., Conte, I., and Costa, N. 2001. Production and characterisation of hydroxyapatite to be used as coating on prostheses via powder metallurgy. *Key Eng. Mater.* 192–195: 175–178.

Davis, J. R. 2004. *Handbook of Thermal Spray Technology*. ASM International. Thermal Spray Society Training Committee, September 2004.

de Lange, G.L., de Putter, C., and Burger, E.H. 1987. The bone-hydroxylapatite interface. In Pizzoferrato, A., Marchetti, P.G., Ravaglioli, A., and Lee, A.J.C. (eds.), *Biomaterials and Clinical Applications, Proceedings of the Sixth Conference for Biomaterials*, Bologna, Italy, 1987, pp. 217–222.

de Putter, C., de Lange, G.L., and de Groot, K. 1987. Permucosal dental implants of dense hydroxylapatite in prosthetic dentistry. In Vincenzini, P. (ed.), *Ceramics in Clinical Applications*. Elsevier Science Publishers, Amsterdam, pp. 275–281.

Deligianni, D.D., Katsala, N.D., Koutsoukos, P.G., and Missirlis, Y.F. 2001. Effect of surface roughness of hydroxyapatite on human bone marrow cell adhesion, proliferation, differentiation and detachment strength. *Biomaterials* 22: 87–96.

Delplanque, J.P., Cai, W.D., Rangel, R.H., and Lavernia, E.J. 1997. Spray atomization and deposition of tantalum alloys. *Acta Mater.* 45: 5233–5243.

Drouin, J.M., Cales, B., Chevalier, J., and Fantozzi, G. 1997. Fatigue behavior of Zirconia hip joint heads: Experimental results and finite element analysis. *J. Biomed. Mater. Res.* 34: 149–155.

Ducheyne, P., Radin, S., and King, L. 1993. The effect of calcium phosphate ceramic composition and structure on in vitro behavior, I. Dissolution. *J. Biomed. Mater. Res.* 27: 25–34.

Dyshlovenko, S., Pateyron, B., Pawlowski, L., and Murano, D. 2004. Numerical simulations of hydroxyapatite powder behavior in plasma jet. *Surf. Coat. Technol.* 179: 110–117.

Dyshlovenko, S., Pawlowski, L., Pateyron, B., Smurov, I., and Harding, J.H. 2006. Modeling of plasma particles interactions and coating growth for plasma spraying of hydroxyapatite. *Surf. Coat. Technol.* 200: 3757–3769.

Eckert, K.-L., Ha, S.W., and Mathey, M. 1995. Ceramic processing of titania for biomedical application. In: Wilson, J., Hench, L.L. and Greenspan, D. (eds.), *Bioceramics*, Volume 8, pp. 447–452.

Espanol Pons, M. 2003. *Developing Hydroxyapatite CAPS Coatings on Metallic Implants for Tissue Replacement*. PhD thesis, Nanyang Technological University, Singapore.

Feng, C.F., Khor, K.A., Liu, E.J., and Cheang, P. 2000. Phase transformations in plasma sprayed hydroxyapatite coatings. *Scr. Mater.* 42: 103–109.

Filiaggi, M.J., Pilliar, R.M., and Coombs, N.A. 1993. Post-plasma-spraying heat treatment of the HA coating/Ti–6Al–4V implant system. *J. Biomed. Mater. Res.* 27: 191–198.

Fruh, H.J., Willmann, G., and Pfaff, H.G. 1997. Wear characteristics of ceramic-on-ceramic for hip endoprostheses. *Biomaterials* 18: 873–876.

Fujisawa, A., Shimotoso, T., and Masuda, S. 1996. The development of zirconia ball for T.H.R. with a high mechanical strength, low phase transformation. *Bioceramics* 9: 495–498.

Gang, J., Morniroli, J.P., and Grosdidier, T. 2003. Nanostructures in thermal spray coatings. *Scr. Mater.* 48: 1599–1604.

Gell, M., Jordan, E.H., Sohn, Y.H., Goberman, D., Shaw, L., and Xiao, T.D. 2001. Development and implementation of plasma sprayed nanostructured ceramic coatings. *Surf. Coat. Technol.* 146: 48–54.

Girardin, E., Millet, P., and Lodini, A. 2000. X-ray and neutron diffraction studies of crystallinity in hydroxyapatite coatings. *J. Biomed. Mater. Res.* 49: 211–215.

Gordon England. 2010. http://www.gordonengland.co.uk/tsc.htm.

Gougeon, P. and Moreau, C. 2001. Simultaneous independent measurement of splat diameter and cooling time during impact on a substrate of plasma-sprayed molybdenum particles. *J. Therm. Spray Technol.* 10: 76–82.

Gross, K.A., Ben-Nissan, B., Walsh, W.R., and Swarts, E. 1998a. Analysis of retrieved hydroxyapatite coated orthopaedic implants. In: Coddet, C. (ed.), *Thermal Spray: Meeting the Challenges of the 21st Century, Proceedings of the 15th International Thermal Spray Conference*, Nice, France, May 1998, pp. 1133–1138.

Gross, K.A. and Berndt, C.C. 1994. In vitro testing of plasma-sprayed hydroxyapatite coatings. *J. Mater. Sci. Mater. Med.* 5: 219–224.

Gross, K.A. and Berndt, C.C. 1998a. Thermal processing of hydroxyapatite for coating production. *J. Biomed. Mater. Res.* 39: 580–587.

Gross, K.A., Berndt, C.C., and Herman, H. 1998b. Amorphous phase formation in plasma-sprayed hydroxyapatite coatings. *J. Biomed. Mater. Res.* 39: 407–414.

Gross, K.A., Gross, V., and Berndt, C.C. 1998c. Thermal analysis of amorphous phases in hydroxyapatite coatings. *J. Am. Ceram. Soc.* 81: 106–112.

Gualtieri, G., Gualtieri, I., and Bettini, N. 1987. Tissue reaction to alumina powder injected into the joints of a pig. In: Pizzoferrato, A., Marchetti, P.G., Ravaglioli, A., and Lee, A.J.C. (eds.), *Biomaterials and Clinical Applications, Proceedings of the Sixth Conference for Biomaterials*, Bologna, Italy, pp. 741–745.

Gui, M. and Suk, B.K. 2001. Aluminum hybrid composite coatings containing SiC and graphite particles by plasma spraying. *Mater. Lett.* 51: 396–401.

Guipont, V., Espanol, M., Borit, F., Llorca-Isern, N., Jeandin, M., Khor, K.A., and Cheang, P. 2002. High-pressure plasma spraying of hydroxyapatite powders. *Mater. Sci. Eng.* A325: 9–18.

Haman, J.D. and Chittur, K.K. 1997. Four point bend testing of calcium phosphate coatings. *Proc. 16th Southern Biomedical Engineering Conf.*, pp. 305–308.

Hardy, D.C.R., Frayssinet, P., and Delince, P.E. 1999. Osteointegration of hydroxyapatite-coated stems of femoral prostheses. *Eur. J. Orthop. Surg. Traumatol.* 9: 75–81.

Harris, D.H. 1990. Overview of problems surrounding the plasma spraying of hydroxyapatite coatings. In: Bernecki, T.F. (ed.), *Thermal Spray Research and Applications, Proceedings of the Third NTSC*, Long Beach, CA, May 1990, pp. 419–423.

Hayashi, K., Inadome, T., Mashima, T., and Sugioka, Y. 1993. Comparison of bone-implant interface shear strength of solid hydroxyapatite and hydroxyapatite-coated titanium implants. *J. Biomed. Mater. Res.* 27: 557–563.

Healy, K.E. and Ducheyne, P. 1992. The mechanisms of passive dissolution of titanium in a model physiological environment. *J. Biomed. Mater. Res.* 26: 319–338.

Heimann, R.B., Kurzweg, H., and Vu, T.A. 1998. Hydroxyapatite-bond coat systems for improved mechanical and biological performance of HIP implants. In: Coddet, C. (ed.), *Thermal Spray: Meeting the Challenges of the 21th Century, Proceedings of the 15th International Thermal Spray Conference*, Nice, France, May 1998, pp. 999–1005.

Heimke, G., Hoedt, B.D., and Schulte, W. 1987. Ceramics in dental implantology, Biomaterials and Clinical Applications. In: Pizzoferrato, A., Marchetti, P.G., Ravaglioli, A., and Lee, A.J.C. (eds.), *Biomaterials and Clinical Applications, Proceedings of the Sixth Conference for Biomaterials*, Bologna, Italy. pp. 93–104.

Hench, L.L. 1987. Cementless fixation. In: Pizzoferrato, A., Marchetti, P.G., Ravaglioli, A., and Lee, A.J.C. (eds.), *Biomaterials and Clinical Applications, Proceedings of the Sixth Conference for Biomaterials*, Bologna, Italy, pp. 23–34.

Hench, L.L. and Ethridge, E.C. 1982. *Biomaterials: An Interfacial Approach*. Academic Press, New York.

Hing, K.A., Best, S.M., and Bonfield, W. 1999. Characterization of porous hydroxyapatite. *J. Mater. Sci.: Mater. Med.* 10: 135–145.

Hossain, M., Irwin, R., Baumann, M.J., and McCabe, L.R. 2005. Hepatocyte Growth Factor (HGF) adsorption kinetics and enhancement of osteoblast differentiation on hydroxyapatite surfaces. *Biomaterials* 26: 2595–2602.

Howard, S.J. and Clyne, T.W. 1991. Interfacial fracture toughness of vacuum-plasma-sprayed coatings. *Surf. Coat. Technol.* 45: 333–342.
Howard, S.J., Phillips, A.J., and Clyne, T.W. 1993. The interpretation of data from the four-point bend delamination test to measure interfacial fracture toughness. *Composites.* 24: 103–112.
Howard, S.J., Tsui, Y.C., and Clyne, T.W. 1994. The effect of residual stresses on the debonding of coatings-I: A model for delamination at a bimaterial interface. *Acta Metall. Mater.*, 42, 2823–2836.
Hwang, K. and Lim, Y. 1999. Chemical and structural changes of hydroxyapatite films by using a sol–gel method. *Surf. Coat. Technol.* 115: 172–175.
Inadome, T., Hayashi, K., Nakashima, Y., Tsumura, H., and Sugioka, Y. 1995. Comparison of bone-implant interface shear strength of hydroxyapatite-coated and alumina-coated implants. *J. Biomed. Mater. Res.* 29: 19–24.
Ishihara, S., Mcevily, A.J., Goshima, T., Kanekasu, K., and Nara, T. 2000. On fatigue lifetimes and fatigue crack growth behavior of bone cement. *J. Mater. Sci. Mater. Med.* 11: 661–666.
Ishikawa, K., Miyamoto, Y., Nagayama, M., and Asaoka, K. 1997. Blast coating method: New method of coating titanium surface with hydroxyapatite at room temperature. *J. Biomed. Mater. Res.* 38: 129–134.
Jarcho, M. 1981. Calcium phosphate ceramics as hard tissue prosthetics. *Clin. Orthop. Relat. Res.* 157: 259–278.
Ji, H. and Marquis, P.M. 1993. Effect of heat treatment on the microstructure of plasma-sprayed hydroxyapatite coating. *Biomaterials* 14: 64–68.
Jiang, X., Sampath, S., and Herman, H. 2001. Grain morphology of molybdenum splats plasma-sprayed on glass substrates. *Mater. Sci. Eng.* A299: 235–240.
Kanagaraja, S., Wennerberg, A., Eriksson, C., and Nygren, H. 2001. Cellular reactions and bone apposition to titanium surfaces with different surface roughness and oxide thickness cleaned by oxidation. *Biomaterials* 22: 1809–1818.
Khor, K.A. and Cheang P. 1994a. Effect of powder feedstock on thermal sprayed hydroxyapatite coatings. In: Berndt, C.C. and Sampath, S. (eds.), *Thermal Spray: Industrial Applications, Proceedings of the Seventh National Thermal Spray Conference*, Boston, MA, pp. 147–152.
Khor, K.A., and Cheang, P. 1994b. Laser post-treatment of thermally sprayed hydroxyapatite coatings. In: Berndt, C.C. and Sampath, S. (eds.), *Thermal Spray: Industrial Applications, Proceedings of the Seventh National Thermal Spray Conference*, Boston, MA, pp. 153–157.
Khor, K.A., Gu, Y.W., and Dong, Z.L. 2000. Plasma spraying of functionally graded yttria stabilized zirconia/NiCoCrAlY coating system using composite powders. *J. Therm. Spray Technol.* 9: 245–249.
Khor, K.A., Li, H., and Cheang, P. 2003a. Characterization of the bone-like apatite precipitated on HVOF sprayed calcium phosphate deposits. *Biomaterials* 24: 769–775.
Khor, K.A., Li, H., and Cheang, P. 2004. Significance of melt-fraction in HVOF sprayed hydroxyapatite particles, splats and coatings. *Biomaterials* 25: 1177–1186.
Khor, K.A., Li, H., Cheang, P., and Boey, S.Y. 2003b. In vitro behavior of HVOF sprayed calcium phosphate splats and coatings. *Biomaterials* 24: 723–735.
Kido, H. and Saha, S. 1998. Effect of HA coating on the dental implants: past, present and future directions. *Proc. 16th Southern Biomedical Engineering Conf.*, pp. 272–275.
Kijk, K., Schaeken, H.G., Wolde, J.G.C., and Jansen, J.A. 1996. Influence of annealing temperature on RF magnetron sputtered calcium phosphate coatings. *Biomaterials* 17: 405–410.
Kim, H., Georgiou, G., Knowles, J.C., Koh, Y., and Kim, H. 2004. Calcium phosphates and glass composite coatings on zirconia for enhanced biocompatibility. *Biomaterials* 25: 4203–4213.
Klein, C.P.A.T., Wolke, J.G.C., de Blieck-Hogervorst, J.M.A., and de Groot, K. 1994. Features of calcium phosphate plasma-sprayed coatings: An in vitro study. *J. Biomed. Mater. Res.* 28: 961–967.
Knabe, C., Howlett, C.R., Klar, F., and Zreiqat, H. 2004. The effect of different titanium and hydroxyapatite-coated dental implant surfaces on phenotypic expression of human bone-derived cells. *J. Biomed. Mater. Res. A* 71: 98–107.
Kokubo, T., Kushitani, H., Sakka, S., Kitsugi, T., and Yamamuro, T. 1990. *J. Biomed. Mater. Res.* 24: 721.

Kozerski, S., Pawlowski L., Jaworski, R., Roudet, F., and Petlt, F. 2010. Two zones microstructure of suspension plasma sprayed hydroxyapatite coatings. *Surf. Coat. Technol.* 204: 1380–1387.

Krauser, J.T. and Berthold, P. 1991. A scanning electron microscopy study of failed root from dental implant. *J. Dental Res.* 70: 274–281.

Kreye, H., Fandrich, D., and Muller, H.-H. 1986. Microstructure and bond strength of WC-Co coatings deposited by hypersonic flame spraying (Jet-Kote process). *Proc. 11th ITSC Montreal*, pp. 121–128.

Kumar, R., Cheang, P., and Khor, K. A. 2003. Radio frequency (RF) suspension plasma sprayed ultra-fine hydroxyapatite (HA)/zirconia composite powders. *Biomaterials* 24: 2611–2621.

Kurzweg, H., Heimann, R.B., Troczynski, T., and Wayman, W.L. 1998. Development of plasma-sprayed bioceramic coatings with bond coats based on titania and zirconia. *Biomaterials* 19: 1507–1511.

Kweh, S.W.K. 2000. Thermal spraying of bioceramics (HA) coatings. Masters in Engineering. School of Mechanical and Production Engineering. Nanyang Technological University.

Kwong, C.H., Burns, W.B., and Cheung, H.S. 1989. Solubilization of hydroxyapatite crystals by marine bone cells, macrophages and fibroblasts. *Biomaterials* 10: 579–584.

Labat, B., Chamson, A., and Frey, J. 1995. Effects of r-alumina and hydroxyapatite coatings on the growth and metabolism of human osteoblasts. *J. Biomed. Mater. Res.* 29: 1397–1401.

Lamy, D., Pierre, A.C., and Heimann, R.B. 1996. Hydroxyapatite coatings with a bond coat of biomedical implants by plasma projection. *J. Mater. Res.* 11: 680–686.

Laurent, P., Ducasse, P., and the ESSOR Group. 1999. Case reports: Total cementless knee prosthesis with hydroxyapatite coating: Results with the Alienor prosthesis after more than 6 years. *Eur. J. Orthop. Surg. Traumatol.* 9: 119–121.

Lausmaa, J., Ask, M., and Rolnnder, U. 1989. Preparation and analysis of Ti and alloyed Ti surfaces used in the evaluation of biological response. In: Hamker, J.S. and Giammara, B.L. (eds.), *Biomedical Materials and Devices.* 110: 647–653.

Lausmaa, J., Mattsson, L., and Rolander, U. 1986. Chemical composition and morphology of titanium surface oxides. *Biomed. Mater.* 55: 351–359.

Leguillon, D. 1997. Influence of micro-voids on toughness of interfaces. In: Rossmanith, H.P. (ed.), *Damage and Failure of Interface.* Balkema, Rotterdam, pp. 113–120.

Leigh, S.H., Lin, C.K., and Berndt, C.C. 1997. Elastic response of thermal spray deposits under indentation tests. *J. Am. Ceram. Soc.* 80: 2093–2099.

Lewis, G. and Mcvay, B. 1998. Effect of thermal spray process for depositing hydroxyapatite coating on a titanium alloy on its fatigue performance. *Proc. 17th Southern Biomedical Engineering Conf.*, pp. 119.

Li, C.J., Ohmori, A., and McPherson, R. 1997. Relationship between microstructure and Young's modulus of thermally sprayed ceramic coatings. *J. Mater. Sci.* 32: 997–1004.

Li, H. 2002. HVOF spraying of hydroxyapatite and hydroxyapatite/titania composites, PhD thesis, Nanyang Technological University, Singapore.

Li, H. 2004. unpublished data.

Li, H. and Khor, K.A. 2006. Characteristics of the nanostructures in thermal sprayed hydroxyapatite coatings and their influence on coating properties. *Surf. Coat. Technol.* 201: 2147–2154.

Li, H., Khor, K.A., and Cheang, P. 2000. Effect of the powders' melting state on the properties of HVOF sprayed hydroxyapatite coatings. *Mater. Sci. Eng. A* 293: 71–80.

Li, H., Khor, K.A., and Cheang, P. 2002a. Properties of heat treated calcium phosphate coatings deposited by high velocity oxy-fuel (HVOF) spray. *Biomaterials* 23: 2015–2112.

Li, H., Khor, K.A., and Cheang, P. 2002b. Titanium dioxide reinforced hydroxyapatite coatings deposited by high velocity oxy-fuel (HVOF) spray. *Biomaterials* 23: 85–91.

Li, H., Khor, K.A., and Cheang, P. 2003. Impact formation and microstructure characterization of thermal sprayed hydroxyapatite/titania composite coatings. *Biomaterials* 24: 949–957.

Li, H., Khor, K.A., and Cheang, P. 2004a. Thermal sprayed hydroxyapatite splats: Nanostrucures, splat formation mechanisms and TEM characterization. *Biomaterials* 25: 3463–3471.

Li, H., Khor, K.A., and Cheang, P. 2006. Effect of steam treatment during plasma spraying on the microstructure of hydroxyapatite (HA) splats and coatings. *J. Therm. Spray Technol.* 15: 610–616.

Li, H., Khor, K.A., and Cheang, P. 2007a. Adhesive and bending failure of thermal sprayed hydroxyapatite coatings: Effect of the nanostructures at interface and crack propagation phenomenon during bending. *Eng. Fract. Mech.* 74: 1894–1903.

Li, H., Khor, K.A., Chen, W.N., Tan, T.L., Pan, H., and Cheang, P. 2007b. Proteomics study of the osteoblast cells proliferated on nanostructured hydroxyapatite coatings. *Key Eng. Mater.* 330–332: 381–384.

Li, H., Khor, K.A., Chow, V., and Cheang, P. 2007c. Nanostructural characteristics, mechanical properties, and osteoblast response of spark plasma sintered hydroxyapatite. *J. Biomed. Mater. Res.* 82A: 296–303.

Li, H., Khor, K.A., Kumar, R., and Cheang, P. 2004b. Characterization of hydroxyapatite/nano-zirconia composite coatings deposited by high velocity oxy-fuel (HVOF) spray process. *Surf. Coat. Technol.* 182: 227–236.

Li, H., Ng, B.S., Khor, K.A., Cheang, P., and Clyne, T.W. 2004c. Raman spectroscopy determination of phases within thermal sprayed hydroxyapatite splats and subsequent in vitro dissolution examination. *Acta Mater.* 52: 445–453.

Li, J., Liao, H., and Hermansson, L. 1996. Sintering of partially-stabilized zirconia and partially-stabilized zirconia-hydroxyapatite composites by hot isostatic pressing and pressureless sintering. *Biomaterials* 17: 1787–1790.

Liao, C., Lin, F., Chen, K., and Sun, J. 1999. Thermal decomposition and reconstitution of hydroxyapatite in air atmosphere. *Biomaterials* 20: 1807–1813.

Liao, H., Normand, B., and Coddet, C. 2000. Influence of coating microstructure on the abrasive wear resistance of WC/Co cermet coatings. *Surf. Coat. Technol.* 124: 235–242.

Lima, R.S., Kucuk, A., and Berndt, C.C. 2001. Integrity of nanostructured partially stabilized zirconia after plasma spray processing. *Mater. Sci. Eng. A* 313: 75–82.

Lin, F., Liao, C., Chen, K., and Sun, J. 2000. Thermal reconstruction behavior of the quenched hydroxyapatite powder during reheating in air. *Mater. Sci. Eng.* C 13: 97–104.

Liu, D.M., Chou, H.M., and Wu, J.D. 1994. Plasma-sprayed hydroxyatptite coating: effect of different calcium phosphate ceramics. *J. Mater. Sci.: Mater. Med.* 5: 147–153.

Lopes, M.A., Santos, J.D., Monteriro, F.J., and Knowles, J.C. 1998. Glass-reinforced hydroxyapatite: A comprehensive study of the effect of glass composition on the crystallography of the composite. *J. Biomed. Mater. Res.* 39: 244–251.

Lopez-Sastre, A., Gonzalo-Orden, J.M., Altonage, J.A.R., Altonaga, J.R., and Orden, M.A. 1998. Coating titanium implants with bioglass and with hydroxyapatite: A comparative study in sheep. *Int. Orthop. (SICOT).* 22: 380–383.

Lugscheider, L., Remer, P., and Nyland, A. 1996. High velocity oxy fuel spraying: An alternative to the established APS-process for production of bioactive coatings. In: Sudarsan, T.S., Khor, K.A., and Jeandin, M. (eds.), *Proceedings of the Tenth International Conference on Surface Modification Technologies*, Singapore, 1996, pp. 717–727.

Luo, Z.S., Cui, F.Z., and Li, W.Z. 1999. Low-temperature crystallization of calcium phosphate coatings synthesized by ion-beam-assisted deposition. *J. Biomed. Mater. Res.* 46: 80–86.

Maxian, S.H., Zawadsky, J.P., and Dunn, M.G. 1993a. In vitro evaluation of amorphous calcium phosphate and poorly crystallized hydroxyapatite coatings on titanium implants. *J. Biomed. Mater. Res.* 27: 111–117.

Maxian, S.H., Zawadsky, J.P., and Dunn, M.G. 1993b. Mechanical and histological evaluation of amorphous calcium phosphate and poorly crystallized hydroxyapatite coatings on titanium implants. *J. Biomed. Mater. Res.* 24: 717–728.

McPherson, R., Gane, N., and Bastow, T.J. 1995. Structural characterization of plasma-sprayed hydroxylapatite coatings. *J. Mater. Sci. Mater. Med.* 6: 327–334.

Meyer, U., and Wiesmann, H.P. 2006. *Bone and Cartilage Engineering*. Springer, Berlin.

Montavon, G., Sampath, S., Berndt, C.C., Herman, H., and Coddet, C. 1995. Effects of vacuum plasma spray processing parameters on splat morphology. *J. Therm. Spray Technol.* 4: 67–74.

Munting, E. 1996. The contributions and limitations of hydroxyapatite coatings to implant fixation: A histomorphometric study of load bearing implants in dogs. *Int. Orthop. (SICOT).* 20: 1–6.

Murakami, T., Higaki, H., and Doe, S. 1996. Friction and wear characteristics of sliding pairs of bioceramics and polyethylene: Influence of aging and lubricants on tribological behavior of tetragonal zirconia polycrystals. *Bioceramics* 9: 499–502.

Murakami, Y. (chief editor). 1992. *Stress Intensity Factors Handbook*, Volume 3. Committee on Fracture Mechanics, The Society of Materials Science, Japan.

Nationalthermalspray.com. http://www.nationalthermospray.com/hvof.htm.

Ogiso, M., Yamamura, M., Kuo, P.T., Borgese, D., and Matsumoto, T. 1998a. Comparative push-out test of dense HA implants and HA-coated implants: Findings in a canine study. *J. Biomed. Mater. Res.* 39: 364–372.

Ogiso, M., Yamashita, Y., and Matsumoto, T. 1998b. Differences in microstructural characteristics of dense HA and HA coating. *J. Biomed. Mater. Res.* 41: 296–303.

Oonishi, H., Miyamoto, S., and Kohda, A. 1987. Hydroxyapatite coating on Ti and Al_2O_3—studies on the biological fixation. In: Pizzoferrato, A., Marchetti, P.G., Ravaglioli, A., and Lee, A.J.C. (eds.), *Biomaterials and Clinical Applications, Proceedings of the Sixth Conference for Biomaterials*, Bologna, Italy, pp. 69–74.

Oonishi, H., Yamamoto, M., Ishimau, H., Tsuji, E., Kushitani, S., Aono, M., and Ukon, Y. 1989. The effect of hydroxyapatite coating on bone growth into porous titanium alloy implants. *J. Bone Jt. Surg.* 10: 213–216.

Park, J.B. 1981. *Biomaterials Science and Engineering.* Plenum Press, New York.

Pasandideh-Fard, M., Pershin, V., Chandra S., and Mostaghimi, J. 2002. Splat shapes in a thermal spray coating process: Simulations and Experiments. *J. Therm. Spray Technol.* 11: 206–217.

Patel, A.M. and Spector, M. 1995. Oxidized zirconium for hemiarthroplasty: An in vitro assessment. *Bioceramics* 8: 169–175.

Patel, A.M. and Spector, M. 1997. Tribological evaluation of oxidized zirconium using an articular cartilage counterface: A novel material for potential use in hemiarthroplasty. *Biomaterials.* 18: 441–447.

Pawlowski, L. 1995. *The Science and Engineering of Thermal Spray Coatings.* John Wiley & Sons, Chichester, United Kingdom.

Pawlowski, L. 2008. *The Science and Engineering of Thermal Spray Coatings*, 2nd Edition. John Wiley & Sons, Chichester, United Kingdom.

Pazzaglia, U.E., Brossa, F., Zatti, G., Chiesa, R., and Andrini, L. 1998. The relevance of hydroxyapatite and spongious titanium coatings in fixation of cementless stems, an experimental comparative study in rat femur employing histological and microangiographic techniques. *Arch. Orthop. Trauma Surg.* 117: 279–285.

Penel, G., Leroy, G., Rey, C., Sombret, B., Huvenne, J.P., and Bres, E. 1997. Infrared and Raman microspectrometry study of fluor-fluor-hydroxy and hydroxyapatite powders. *J. Mater. Sci. Mater. Med.* 8: 271–277.

Piveteau, L.D., Girona, M.I., Schlapbach, L., Barbous, P., Boilot, J.-P., and Gasser, B. 1999. Thin films of calcium phosphate and titanium dioxide by a sol–gel route: A new method for coating medical implants. *J. Mater. Sci. Mater. Med.* 10: 161–164.

Radin, S., and Ducheyne, P. 1992. The effect of plasma sprayed induced changes in the characteristics on the in vitro stability of calcium phosphate ceramics. *J. Mater. Sci.* 3: 33–42.

Ramachandran, K., Selvarajan, V., Ananthapadmanabhan, P.V., and Sreekumar, K.P. 1998. Microstructure, adhesion, microhardness, abrasive wear resistance and electrical resistivity of the plasma sprayed alumina and alumina-titania coatings. *Thin Solid Films.* 315: 144–152.

Ranz, X., Pawlowski, L., and Sabatier, L. 1998. Phases transformations in laser treated hydroxyapatite coatings. In: Coddet, C. (ed.), *Thermal Spray: Meeting the Challenges of the 21th Century, Proceedings of the 15th International Thermal Spray Conference*, Nice, France, pp. 1343–1349.

Rao, R.R. and Kannan, T.S. 2002. Synthesis and sintering of hydroxyapatite-zirconia composites. *Mater. Sci. Eng.* C20: 187–193.

Reis, R.L. and Monteiro, F.J. 1996. Crystallinity and structural changes in HA plasma-sprayed coatings induced by cyclic loading in physiological media. *J. Mater. Sci.: Mater. Med.* 7: 407–411.

Reser, M.K., American Ceramic Society. 1983. *Phase Diagrams for Ceramists,* Volume 5, American Ceramic Society, Washington, DC.

Rey, C., Freche, M., Heghebaert, M., Heuughebaert, J.C., Lacout, J.L., Lebugle, A., Szilagyi, J., and Vignoles, M. 1991. Apatite Chemistry in Biomaterials, Shaping, and Biological Behaviour. In: Bonfield, W., Hasrings, G.W., and Tanner, K.E. (eds.), *Bioceramics, Volume 4,* 4th International Symposium on Ceramics in Medicine, London, UK.

Rohanizadeh, R., Trecant-Viana, M., and Daculsi, G. 1999. Ultrastructural study of apatite precipitation in implanted calcium phosphate ceramic: Influence of the implantation site. *Calcif. Tissue Int.* 64: 430–436.

Rose, F.R., Cyster, L.A., Grant, D.M., Scotchford, C.A., Howdle, S.M., Kevin, K.M., and Shakesheff, M. 2004. In vitro assessment of cell penetration into porous hydroxyapatite scaffolds with a central aligned channel. *Biomaterials* 25: 5507–5514.

Ruan, L., Wang, X., and Li, L. 1996. Structural analysis of new crystal phase for calcium phosphate in AL-A phase transition. *Mater. Res. Bull.* 31: 1207–1212.

Sampath, S. and Herman, H. 1996. Rapid solidification and microstructure development during plasma spray deposition. *J. Therm. Spray Technol.* 5: 445–456.

Sampath, S. and Jiang, X. 2001. Splat formation and microstructure development during plasma spraying: Deposition temperature effects. *Mater. Sci. Eng. A* 304–306: 144–150.

Schroeder, M. and Unger, R. 1997. Thermal spray coatings replace hard chrome. *Adv. Mater. Process.* 152: 19–21.

Sevostianov, I. and Kachanov, M. 2000. Modeling of the anisotropic elastic properties of plasma-sprayed coatings in relation to their microstructure. *Acta Mater.* 48: 1361–1370.

Shaw, L.L., Barber, B., Jordan, E.H., and Gell, M. 1998. Measurements of the interfacial fracture energy of thermal barrier coatings. *Scr. Mater.* 39: 1427–1434.

Shen, T.D., Koch, C.C., Tsui, T.Y., and Pharr, G.M. 1995. On the elastic moduli of nanocrystalline Fe, Cu, Ni, and Cu-Ni alloys prepared by mechanical milling/alloying. *J. Mater. Res.* 10: 2892–2896.

Shirkhanzadeh, M. 1994. X-ray diffraction and Fourier transform infrared analysis of nanophase apatite coatings prepared by electrocrystallization. *Nanostruct. Mater.* 4: 677–684.

Shirkhanzadeh, M. 1995. Calcium phosphate coatings prepared by electrocrystallization from aqueous electrolytes. *J. Mater. Sci.: Mater. Med.* 6: 90–93.

Sih, G.C. 1991. *Mechanics of Fracture Initiation and Propagation.* Kluwer Academic Publishers, Culembourg, The Netherlands.

Silva, C.C., Thomazini, D., Pinheiro, A.G., Lanciotti, F., Sasaki, J.M., Góes, J.C., and Sombra, A.S.B. 2002. Optical properties of hydroxyapatite obtained by mechanical alloying. *J. Phys. Chem. Solids.* 63: 1745–1757.

Silver, F.H. and Christiansen, D.L. 2000. *Biomaterials Science and Biocompatibility.* Springer–Verlag, New York.

Soga, N. 1982. Three-band theory and elastic moduli of glass. *J. Non-Cryst. Solids.* 52: 365–375.

Sordelet, D.J., Besser, M.F., and Logsdon, J.L. 1998. Abrasive wear behavior of Al–Cu–Fe quasicrystalline composite coatings. *Mater. Sci. Eng.* A255: 54–65.

Stein, G.S. and Lian, J.B. 1993. *Endocrine Rev.* 14: 424–442.

Steinhauser, S. and Wielage, B. 1997. Composite coatings: Manufacture, properties and application. *Proc. 10th Conf. on Surf. Modif. Technol.*, Singapore, pp. 436–450.

Stubican, V.S. 1988. Phase equilibria and metastabilities in the systems ZrO_2–MgO, ZrO_2–CaO, and ZrO_2–Y_2O_3. In: Somiya, S., Yamamoto, N., Hanagida, H. (eds.), *Advances in Ceramics, Volume 24A, Science and Technology of Zirconia III,* The American Ceramic Society, Inc., Ohio, pp. 71–82.

Sturgeon, A.J. and Harvey, M.D.F. 1995. High velocity oxyfuel spraying of hydroxyapatite. *Proc. ITSC'95,* Kobe, May 1995, pp. 933–938.

Suchanek, W., Yashima, M., Kakihana, M., and Yoshimura, M. 1997. Hydroxyapatite ceramics with selected sintering additives. *Biomaterials* 18: 923–933.

Sulzemetco.com. http://www.sulzermetco.com/desktopdefault.aspx/tabid-1741/3381_read-5289.

Suominen, E., Aho, A.J., Vedel, E., Kangasniemi, I., Uusipaikka, E., and Yli-Urpo, A. 1996. Subchondral bone and cartilage repair with bioactive glasses, hydroxyapatite, and hydroxyapatite-glass composite. *J. Biomed. Mater. Res.* 32: 543–551.

Szivek, J.A., Anderson, P.L., Dishongh, T.J., and de Young, D.W. 1996. Evaluation of factors affecting bonding rate of calcium phosphate ceramic coatings for in vivo strain gauge attachment. *J. Biomed. Mater. Res.* 33: 121–132.

Tadnno, S.T., Shibano, M., and Ukai, J. 1997. Residual stress evaluation of hydroxyapatite coating Ti implant. *J. Solid Mech. Strength Mater.* 40: 328–335.

Thomas, K.A., Kay, J.F., Cook, S.D., and Jarcho, M. 1987. The effect of surface macrotexture and hydroxylapatite coating on the mechanical strengths and histologic profiles of titanium implant materials. *J. Biomed. Mater. Res.* 21: 1395–1414.

Thorpe, R., Kopech, H., and Gahne, N. 2000. HVOF thermal spray technology. *Adv. Mater. Process.* 157: 27–29.

Tjong, S.C. and Chen, H. 2004. Nanocrystalline materials and coatings. *Mater. Sci. Eng. R: Rep.* 45: 1–88.

Tong, W., Chen, J., Li, X., Cao, Y., Yang, Z., Feng, J., and Zhang, X. 1996. Effect of particle size on molten states of starting powder and degradation of the relevant plasma-sprayed hydroxyapatite coatings. *Biomaterials* 17: 1507–1513.

Tong, W., Yang, Z., Zhang, X., Yang, A., Feng, J., Cao, Y., and Chen, J. 1998. Studies on diffusion maximum in x-ray diffraction patterns of plasma-sprayed hydroxyapatite coatings. *J. Biomed. Mater. Res.* 40: 407–413.

Toni, A., Pizzoferrato, A., and Venturini, A. 1987. Experimental bone ingrowth study of 3-D porous ceramic coating (poralo) for cementless HIP prosthesis. In: Pizzoferrato, A., Marchetti, P.G., Ravaglioli, A., and Lee, A.J.C. (eds.), *Biomaterials and Clinical Applications, Proceedings of the Sixth Conference for Biomaterials*, Bologna, Italy, pp. 57–62.

Tranquilli, P.L., Merolli, A., Palmacci, O., Gabbi, C., Cacchioli, A., and Gonnizzi, G. 1994. Evaluation of different preparations of plasma-spray hydroxyapatite coating on titanium alloy and duplex stainless steel in the rabbit. *J. Mater. Sci.: Mater. Med.* 5: 345–349.

Trentani, C., Montagnani, A., and Vicent, G. 1987. Ten year follow up of uncemented total HIP prosthesis with alumina acetabulum and titanium femoral stem by plasma jet technique. In: Pizzoferrato, A., Marchetti, P.G., Ravaglioli, A., and Lee, A.J.C. (eds.), *Biomaterials and Clinical Applications, Proceedings of the Sixth Conference for Biomaterials*, Bologna, Italy, pp. 177–182.

Tsui, Y.C., Doyle, C., and Clyne, T.W. 1998. Plasma sprayed hydroxyapatite coatings on titanium substrates: Part 2. Optimization of coating properties. *Biomaterials* 19: 2023–2043.

van Dijk, K., Gupta, V., Yu, A.K., and Jansen, J.A. 1998. Measurement and control of interface strength of RF magnetron-sputtered Ca–PO coatings on Ti–6Al–4V substrate using a laser spallation technique. *J. Biomed. Mater. Res.* 41: 624–632.

Vijayaraghavan, T.V. and Bensalem, A. 1994. Electrodeposition of apatite coating on pure titanium and titanium alloys. *J. Mater. Sci. Lett.* 13: 1782–1785.

Vogel, J., Russel, C., and Guntheer, G. 1996. Characterization of plasma-sprayed hydroxyapatite by P-MAS-NMR and the effect of subsequent annealing. *J. Mater. Sci.: Mater. Med.* 7: 495–499.

Vu, T.A. and Heimann, R.B. 1997. Influence of the CaO/TiO_2 ratio on thermal stability of hydroxyapatite in the system $Ca_5(PO_4)_3OH$–CaO–TiO_2. *J. Mater. Sci. Lett.* 16: 1680–1682.

Vu, T.A., Heimann, R.B., and Freiberg. 1996. Improvement of the adhesion of bioactive plasma sprayed coatings. Thermal Spray Conference, Essen, pp. 178–181.

Wang, B.C., Chang, E., Yang, C.Y., Tu, D., and Tsai, H. 1993a. Characteristics and osteoconductivity of three different plasma-sprayed hydroxyapatite coatings. *Surf. Coat. Technol.* 58: 107–117.

Wang, B.C., Lee, T.M., Chang, E., and Yang, C.Y. 1993b. The shear strength and failure mode of plasma-sprayed hydroxyapatite coating to bone: The effects of coating thickness. *J. Biomed. Mater. Res.* 27: 1315–1327.

Wang, H., Xia, W., and Jin, Y. 1996. Study on abrasive resistance of Ni-based coatings with a WC hard phase. *Wear* 195: 47–52.

Wang, J., Layrolle, P., Stigter, M., and de Groot, K. 2004. Biomimetic and electrolytic calcium phosphate coatings on titanium alloy: Physicochemical characteristics and cell attachment. *Biomaterials* 25: 583–592.

Wang, M., Yang, X.Y., Khor, K.A., and Wang, Y. 1999. Preparation and characterization of bioactive monolayer and functionally graded coatings. *J. Mater. Sci. Mater. Med.* 10: 269–273.

Wang, S., Lacefield, W.R., and Lemons, J.E. 1996. Interfacial shear strength and histology of plasma sprayed and sintered hydroxyapatite implants in vivo. *Biomaterials* 17: 1965–1970.

Wang, Y., Khor, K.A., and Cheang, P. 1998. Thermal spraying of functionally graded calcium phosphate coatings for biomedical implants. *J. Therm. Spray Technol.* 7: 50–57.

Webster, T.J. and Ejiofor, J.U. 2004. Increased osteoblast adhesion on nanophase metals: Ti, Ti6Al4V, and CoCrMo. *Biomaterials* 25: 4731–4739.

Webster, T.J., Siegel, R.W., and Bizios, R. 1999. Osteoblast adhesion on nanophase ceramics. *Biomaterials* 20: 1221–1227.

Wei, M., Ruys, A.J., Milthorpe, B.K., Sorrell, C.C., and Evans, J.H. 2001. Electrophoretic deposition of hydroxyapatite coatings on metal substrates: A nanoparticulate dual-coating approach. *J. Sol–Gel Sci. Technol.* 21: 39–48.

Wei, M., Ruys, A.J., Swain, M.V., Kim, S.H., Milthorpe, B.K., and Sorrell, C.C. 1999. Interfacial bond strength of electrophoretically deposited hydroxyapatite coatings on metals. *J. Mater. Sci.: Mater. Med.* 10: 401–409.

Wen, J., Leng, Y., Chen, J., and Zhang, C. 2000. Chemical gradient in plasma-sprayed HA coatings. *Biomaterials* 21: 1339–1343.

Weng, J., Liu, X., Zhang, X., and Ji, X. 1994. Thermal decomposition of hydroxyapatite structure induced by titanium and its dioxide. *J. Mater. Sci. Lett.* 13: 159–161.

Weng, W. and Baptista, J.L. 1998. Sol–gel derived porous hydroxyapatite coatings. *J. Mater. Sci. Mater. Med.* 9: 159–163.

Williams, D. F. 1981. *Biocompatibility of Clinical Implant Materials.* Vol. I, p. 9. Williams, D.F. (ed.). CRC Press, Boca Raton, FL.

Williams, K.R. and Blayney, A.W. 1987. An electron and optical microscopy study of implants in the rat middle ear: Comparison of several ceramics. In: Vincenzini, P. (ed.), *Ceramics in Clinical Applications*. Elsevier Science Publishers, pp. 265–274.

Wise, D.L., Trantolo, D.J., Lewandrowski, K., Gresser, J.D., Cattaneo, M.V., and Yaszemski, M.J. (eds.). 2000. Biomaterials engineering and devices: Human applications. *Volume 2: Orthopedic, Dental, and Bone Graft Applications*. Humana Press, Totowa, NJ.

Xie, J.W., Baumann, M.J., and McCabe, L.R. 2004. Osteoblasts respond to hydroxyapatite surfaces with immediate changes in gene expression. *J. Biomed. Mater. Res. A* 71: 108–117.

Xu, J.L., Khor, K.A., Gu, Y.W., Kumar, R., and Cheang, P. 2005. Radio frequency (RF) plasma spheroidized HA powders: Powder characterization and spark plasma sintering behavior. *Biomaterials* 26: 2197–2207.

Yamashita, K., Arashi, T., Kitagaki, K., Yamada, S., and Ogawa, K. 1994. Preparation of apatite thin films through RF-sputtering from calcium phosphate glasses. *J. Am. Ceram. Soc.* 77: 2401–2407.

Yang, C.Y., Lin, R.M., Wang, B.C., Lee, T.M., Chang, E., Hang, Y.S., and Chen, P.Q. 1997. In vitro and in vivo mechanical evaluations of plasma-sprayed hydroxyapatite coatings on titanium implants: The effect of coating characteristics. *J. Biomed. Mater. Res.* 37: 335–345.

Yang, C.Y., Wang, B.C., Chang, E., and Wu, J.D. 1995. The influences of plasma spraying parameters on the characteristics of hydroxyapatite coatings: a quantitative study. *J. Mater. Sci.: Mater. Med.* 6: 249–257.

Yang, Y.C. 2007. Influence of residual stress on bonding strength of the plasma-sprayed hydroxyapatite coating after the vacuum heat treatment. *Surf. Coat. Technol.* 201: 7187–7193.

Yankee, S.J., Pletka, B.J., Luckey, H.A., and Johnson, W. 1990. Processes for fabricating hydroxyapatite coatings for biomedical applications. In: Bernecki, T.F. (ed.), *Thermal Spray Research and Applications, Proceedings of the Third NTSC*, Long Beach, CA, May 1990, pp. 433–438.

Yoshikawa, T., Ohgushi, H., and Tamai, S. 1996. Immediate bone forming capability of prefabricated osteogenic hydroxyapatite. *J. Biomed. Mater. Res.* 32: 481–492.

Yoshinari, M., Ohtsuka, Y., and Derand, T. 1994. Thin hydroxyapatite coating produced by the ion beam dynamic mixing method. *Biomaterials*. 15: 529–535.

Yosomiya, R., Morimoto, K., and Nakajima, A. editors. 1990. *Adhesion and Bonding in Composites.* Marcel Dekker Inc.

Zhou, J., Zhang, X., Chen, J., Zeng, S., and de Groot, K. 1993. High temperature characteristics of synthetic hydroxyapatite. *J. Mater. Sci. Mater.* Med. 4: 83–85.

5

Nanostructured Titania Coatings for Biological Applications: Fabrication and Characterization

Yunchang Xin and Paul K. Chu

CONTENTS

Introduction

Since the interactions between artificial biomaterial and biological tissues occur mainly at their interface, the surface properties of biomaterials such as topography, roughness, chemistry, and physical characteristics exert a large influence on their biological response. On the other hand, nanomaterials can mimic the surface properties (including topography, energy, etc.) of natural tissues and may provide the preferred environment for tissue growth (Zhang and Webster 2007). There is increasing evidence that nanoscaled topography can enhance the activity of alkaline phosphate (ALP), accelerate hydroxyapatite (HA) nucleation and growth, and promote osteoblast adhesion and proliferation. Nanoporous structures have been observed to not only accelerate HA growth and improve adhesion and proliferation of osteoblasts, but also enhance biological fixation of the implants to the natural tissues (Sun et al. 2007; Popat et al. 2007a; Yao et al. 2006, 2008; Karlsson et al. 2003; Khang et al. 2008a; Khang et al. 2008b; Ruckh et al. 2009). These results suggest that if the surface architecture can be further refined, optimization of the various cell/matrix/substrate interactions and gene expression on the nanoscale can be accomplished (Nanci et al. 2006).

Biocompatible titania possesses excellent tribological performance and good corrosion resistance. The abundant Ti–OH groups on the surface can immobilize various functional substances. Owing to the nanosize effect, a nanostructured titania coating is a desirable candidate on biological devices. In this chapter, the strategies pertaining to the fabrication of various TiO_2 nanostructured coatings including nanotube arrays, nanoporous structures, and nanocrystalline films are reviewed. Structure characterization of the derived nanopatterns is described and the biological performance and applications of these nanosized titania coatings are succinctly discussed. Finally, the future trend of titania coating is discussed.

Titania

Titania is an n-type semiconductor and the conductivity decreases with O_2 partial pressure at temperature above 600°C. The activation energy for electronic conductivity is found to be 1.75 eV and the band gap energy is reported to be 3.05 eV. Rutile, anatase, and brookite constitute the three main phases of TiO_2. There are three main crystal faces in the rutile structure in which two of them, (110) and (100), possess quite low energy. The most thermally stable one is (110) in which an O atom is connected to two Ti atoms. The Ti atoms are 6-coordinated. (001) is less thermally stable and restructures above 475°C. There are 5-coordinate Ti atoms parallel to the rows of bridging O (Ramamoorthy et al. 1994). The two low-energy faces in the anatase structure are (101) and (001). The (101) face is the most prevalent one in anatase nanoscrystals and is corrugated with 5-coordinate Ti atoms (Burnside et al. 1998). In the brookite phase, the order of stability of the crystal faces is (010) < (110) < (100) (Beltran et al. 2006; Fujishima et al. 2008). The stability of the various nanoscaled titania phases is believed to be size-dependent. Rutile is the most stable phase when the particle size is above 35 nm. Below 11 nm, anatase is more stable. Brookite is found to be the most stable for particle size ranging from 11 to 35 nm (Zhang and Banfield 2000; Shklover et al. 1997; Fujishima et al. 2008).

Good biocompatibility of titania has been demonstrated in many in vivo and in vitro experiments (Erli et al. 2006; Li et al. 2004; Khang et al. 2008b). Titania coatings also possess ultrahigh hardness, excellent tribology behavior, as well as good corrosion resistance (Liu and Ding 2002; Zhao et al. 2007). TiO_2 is well known for its photocatalytical properties. The photogenerated charge carriers from reactive oxygen species include O_2^- and $OH^\bullet$ radicals. Matasunaga et al. demonstrate that UV-irradiated platinized TiO_2 powders can kill bacteria in an aqueous environment (Matsunaga et al. 1985). Titania is now becoming a desirable candidate as functional coatings and materials on biomedical devices.

Fabrication and Characterization of Nanostructured Titania Coatings

Fabrication of Titania Nanotube Arrays

A highly ordered and vertically oriented titania nanotubes array has been fabricated by simple anodization of pure titanium and its alloys in various solutions. This nanoscaled topography constitutes a materials architecture that offers a large surface area without concomitant reduction in the geometric and structural order (Doohun et al. 2008; Grimes and Mor 2009). The anodization process is economical, easy to operate, and capable of processing targets with complex shapes. The geometry of the titania nanotube such as tube length, tube diameter, tube spacing, wall thickness, and bonding strength can be precisely designed and controlled by modifying the processing parameters. This nanoscaled architecture has aroused increasing attention in applications such as filtration, drug delivery, and so forth.

Equipment for Anodization

Anodization is an electrolytic process that generates a protective or decorative oxide film on a metallic surface. Electrochemical anodization of titanium is usually carried out in an aqueous electrolyte using a cell with the titanium sheet as the anode and a Pt or graphite sheet as the cathode. Figure 5.1 illustrates a typical electrochemical anodization apparatus. The applied voltage forces the electron to the positive anode and surface metal atoms are exposed to oxygen ions within the electrolyte. These metal atoms and oxygen react and become an intrinsic part of the oxide layer. Initially, the increased voltage generates no additional current flow until a threshold is reached where the electric field intensity in the barrier is sufficient to force oxygen ions to diffuse across it and generate an ionic current. The oxygen ions react with the metal and thicken the oxide layer. This process goes on until the maximum applied voltage is reached, above which no desired reactions become obvious. Two processing modes, namely constant current mode and constant voltage mode, are commonly used (Grimes and Mor 2009).

Background of Titania Nanotubes

From an historical perspective, fabrication of titania nanotubes has gone through four generations. In 2001, Gong et al. fabricated the first generation of titania nanotube arrays up to 500 nm in length by electrochemical oxidation of pure titanium in an aqueous HF

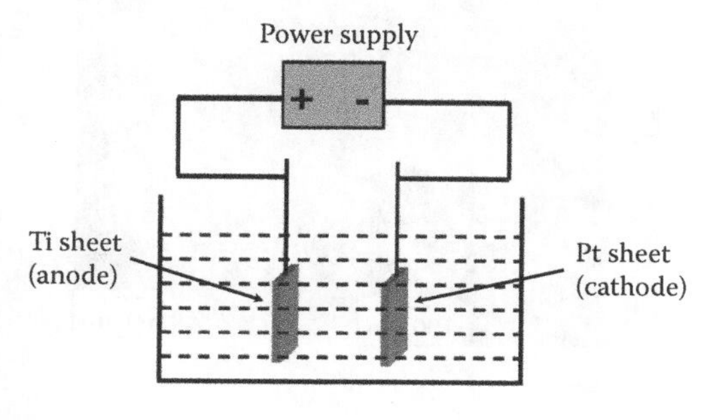

FIGURE 5.1
Scheme of typical electrochemical anodization cell for fabrication of titania nanotube arrays.

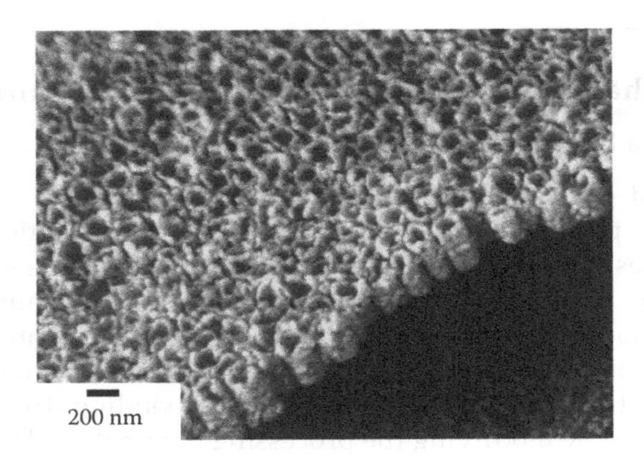

FIGURE 5.2
SEM micrograph of first-generation nanotubes on surface and cross section. (From Gong et al., *J. Mater. Res.*, 16, 3331–3334, 2001. With permission.)

electrolyte. The typical surface and cross-sectional morphologies are depicted in Figure 5.2 (Gong et al. 2001). Recently, Allam and Grimes (2008a) reported successful fabrication of titania nanotubes 2.5 μm long by using an Fe cathode. The second-generation fabrication feature increased nanotube lengths to several micrometers and growth rates of around 0.25 μm/h. This is accomplished by adjusting the pH of both the aqueous KF and NaF electrolytes to reduce the chemical dissolution rate of oxide (Michailowski et al. 2001). The representative morphology of these second-generation titania nanotube arrays is displayed in Figure 5.3. The third-generation synthesis employs organic electrolytes such as ethylene

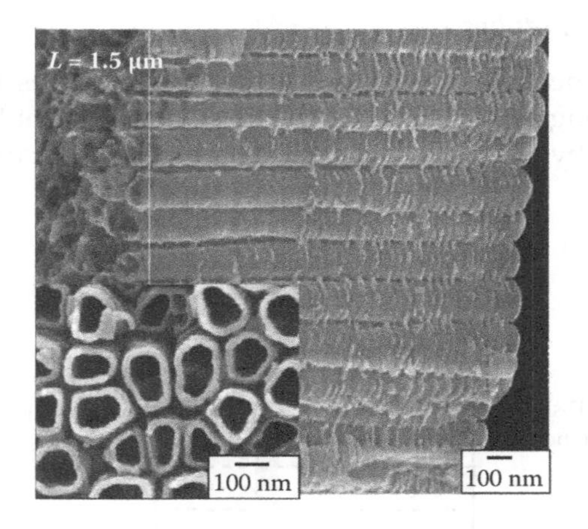

FIGURE 5.3
Lateral and cross-sectional views of second-generation titania nanotubes. (From Cai et al., *J. Mater. Res.*, 20, 230–236, 2005. With permission.)

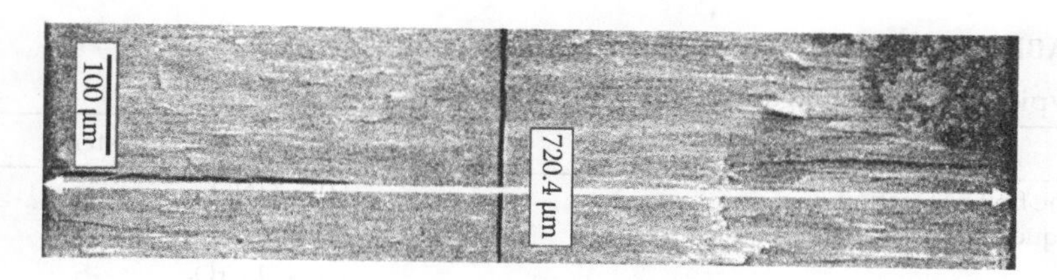

FIGURE 5.4
Cross-sectional views of a 720-μm-thick membrane synthesized using a fixed 60 V potential for double-sided anodization of Ti plate. (From Prakasam et al., *J. Phys. Chem. C*, 111, 7235–7241, 2007. With permission.)

glycol (EG), di–ethylene glycol, formamide (FA), *N*–methyformamide (NMF), and diethyl sulfoxide (DMSO) in combination with HF, KF, NaF, NH_4F, or $BnMe_3NF$ to provide fluoride ions to produce nanotube arrays with lengths up to 1000 μm (Michailowski et al. 2001; Jung et al. 2002, Kobayashi et al. 2002; Cai et al. 2005). A typical morphology of this type of titania nanotube arrays is presented in Figure 5.4. The fourth-generation fabrication technique utilizes nonfluoride-based anodization electrolytes (Grimes and Mor 2009) and a representative example is shown in Figure 5.5. Some important electrolytes used in the fabrication of the four generations of nanotube arrays are summarized in Table 5.1.

Mechanism of Nanotube Array Formation

The key processes in the growth of nanotube arrays are:

1. Growth of oxide at the metal surface due to reactions between the metal and O or OH^- ions
2. Migration of the metal ions through the metal to the metal/oxide interface
3. Field-assisted dissolution of oxide at the oxide/electrolyte interface
4. Chemical dissolution of the metal/oxide in the acidic electrolyte

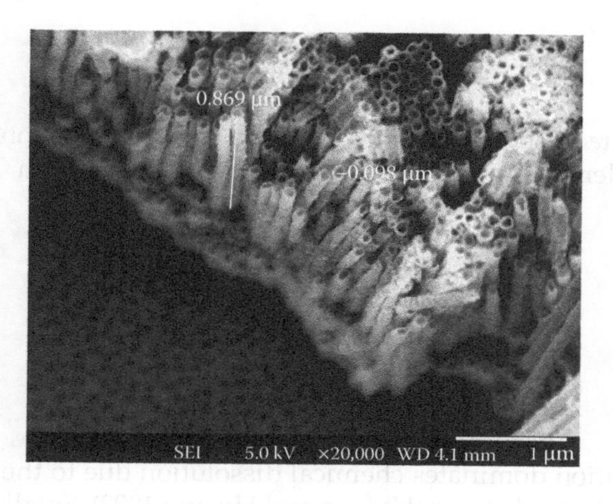

FIGURE 5.5
Representation of SEM morphology of fourth generations of nanotube arrays fabricated in HCl electrolytes. (From Allam et al., *J. Mater. Chem.*, 18, 2341–2348, 2008b. With permission.)

TABLE 5.1

Typical Electrolytes Four-Generation Synthesis of Titania Nanotubes

	Electrolyte Systems
The first generation (aqueous electrolyte)	$HF + HNO_3$
	$HF + H_2SO_4$
	$HF + H_2CrO_7$
	$NH_4F + CH_3COOH/H_2SO_4$
	$HF + H_3PO_4$
The second generation (buffered electrolyte)	Citric acid + NaF + Na_2SO_4
	Citric acid+ KF + Na_2SO_4
The third generation (polar organic electrolyte)	Formamide + dimethyl
	Dimethly sulfoxide
	Ethylene glycol
	Glycerol + NH_4F
	Methanol + H_2O +HF
The fourth generation (nonfluoride-based electrolyte)	HCl
	H_2O_2
	HCl + H_2O_2

Source: Grimes, C.A., Mor, C.K., *TiO_2 Nanotube Arrays. Synthesis, Properties, and Applications*, Springer Science, New York, NY, 2009; Allam et al., *J. Mater. Chem.*, 18, 2341–2348, 2008b; Prakasam et al., *J. Phys. Chem. C*, 111, 7235–7241, 2007; Christophersen et al., *Phys. Status Solid A*, 197, 34–38, 2003; Liu et al., *J. Phys. Chem. C*, 112, 253–259, 2008a; Paulose et al., *J. Phys. Chem. B*, 110, 16179–16184, 2006; Shankar et al., *J. Phys. Chem. C*, 111, 21–26, 2007; Yoriya et al., *J. Phys. Chem. C*, 111, 13770–13776, 2007; Yoriya et al., *J. Mater. Chem.*, 18, 3332–3336, 2008; Richter et al., *J. Mater. Res.*, 22, 1624–1631, 2007a; Richter et al., *Adv. Mater.*, 19, 946–948, 2007b; Chen et al., *Thin Solid Films*, 515, 8511–8514, 2007; Allam, N.K., Grimes, C.A., *J. Phys. Chem. C*, 111, 13028–13032, 2007. With permission.

As anodization commences, Ti^{4+} ions react with oxygen ions in the electrolyte and the oxide layer uniformly spreads across the surface. The reaction is shown below (Jaroenworaluck et al. 2007):

$$Ti + H_2O \rightarrow TiO_2 + 2H_2 \tag{5.1}$$

Fluoride ions can attack the oxide and hydrated layer, or the ions are moved across the anodic layer under the applied electric field and interact with Ti^{4+} as shown below (Lohrengel 1993):

$$TiO_2 + 6F^- + H^+ \rightarrow TiF_6^{2-} + 2H_2O \tag{5.2}$$

$$Ti(OH)_4 + 6\,F^- \rightarrow TiF_6 + 4OH^- \tag{5.3}$$

$$Ti^{4+} + 6F^- \rightarrow TiF_6^{2-} \tag{5.4}$$

Field-assisted dissolution dominates chemical dissolution due to the relatively large electric field across the thin oxide layer (Hwang and Hwang 1993). Small pits form from localized dissolution of the oxide and serve as the pore formation centers. The pores grow due to the inward movement of the barrier layer (Pakes et al. 2003). Ti^{4+} ions move from the metal to the oxide/electrolyte interface and dissolve in the electrolyte. The growth rate of oxide at the metal and oxide interface and the dissolution rate of oxide at the pore-bottom/electrolyte interface are ultimately equal. Therefore, the thickness of the barrier remains unchanged, although it migrates further into the metal leading to increasing tube length. The SEM results demonstrate that formation of small pits at the interpore region eventually leads to pore separation and tube formation. The thickness of the nanotubes ceases to increase when chemical dissolution of the oxide at the mouth of the tube equals to the rate of inward movement of the metal/oxide interface. This process is schematically illustrated in Figure 5.6 (Grimes and Mor 2009).

Chemical dissolution plays a key role in the formation of self-organized nanotube arrays. It reduces the thickness of the oxide layer (barrier layer) and keeps the electrochemical etching active. No nanotubes can be fabricated when chemical dissolution is too high or too low. The electrochemical dissolution rates depend on the applied potential as well as electrolyte concentrations. When electrochemical etching proceeds faster than chemical dissolution, the thickness of the barrier layer increases leading to reduced electrochemical etching to the rate determined by the chemical dissolution. In the F^- containing system, the chemical dissolution rate is controlled by the F^- concentration and pH of the electrolyte. Chemical dissolution increases with increased F^- and H^+ concentration. The anodization potential at which nanotubes form is related to the F^- concentration, with higher potentials required for an electrolyte with higher F^- concentration (Grimes and Mor 2009).

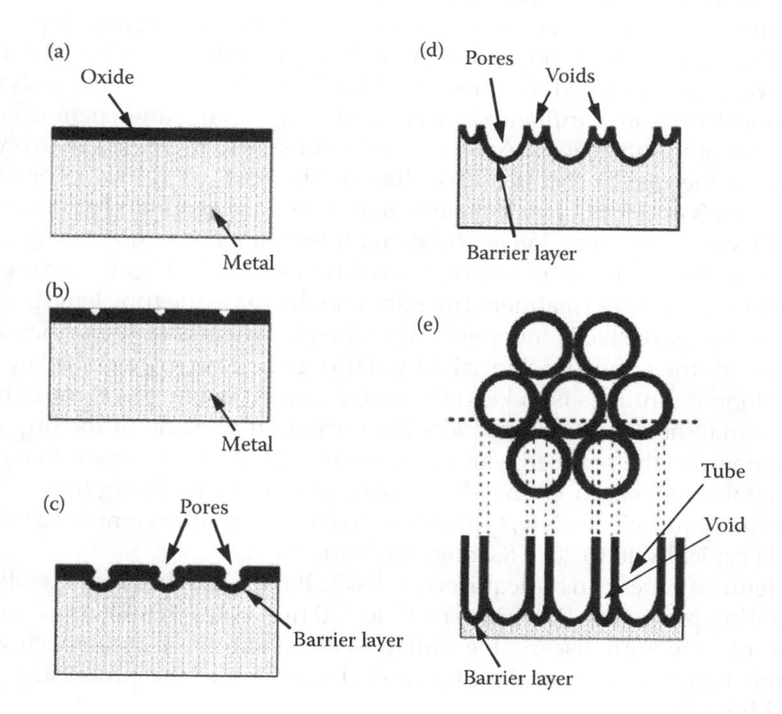

FIGURE 5.6
Schematic illustration of nanotube formation process. (a) Oxide layer formation, (b) pit formation on oxide layer, (c) growth of pit into scallop shaped pores, (d) metallic region between pores undergoes oxidation and field assisted dissolution, and (e) fully developed nanotubes with a corresponding top view. (From Grimes, C.A., Mor, C.K., *TiO_2 Nanotube Arrays. Synthesis, Properties, and Applications*, Springer Science, New York, NY, 2009. With permission.)

In an organic electrolyte system, water usually serves as the source of O. The exact mechanism is not yet well understood (Melody et al. 1998). There is evidence of OH^- injection from the electrolyte into the oxide layer during anodization. If more water is present, hydroxyl groups are injected into the oxide layer and influence the structure sufficiently to impede ion transport through the barrier layer. When less water is used, it is difficult to extract oxygen or hydroxyl ions from the solution, and the growth rate of the overall oxide film is reduced. The barrier layer possesses increased ionic conductivity caused by non-stoichiometry due to the insufficient supply of OH^- (Grimes and Mor 2009).

Geometry Control of Titania Nanotube Arrays

The geometrical features of the nanotube arrays can be controlled by parameters including applied potential, electrolyte composition, conductivity, and viscosity, as well as treatment duration and temperature. Furthermore, chemical dissolution and electrochemical etching are critical factors in the growth of nanotube arrays and the electrolyte temperature influences the rate of both etching processes. In an HF-base electrolyte, a low temperature tends to increase the wall thickness and reduce the tube length (Mor et al. 2005). It has been shown that the cathode materials play a significant role in the appearance of surface precipitates. An overpotential is referred to the excess potential required for discharge of an ion at the electrode above the equilibrium potential of the electrode. The overpotential at the cathode is a critical factor affecting the dissolution kinetics of the Ti anode and in turn the activity of the electrolyte and morphology of the architecture. Up to now, foils of Pt, Pd, Ni, Fe, Co, Cu, Ta, W, Sn, and Al as well as graphite sheets have been used and the details have been described (Grimes and Mor 2009). In buffered electrolyte systems, the pH of the electrolyte also influences electrochemical etching and chemical dissolution due to hydrolysis of titanium ions. An enhanced pH leads to increased hydrolysis, subsequently reducing the rate of chemical dissolution. The best pH values to produce longer tubes are between 3 and 5. Shorter but clean nanotubes are generated at lower pH values and higher pH values produce longer tubes with unwanted precipitates. Alkaline solutions do not favor the formation of self-organized nanotubes. In highly acidic electrolytes, for example, $pH < 1$, a longer treatment time does not increase the tube length. At a specific applied voltage, the pore size is independent of the pH whereas at a specific pH, the pore size increases with the applied potential. In polar organic electrolytes, the key to successful growth of long nanotubes is to keep the water content below 5%. Compared to water, the reduced availability of oxygen reduces the formation of oxide in the organic electrolyte. At the same time, the reduced water content retards chemical dissolution of the oxide in a fluoride-containing solution, thereby benefiting formation of long tubes. The applied voltage range in organic electrolyte, typically 10 to 60 V, is broader compared to that in NaF or KF which is typically 10 to 30 V (Grimes and Mor 2009).

Virtually identical tubes can be acquired in dissimilar electrolytes by controlling the different anodization processes. Pore sizes of 12 to 350 nm, outer diameters of 48 to 256 nm, wall thickness of 5 nm with discernable wall to 34 nm, and tube-to-tube spacing from adjacent to micrometers can be controlled by careful selection of the processing parameters (Grimes and Mor 2009).

Structure Characterization of Titania Nanotube Arrays

The typical morphology of titania nanotube arrays is shown in Figure 5.7. Vertically oriented nanotube arrays attach to the substrate with an open top and the bottom is closed

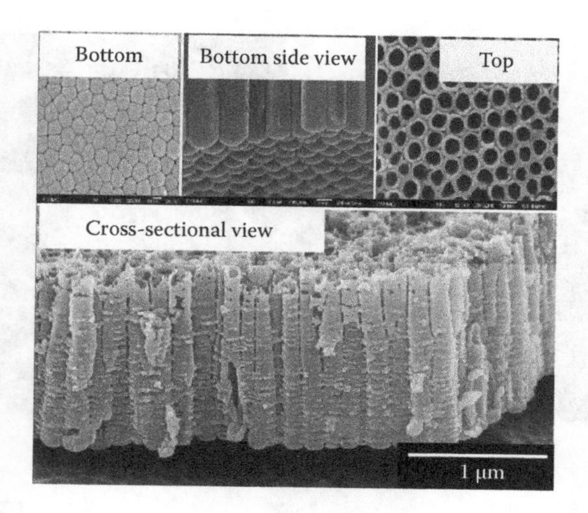

FIGURE 5.7
Morphologies of TiO_2 nanotube arrays acquired by anodization of Ti. Upper images are architecture from anodization in ethylene glycol electrolyte; lower image is architecture from Ti anodization in an aqueous KF bath. (From Grimes, C.A., Mor, C.K., *TiO_2 Nanotube Arrays. Synthesis, Properties, and Applications*, Springer Science, New York, NY, 2009. With permission.)

by a barrier layer of metal oxide. Both well-separated, stand-alone nanotubes and densely packed arrays can be acquired by using different electrolytes.

Generally, the as-prepared titania nanotubes are amorphous as suggested by both x-ray diffraction (XRD) and selection area diffraction (SAD) patterns. As shown in Figure 5.8, only peaks from crystalline titanium are present in the spectrum acquired after anodization in the NaF +Na_2SO_4 electrolyte. Nguyen has systematically studied the detailed structure of titania nanotubes using TEM and high-resolution TEM (HR–TEM). The nanotube is fabricated in an ethylene glycol solution containing 0.5 wt.% NH_4F at a constant potential of 20 V for 1 h (Nguyen et al. 2009). As shown in cross-sectional TEM pictures in Figure 5.9, the tubes are always oriented perpendicular to the metal surface. Adjacent tubes are connected by ridges that run perpendicular to the tube length. In addition, a barrier layer

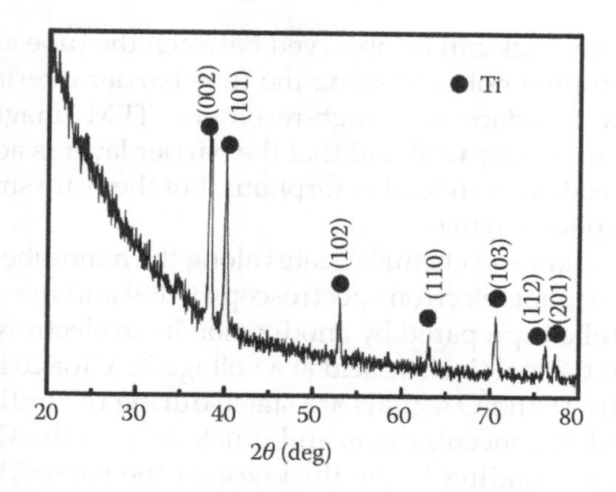

FIGURE 5.8
XRD pattern of titania nanotube arrays acquired by anodization in electrolyte containing 0.1 m/L NaF and 1 M/L Na_2SO_4 at 20 V for 2 h.

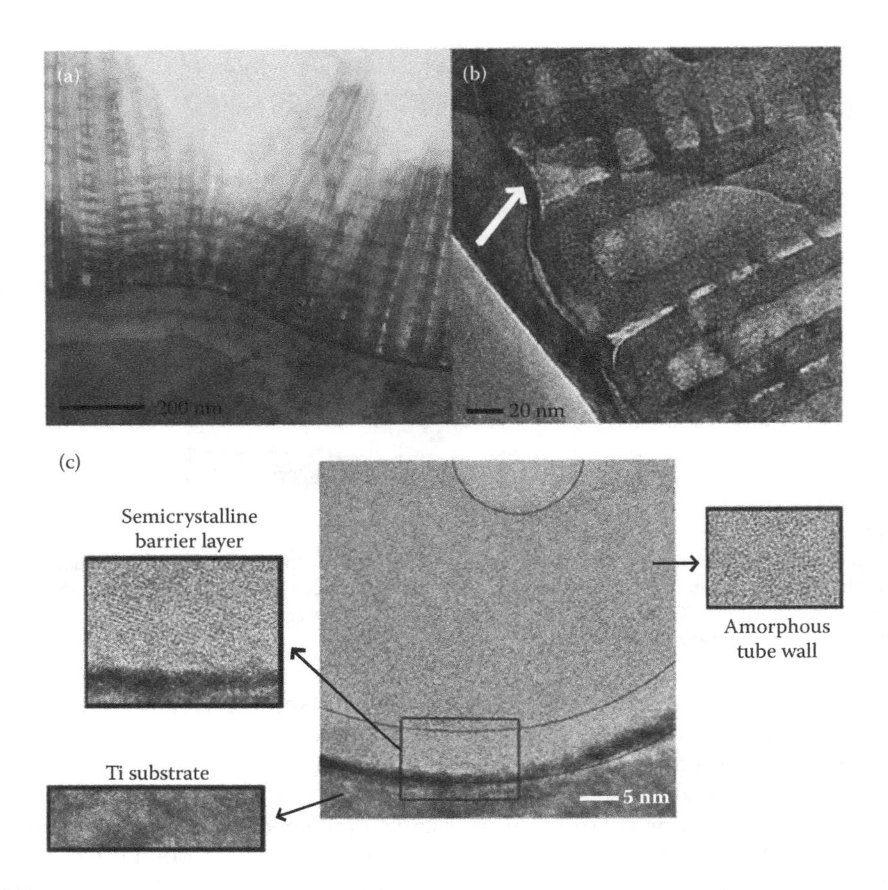

FIGURE 5.9
TEM views at various sites of the nanotube (a) and (b) are cross-section views; (c) HRTEM image of Ti substrate barrier layer and nanotube oxide. (From Nguyen et al., *Electrochim. Acta*, 54, 4340–4344, 2009. With permission.)

approximately 5 to 10 nm thick can be observed between the tube and metal (Figure 5.9b). This barrier layer is sculpted not only along the tube barrier interface, but also along the barrier/metal substrate interface. The high-resolution TEM images disclose the amorphous structure of the nanotube wall and that the barrier layer is actually semicrystalline in nature. Most of the oxides are indeed amorphous, but there are small crystalline regions embedded in the amorphous matrix.

The elemental distribution and chemical states along the nanotube length of titania nanotube are studied by x-ray photoelectron spectroscopy (XPS) and the results are presented in Figure 5.10. This nanotube is prepared by anodization in an electrolyte containing 1 mol/L Na_2SO_4, 0.1 mol/L NaF, 0.2 mol/L citric acid at a voltage 20 V for 20 h. The surface contains a high content of O. The Ti and O signals are stable during the initial 6 min of sputtering. Progressively increased Ti concentrations and quick drop in the O content are observed after about 58 min corresponding to the thickness of the barrier layer formed by anodization. The Ti 2p signal in the surface region only consists of one chemical state, Ti^{4+}/TiO_2. After sputtering for about 6 min, peaks corresponding to Ti^{2+}/TiO and Ti^{3+}/Ti_2O_3 also appear. When the sputtering time reaches about 70 min, a high Ti content is observed

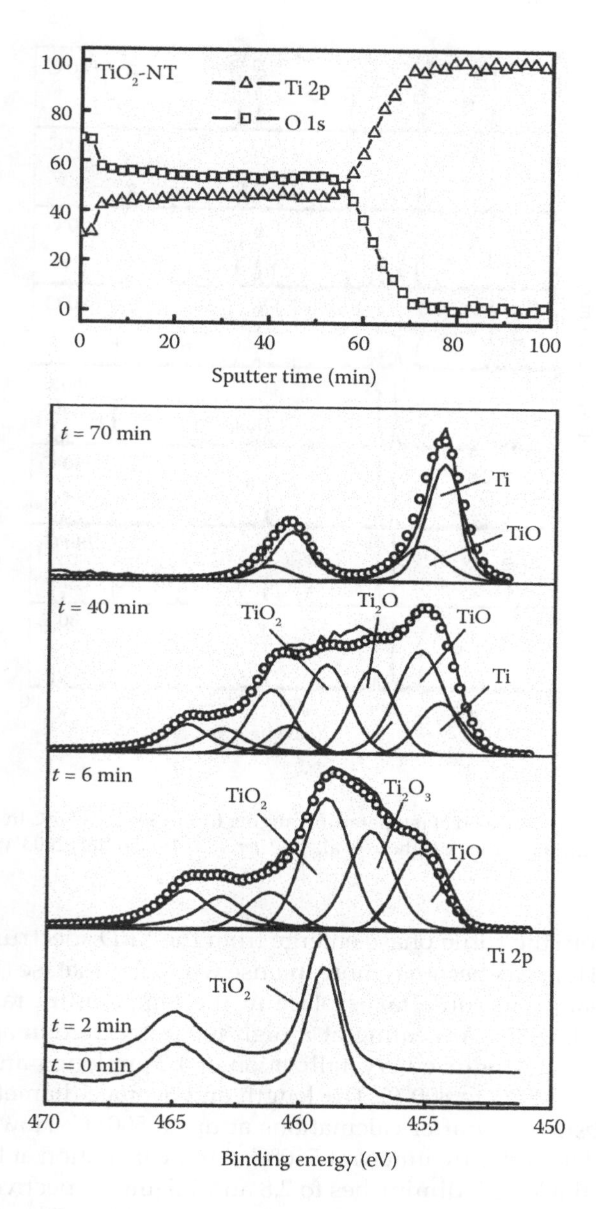

FIGURE 5.10
XPS depth profile of Ti and O and fine scanning spectra of Ti 2p in titania nanotube acquired by anodization in electrolyte containing 0.1 m/L NaF, 0.2 mol/L, citric acid, and 1 M/L Na_2SO_4 at 20 V for 2 h (sputtering rate is about 20 nm/min referenced to that SiO_2).

together with a small amount of Ti^{2+}/TiO as shown in the spectrum. The XPS results suggest that insufficient oxidization takes place during anodization of pure titanium and the anodized nanotubes consist of not only titania but also other forms of titanium oxides such as Ti_2O_3 and TiO.

Crystalline titania nanotubes can be obtained by annealing in oxygen or air. As shown in Figure 5.11, peaks from the anatase phase begin to appear at about 280°C. At temperatures

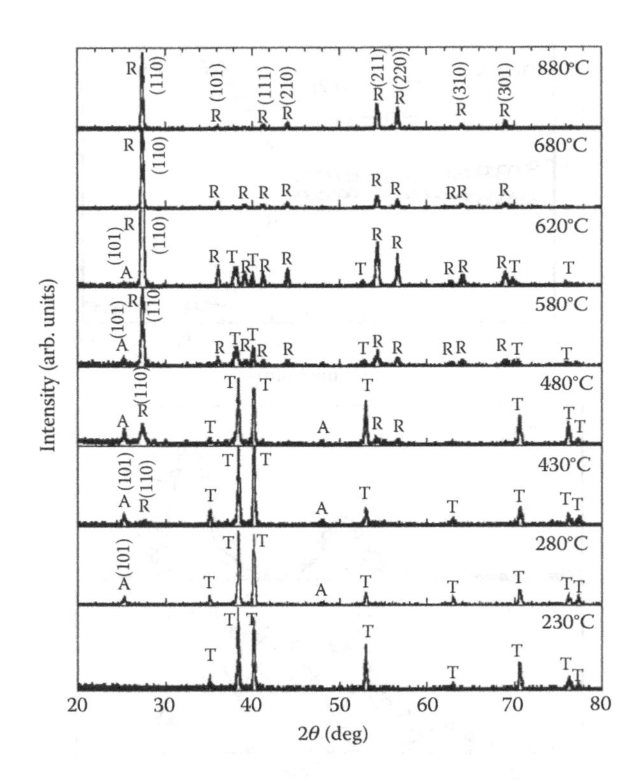

FIGURE 5.11
XRD patterns of the nanotube annealed at temperature ranging from 230°C to 880°C in oxygen ambient for 3 h. A, anatase; R, rutile; T, titanium. (From Varghese et al., *J. Mater. Res.*, 18, 156–165, 2003. With permission.)

near 430°C, peaks from the rutile phase emerge from the XRD spectrum. Above this temperature, the rutile (110) peak becomes more intense while the anatase (101) peak is weaker. Complete transformation to rutile takes place in the temperature range from 620°C to 680°C (Varghese et al. 2003). Annealing at a high temperature damages the nanotubes. Yang and coworkers had conducted crystallization of 4.2-μm long nanotubes with a pore size of about 80 nm at 300°C to 800°C. The length and average diameter of the nanotube are not changed substantially after calcinations at up to 500° C. However, the nanotube length decreases to 3 μm after treatment at 550°C. After calcination at higher temperature of 600°C and 700°C, the length diminishes to 2.8 and 1.5 μm, respectively. At 700°C, small protrusions occur through the nanotubes leading to cracking. The nanotube structure completely collapses when calcinated at 800°C (Yang et al. 2008a).

Biological Performance and Applications

Cell Response to Titania Nanotubes

The geometry of titania nanotubes that can be tailored influences the cell response. Popat and coworkers have carried out systematical investigation on the cell response for engineered titania nanotube arrays. A nanotube array about 80 nm in diameter and 500 nm in length is used. Progressively enhanced cell proliferation and ALP activity are observed compared to pure titanium. No adverse immune response occurs under in vivo conditions

(Popat et al. 2007a). However, the difference between this nanoscaled topography and dense titania films is not given. Park et al. have systematically investigated the influence of the pore size of the nanotube on the cell response. Titania nanotube arrays with diameters ranging from 15 to 100 nm are prepared by controlling the applied potential. The morphology of the as-prepared titania nanotube arrays is exhibited in Figure 5.12. Cell adhesion and spreading are highest on the 15-nm tubes and decline significantly for larger pore size. Cell growth experiments conducted on the 30-nm and smaller diameter nanotubes show extensive formation of paxillin-positive focal contact to which actin stress fibers are anchored and the cells have a highly migratory morphology with long protrusions (Park et al. 2009; Park et al. 2007). An enhanced cell migration behavior has been reported on titania nanotube arrays by Brammer et al. (2008). Cell differentiation of mesenchymal stem cells into osteogenic lineages has been observed and osteocalcin immunofluorescence is the highest on the 15-nm tubes but severely impaired on the 100-nm nanotubes. The most remarkable discovery is the strong induction of apoptosis on the 100-nm tubes (Park et al. 2007). As the predicted surface occupancy size by the head of an integrin heterodimer consisting of a β-propeller of the R-chain and the domain of β-chain is about 10 nm (Takagi et al. 2002), it is believed that 15 to 20 nm spacing allows or force clustering of integrins into the nearly closest spacing possible resulting in optimal integrin activation.

Bioactivity/Bone Conductivity

Bioactivity or named bone conductivity is referred to as the capability that the materials can induce growth of bone like HA from body fluids. This performance can be evaluated both in vivo and in vitro. Tsuchiya has reported HA growth behavior on anodic titania nanotubes. Their study demonstrates that apatite formation on titania nanotubes depends on the nanotube length and crystallographic phase of titania. The 500-nm-long nanotube hardly induces precipitation of apatite, while a thick HA layer forms on the 2.5-μm-long nanotube after soaking in SBF for 2 weeks. It has been reported that a crystalline structure greatly affects the bioactivity of titania nanotubes. Anatase or anatase and rutile structures can induce more effective apatite growth on the nanotubes. It is interesting that the

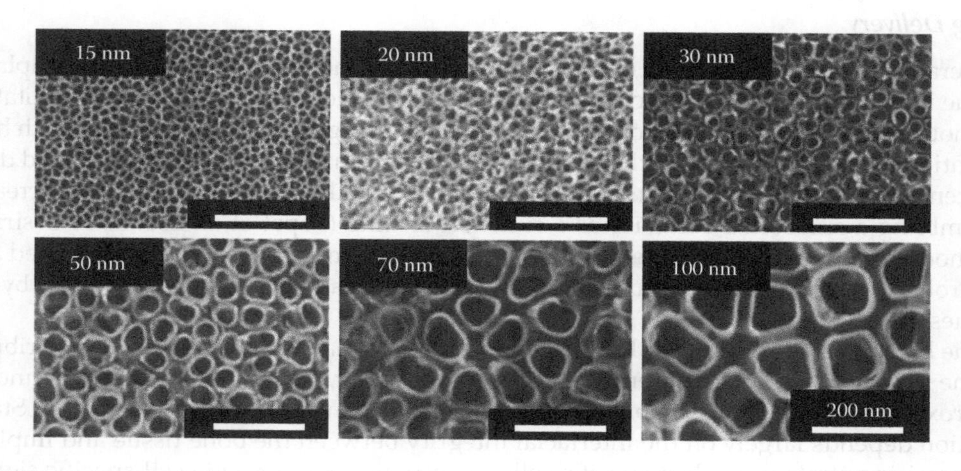

FIGURE 5.12
SEM views of a highly ordered titanitube with various pore sizes between 15 and 100 nm fabricated by tailoring applied potentials ranging from 1 to 20 V. (From Park et al., *Nano Lett.*, 7, 1686–1691, 2007. With permission.)

500-nm-long crystalline nanotubes can also induce growth of HA rapidly. Both the Ti–OH and crystallography influence the bioactivity of titania nanotubes (Tsuchiya et al. 2006).

Kunze et al. have uncovered more details about the precipitation process of HA on titania nanotube arrays. During the early stages of apatite nucleation, more Ca and P are found on the nanotubes than on flat TiO_2. Initial nucleation proceeds better on unannealed substrates than that on the annealed one on account of a higher degree of hydration. The crystallography does not appear to play a major role in the initial stage of apatite formation and it is believed that there are similar nucleation mechanisms for crystalline and on amorphous nanotubes. At the later stage of precipitation, the crystallography of the substrate plays an important role in homogeneous apatite formation as stable growth can only proceed on a crystalline substrate surface. It has also been found that titania nanotubes promote formation of very thick apatite films, whereas thin but incompletely closed precipitated layers form on the compact TiO_2 surface (Julia et al. 2008).

It has been found that titania nanotubes enhance apatite deposition from simulated body fluids (SBFs) compared to compact TiO_2 layer. A possible reason is the higher nucleation rates on titania nanotubes than on a flat surface. This mainly results from the higher specific surface area that provides a larger amount of OH^- on the surface. The surface area in a titania nanotube 1.66 μm long, 100 nm in diameter, and 20 nm thick (wall thickness) is about 45 times larger than that of a flat surface. The TiO_2/solution interface has positively polarized titanium and negatively polarized oxygen sites. In body fluids, OH^- can adsorb onto the TiO_2 surface and Ti–OH forms at the solid–liquid interface. The Ti–OH groups are acidic or basic depending on the pH of the surrounding solution. The isoelectric point at which the surface shows zero charge corresponds to a pH of about 5.4 for titanium oxide. In a physiological pH of about 7.4, the surface is slightly negatively charged due to the presence of deprotonated acidic hydroxides. This negatively charged surface attract cations such as Ca^{2+} followed by the arrival of HPO_4^{2-} or $H_2PO_4^-$, resulting in nucleation of HA. The HA will grow by consuming Ca and P from the SBFs. In addition, faster and better nucleation on the nanotubes may stem from the fact that the ions from the SBFs have better access to the nanotubular surface because they can diffuse into the channels and form nuclei uniformly over the walls.

Drug Delivery

Generally, orally supplemented or injection of drugs cannot effectively reach the implant–tissue interface, particularly necrotic or vascular tissues left after surgery. This limitation cannot be overcome by increasing the doses because of organ toxicity associated with high quantities of certain drugs. On the other hand, oral administration leads to increased drug concentration in the blood plasma immediately after intake but it subsequently decreases resembling a sinusoidal behavior as a function of time (Popat et al. 2007b). A desirable method is to effectively load the drug on the surface of implants to achieve sustained and controlled release of the drug so that the released drug can be effectively absorbed by the tissues in the vicinity directly.

The high specific area and hollow tubular structure of nanotubes are desirable attributes in the drug loading and delivery platform. In particular, the TiO_2 surface has abundant hydroxyl groups that can enable immobilization of many functional substances. Stable fixation depends largely on the interfacial integrity between the bone tissue and implant. A promising strategy to elicit specific cellular response is to provide cell-specific signals to control and improve the osseointegration of implants. RGD peptides, growth factor including transforming growth factor–β (TGF–β), bone morphogenetic proteins (BMPs), insulin-like growth factors (IGFs), fibroblast growth factors (FGFs), bone morphogenetic protein–2 (BMP–2), bovine serum albumin (BSA), and lysozyme (LYS) have been investigated as model proteins for the loading and release efficiency from nanotube platforms. BSA is a large molecule with a net negative charge at neutral pH as opposed to LYS, which is smaller in size with a net positive charge at neutral pH. Nanotubes can be filled with BSA and LYS by the simplified lyophilization method. The release characteristics of BSA and LYS are studied in PBS (pH = 7) and acetate buffer (pH = 4.5). When loaded with 200 to 800 μg of BSA and LYS, approximately 60% to 80% of the protein is retained in the nanotubes after washing regardless of the initial loading. As expected, slower and sustained release from nanotubes takes place. The release curves also suggest that leaching rate of the positively charged LYS is much slower than that of negatively charged BSA. This is believed to stem from the difference between the negatively and positively charged proteins interacting with the surface charges of the nanotube interface. There are stronger electrostatic interactions between the positive charged LYS and negatively charged nanotube surface (Popat et al. 2007b).

The release of functional substances using the above method can only be sustained for h. In order to be clinically useful, drug release from implants should last for days or weeks. The release rate of drugs can be tailored by changing the length and diameter of the nanotubes. Using titania nanotubes with variable diameters from 100 to 300 nm and lengths from 1 μm and 5 μm, paclitaxel (with hydrodynamic radius about 0.5 nm) elution in PBS at 37°C from nanotube arrays suggests that the maximum drug release is reached at approximately 2 weeks. The release of drug as a function of time is presented in Figure 5.13. With the same nanotube pore size, the nanotube length profoundly affects the total drug elution. The 1-μm-long nanotube holds less than half the amount of drug compared to a 5-μm-long nanotube. The drug delivery dependence on the nanotube dimensions shows that the nanotopography of the tubes is directly responsible for the drug elution behavior. Elution is largely insensitive to the tube diameter, but rather to the total length of nanotube. Elution measurements of large molecule BSA have been performed and the results indicate elution durations on the order of months. Larger diameter nanotubes elute less drug than 100-nm nanotubes with the same length (Peng et al. 2009).

Song et al. (2009) have recently developed an actively controllable drug delivery system based on titania nanotubes. The amphiphilic TiO_2 nanotube serves as the controllable drug release system based on a hydrophobic cap on a hydrophilic titania nanotube. This

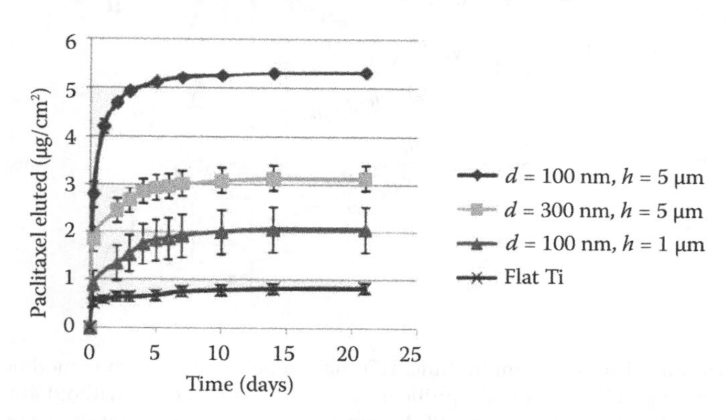

FIGURE 5.13
Paclitaxel elutions for nanotube arrays of various dimensions. (From Peng et al., *Nano Lett.*, 9, 1932–1936, 2009. With permission.)

hydrophobic cap prevents uncontrolled leaching of the hydrophilic drugs into the aqueous environment. By exploiting the photocatalytic properties of TiO_2 for UV induced chain scission of the attached organic monolayer, the cap can be removed and highly controlled release of drugs is achieved. Figure 5.14 schematically describes the procedures to fabricate amphiphilic TiO_2 nanotubes and the drug loading methods. The procedures begin with an anodization step followed by hydrophobic surface modification. Afterward, a second tube (hydrophilic) layer is grown underneath the first one by a second anodization process. The first layer is grown in an electrolyte containing glycerol/water/NH_4F to a thickness of about 750 nm and a diameter of 90 nm. Subsequently, a hydrophobic monolayer of octadecylphosphonic acid (OPDA) is attached to the tube wall. The nanotube is then anodized again in an ethylene glycol/NH_4F electrolyte. The second layer consists of 1-μm-

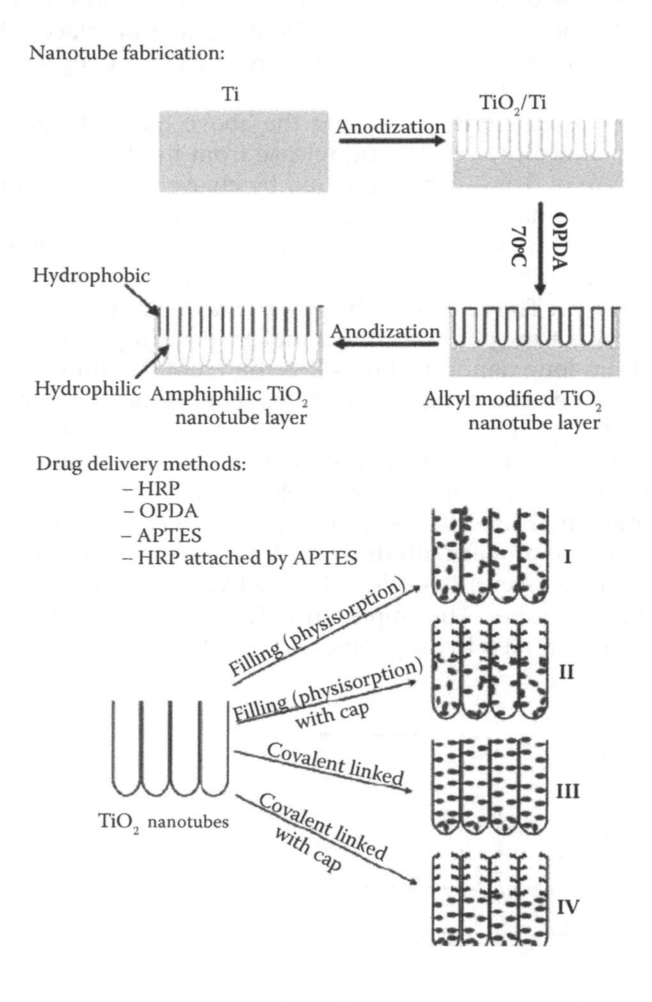

FIGURE 5.14
Scheme of procedure for fabricating amphiphilic TiO_2 nanotube layers and four methods for drug loading using horseradish peroxide (HRP) as a hydrophilic model drug (I) immersion without any TiO_2 surface modification (for reference), (II) immersion after OPDA modification in upper nanotube layer (hydrophobic cap), (III) covalently attached HRP over entire nanotube layers, and (IV) OPDA cap in upper nanotube layer and covalently attached HRP in lower nanotube layer. (From Song et al., *J. Am. Chem. Soc.*, 131, 4230–4232, 2009. With permission.)

long tubes with a diameter of about 90 nm. The grafted OPDA monolayer after the first step of anodization generates a hydrophobic top on the tube. After the second anodization step, a new hydrophilic surface is created. Four loading methods have been developed. Unmodified nanotubes are loaded by simple immersion in the drug system to allow free and physisorbed drug molecules inside the tube. In the second approach, capped tubes are exposed to the drug solution with DMSO, which acts as a surfactant. This approach leads to free HRP molecules in the lower part of the tubes. After evaporation of DMSO, the drugs are trapped by the hydrophobic cap. The drugs are grafted onto the hydrophilic tube walls by an APTES/vitamin C monolayer linker. The fourth approach combines approaches 2 and 3 resulting in loading of the drugs to the lower part of the nanotubes. Different release curves in the phosphate buffering solution (PBS) are obtained. Quick and uncontrolled release is observed in nanotubes loading by approach 1. Almost 90% of the drug is released during the first 1 min. With regard to the OPDA-capped nanotube and surface-linked drug nanotube, the release rate can be adjusted by UV irradiation. Strong UV irradiation yields a faster release rate. The amphiphilic nanotube layer with OPDA and covalently linked drugs allows controllable release.

Mg, Zn, and Sr are important biological elements. By a simple hydrothermal treatment, titania nanotubes can be transformed into crystalline $SrTiO_3/MgTiO_3/ZnTiO_3$ nanotube arrays. More detailed information about the $SrTiO_3$ nanotubes can be found in (Xin et al. 2009). This $SrTiO_3$ or ($MgTiO_3$ and Zn TiO_3) can leak Sr (Mg, Zn) slowly for a prolonged period by slow dissolution and ion exchange. After the hydrothermal treatment, the nanotube architecture is retained. A representative morphology of the $SrTiO_3$ nanotubes arrays prepared by the hydrothermal treatment in 0.02 mol/L $Sr(OH)_2$ is shown in Figure 5.15. As $Mg(OH)_2$ and $Zn(OH)_2$ are nearly insoluble, transformation from titania nanotube to $MgTiO_3$ nanotubes can be realized in two steps—hydrothermal treatment in a diluted NaOH solution forming the Na_2TiO_3 nanotube arrays and subsequent ion exchange reaction of the derived Na_2TiO_3 in the $MgCl_2$ or $ZnCl_2$ solution. It should be kept in mind that the NaOH solution should not be too concentrated, as a high content of OH^- destroys the tubular structure. Generally, the NaOH concentration does not exceed 0.05 mol/L. The nanotube arrays are capable of leaching biological elements but also leave room for loading

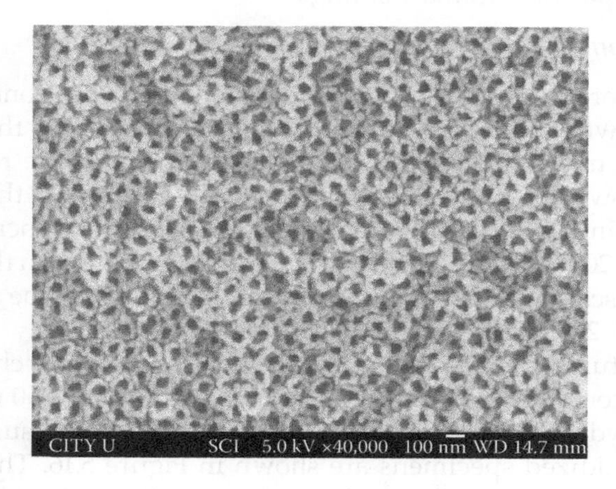

FIGURE 5.15
SEM micrograph of $SrTiO_3$ nanotube arrays fabricated by hydrothermal treatment titania nanotube arrays in 0.02 mol/L $Sr(OH)_2$ solution.

other functional substances. In addition, the well-retained nanotube arrays also retain the scale effects on the biological response.

The success of implants depends not only on the bone-implant integration process, but also a sterile environment around the implant preventing bacterial infection. In fact, bacterial infection is one of the most common problems after orthopedic surgery and can result in serious and life-threatening conditions such as osteomyelitis. Acute infection or chromic osteomyelitis develops in as many as 5% to 33% of implant surgeries (Popat et al. 2007c; Sujata 2005; Wong and Bronzino 2007). Hence, antibiotic treatment is usually prescribed to patients to prevent any complications that may arise after implant surgery. In situ loading of antibiotic substances (gentamicin, Ag and Cu elements) on titanium nanotube is a desirable solution. In the work of Popat et al. (2007c), gentamicin is filled by a simplified lyophilization method. The gentamicin solution is prepared in a phosphate buffering solution and introduced onto the nanotube surface to ensure even coverage. Afterward, the surface is dried under vacuum at room temperature for 2 h. The above process is repeated several times. Finally, PBS is used to remove the excess drugs. It has been found that the gentamicin-loaded nanotubes are effective in minimizing initial bacterial adhesion. Cell cultures up to 7 days also suggest higher cell adhesion and proliferation compared to titanium surfaces. Gibbins et al. have loaded silver on titania nanotubes by electrodeposition and the antibiobacterial properties and biocompatibility are examined; 99% of bacteria are killed. However, the TiO_2 nanotube surfaces with and without silver show good cell-to-cell attachment, high cell proliferation, and enhanced bone cell-material interactions in comparison to the Ti control (Das et al. 2008).

Surface modification with the nanotube layers may be particularly desirable as it not only enhances the mechanical properties, biocompatibility, and bioactivity of the medical implants by controlling the geometry, but also offers the opportunity to additionally regulate the cell response by loading biologically active signaling molecules. In conclusion, by tailoring the geometry and functionalization, TiO_2 nanotubes can be designed to support functions of osteoblasts including differentiation and are useful in coatings on osteointegrative implants.

Fabrication of Nanoporous Titania Coatings

Fabrication of Interconnected Porous Coating

An interconnected porous structure on the micrometer scale can contain living bone cells leading to tissue growth and enhanced bonding strength between the implants and adjacent bone tissues. A nanoscaled porous structure cannot provide room for living cells. However, it can allow filopodia of the growing cells to go into the nanoscaled pores, producing a locked-in cell structure that in the long term can increase the stability of implants (Oh and Jin 2006). There has been more evidence that when the surface roughness approaches the nanoscale, many surprising biological benefits can be achieved (Popat et al. 2007a; Brammer et al. 2008; Nanci et al 1998; de Oliveira et al. 2004).

A porous nanotextured surface can be fabricated by controlled chemical oxidiation of Ti in an electrolyte containing a mixture of H_2SO_4 and H_2O_2 (50:50 of 37 N sulfuric acid and 30% aqueous hydrogen peroxide). The SEM pictures of the surface morphology of the untreated and oxidized specimens are shown in Figure 5.16. The untreated samples show a very smooth surface at high magnification and a distinctive nanotexture characterized by nanopits formed after chemical oxidization. The inset in Figure 5.16b reveals 3-D spongelike porosity with a 22 ± 0.5 nm average diameter of the nanopits. The surface of the

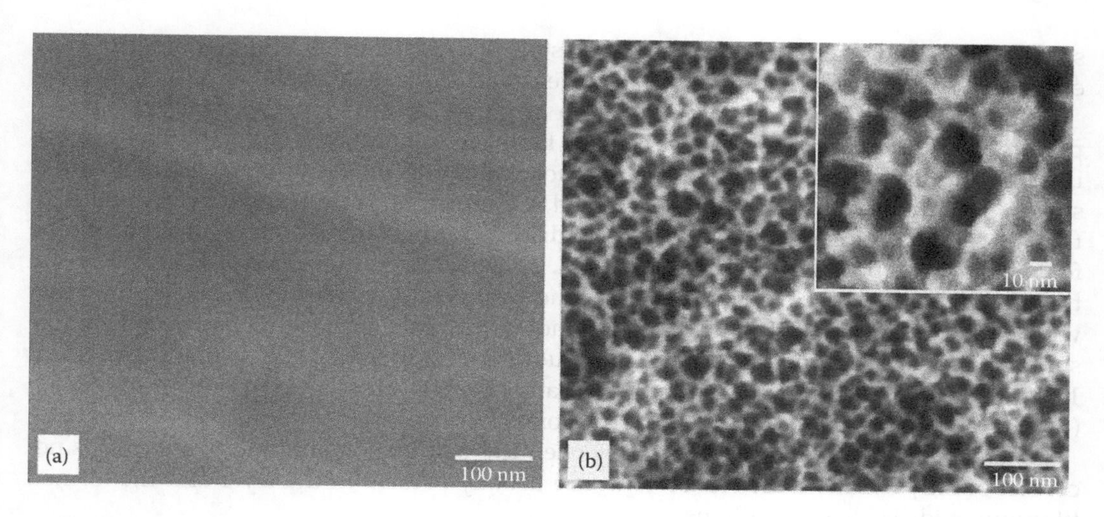

FIGURE 5.16
SEM micrographs of the control (a) and the chemical oxidized pure Ti (b). (From Nanci et al., *Surf. Sci.*, 600, 4613–4621, 2006. With permission.)

oxide layer is nearly TiO_2, as suggested by the XPS results. XRD results further show that the formed layer is mainly amorphous. In fact, oxide layers formed by chemical oxidization or electrochemical oxidization are usually amorphous (Nanci et al. 2006).

Variola et al. have produced a nonporous structure in Ti–6Al–4V alloy as shown in Figure 5.17 (Variola et al. 2008). As this alloy consists of two phases, different etching behavior is observed. The β phase tends to form the nanotexture morphology more quickly. However, after about 2 h of etching, the nanoscaled morphologies in the β and α phase grains become similar. That is, a uniform nanopit surface is formed. As etching proceeds, the diameter of pits increases slightly. It has also been demonstrated that the nanoporous

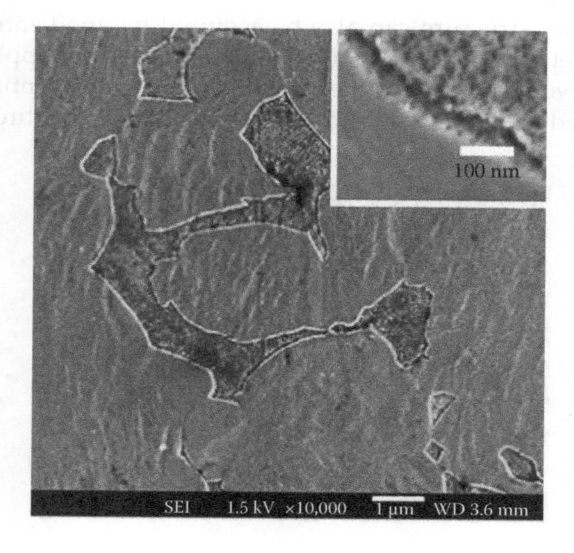

FIGURE 5.17
Morphology of nanoporous structure on Ti–6Al–4V alloy fabricated by etching in HNO_3 for electrolyte containing H_2SO_4 and H_2O_2 for 30 min. (From Variola et al., *Biomaterials*, 29, 1285–1298, 2008. With permission.)

surface selectively promotes the growth of osteoblasts while inhibiting that of fibroblasts, effectively realizing regulation of the activities of cells in a biological environment.

Besides chemical oxidization, anodization of pure titanium can also generate a nanoporous titanium oxide layer. Shih et al. have fabricated multinanoporous titania by anodization in an NaOH solution. The surface morphology of the multinanoporous titania is shown in Figure 5.18. A pretreatment named cathodization is performed before anodization. By cathodization in H_2SO_4, titanium hydride is formed and it is claimed to benefit the formation of the porous structure (Shih et al. 2007). XPS depth profiles of Ti and O reveal that the thickness of the oxide layer with cathodization (300 nm) is much thicker than that without cathodization (200 nm). Here, it is noted that the mechanically polished sample suffers from acid pickling (2% ammonium fluoride, a solution of 2% hydrofluoric acid, and 10% nitric acid at room temperature for 60 s.) and chemical etching (HF (2 vol.%) and HNO_3 (4 vol.%) at room temperature for several seconds).

Generally, the oxide layer fabricated by chemical oxidization and anodization does not consist of only titania. Both TiO or Ti_2O_3 are usually present in the layer and the formed titanium oxide is also amorphous.

Nanonetworked Titania Coatings

There is an interesting type of nanoscaled porous structure of titania, namely the nanonetwork. This structure can be fabricated by galvanic–static anodization in a highly concentrated NaOH solution (Chiang et al. 2009; Yang et al. 2009). The typical morphology of the nanoscaled network is shown in Figure 5.19. A multilayered network structure with lateral pore size of about 65 ± 33 nm is observed. The thickness of the grid ranges from 5 to 30 nm. It is also found that a higher anodization current results in a greater lateral pore size. XRD results indicate that the network is composed of mainly anatase TiO_2. Subsequent in vitro experiments disclose good bioactivity. This morphology also stimulates human bone marrow mesenchymal stem cells growth as demonstrated by in vitro and in vivo experiments.

This kind of network structure can also be acquired by anodization in the potentiostatic mode (Huang et al. 2004). The pore size depends on the applied voltage but the wall thickness is not very sensitive to the potential. At larger potentials, the thickness of oxide layer is increased. A similar morphology can be obtained by direct exposure of pure

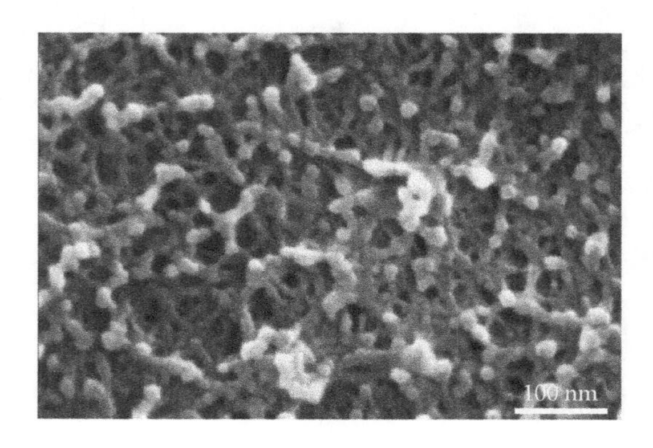

FIGURE 5.18
Surface morphology of Ti with 15 A/cm² anodization and 5 A/cm² cathodic pretreatments. (From Shih et al., *Appl. Surf. Sci.*, 253, 3678–3682, 2007. With permission.)

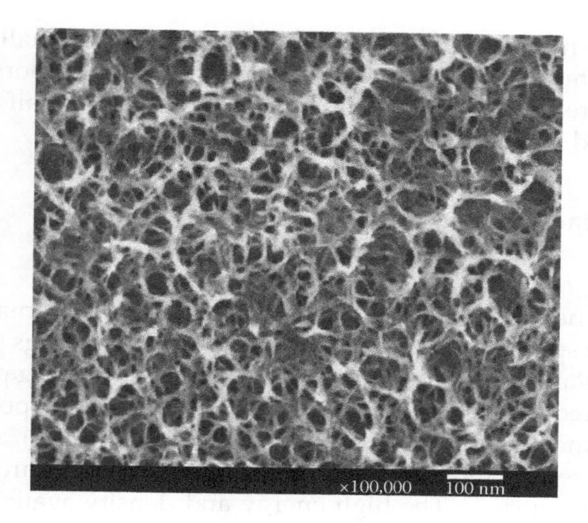

FIGURE 5.19
A typical SEM view of nanonetwork titania coating on titanium fabricated by anodization in high concentration of NaOH solution. (From Yang et al., *J. Alloy. Compd.*, 479, 642–647, 2009. With permission.)

Ti to a concentrated NaOH solution. Figure 5.20 shows the cross-sectional view of this type of porous structure. The pore size increases with the NaOH concentration but it is not affected much by the treatment time (1.5–15 M/L). The pore size is also progressively enhanced compared to the anodization method. TEM view discloses that the net has a nanotubular structure 200 to 300 nm long and about 10 nm in diameter. SAD patterns

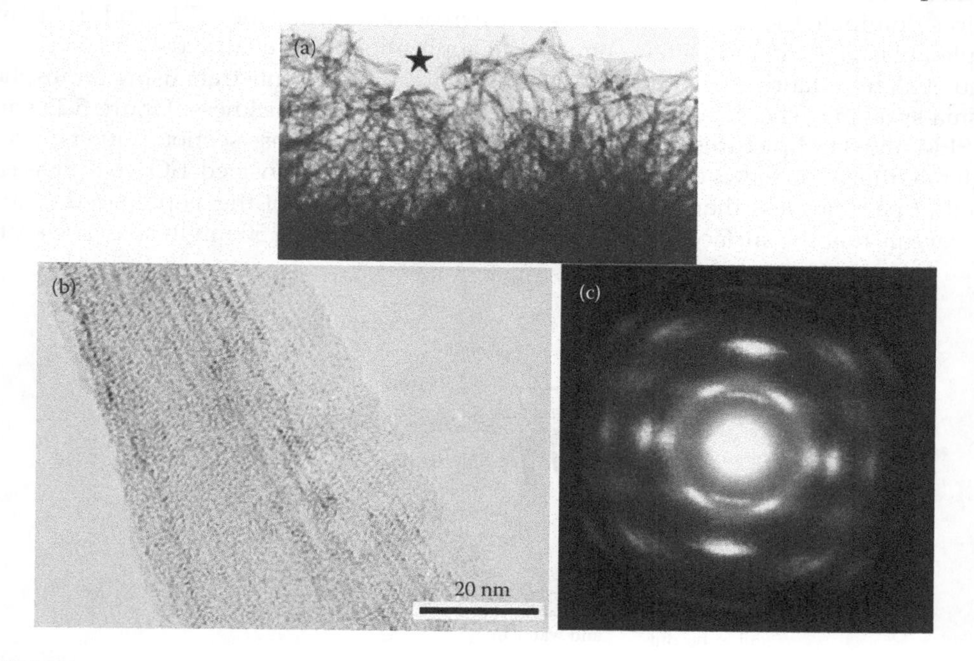

FIGURE 5.20
TEM views of one type of network structure on pure Ti after exposure in concentrated KOH for 10 h. (a) Cross-section views, (b) views of single net, and (c) SAD pattern of single net in (b). (From Lee et al., *Curr. Appl. Phys.*, 9, e266–e269, 2009. With permission.)

suggest that the net is nanocrystallined K_2TiO_3 (Lee et al. 2009). Usually, the network structure obtained by chemical treatment needs a processing time of more than 10 h, whereas the electrochemical treatment can be completed in no more than half an hour. In addition, the pore size achieved by anodization is much smaller.

Fabrication of Compact Nanocrystalline Titania Coatings

Plasma Spraying

Titania coating with nanosized particles can be fabricated by plasma spraying. Both cold spraying and plasma spraying can produce nanocrystalline coatings (Zhu and Ding 2000). Usually, nanosized titania powders are utilized during the spraying process. The particles size in the as-deposited coating depends mainly on the size of the powders.

Plasma spraying includes atmospheric plasma spraying (APS) and vacuum plasma spraying (VPS). Figure 5.21 illustrates this process. An electrical arc is used to melt and spray materials onto a surface. The high energy and density available in the plasma jet make it one of the popular thermal spraying techniques. The density, temperature, and velocity of the plasma plume are crucial to the formation of coatings. The temperature of the plasma depends mainly on the degree of ionization which in turn is determined by the type of plasma gas and parameters of the plasma. At present, gases such as Ar, He, N_2, and H_2 are commonly used in a plasma torch. To ensure environmental inertness, a mixture of argon and hydrogen is commonly used. Formation of the plasma sprayed coating consists of three stages: (1) melting and accelerating of the particle from the supplier, (2) transportation of the powder to the plasma torch, and (3) interaction between the molten materials and plasma beam and surrounding atmosphere. Currently, DC plasma arc devices dominate the commercial market, whereas radio frequency (RF) and inductively coupled plasma (ICP) have a few commercial applications (Liu et al. 2004).

Liu et al. have fabricated nano-TiO_2 coatings on Ti–6Al–4V substrate using atmospheric plasma spraying. The deposited coating is about 100 μm in thickness. Figure 5.22 shows the SEM and TEM pictures of the surface morphology and cross section (Liu et al. 2005). High magnification views of the SEM picture show that the nanosized TiO_2 coating is composed of particles less than 50 nm in size. TEM observation of the as-prepared coatings also reveals that the surface mainly consists of grains less than 50 nm in size. The coating

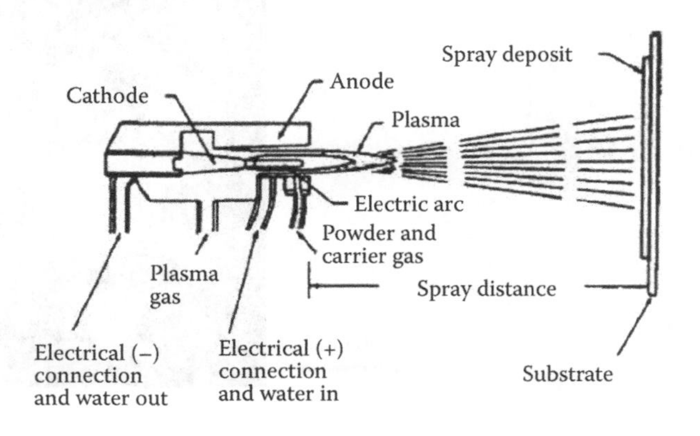

FIGURE 5.21
Schematic illustration of plasma-spraying technique. (From Liu et al., *Mater. Sci. Eng.*, R 47, 49–121, 2004. With permission.)

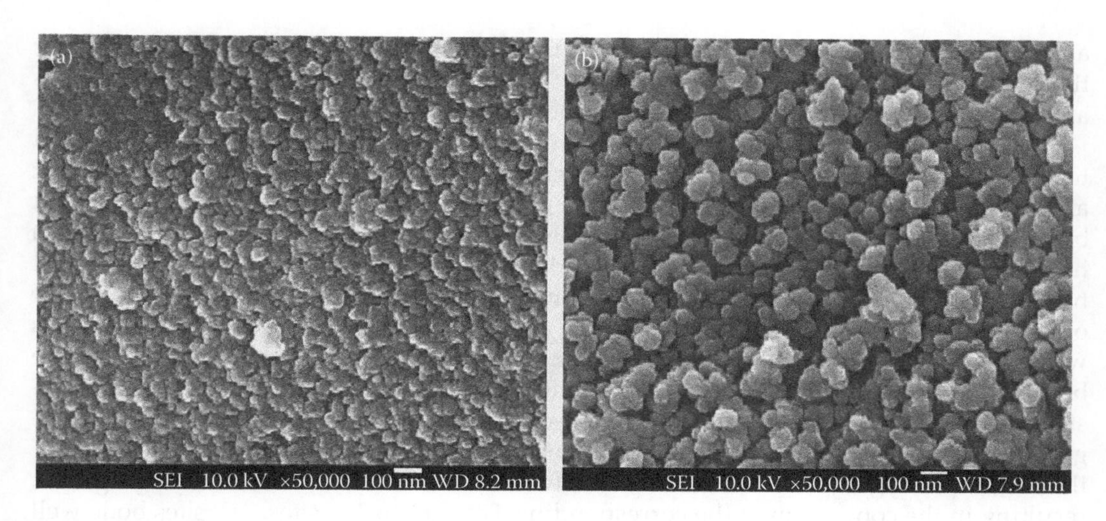

FIGURE 5.22
SEM micrographs of nanosized titania coating on pure titanium prepared by plasma spraying. (a) Low magnification, (b) high magnification. (From Liu et al., *Biomaterials*, 26, 6143–6150, 2005. With permission.)

is composed of two layers. The outer layer is about 500 nm thick with grains size of less than 50 nm, whereas the interior layer contains columnar grains with size ranging from 100 to 200 nm, as shown in Figure 5.23b. The SAD pattern discloses a crystalline structure of the TiO_2. XRD results further confirm that the coating mainly consists of rutile titania with a small amount of anatase and TiO_{2-x} suboxide.

Fan et al. have also successfully prepared nanosized titania coatings using vacuum cold spraying. This system is composed of a vacuum chamber and vacuum pump, an aerosol room, an accelerating gas feeding unit, a particle-accelerating nozzle, a two-dimensional work table, and the control unit. TiO_2 particles are accelerated by high-pressure He gas and

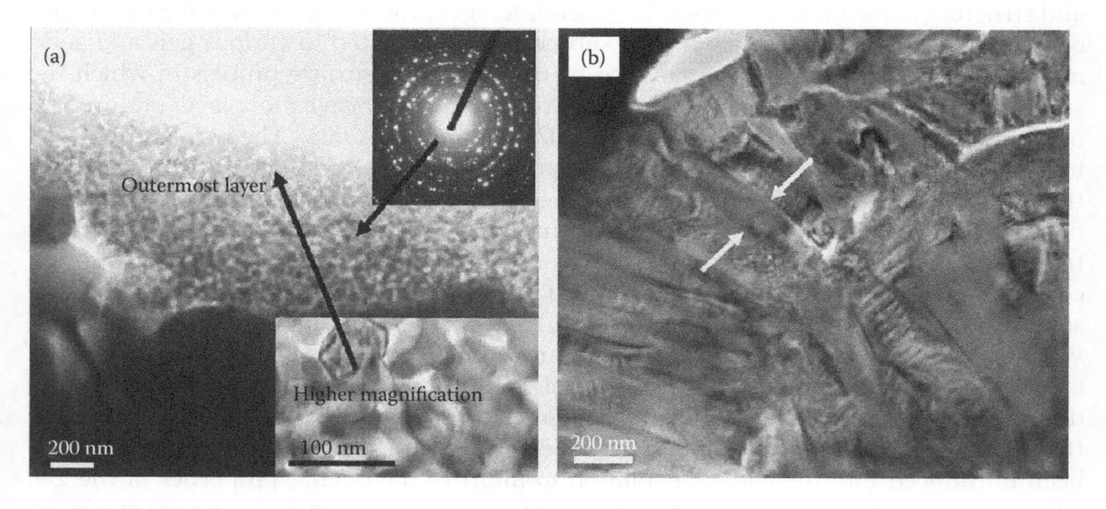

FIGURE 5.23
TEM views of cross section of nanosized titania coating fabricated by plasma spraying and SAD pattern at selected region. (From Liu et al., *Biomaterials*, 26, 6143–6150, 2005. With permission.)

a coating with 25-nm particle size and 40 μm thick is deposited. It is found that the smaller the particle size in the powder, the denser is the coatings (Fan et al. 2006). As the coatings are deposited at a low temperature, poor bonding strength is suspected.

The plasma-sprayed coatings deposited on stainless and titanium alloys are intended to enhance the bioactivity and tribological performance. In the study conducted by Liu et al. (2005), an HA layer about 20 μm thick are grown on the nanosized coatings fabricated by plasma spraying after exposure in simulated body fluids for 4 weeks. Liu et al. (2008b) have tried to further modify the as-prepared coating by ultraviolet light irradiation and hydrogen plasma immersion ion implantation. These two treatments increase the amount of Ti–OH groups that are considered to play an important role in the growth of HA. It is widely accepted that the atomic coordination on the TiO_2 surface differs from that in the bulk due to truncation of atomic arrangements on the surface. The perfect surface is constructed from 5-coordinated Ti atoms and 3-coordinated O atoms, which are more energetically reactive than the 6-coordinated Ti and 3-coordinated O atoms in the bulk. By UV illumination, oxygen vacancies are most likely created at the 2-coordinated bridging sites, resulting in the conversion of the corresponding Ti^{4+} sites to Ti^{3+} sites. Ti^{3+} sites bode well for dissociation of water that is absorbed from the atmosphere (Hugenschmidt et al. 1994). This leads to an abundance of Ti–OH groups at the bridging oxygen sites on the surface of titania coating. The reactions can be explained as follows:

$$2Ti^{4+} + O_O + h\upsilon \rightarrow 2Ti^{3+} + V_O + 1/2O_2,$$

$$Ti^{3+} + H_2O \rightarrow Ti^{4+} - OH + 1/2H_2.$$

Sol–Gel Processing

The sol–gel process can be employed to fabricate metal oxide and ceramic materials with high purity and high homogeneity. This technique allows good control of the composition and structure at the molecular level. In general, sol–gel processing involves the generation of a colloidal suspension (sol), which is subsequently converted to various gels and solid materials. Thin sol–gel coatings can also be obtained by a surface process in which the sol–gel reaction proceeds only on the surface of substrate to form a monolayer of thin TiO_2 on each circle (Ichinose et al. 1996; Chen 2007; Biju and Jain 2008). The process proceeds in a sequential manner involving chemisorption to an OH^- functionalized surface in a titanium alkoxide solution followed by rinsing, hydrolysis, and drying of the film. A calcination treatment may be needed if a denser, more crystalline coating is desired. This heat treatment can also remove organic groups from the coating. This process is readily applicable to any hydroxylated surface using metal alkoxide to react with hydroxyl groups. The sol–gel process can be conducted separately. That is, each different cycle allows the individual layer to be nanostructured (Acharya and Kunitake 2003; He et al. 2002; Advincula et al. 2006). As coatings produced by the sol–gel process are usually prone to cracking during densification and crystallization, chemicals such as PEG, polyvinyl alcohol (PVA) (Larbot et al. 1988), and hydroxypropyl–cellulose (HPC) (Lucic and Turkovi 2002) have been introduced into the colloidal solution to improve the drying properties of the gel, adjust the viscosity of sol, and increase the strength of the materials to prevent crack formation (Larbot et al. 1988; Maria et al. 2006). The coatings produced by the sol–gel method have abundant hydroxyl groups and possess the desirable capability of inducing growth of HA or formation of mineralized matrix by osteoblasts (Wu et al. 2002). The most frequently used sols are obtained by hydrolyzing acetic acid and acetilacetone complexed titanium alkoxides. Shimizu et al. have successfully fabricated anatase titania thin films on glass and various organic substrates at 40°C to 70°C using aqueous solutions of titanium tetrafluoride (TiF_4) (Shimizu et al. 1999). Wu et al. have also fabricated anatanse titania coatings on titanium. In vitro experiments disclose that the coatings have good bone bonding ability (Wu et al. 2002).

Controlling the grains size of the titania particles can be accomplished by two techniques. The most frequently used method to suppress the agglomeration and growth of nanoparticles is the substitution of the surface hydroxyl groups by other functional groups such as organic complex molecules that do not condense like OH^- and that can eventually provide the redispersibility of the powdered xerogel (Kaminski et al. 2005). Nevertheless, subsequent heat treatments that should be carried out in order to remove the organic groups may strongly affect the regular nanostructure of the prepared film.

Shen et al. (2005) have reported the fabrication of hydrophobic nanoporous titania by the sol–gel and dip method. However, it is generally accepted that a hydrophilic surface benefits cell attachment but the biological performance of a hydrophobic surface is unknown. It is noted that this hydrophobic surface can greatly improve the corrosion resistance of the coated metal as demonstrated by Shen et al. (2005). As the titania coatings produced by the sol–gel method are usually prone to cracking during densification and crystallization, immersion in boiling water for 5 to 10 min can alleviate the problem, and the morphologies of the coating before and after exposure in water are exhibited in Figure 5.24. Kuyyadi has fabricated nanocrystalline titania coatings using titanium isopropoxide $\{Ti(OC_3H_7)_4\}$ and ethanol. Water is added for hydrolysis and polycondensation and nitric acid is used to control precipitation (Biju and Jain 2008). The coating is then annealed and Figure 5.25 shows the typical morphology of the sol–gel coating after heating at 550°C. The anatase titania coating with a grain size of about 25 nm is observed from the picture and the grain size increases with sintering temperature.

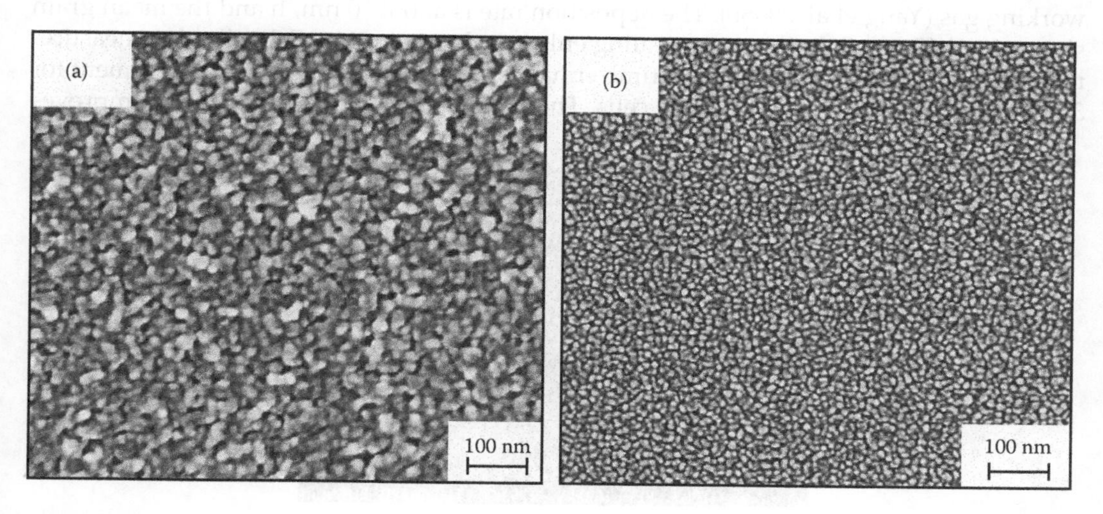

FIGURE 5.24
SEM images of nano-TiO_2 coated 316L stainless steel by sol–gel processing (a) before hydrothermal posttreatment and (b) after hydrothermal treatment. (From Shen et al., *Electrochim. Acta*, 50, 5083–5089, 2005. With permission.)

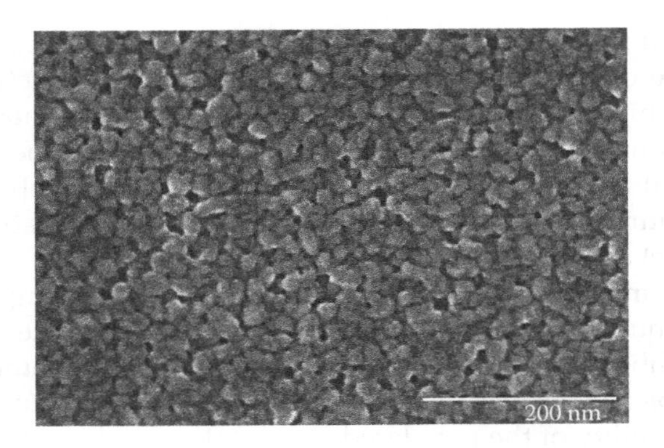

FIGURE 5.25
SEM micrograph of nanocrystalline titania coating fabricated sol–gel-derived coating after annealing at 550°C. (From Biju, K.P., Jain, M.K., *Thin Solid Films*, 516, 2175–2180, 2008. With permission.)

Physical Vapor Deposition

Physical vapor deposition (PVD) is a powerful technique to fabricate hydrophilic nano-TiO_2 coatings. Magnetron sputtering offers uniform deposition and precise control of the deposition rate. High quality of nanocrystalline TiO_2 coatings can be produced by careful control of the processing parameters. As reported by Ye et al. (2007), a TiO_2 target is used and annealing can transform the amorphous titania into a crystalline coating. However, a low heating rate can prevent film cracking. As shown in Figures 5.26 and 5.27, the water contact angle is progressively influenced by the treatment temperature. The mean diameter of the grain is about 30 nm. The annealing temperature influences the final grain size. Generally, a higher temperature induces a larger grain size and the contact angle drops, but from about 600°C the contact angle is nearly independent of the processing temperature.

A pure Ti target can also be used as the target and a mixture of Ar and O_2 serves as the working gas (Yang et al. 2008b). The deposition rate is about 70 nm/h and the mean grain size around 40 nm. Subsequent annealing enlarges the grain size. Cell adhesion measurement shows that the longer heating time enhances cell adhesion and a heat treatment for 3 h increases the ALP activity of the cells. The nanoscaled coating significantly improves

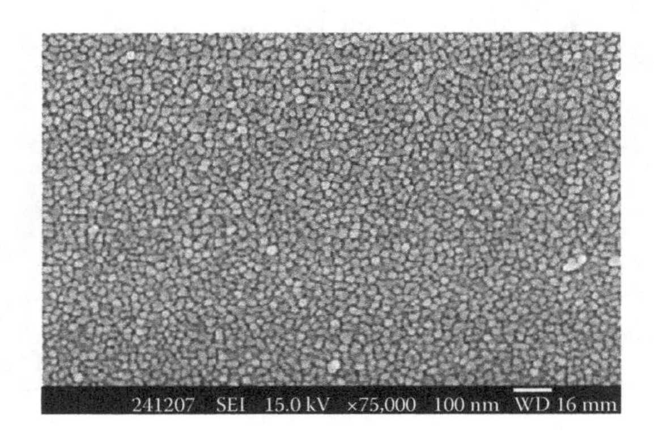

FIGURE 5.26
Surface morphology of TiO_2 thin film prepared by RF magnetron sputtering with annealing treatment at 200°C. (From Ye et al., *Vacuum*, 81, 627–631, 2007. With permission.)

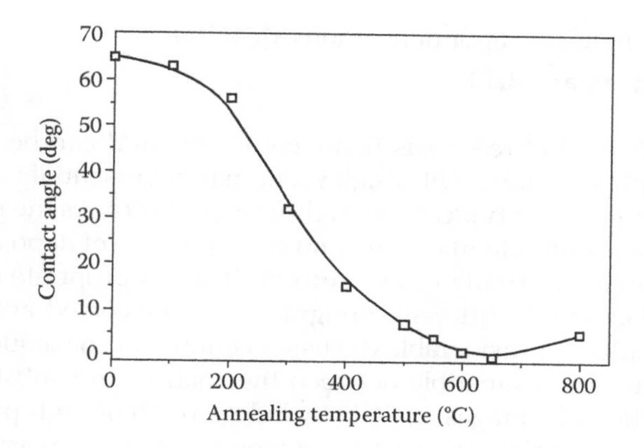

FIGURE 5.27
Relationship between water contact angles and annealing temperature of TiO_2 film fabricated by RF magnetron sputtering. (From Ye et al., *Vacuum*, 81, 627–631, 2007. With permission.)

cell adhesion in the first hour. However, the cell proliferation and differentiation behavior is similar on the nanoscale surface and microscale Ti control.

Chemical Vapor Deposition

Chemical vapor deposition is a chemical process to fabricate pure and high-performance solid materials. This process is common in the fabrication of functional films. Figure 5.28 depicts the schematic of a CVD apparatus. In a typical CVD process, the substrate is exposed to one or more volatile precursors that react and/or decompose on the substrate surface to conduct deposition. The volatile by-products are removed by the gas flow through the reaction chamber. Various monocrystalline, polycrystalline, amorphous, and epitaxial layers can be produced. The CVD process can be performed at atmospheric pressure and ultrahigh vacuum below 10^{-8} Pa. There are many types of CVD processes such as (Seifried et al. 2000):

- Atmospheric-pressure chemical vapor deposition (APCVD)
- Low-pressure chemical vapor deposition (LPCVD)
- Plasma-assisted (enhanced) chemical vapor deposition (PACVD, PECVD)
- Photochemical vapor deposition (PCVD)
- Laser chemical vapor deposition (LCVD)

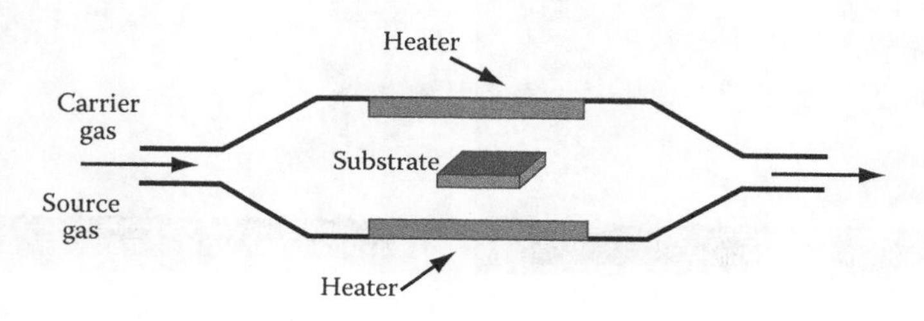

FIGURE 5.28
Schematic layout of CVD equipment.

- Metal-organic chemical vapor deposition (MOCVD)
- Chemical beam epitaxy (CBE)

Compared to PVD, a CVD reactor is relatively simple and can be scaled up easily to accommodate multiple substrates. Ultrahigh vacuum is not essential for CVD and changes and addition of precursors are typically straightforward tasks. As the process is gas phase in nature, and gives a uniform temperature and concentration of deposition species within the chamber, deposition is usually quite uniform. If the appropriate coating powders or gases are used, surfaces with different topography can be coated evenly. The high temperature in CVD results in considerable diffusion action and consequently, if the thermal expansion coefficients are compatible between the coating and substrate, film adhesion will be excellent. Other advantages of CVD include growth of high-purity films (Seifried et al. 2000). The source materials are usually transported by the carrier gas to the chamber. When heated to certain temperature, the substances decompose and reactions take place on the substrate. At the same time, the by-products are flushed out of the chamber by the carrier gas. The mechanism for CVD growth is generally complex. In some cases, small molecular clusters, as well as small molecules, have been identified as the growth species (Seifried et al. 2000; Md et al. 2009; Wavhal et al. 2009).

Evans and Sheel have fabricated thin titania films on stainless steel using APCVD with different precursors (TTIP and $TiCl_4$). Fairly spherical grains are observed in Figure 5.29, which also shows the SEM pictures of titania coatings produced using different source materials. The two coatings are found to possess antibacterial properties (Evans and Sheel 2007). On a time scale between 120 and 180 min, 100% of the bacteria can be killed.

Titanium tetrachloride and ethyl acetate are usually used as precursors in the fabrication of titania films. TTIP ($Ti(OC_3H_7)_4$) is usually used in MOCVD (Backman et al. 2005). Oxygen is used as the carrier gas to transport the reagent gas to the reaction chamber. The processing conditions dramatically influence the structure of the coating. The TTIP is thermally decomposed as shown below when heated to 400°C (Fictorie et al. 1994):

$$\text{TTIP} \rightarrow TiO_2 + 4C_3H_6 + 2H_2O$$

$$TiCl4 + O_2 \rightarrow TiO_2 + 2Cl_2$$

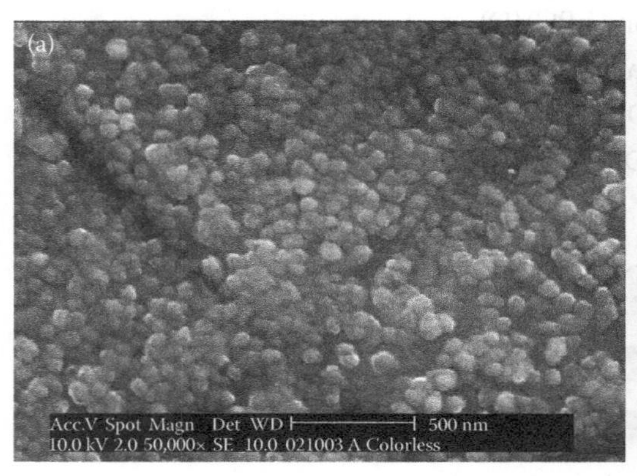

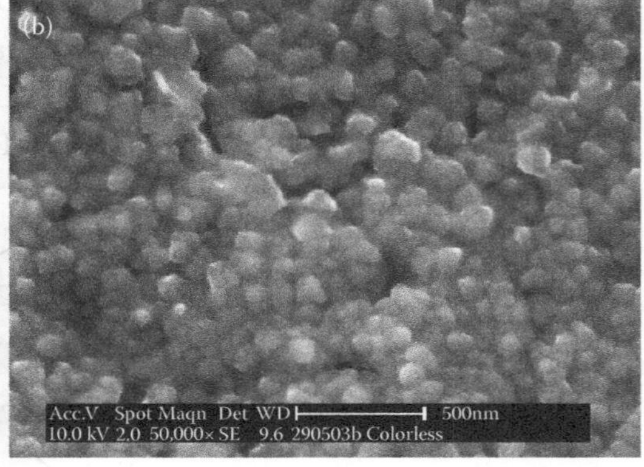

FIGURE 5.29
SEM images of TiO_2 deposited directly on stainless steel using TTIP (a) at 500°C and (b) $TiCl_4$ at 650°C. (From Evans P., Sheel, D.W., *Surf. Coat. Technol.*, 201, 9319–9324, 2007. With permission.)

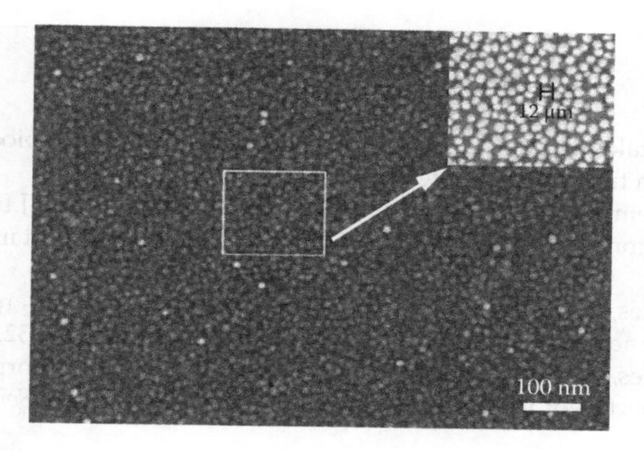

FIGURE 5.30
SEM micrograph of calcined nanocrystalline TiO_2 thin film. Inset shows high magnification image at selected area marked by a white rectangle. (From Liu et al., *J. Non-Cryst. Solids*, 352, 2284–2287, 2006. With permission.)

The slower growth rate may favor evolution of larger crystal grains. At a high deposition temperature, the coatings are generally crystalline. The exact structure (rutile or anatase) depends on the reaction temperature. A titania coating with uniform morphology and narrow crystallite size distribution is obtained by using $TiCl_4$ as the inorganic source and triblock copolymer $EO_{20}PO_{70}EO_{20}$ (Pluronic P123, EO = ethylene oxide) as the uniform-structure-directing agent. Their method is based on the evaporation-induced assembly (EIA) approach for the titania thin films synthesis. The EIA method combines the advantages of sol–gel dip coating and organic–inorganic cooperative assembly technique (Liu et al. 2006). Figure 5.30 shows the representative SEM pictures of the coatings. Uniform nanocrystalline titania coatings are shown. The grains size is about 12 nm in diameter. XRD patterns acquired from the coating after annealing at 400°C reveal an anatase crystalline structure. For more details about the method and preparation procedure, please refer to Liu et al. (2006).

A modified CVD method called chemistry vapor synthesis (CVS) has been developed. CVS is performed at a higher processing temperature and precursor partial pressure as well as for a longer time than common CVD. It can produce particle- and void-free films. Thick nanocrystalline CVS films exhibiting a noncolumnar morphology have also been fabricated under conditions intermediate to that of CVD and CVS. Here, both nanoparticles and molecular species are used for the film formation (Seifried et al. 2000).

Conclusion

Nanoscaled titania coatings possess excellent mechanical properties and good biocompatibility, thereby making them desirable in biological coatings and materials. The nanoscaled topography may also provide additional biological benefits to natural tissues. Among the various types of nanoscaled titania coatings, well-ordered titania nanotube arrays fabricated by anodization are attracting increasing attention. Various applications pertaining to drug delivery, biosensing, and so forth are proposed and being developed. In the future, precise design of various nanoscaled titania patterns on biological devices is called for and so more systematic and fundamental investigations on the effects and corresponding mechanism of nanosized titania coatings on biological tissues are necessary.

References

Acharya, G. and Kunitake, T. 2003. A general method for fabrication of biocompatible surfaces by modification with titania layer. *Langmuir* 19:2260–2266.

Advincula, M.C., Rahemtulla, F.G., Advincula, R.C., Ada, E.T., Lemons, J.E., and Bellis, S.L. 2006. Osteoblast adhesion and matrix mineralization on sol–gel-derived titanium oxide. *Biomaterials* 27:2201–2212.

Allam, N.K. and Grimes, C.A. 2007. Formation of vertically oriented TiO_2 nanotube arrays using a fluoride free HCl aqueous electrolyte. *J. Phys. Chem. C* 111:13028–13032.

Allam, N.K. and Grimes, C.A. 2008a. Effect of cathode material on the morphology and photoelectrochemical properties of vertically oriented TiO_2 nanotube arrays. *Sol. Energy Mater. Sol Cells* 92:1468–1475.

Allam, N.K., Shankar, K., and Grimes, C.A. 2008b. Photoelectrochemical and water photoelectrolysis properties of ordered TiO_2 nanotubes fabricated by Ti anodization in fluoride-free HCl electrolytes. *J. Mater. Chem.* 18:2341–2348.

Backman, U., Auvinen, A., and Jokiniemi, J.K. 2005. Deposition of nanostructured titania films by particle-assisted MOCVD. *Surf. Coat. Technol.* 192:81–87.

Beltran, A.L., Gracia, J., and Andres, J. 2006. Density functional theory study of the brookite surfaces and phase transitions between natural titania polymorphs. *J. Phys. Chem. B* 110:23417–23423.

Biju, K.P. and Jain, M.K. 2008. Effect of crystallization on humidity sensing properties of sol-gel derived nanocrystalline TiO_2 thin films. *Thin Solid Films* 516:2175–2180.

Brammer, K.S., Oh, S.H., Gallagher, J.O., and Jin, S.H. 2008. Enhanced cellular mobility guided by TiO_2 nanotube surfaces. *Nano Lett.* 8:786–793.

Burnside, S.D., Shklover, V., and Barbe C., et al. 1998. Self-organization of TiO_2 nanoparticles in thin films. *Chem. Mater.* 10:2419–2425.

Cai, Q., Paulose, M., Varghese, O.K., and Grimes, C.A. 2005. The effect of electrolyte composition on the fabrication of self-organized titanium oxide nanotube arrays by anodic oxidation. *J. Mater. Res.* 20:230–236.

Chen, X., Schriver M., Suen. T, and Mao, S.S. 2007. Fabrication of 10 nm diameter TiO_2 nanotube arrays by titanium anodization. *Thin Solid Films* 515:8511–8514.

Chiang, C.Y., Chiou, S.H., and Yang, W.E., et al. 2009. Formation of TiO_2 nano-network on titanium surface increases the human cell growth. *Dent. Mater.* 25:1022–1029.

Christophersen, M., Carstensen, J., Voigt, K., and Foll, H. 2003. Organic and aqueous electrolytes used for etching macro- and mesoporous silicon. *Phys. Status Solid A* 197:34–38.

Das, K., Bose, S., Bandyopadhyay, A., Karandikar, B., and Gibbins, B.L. 2008. Surface coatings for improvement of bone cell materials and antimicrobial activities of Ti implants. *J. Biomed. Mater. Res.* 87:455–460.

de Oliveira, P.T. and Nanci, A. 2004. Nanotexturing of titanium-based surfaces upregulates expression of bone sialoprotein and osteopontin by cultured osteogenic cells. *Biomaterials* 25:403–413.

Doohun, K., Fujimoto, S., Schmuki, P., and Tsuchiya, H. 2008. Nitrogen doped anodic TiO_2 nanotubes grown from nitrogen-containing Ti alloys. *Electrochem. Commun.* 10:910–913.

Erli, H.J., Ruger, M., and Ragoss, C., et al. 2006. The effect of surface modification of a porous TiO_2/perlite composite on the ingrowth of bone tissue in vivo. *Biomaterials* 27:1270–1276.

Evans, P. and Sheel, D.W. 2007. Photoactive and antibacterial TiO_2 thin films on stainless steel. *Surf. Coat. Technol.* 201:9319–9324.

Fan, S.Q., Yang, G.J., Li, C.J., Liu, G.J., Li, C.X., and Zhang, L.Z. 2006. Characterization of microstructure of nano-TiO_2 coating deposited by vacuum cold spraying. *J. Therm. Spray Technol.* 15:513–517.

Fictorie, C.P., Evans, J.F., and Glandfelter, W.L. 1994. Kinetic and mechanistic study of the chemical-vapor-deposition of titanium-oxide thin-films using tetrakis-(isopropoxo)-titanium. *J. Vac. Sci. Technol. A* 12:1108–1113.

Fujishima, A., Zhang, X.T., and Tryk, D.A. 2008. TiO_2 photocatalysis and related surface phenomena. *Surf. Sci. Rep.* 63:515–582.

Gong, D., Grimes, C.A., and Varghese, O.K., et al. 2001. Titanium oxide nanotube arrays prepared by anodic oxidation. *J. Mater. Res.* 16:3331–3334.

Grimes, C.A. and Mor, C.K. 2009. TiO_2 *Nanotube Arrays. Synthesis, Properties, and Applications.* New York: Springer Science.

He, J.H., Ichinose, I., Fujikawa, S., Kunitake, T., and Nakao, A. 2002. A general, efficient method of incorporation of metal ions into ultrathin TiO_2 films. *Chem. Mater.* 14:3493–3500.

Huang, H.H., Pan, S.J., Lai, Y.J., Lee, T.H., Chen, C.C., and Lu, F.H. 2004. Osteoblast-like cell initial adhesion onto a network-structured titanium oxide layer. *Scr. Mater.* 51:1017–1021.

Hugenschmidt, M.B., Gameble, L., and Campbell, C.T. 1994. The interaction of H_2O with a TiO_2 (110) surface. *Surf. Sci.* 302:329–340.

Hwang, B.J. and Hwang, J.R. 1993. Kinetic-model of anodic-oxidation of titanium in sulfuric acid. *J. Appl. Electrochem.* 23:1056–1062.

Ichinose, I., Senzu., H., and Kunitake, T. 1996. Stepwise adsorption of metal alkoxides on hydrolyzed surfaces: A surface sol–gel process. *Chem. Lett.* 25:831–832.

Jaroenworaluck, A., Regonini, D., Bowen, C.R., Stevens, R., and Macro, D.A. 2007. Micro and nanostructure of TiO_2 anodised films prepared in a fluorine-containing electrolyte. *J. Mater. Sci.* 42:6729–6734.

Julia, K., Lenka, M., Jan, M.M., Peter, G., Patrik, S., and Frank, A.M. 2008. Time-dependent growth of biomimetic apatite on anodic TiO_2 nanotubes. *Electrochim. Acta* 53:6995–7003.

Jung, J.H., Kobayashi, H., van Bommel, K.J.C., Shinkai, S., and Shimizu, T. 2002. Creation of novel helical ribbon and double-layered nanotube TiO_2 structures using an organogel template. *Chem. Mater.* 14:1445–1447.

Kaminski, R.C., Pulcinelli, S.H., Craievich, A.F., and Santilli, C.V. 2005. Nanocrystalline anatase thin films prepared from redispersible sol–gel powders. *J. Eur. Ceram. Soc.* 25:2175–2180.

Karlsson, M., Palsgard, E., Wilshaw, P.R., and Di Silvio, L. 2003. Initial in vitro interaction of osteoblasts with nano-porous alumina. *Biomaterials* 24:3039–3046.

Khang, D., Lu, J., Yao, C., Haberstroh, K.M., and Webster, T.J. 2008a. The role of nanometer and submicron surface features on vascular and bone cell adhesion on titanium. *Biomaterials* 29:970–983.

Khang, D., Park, G.E. and Webster, T.J. 2008b. Enhanced chondrocyte densities on carbon nanotube composites: The combined role of nanosurface roughness and electrical stimulation. *J. Biomed. Mater. Res. A* 86A:253–260.

Kobayashi, S., Hamasaki, N., Suzuki, M., Kimura, M., Shirai, H., and Hanabusa, K. 2002. Preparation of helical transition-metal oxide tubes using organogelators as structure-directing agents. *J. Am. Chem. Soc.* 124:6550–6551.

Larbot, A., Fabre, J.P., Guizard, C., and Cot, L. 1988. Inorganic membranes obtained by sol-gel techniques. *J. Membr. Sci.* 39:203–212.

Lee, S., Takai, M., Kim, H., and Ishihara, K. 2009. Preparation of nano-structured titanium oxide film for biosensor substrate by wet corrosion process. *Curr. Appl. Phys.* 9:e266–e269.

Li, L.H., Kong, Y.M., and Kim, H.W., et al. 2004. Improved biological performance of Ti implants due to surface modification by micro-arc oxidation. *Biomaterials* 25:2867–2875.

Liu, K.S., Zhang, M.L., Shi, K.Y., Zhou, W., and Fu, H.G. 2006. Uniform TiO_2 thin films with anatase nanocrystallites synthesized through evaporation-induced assembly. *J. Non-Cryst. Solids* 352:2284–2287.

Liu, X.Y., Chu, P.K., and Ding, C.X. 2004. Surface modification of titanium, titanium alloys, and related materials for biomedical applications. *Mater. Sci. Eng. R* 47:49–121.

Liu, X.Y. and Ding, C.X. 2002. Plasma sprayed wollastonite/TiO_2 composite coatings on titanium alloys. *Biomaterials* 23:4065–4077.

Liu, X.Y., Zhao, X.B., Fu, R.K.Y., Ho, J.P.Y., Ding, C.X., and Chu, P.K. 2005. Plasma-treated nanostructured TiO_2 surface supporting biomimetic growth of apatite. *Biomaterials* 26:6143–6150.

Liu, Z., Zhang, X., and Nishimoto, S., et al. 2008a. Highly ordered TiO_2 nanotube arrays with controllable length for photoelectrocatalytic degradation of phenol. *J. Phys. Chem. C* 112:253–259.

Liu, X.Y., Zhao, X.B., and Li, B., et al. 2008b. UV-irradiation-induced bioactivity on TiO_2 coatings with nanostructural surface. *Acta Biomater.* 4:544–552.

Lohrengel, M.M. 1993. Thin anodic oxide layers on aluminum and other valve metals—high-field regime. *Mater. Sci. Eng. R* 11:243–294.

Lucic, M. and Turkovi, L.A. 2002. Small-angle X-ray scattering and wide-angle X-ray diffraction on thermally annealed nanostructured TiO_2 films. *Thin Solid Films* 419:105–113.

Maria, C.A., Firoz, G.R., Rigoberto, C.A., Earl, T.A., Jack, E.L., and Susan, L.B. 2006. Osteoblast adhesion and matrix mineralization on sol–gel-derived titanium oxide. *Biomaterials* 27:2201–2212.

Matsunaga, T., Tomoda, R., Nakajima, T., and Wake, H. 1985. Photoelectrochemical sterilization of microbial-cells by semiconductor powders. *FEMS Microbiol. Lett.* 29:211–214.

Md, I.A., Bhattacharya, S.S., and Hahn, H. 2009. Structure, thermal stability, and optical properties of boron modified nanocrystalline anatase prepared by chemical vapor synthesis. *J. Appl. Phys.* 105:113526.

Melody, B., Kinard, T., and Lessner, P. 1998. The non-thickness-limited growth of anodic oxide films on valve metals. *Electrochem. Solid State Lett.* 1:126–129.

Michailowski, A., AlMawlwai, D., Cheng, G.S., and Moskovits, M. 2001. Highly regular anatase nanotubule arrays fabricated in porous anodic templates. *Chem. Phys. Lett.* 349:1–5.

Mor, G.K., Shankar, K., Paulose, M., Varghese, O.K., and Grimes, C.A. 2005. Enhanced photocleavage of water using titania nanotube arrays. *Nano Lett.* 5:191–195.

Nanci, A., Ji-Hyun, Y., and Bernard, C., et al. 2006. Characterization of a bioactive nanotextured surface created by controlled chemical oxidation of titanium. *Surf. Sci.* 600:4613–4621.

Nanci, A., Wuest, J.D., and Peru, L., et al. 1998. Chemical modification of titanium surfaces for covalent attachment of biological molecules. *J. Biomed. Mater. Res.* 40:324–335.

Nguyen, Q.A.S., Yash, V.B., Radmilovic, V.R., and Devine, T.M. Structural study of electrochemically synthesized TiO_2 nanotubes via cross-sectional and high-resolution TEM. *Electrochim. Acta* 54:4340–4344.

Oh, S. and Jin, S. 2006. Titanium oxide nanotubes with controlled morphology for enhanced bone growth. *Mater. Sci. Eng. C* 26:1301–1306.

Pakes, A., Thompson, G.E., Skeldon, P., and Morgan, P.C. 2003. Development of porous anodic films on 2014-T4 aluminium alloy in tetraborate electrolyte. *Corros. Sci.* 45:1275–1287.

Park, J., Bauer, S., Schlegel, K.A., Neukam, F.W., von der Mark, K., and Schmuki, P. 2009. TiO_2 nanotube surfaces: 15 nm—An optimal length scale of surface topography for cell adhesion and differentiation. *Small* 5:666–671.

Park, J., Bauer, S., von der Mark, K., and Schmuki, P. 2007. Nanosize and vitality: TiO_2 nanotube diameter directs cell fate. *Nano Lett.* 7:1686–1691.

Paulose, M., Shankar, K., and Yoriya, S., et al. 2006. Anodic growth of highly ordered TiO_2 nanotube arrays to 134 μm in length. *J. Phys. Chem. B* 110:16179–16184.

Peng, L.L., Mendelsohn, A.D., LaTempa, T.J., Yoriya, S., Grimes, C.A., and Desai, T.A. 2009. Long-term small molecule and protein elution from TiO_2 nanotubes. *Nano Lett.* 9:1932–1936.

Popat, K.C., Leoni, L., Grimes, C.A., and Desai, T.A. 2007a. Influence of engineered titania nanotubular surfaces on bone cells. *Biomaterials* 28:3188–3197.

Popat, K.C., Eltgroth, M., LaTempa, T.J., Grimes, C.A., and Desai, T.A. 2007b. Titania nanotubes: A novel platform for drug-eluting coatings for medical implants? *Small* 3:1878–1881.

Popat, K.C., Eltgroth, M., LaTempa, T.J., Grimes, C.A., and Desai, T.A. 2007c. Decreased *Staphylococcus epidermis* adhesion and increased osteoblast functionality on antibiotic-loaded titania nanotubes. *Biomaterials* 28:4880–4888.

Prakasam, H.E., Shankar, K., Paulose, M., and Grimes, C.A. 2007. A new benchmark for TiO_2 nanotube array growth by anodization. *J. Phys. Chem. C* 111:7235–7241.

Ramamoorthy, M., Vanderbilt, D., and King-Smith, R.D. 1994. First-principles calculations of the energetics of stoichiometric TiO_2 surfaces. *Phys. Rev. B* 49:16721.

Richter, C., Panaitescu, E., Willey, R., and Menon, L. 2007a. Titania nanotubes prepared by anodization in fluorine-free acids. *J. Mater. Res.* 22:1624–1631.

Richter, C., Wu, Z., Panaitescu, E., Willey, R., and Menon, L. 2007b. Ultra-high aspect ratio titania nanotubes. *Adv. Mater.* 19:946–948.
Ruckh, T., Porter, J.R., Allam, N.K., Feng, X.J., Grimes, C.A., and Popat, K.C. 2009. Nanostructured tantala as a template for enhanced osseointegration. *Nanotechnology* 20:45102.
Seifried, S., Winterer, M., and Hahn, H. 2000. Nanocrystalline titania films and particles by chemical vapor synthesis. *Adv. Mater.* 6:239–244.
Shankar, K., Mor, G.K., Fitzgerald, A., and Grimes, C.A. 2007. Cation effect on the electrochemical formation of very high aspect ratio TiO_2 nanotube arrays in formamide–water mixtures. *J. Phys. Chem.* C 111:21–26.
Shen, G.X., Chen, Y.C., Lin, L., Lin, C.J., and Scantlebury, D. 2005. Study on a hydrophobic nano-TiO_2 coating and its properties for corrosion protection of metals. *Electrochim. Acta* 50:5083–5089.
Shih, Y.H., Lin, C.T., Liu, C.M., Chen, C.C., Chen, C.S., and Ou, K.L. 2007. Effect of nano-titanium hydride on formation of multi-nanoporous TiO_2 film on Ti. *Appl. Surf. Sci.* 253:3678–3682.
Shimizu, K., Imai, H., Hirashima, H., and Tsukuma, K. 1999. Low-temperature synthesis of anatase thin films on glass and organic substrates by direct deposition from aqueous solutions. *Thin Solid Films* 351:220–224.
Shklover, V., Nazeeruddin, M.K., and Zakeeruddin, S.M., et al. 1997. Structure of nanocrystalline TiO_2 powders and precursor to their highly efficient photosensitizer. *Chem. Mater.* 9:430–439.
Song, Y.Y., Schmidt-Stein, F., Bauer, S., and Schmuki, P. 2009. Amphiphilic TiO_2 nanotube arrays: An actively controllable drug delivery system. *J. Am. Chem. Soc.* 131:4230–4232.
Sujata, V.B. 2005. *Biomaterials*. Harrow: Alpha Science International.
Sun, W., Puzas J.E., Sheu T.J., Liu, X., and Fauchet, P.M. 2007. Nano-to microscale porous silicon as a cell interface for bone-tissue engineering. *Adv. Mater.* 19:921–924.
Takagi, J., Petre, B.M., Walz, T., and Springer, T.A. 2002. Global conformational rearrangements in integrin extracellular domains in outside-in and inside-out signaling. *Cell* 110:599–611.
Tsuchiya, H., Macak, J.M., and Muller, L., et al. 2006. Hydroxyapatite growth on anodic TiO_2 nanotubes. *J. Biomed. Mater. Res. A* 77A:534–541.
Varghese, O.K., Gong, D., Paulose, M., Ong, K.G., Grimes, C.A., and Dickey, E.C. 2003. Crystallization and high-temperature structural stability of titanium oxide nanotube arrays. *J. Mater. Res.* 18:156–165.
Variola, F., Yi, J.H., Richert, L., Wuest, J.D., Rosei, F., and Nanci, A. 2008. Tailoring the surface properties of Ti6Al4V by controlled chemical oxidation. *Biomaterials* 29:1285–1298.
Wavhal, D.S., Goyal, S., and Timmons, R.B. 2009. Synthesis of electrically conducting tin films by low-temperature, plasma-enhanced CVD. *Chem. Mater.* 21:4442–4447.
Wong, J.Y. and Bronzino, J.D. 2007. *Biomaterials*. Boca Raton: CRC Press.
Wu, J.M., Hayakawa, S., Tsuru, K., and Osaka, A. 2002. In vitro bioactivity of anatase film obtained by direct deposition from aqueous titanium tetrafluoride solutions. *Thin Solid Films* 414:275–280.
Xin, Y.C., Jiang, J., Huo, K.F., Hu, T., and Chu, P.K. 2009. Bioactive $SrTiO_3$ nanotube arrays: Strontium delivery platform on Ti-based osteoporotic bone implants. *ACS Nano* 3:3228–3234.
Yang, W.E., Hsu, M.L., Lin, M.C., Chen, Z.H., Chen, L.K., and Huang, H.H. 2009. Nano/submicron-scale TiO_2 network on titanium surface for dental implant application. *J. Alloys Compd.* 479:642–647.
Yang, Y., Wang, X., and Li, L. 2008a. Crystallization and phase transition of titanium oxide nanotube arrays. *J. Am. Ceram. Soc.* 91:632–635.
Yang, Y.Z., Park, S.W., Liu, Y.X., et al. 2008b. Development of sputtered nanoscale titanium oxide coating on osseointegrated implant devices and their biological evaluation. *Vacuum* 83:569–574.
Yao, C., Slamovich, E.B., and Webster, T.J. 2008. Enhanced osteoblast functions on anodized titanium with nanotube-like structures. *J. Biomed. Mater. Res. A* 85A:157–166.
Yao, C. and Webster, T.J. 2006. Anodization: A promising nano-modification technique of titanium implants for orthopedic applications. *J. Nanosci. Nanotechnol.* 6:2682–2692.
Ye, Q., Liu, P.Y., Tang, Z.F., and Zhai, L. 2007. Hydrophilic properties of nano-TiO_2 thin films deposited by RF magnetron sputtering. *Vacuum* 81:627–631.

Yoriya, S., Mor, G.K., Sharma. S., and Grimes. C.A. 2008. Synthesis of ordered arrays of discrete, partially crystalline titania nanotubes by Ti anodization using diethylene glycol electrolytes. *J. Mater. Chem.* 18:3332–3336.

Yoriya, S., Paulose, M., Varghese, O.K., Mor, G.K., and Grimes, C.A. 2007. Fabrication of vertically oriented TiO_2 nanotube arrays using dimethyl sulfoxide electrolytes. *J. Phys. Chem. C.* 111:13770–13776.

Zhang, H. and Banfield, J.F. 2000. Understanding polymorphic phase transformation behavior during growth of nanocrystalline aggregates: Insights from TiO_2 *J. Phys. Chem. B* 104:3481–3487.

Zhang, L.J. and Webster, T.J. 2007. Nanotechnology and nanomaterials: Promises for improved tissue regeneration. *Nano Today* 4:66–80.

Zhao, X.B., Liu, X.Y., Ding, C.X., and Chu, P.K. 2007. Effects of plasma treatment on bioactivity of TiO_2 coatings. *Surf. Coat. Technol.* 201:6878–6881.

Zhu, Y.C. and Ding, C.X. 2000. Characterization of plasma sprayed nano-titania coatings by impedance spectroscopy. *J. Eur. Ceram. Soc.* 20:127–132.

6

Hydrothermal Crystallization with Microstructural Self-Healing Effect on Mechanical and Failure Behaviors of Plasma-Sprayed Hydroxyapatite Coatings

Chung-Wei Yang and Truan-Sheng Lui

CONTENTS

Introduction

With the same chemical and crystallographic structure as the major inorganic constituents of human bone, teeth, and hard tissues, hydroxyapatite ($Ca_{10}(PO_4)_6(OH)_2$; HA) is a widely used calcium phosphate bioceramic, which is considered an excellent bone substitute [1,2] in dentistry and orthopedics because of its favorable bioactive properties and excellent osteoconductivity [3–5]. Like other calcium phosphate biomaterials, HA is an osteoconductive biomaterial that allows the formation of bone on its surface by serving as a scaffold or a template. The advantages for the use of HA include (1) faster stabilization, rapid fixation, and stronger chemical bonding between the host bone and the implant

[4,6,7], and (2) increased uniform bone ingrowth and ongrow the bone–implant interface. Therefore, HA has been generally acknowledged as an excellent bone substitute [1,2] because of its ability to reduce the healing time after reconstructive surgery and extend the functional life of the prosthesis.

During various clinical dental and orthopedic applications for the repair of bone defects and immediate tooth root replacement, crystalline HA obtained through hot-pressing or other conventional sintering processes were used as bulk implants. The bulk HA implants generally show the maximum porosity less than 5% by volume with the micropores size less than 1 μm in diameter [8,9], and they are also called dense HA. Although the crystalline dense HA exhibits higher flexural strength (about 115–200 MPa) [10] than the human cortical bone (about 15–150 MPa) [11], the fracture toughness of the dense HA sintering bulks (about 1.0 MPa $m^{1/2}$) is much lower than the human cortical bone (about 2–12 MPa $m^{1/2}$) [11]. Dense HA is brittle and relatively weak compared with common implant metals, alloys, and high-strength ceramics. In spite of the good biocompatibility and osteoconductivity of HA, the limitations for the usage of the dense HA sintering bulks for bone replacement are their low fracture toughness and bending strength under load-bearing situations [12–14]. In the biomedical fields, bioactive ceramics have often been used as coatings to modify the surface of bioinert metallic implants and in some cases to create an entirely new surface that gives the implant properties quite different from the uncoated implants. Figure 6.1 illustrates the artificial Ti–6Al–4V stem and the acetabular cup with an HA-coated surface for the joint replacement of total hip prosthesis.

The concept to design a surface biological fixation for orthopedic joint implants such as a total hip prosthesis has been achieved by the bone ingrowth and bone apposition methods. Investigations for calcium phosphate ceramic coatings on metallic implants started with the observation that HA in the pores of a metal implant with a porous coating would significantly affect the rate and vitality of bone ingrowth into the pores [15]. HA is extensively applied for the purpose of improving the bioactivity of these bioinert metal implants including the stem and the acetabular cup. Therefore, the combination of high-strength metallic substrates with osteoconductive properties of bioceramic ceramics makes HA-coated titanium implants attractive for the load-bearing situations in orthopedic and dental surgery. In addition to enabling earlier stabilization of the implant in surrounding bone, using an HA coating extends the functional life of the prosthesis and improves the adhesion of the prosthesis to the bone. Animal studies have indicated that HA-coated titanium implants showed higher push-out strength compared to uncoated titanium implants [16–19], and postmortem studies reported direct bone contact with implants without a fibrous tissue interface in patients who had successful HA-coated total hip arthroplasties [20,21]. Moreover, the bone bonding capacity of the HA coatings can help cementless fixation of orthopedic prostheses. It has been shown that the skeletal bonding is enhanced immediately after implantation [22–24].

There are many coating techniques available for applying HA onto metallic substrates, including plasma spraying, chemical vapor deposition (CVD), RF sputtering coating, sol–gel coating, electrochemical deposition, electrophoresis, and biomimetic coating methods [25–32]. Compared with these techniques, plasma-sprayed HA coatings (HACs) deposited on metallic implants, which is a state-of-the-art and extensively used process in commercial products, can exhibit enhanced interfacial strength and tend to avoid the inherent mechanical property limitations of HA without any significant loss in biocompatibility [33,34]. Reports on the short-term to medium-term results of implantation of HA-coated femoral stems have been encouraging [17,23,35–37]. Among the various biocompatible metals, Ti–6Al–4V alloy used as a metallic substrate is more favorable compared to other

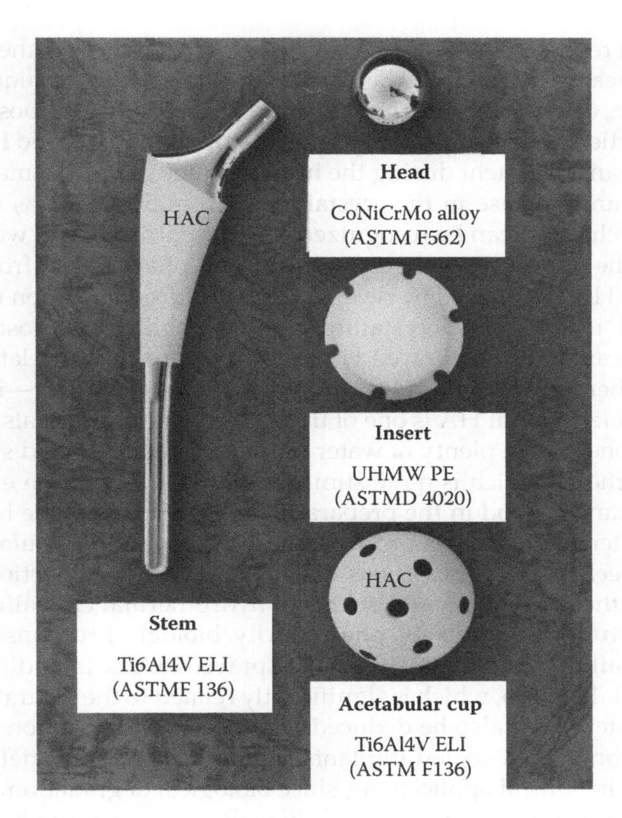

FIGURE 6.1
Artificial total hip prosthesis includes stem, head insert, and acetabular cup.

alloys because of the compatibility between elastic moduli of bone and that of the Ti alloy is important in order to avoid a difference in deformation between bone and the implant when stress is applied. Therefore, clinical application of plasma-sprayed HACs on Ti–6Al–4V alloy has the potential as an implant material not only because HA can bond physicochemically with surrounding bone [4,17,38] and promote bone growth onto its surface [39–41], but also due to the excellent corrosion resistance and lower elastic modulus of Ti alloy compared to 316L stainless steel and cobalt chromium alloys [42–44].

However, the high temperature and enthalpy employed during the plasma-spraying process will result in large-scale dehydroxylation and decomposition effects of crystalline HA phase within the sprayed coatings [45,46]. Plasma-sprayed HACs with a higher content of impurity phases and amorphous calcium phosphate will increase higher dissolution rate than crystalline HA in aqueous solutions and body fluids. It results in some problems with decreasing the structural homogeneity and the degradation of mechanical properties in the firm fixation between the implant and surrounding bone tissue [47,48]. Furthermore, clinical studies have indicated that the release of particles and subsequent inclusion will result in fretting and abrasive wear behaviors between the implants and the surrounding bone [21,49–51]. Therefore, decreasing the content of impurity phases and amorphous calcium phosphate are rather important for the long-term biological stability of plasma-sprayed HACs.

Referring to past reports, it has been generally recognized that postheat treatments such as air or vacuum heat treatments, spark plasma sintering (SPS) technique, and hydrothermal treatments, etc., can significantly help to improve the phase composition, crystallinity, mechanical properties, and biological responsibility of plasma-sprayed HACs [16,45,52–65]. In addition, the steam treatment during the in-flight stage of the plasma spraying can also result in a significant increase in the crystallinity (from 58% to 79%) of plasma-sprayed HACs [66]. The mechanism can be recognized that the entrapping of water molecules into HA droplets and the improvement in crystallinity and phase purity from amorphous calcium phosphate to HA is achieved by reversing the HA decomposition through providing extra OH^-. Overall, the degree of crystallinity, phase stability, and postheat treatments of calcium phosphate and plasma-sprayed HACs—which are closely related to heating temperatures, atmosphere, water molecules, and partial steam pressure—is presented in the next section. Considering that HA is one of the natural apatite minerals and the phase stability in an atmosphere with plenty of water molecules and saturated steam pressure, the hydrothermal synthesis, which is quite similar to mineral formation environment in the earth, is an important method in the preparation of HA crystals. The hydrothermal technique and hydrothermal materials processing are becoming a popular field of research for scientists and technologists of various disciplines. Therefore, Sections 6.3 and 6.4 will specifically reveal the advantages and effects of hydrothermal crystallization on improving the microstructural homogeneity, phase purity, biological responses, adhesive bonding strength, and failure mechanism of plasma-sprayed HACs. In addition, the kinetics of hydrothermal crystallization, which is significantly related to the saturated steam pressure in a hermetical system, will also be deduced and discussed in Section 6.3. The reliability and failure behaviors of HA-coated implants should be studied in detail to ensure their long-term stability in clinical applications, since biological degradation and failure of artificial joints that result from dissolution and dissociation may occur during the period of implantation. Thus, knowledge of statistical analysis of the reliability engineering by the Weibull model will be represented in Section 6.5. Meanwhile, the failure probability density function, cumulative failure probability, failure rate, and reliability functions, which correlate with the cohesive strength of coatings and the adhesive strength of a coating to a metal substrate, will also be reviewed in this section.

Characteristics of HA Coatings

Phase Stability of the Crystalline HA Powders

Pure HA has a theoretical composition of 39.68 wt.% Ca element, 18.45 wt.% of P element, a Ca/P weight ratio of 2.151, and a Ca/P molar ratio of 1.667. According to criterion of ASTM F1185-88, the acceptable composition for commercial HA powder should be a minimum value of 95 wt.% HA purity, as established by x-ray diffraction analysis. HA can be produced by using a variety of methods, and the characteristics of raw HA powders have significant effects on the subsequent products with HA being in the form of dense or porous bulks and in coatings. In biological and clinical applications, HA bulks and HA-coated implants are often immersed and applied in solutions or in the body fluids. Thus, the stability of HA bulks and coating implants is significantly affected by the environmental temperatures and the pH values.

Generally, high-purity HA powder is soluble in acid solution, insoluble in alkaline solution, and slightly soluble in water. Also, the solubility of crystalline HA is varied with the presence of amino acids, proteins, enzymes, and other organic compounds. The dissolution rate also depends on the particle size and the shape of HA granules and the porosity, crystal size, and crystallinity of HA implants. As indicated by Driessens [67], there are only two calcium phosphate compounds that are stable at room temperature when in contact with aqueous solutions. It is the pH value of the solution that determines which one is stable. At a pH value lower than 4.2, the component $CaHPO_4{\cdot}2H_2O$ (dicalcium phosphate) is the most stable phase, while at a pH value higher than 4.2, well-crystallized HA is a stable phase. In addition, Adam et al. found that the surface of tricalcium phosphate ($Ca_3(PO_4)_2$, TCP) and tetracalcium phosphate ($Ca_4P_2O_9$, TP) compounds will be coated with thin HA layers through the phase transformation at a suitable pH value [68], and these reactions can be represented as follows [69].

$$4Ca_3(PO_4)_2 \rightarrow Ca_{10}(PO_4)_6(OH)_2 + 2Ca^{2+} + 2HPO^{4-} \quad (6.1)$$

$$3Ca_4P_2O_9 + 3H_2O \rightarrow Ca_{10}(PO_4)_6(OH)_2 + 2Ca^{2+} + 4OH^- \quad (6.2)$$

The in vitro dissolution properties of crystalline HA depend on several factors, such as the type and concentration of the buffered or unbuffered solutions, pH of the solutions, degree of saturation, solid/solution ratio, the length of suspension in solutions, and the crystallinity of the HA [70–74]. In the case of ceramic HA bulks, the degree of porosities, defect structure, the amount, and the type of other calcium phosphate phases present also display significant influences. The extent of dissolution of the ceramic HA bulk is less in lactic acid buffer compared to that in acetic acid buffer [75]. For the crystalline HA powders containing other calcium phosphate phases, the extent of dissolution will be affected by the type and the amount of non-HA phases. According to previous studies made by Ducheyne et al. [76] and Radin and Ducheyne [77], the evaluation of dissolution rate for the nonwell-crystallized HA, α-TCP, β-TCP, T,P and crystallized HA were measured in 0.05 mol Tris(hydroxy)methylaminomethane-HCl buffered solution at pH 7.3, 37°C for immersion time periods ranging from 15 min to 72 h. The results indicated that the concentration of dissolved Ca^{2+} reaches saturation (about 1.5 mM) for TP in a few minutes immersion, and the value significantly exceeds that of β-TCP ($[Ca^{2+}]$ is about 1×10^{-1} mM) and crystalline HA ($[Ca^{2+}]$ is less than 1×10^{-1} mM) after 24 h immersion. Comparing the dissolution rate of β-TCP with α-TCP, the dissolution rate of β-TCP is about four times larger than that of α-TCP. Therefore, it can be recognized that the dissolution rate of various monophasic calcium phosphate compounds decreased in the following order [76–78]:

Amorphous HA > TP > α-TCP > β-TCP > crystalline HA

In addition, the results of previous studies also showed that the values of solubility product (K) for β-TCP and crystalline HA powder are 1.2×10^{-29} $mol^5\ l^{-5}$ and 3.04×10^{-59} $mol^9\ l^{-9}$ at 25°C, respectively [79,80]. Thus, when HA bulks or HA-coated implants, which have a low crystallinity and high impurity phase content, are implanted, it may result in the dissolution, degradation of mechanical properties, and the dissociation of implants [47,48,76]. Therefore, the degree of crystallinity, phases, and chemical compositions of ceramic HA bulks and HA-coated implants must be controlled in order to maintain long-term stability in the body fluid after implantation.

The thermal stability of crystalline HA is rather complicated. Figure 6.2 shows the phase diagrams of $CaO–P_2O_5$ system [81] at high temperature without water present (Figure 6.2a) and with a partial water vapor pressure of 500 mmHg (Figure 6.2b). Various calcium phosphate compounds can be found at high temperatures, such as α-C_3P (α-TCP), C_4P (TP), monetite (C_2P), and mixtures of CaO and C_4P. It can be seen that crystalline HA is not stable when the ambient atmosphere contains no water. If the partial water vapor pressure is increased, then the crystalline HA becomes a stable phase and it can be found in the phase diagram, as shown in Figure 6.2b. Previous studies reported that the partial dehydration of HA significantly occurred at a temperature higher than 900°C [82], and the oxyhydroxyapatite (OHA) in the form of $Ca_{10}(PO_4)_6(OH)_{0.8}O_{0.6}\cdot V_{0.6}$ may occur when the heating temperature is higher than 1100°C. With increasing heating temperatures higher than 1300°C, the HA would decompose and the apatite structure changes to a new space group with the appearance of α-TCP and TP according to the reaction shown in Equation 6.3 [83]. The α-TCP is resulted from the transformation of β-TCP at temperatures above 1300°C, and the reaction shown in Equation 6.3 is followed by the reaction shown in Equation 6.4. Thus, it is generally recognized that the highest temperature of HA without phase decomposition is about 1300°C in an ambient atmosphere that contains no water.

$$Ca_{10}(PO_4)_6(OH)_2 \rightarrow 2\alpha\text{-}Ca_3(PO_4)_2 + Ca_4P_2O_9 + H_2O \quad (6.3)$$

$$Ca_4P_2O_9 \rightarrow \alpha\text{-}Ca_3(PO_4)_2 + CaO \quad (6.4)$$

The importance of partial water vapor pressure is shown more clearly in Figure 6.3, which reveals the influence of water vapor pressure on the phase stability of HA. At 1300°C

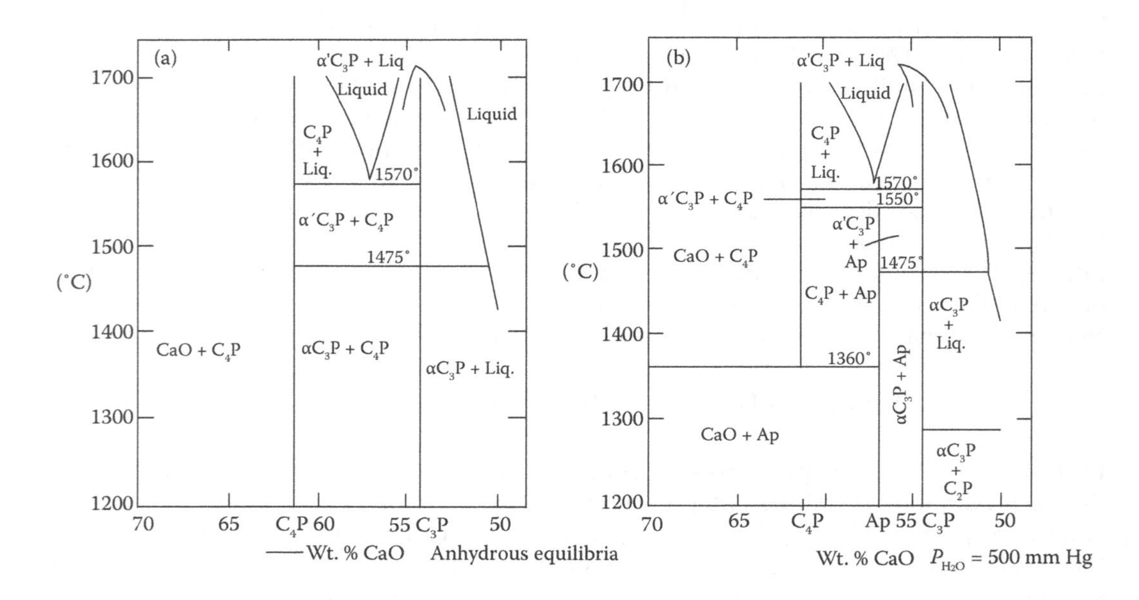

FIGURE 6.2
Phase diagram of the system $CaO–P_2O_5$ at high temperature: (a) no water present and (b) partial water vapor pressure of 500 mmHg. (From Gross et al., *J. Biomed. Mater. Res.*, 39, 580–587, 1998. With permission.)

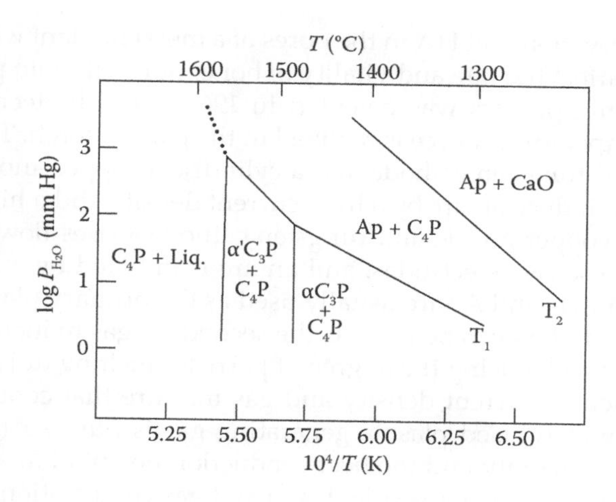

FIGURE 6.3
Influence of ambient water vapor pressure on phase compositions of calcium phosphate. (From Gross et al., *J. Biomed. Mater. Res.*, 39, 580–587, 1998. With permission.)

(or 10^4/T for Equation 6.4), this diagram shows the stable phases are α-TCP and TP when the water vapor pressure is 1 mmHg (log $P_{H_2O} = 0$). The stable phases are HA + TP, and HA + CaO at partial water vapor pressures of about 10 mmHg (log $P_{H_2O} = 1$) and 100 mmHg (log $P_{H_2O} = 2$), respectively. It reveals that a higher partial water vapor pressure can help to maintain and replenish the OH^- groups within the HA crystal structure, and to increase the phase-stabilized temperature of HA. Applying a steam atmosphere or a high steam pressure is an effective method to maintain high thermal stability of HA during the manufacturing process [84]. For a calcium phosphate compound with a Ca/P ratio exceeding HA by only a few percent, stable phases would be changed between α-TCP, TP, HA, and CaO. When the partial water vapor pressure is presented, the formation of the α-CP, β-TCP, and TP phases will be minimized and HA will be the more stable phase below 1550°C [8,12], as shown in Figure 6.2b. But HA becomes unstable and it will still decompose into α-TCP and TP following the reaction shown in Equation 6.3 at temperatures higher than 1550°C.

Plasma-Sprayed HACs

Thermal spray processing has been applied for many years to deposit layer coatings for various purposes such as wear resistance, thermal barrier coatings (TBCs), biocompatibility, and so forth. The major advantages of the thermal spray processes are the ability to apply a wide variety of compositions, including most metallic and ceramic materials, without significantly heating substrate surface to be coated [85]. The main thermal spray techniques include flame spraying, atmospheric plasma spraying (APS), vacuum plasma spraying (VPS), high velocity oxygen fuel (HVOF) spraying, arc metallization, and detonation gun spraying. Among these techniques, the plasma spraying process is becoming the extensively applied technique of the thermal spraying methods and is commonly used to deposit HA into dental implants and orthopedic prostheses. Investigations into some calcium phosphate compounds and HA coatings on metallic implants, such as Ti–6Al–4V, started with the observation that HA in the pores of a metal implant with a porous coating would significantly affect the rate and vitality of bone ingrowth onto pores [15,86].

The plasma spraying process was patented in 1960s, and the technical utilization of plasma as a high-temperature source is realized in the plasma torch. The plasma gun consists of a cone-shaped tungsten cathode and a cylindrical copper anode. The principle of plasma spraying is to induce an arc by a high current density and a high electric potential between the anodic copper nozzle and tungsten cathode. Gases flow through the annular space between these two electrodes, and an arc is initiated by a high-frequency discharge. Noble gases of He and Ar are usually used as the primary plasma-generating gas. Diatomic gases of H_2 and N_2 can be used as the secondary gas to increase the enthalpy of plasma flame. Factors influencing the degree of particles melting during plasma spraying include variables such as current density and gas mixture that control the temperature of the plasma. The widely used plasma-generating gas is pure Ar (purity <99.95 wt.%). Since the thermal conductivity and the heat conduction potential for diatomic gases such as H_2 and N_2 are much higher than Ar [87], a mixed gas composition with Ar and H_2/N_2 gives quite a hotter plasma torch than 100% Ar gas. When well-crystallized HA powders are injected into the high-temperature plasma flame (normally in the range of 1×10^4 to 1.5×10^{4}°C), small granules will be evaporated in the flame, and larger particles are melted or partially melted quickly by the high-temperature plasma flame. Then these melted droplets are accelerated to about 200 m/s before impacting the substrate [88,89]. The high-impact velocity supplies high kinetic energy, which is expended in spreading the molten or semimolten droplets and creating a lamellar microstructure. In addition, the high cooling rate upon impact is estimated to be of the order of 10^6 to 10^8 K s^{-1} [90]. Therefore, the large contact area with the substrate and the rapid solidification result in producing amorphous calcium phosphate (ACP) component within coatings, and it is more commonly found at the coating/substrate interface.

Since the plasma spraying process involves high temperature and rapid solidification, it will result in the dehydroxylation and decomposition of HA and the formation of an amorphous structure within coatings. This decomposition sequence occurs in these steps [91,92]:

$$Ca_{10}(PO_4)_6(OH)_2 \rightarrow Ca_{10}(PO_4)_6(OH)_{2-2x}O_xV_x + xH_2O \tag{6.5}$$

$$Ca_{10}(PO_4)_6(OH)_{2-2x}O_xV_x \rightarrow Ca_{10}(PO_4)_6O_xV_x + (1-x)H_2O \tag{6.6}$$

$$Ca_{10}(PO_4)_6O_xV_x \rightarrow 2\alpha\text{-}Ca_3(PO_4)_2 + Ca_4P_2O_9 \tag{6.7}$$

$$\alpha\text{-}Ca_3(PO_4)_2 \rightarrow 3CaO + P_2O_5 \tag{6.8}$$

$$Ca_4P_2O_9 \rightarrow 4CaO + P_2O_5 \tag{6.9}$$

The symbol "V" in the formulas of oxyhydroxyapatite ($Ca_{10}(PO_4)_6(OH)_{2-2x}O_xV_x$, OHA) and oxyapatite ($Ca_{10}(PO_4)_6O_xV_x$, OA) refers to lattice vacancies in positions of the OH^- groups along the crystallographic *c*-axis in the structure of HA. Thus, the x-ray pattern of a plasma-sprayed HA coating shows the presence of α-TCP, β-TCP, TP, and CaO phases in addition to crystalline HA. The reduction in peak intensity and peak broadening of HA peaks provide an evidence for the formation of ACP. The formation of these additional phases is a result of the extreme temperature of plasma flame and rapid cooling and highly reactive atmospheres that favor nonequilibrium and metastable structures.

When OA appears to be stable in the absence of water vapor environment, it will readily retransform to HA according to the reaction [93,94]

$$O^{2-}\text{ (solid)} + V\text{ (solid)} + H_2O\text{ (gas)} \rightarrow 2OH^-\text{ (solid)} \quad (6.10)$$

The equilibrium temperature of the reaction shown in Equation 6.7 is determined by the temperature of incongruent melting of HA at 1570°C [95]. Based on the decomposition sequence, a model has been developed [91,96,97] that shows the in-flight evolution of calcium phosphate phases, as represented in Figure 6.4. It shows that the inner core, which is still at a temperature below 1550°C, consists of HA, OHA, and OA as stable phases during the short residence time of HA particles in the plasma flame (reactions shown in Equations 6.5 and 6.6). The second shell of Figure 6.2b, which is heated to temperatures of 1360°C to 1570°C, just below the incongruent melting temperature of HA. It undergoes a solid state decomposition to a mixture of α-TCP and TP. The third shell was heated to temperatures above 1570°C following the reaction shown in Equation 6.7. The outer shell is composed of CaO and a melt whose Ca/P ratio shifts by continuous evaporation of P_2O_5 along the liquids of the phase diagram (Figure 6.2) toward CaO-richer phases following reactions shown in Equations 6.8 and 6.9. While impacting at the substrates, this molten phase solidifies to produce ACP with various Ca/P ratios [92,102].

X-ray diffraction (XRD) has been widely used for determining the phase composition, phase content, and crystal structure of plasma-sprayed HACs, as well as for estimating the index of crystallinity and identifying other calcium phosphate compounds generated as a result of the high-temperature spraying process. Figure 6.5 shows the x-ray diffraction patterns of the well-crystallized HA powders (Figure 6.5a) and the plasma-sprayed HACs (Figure 6.5b). The difference in the phase composition and crystallinity between well-crystallized HA and plasma-sprayed HACs are quite evident. The peak intensity of HA phase is significantly decreased after plasma spraying. In addition, it can be seen that a fairly high content of ACP and other impurity phases including TCP, TP, and CaO are represented in the plasma-sprayed HACs besides the desired HA phase. The reduction

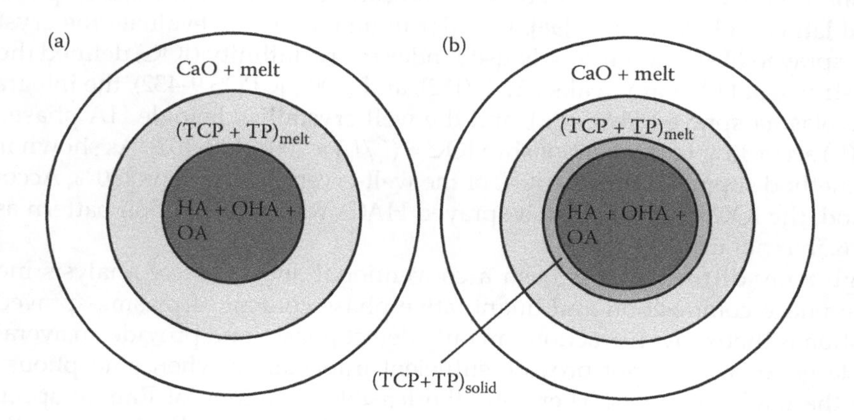

FIGURE 6.4
Schematic model of thermal decomposition of a spherical HA particle subjected to high temperature in a plasma flame at (a) a partial water vapor pressure of about 500 mmHg and (b) a partial water vapor pressure of about 10 mmHg. (From Heimann, R.B., *Surf. Coat. Technol.*, 201, 2012–2019, 2006. With permission.)

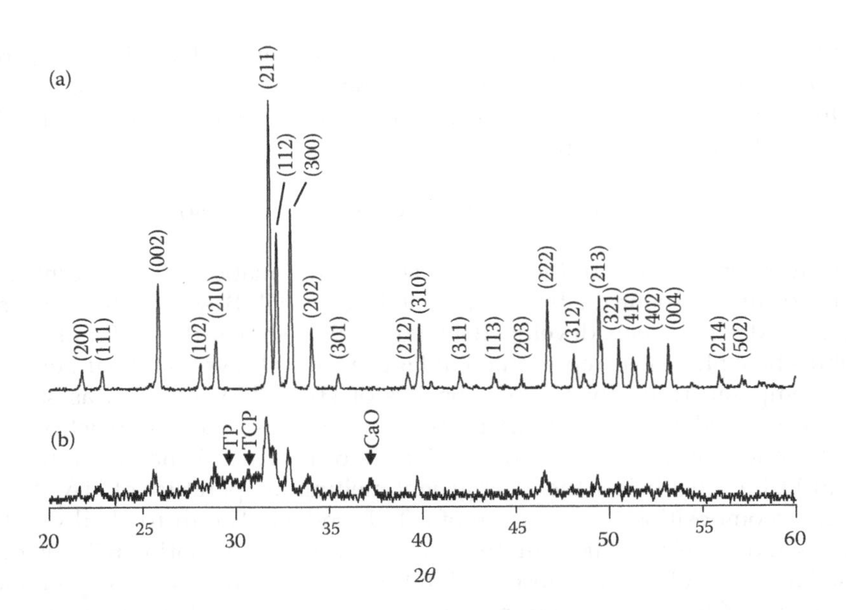

FIGURE 6.5
X-ray diffractions of (a) well-crystallized HA powder and (b) plasma-sprayed HACs.

in peak intensity and peak broadening of HA peaks suggest the formation of ACP [103]. The formation of these phases is a result of HA phase decomposition and dehydroxylation affected by extreme temperatures of plasma flame, rapid solidification, and highly reactive atmospheres that favor nonequilibrium or metastable structures according to the reactions described before. Plasma-sprayed HACs typically have high defect contents, amorphous components, and residual stresses, which result in a broadening of the x-ray diffraction peaks. In addition to providing the variation in phase composition, another material characteristic of plasma-sprayed HACs obtained through the x-ray diffraction analysis is the index of crystallinity. The crystallinity has been defined in different ways for biomedical applications, and it was initially used as an indication of the crystal size or perfection of the crystal lattice in HA crystals [98]. In order to quantitatively evaluate the crystallinity of plasma-sprayed HACs, a commonly used index of crystallinity (IOC) defined the ratio of the three strongest HA main peaks ((211), (112), and (300), JCPDS 9-432), the integral intensity of the plasma-sprayed HACs (I_c), and the well-crystallized single HA phase starting powders (I_p) according to the relationship $IOC = (I_c/I_p) \times 100\%$ [99–102]. As shown in Figure 6.5a, this method supposes that the IOC of the well-crystallized HA is 100%. According to this method, the IOC value of plasma-sprayed HACs with a diffraction pattern as shown in Figure 6.5b is about 20.3% [101].

Although x-ray diffraction has been a conventional and effective analysis method to obtain the phase composition and quantitative phase content of plasma-sprayed HACs, the limitation is that x-ray diffraction can only detect phases and provide an average value within a large area. It cannot provide sufficient information when amorphous components are the major products. Therefore, the feasible technique of Raman spectroscopy provides another way to reinforce the application of the x-ray diffraction method. The Raman spectroscopy can provide information on the short and intermediate range ordering in the solids and it allows a direct and nondestructive detection from the sample surface. Since both in vitro and in vivo biological properties of plasma-sprayed HACs are significantly dependent on the phases, detailed microstructure information such as the individual thermal-sprayed splats acquired with the Raman spectroscopy is important. Studies on thermal-sprayed splats can help to establish the understanding of individual splat's contribution to the phase composition of the thermal-sprayed coatings. In addition, the crystallinity of plasma-sprayed HACs and phase composition at various locations within individual thermal-sprayed HA splats have been quantitatively determined by the Raman spectroscopy analysis [66,94,104,105].

In addition to evaluating the index of crystallinity, it is also important to quantify the phase composition of amorphous component, crystalline HA, and other calcium phosphate phases of plasma-sprayed HACs by quantitative XRD analysis through the internal and external standards. However, pure phases and mixtures with different compositions are needed for establishing the calibration curves, and ACP is not easy to isolate and quantify. Thus, the lack of full quantification and its long task of obtaining calibration curves makes this technique unpopular. To fully determine the phase composition and quantify the amount of decomposed phases, including the amorphous component, of the as-sprayed coatings, the Rietveld method of structure determination from x-ray and neutron powder diffraction patterns is another effective way and has widely been used to study calcium phosphate compounds [60,106–111]. The Rietveld method creates an effective separation of the overlapping data from x-ray and neutron diffraction patterns, thereby allowing an accurate determination of the structure. This method has been successful and today, the structure of materials in the form of powders is being determined. In addition, a more widely used application of the Rietveld method is in determining the components of chemical mixtures. The conventional quantitative phase analysis (QPA), which is carried out using relative peak height ratios of HA and other phases involved by the Rietveld method provides a powerful tool that offers the user simultaneous quantitative phase determination of multiphase systems containing amorphous content. The quantitative analysis results of crystalline HA, amorphous, and various calcium phosphate phases plasma-sprayed and crystallized HACs will be represented in the next section.

Figure 6.6a shows the surface morphology of the plasma-sprayed HACs. It displays a typical microstructural feature, which is composed of completely molten splats (indicated by arrows), accumulated partially molten splats (marked by the circle), and thermal-induced

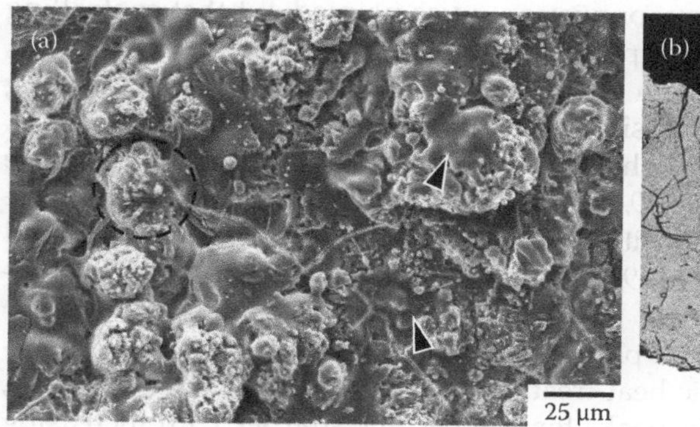

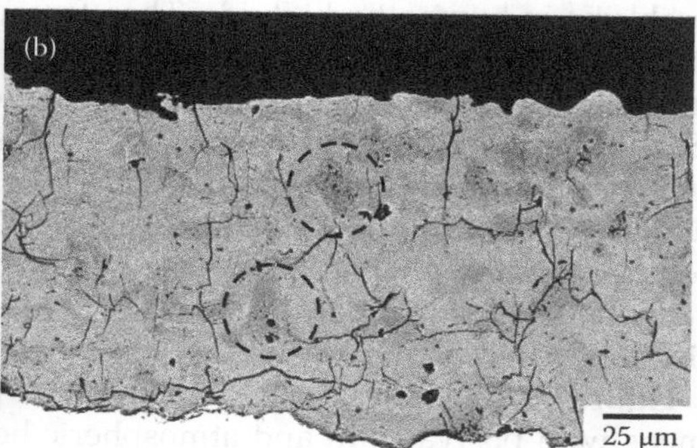

FIGURE 6.6
Typical plasma-sprayed HACs microstructural features for (a) surface morphology with microcracks, accumulated splats (marked by circles), and molten splats (indicated by arrows). (b) Cross-sectional microstructure showing spraying defects including pores and microcracks. Circle marks residual partial molten particle within plasma-sprayed HACs.

microcracks resulting from thermal contraction during the rapid cooling stage after plasma spraying. The cross-sectional feature of the plasma-sprayed HACs is shown in Figure 6.6b. According to the quantitative calculation by an image analyzer OPTIMAS 6.0 [63,64,101], the spraying defects content (in volume %), including microcracks and pores within the entire cross-sectional area of HACs, is about 4% for plasma-sprayed HACs in the case of Figure 6.6b. Although the plasma-sprayed coatings possess inevitable spraying defects, including pores and thermal-induced microcracks, they can be subjected to high densification due to the unapparent lamellar structure. Since the structural density of plasma-sprayed coatings is significantly affected by the variation of spraying parameters such as plasma gas flow rate ($l\ min^{-1}$), plasma power (kW), powder feed rate, surface speed, standoff distance, and so forth, the coating microstructure displayed in Figure 6.6b can be recognized as a dense HA coating (following the definition of the maximum porosity less than 5% by volume [8,9]) obtained from an appropriate spraying parameter. Besides the microstructural defects, a noteworthy feature with a mixture of dark gray and light gray regions is observed within plasma-sprayed HACs, as shown in Figure 6.6b. This distinguishable color contrast is resulted from the difference between amorphous and crystalline area of the coatings [102]. Other phases may be present in small quantities, but they cannot be distinguished from HA. During plasma spraying, the unmolten and partially molten particles are transferred to coatings with a morphology representative of the starting powders. Therefore, these dark gray regions marked by circles can be thought of as the crystalline region from the residual partially molten particles within plasma-sprayed HACs. This phenomenon is important in the performance of the HA coatings because the dissolution of amorphous regions could lead to failure for implants after a period of implantation. Therefore, it is possible to increase the crystallinity and in some cases the bonding strength of plasma-sprayed HACs by performing postheat treatments.

Crystallization of Plasma-Sprayed HACs during Heat Treatments

Referring to the reports about HA, many researchers have investigated the material and medical properties of plasma-sprayed HACs in the past 10 years. Amorphous calcium phosphate (ACP) is thermodynamically metastable and impurity calcium phosphate (including TCP, TP, and CaO, called the impurity phases) is undesirable for its dissolution problems in human body fluids. Therefore, previous studies pointed out that controlling spraying parameters [112] or performing appropriate thermal treatments (in vacuum, in an atmosphere with moisture or steam pressure and the spark plasma sintering (SPS) technique) are available methods that significantly promote the HA crystallization, improve the crystallinity and dissolution behaviors of coatings, and enhance the surface activity to the growth of apatite layers [16,59,65,66,99,113–115]. Additionally, reports have focused on the changes in phase composition, microstructural homogenization, and reduction in residual porosity of HACs [55–59,63,101], as well as the mechanism of crystallization of the coating layers [116].

Figure 6.7 illustrates the XRD patterns of plasma-sprayed HA-coated Ti–6Al–4V specimens with postvacuum and atmospheric heat treatments at 400°C, 500°C, 600°C, 700°C, and 800°C. The three strongest HA main peaks tend to become sharper with increasing heating temperatures, revealing that the plasma-sprayed HACs possess different degrees of crystallization after postheat treatment. For the atmospheric heat-treated HACs, the partial water vapor pressure of atmospheric moisture can help to recover and promote the reconstitution of TCP, TP, and ACP into crystalline HA. However, the vacuum heat-treated specimens possess more TCP and TP than the atmospheric heat-treated specimens.

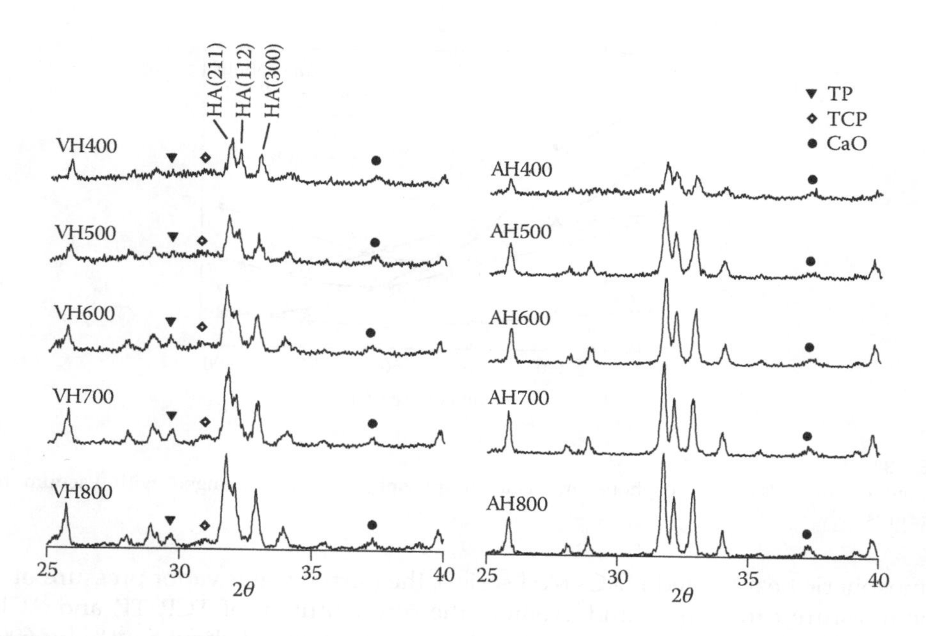

FIGURE 6.7
X-ray diffraction patterns of plasma-sprayed HACs with applying postvacuum heat treatment (VH series) and atmospheric heat treatment (AH-series) at 400°C to 800°C. (From Yang, C.W. and Lui, T.S., *Mater. Trans.*, 48(2), 211–218, 2007. With permission.)

According to the phase diagram of CaO–P_2O_5 system as shown in Figure 6.2, since there is a lack of ambient partial water vapor pressure during vacuum heating, TCP and TP phases cannot be eliminated without the replenishment of OH^- groups. In addition, the CaO remained within both of the heat-treated HACs because it cannot easily be converted into HA if the ambient heating atmosphere is without abundant H_2O molecules [54,59].

Heat treatment is recognized as a proven process of controlling the amount of amorphous calcium phosphate and quantification of the amorphous component has also been attempted by many studies [45,60,64,101,108–111,117]. In order to evaluate the content of ACP and other impurity phases displayed in Figure 6.7, the internal standard method [118] is one of the most common methods to quantitatively determine the fluctuation of phase composition within the heat-treated HACs. The integral intensity of known weight percent pure Si powder added in the specimens is taken as the internal standard. Wang et al. [45] and Chou and Chang [117] have established the calibration curves for calculating the content of ACP, TCP, TP, and CaO phases. The main peak integral intensity ratio between TCP, TP, CaO, and HA phase from various XRD patterns of heat-treated HACs are compared to the calibration curves and the concentrations (in wt.%) of these phases in various coatings are calculated. Figure 6.8 shows the impurity phase content at different temperatures for the vacuum heat-treated HACs (VH series). The impurity phases generally tend to decrease when the increased heating temperature reaches 600°C, at which the HACs contains the lowest content (about 20.3 wt.%) of total impurity phases. There is also a continuous decrease in amorphous content with increasing temperatures. However, when the heating temperature rises to a temperature range of 600°C to 800°C in vacuum, a significant increasing trend of impurity phases content (mostly TP and CaO phases) resulting from the decomposition of HA [54,101] can be recognized as the temperature increases further, resulting in greater total impurity phases about 26.1 wt.% at 800°C. For

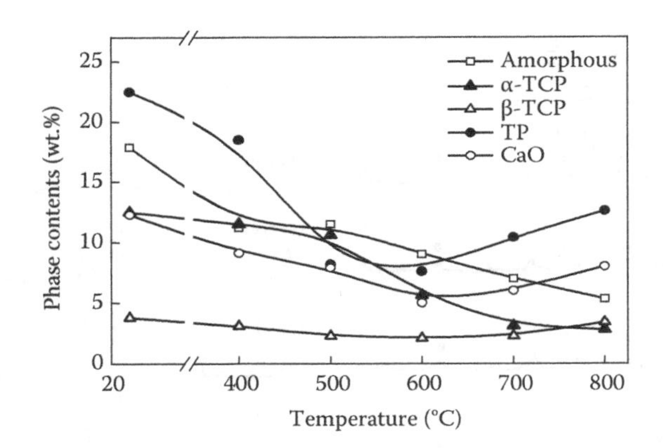

FIGURE 6.8
Phase content (in wt.%) of amorphous and calcium phosphate phases changed with vacuum heating temperatures.

the atmospheric heat-treated HACs (AH series), the partial water vapor pressure of atmospheric moisture can recover and promote the reconstitution of TCP, TP, and ACP into crystalline HA. The residual compound with a phase content of about 5 wt.% for 600°C to 800°C atmospheric heat-treated HACs is thought of as CaO [119]. Referring to the previous presentation in Section 6.2.2, the Rietveld analysis method with QPA is another effective way to determine the phase content of the plasma-sprayed and heat-treated HACs. Since the heat during plasma spraying and crystallization processes is difficult to ascertain, the quantity of ACP is not easy to determine in relation to the heat liberated. Therefore, the Rietveld analysis method with QPA provides a powerful way to completely quantify the associated amorphous component and crystalline phases within a multiphase system for any thermally treated material [60,108,109]. Figure 6.9 illustrates the variation in phase composition of plasma-sprayed powders with changing a series of plate power, which is determined by the QPA technique via Rietveld method [60]. It can be seen that the phase content of crystalline HA, ACP, and other impurity phases, including α-TCP, β-TCP, TP,

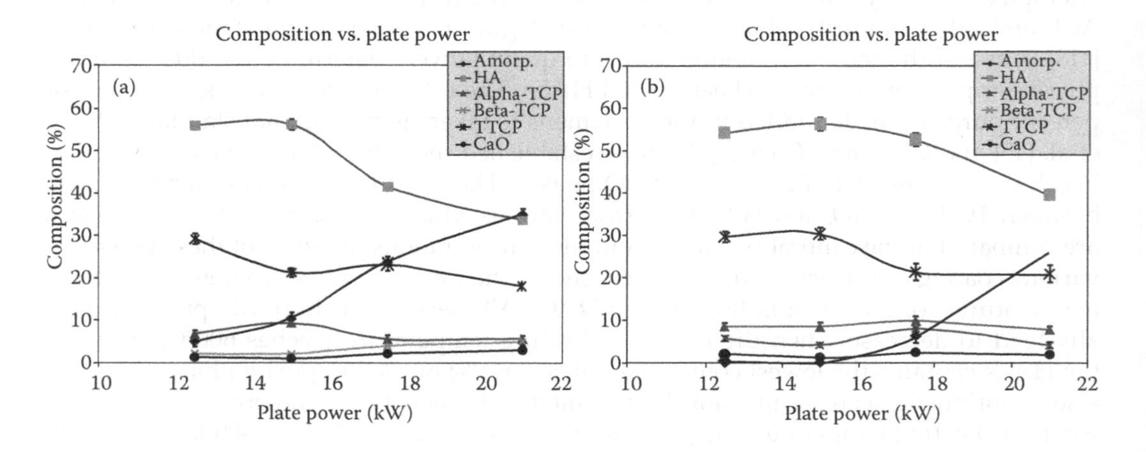

FIGURE 6.9
Phase composition of plasma-sprayed powders determined by quantitative phase analysis (QPA) technique via Rietveld method of (a) 7 wt.% and (b) 14 wt.% HA suspension feedstock for changing a series of plate power.

and CaO, are obtained. The phase decomposition during plasma spraying is quantitatively demonstrated and the amorphous content increased substantially at higher powers.

Because the crystallization of plasma-sprayed HACs is usually accompanied with a change in the coating dimensions, the variation in microstructure during heat treatments can be clarified through thermal dilatometry. In order to exclude the influence of metallic substrate and interfacial reaction between HA/Ti of the HA-coated Ti–6Al–4V specimens, only plasma-sprayed HAC test pieces of dimensions 20 (l) × 3 (w) × 3 (t) mm^3 without Ti substrate are used for thermal dilatometry analysis by a dilatometer. The heating conditions are the same as the above-mentioned temperatures with a heating rate of 10°C/min, followed by furnace cooling after holding for 3 h. The dilatation curve of HACs during heating process is shown in Figure 6.10, which can be divided into three regions of markedly different slopes. The increased dilatation approaches linearity in the temperature intervals of 100°C to 400°C (region I). The linear increased dilatation represents that just a thermal expansion effect on the HACs during heating in temperature interval 100°C to 400°C, and the coefficient of thermal expansion (CTE, α) of sprayed HA coating layer can be suggested about 15.6 × 10^{-6} °C^{-1} calculated from the slope.

Besides thermal expansion effect in region II, however, the dilatation decreases in a nonlinear manner at heating temperatures from above 400°C to 700°C should be correlated with the main temperature interval for the crystallization of plasma-sprayed HACs. When the HA crystallization effect with a fair amount of volume contraction is larger than the thermal expansion of coatings in this region, the dilatation $\delta L/L_o$ (or the slope of the dilatation curve) decreased and even becomes a negative value, especially during the 500°C to 700°C heating interval. Combined with quantitative analysis as shown in Figure 6.8, the evidence is that an apparent change in phase content and crystallinity within this temperature interval. Although the investigations by Feng et al. [61] and Gross et al. [116] indicated that the crystallization has been identified as taking place at about 400°C, but the main HA crystallization region of the HACs should be suggested over 500°C heating temperatures. As the heating temperature approaches to 700°C, there is also a dilatation balance between crystallization and thermal expansion of HACs. Thus, the dilatation curve displays a linear thermal expansion larger than crystallization contraction over 700°C heating temperatures in region III.

Figure 6.11 also illustrates the thermal dilatometry curves for the HACs without Ti–6Al–4V, heating at 400°C, 500°C, 600°C, 700°C, and 800°C, respectively. They all show

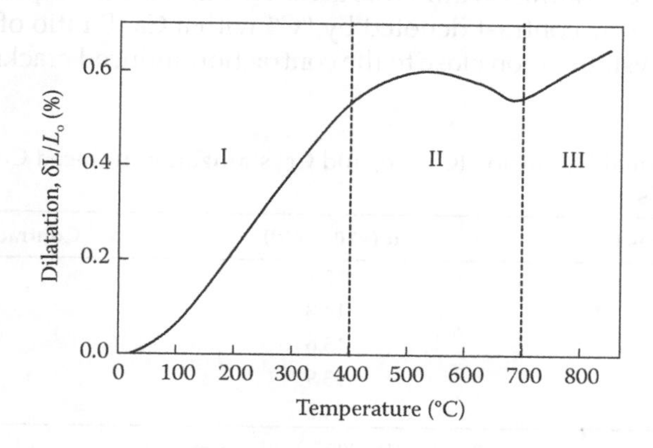

FIGURE 6.10
Dilatation curve of plasma-sprayed HACs for a single heating process through thermal dilatometry.

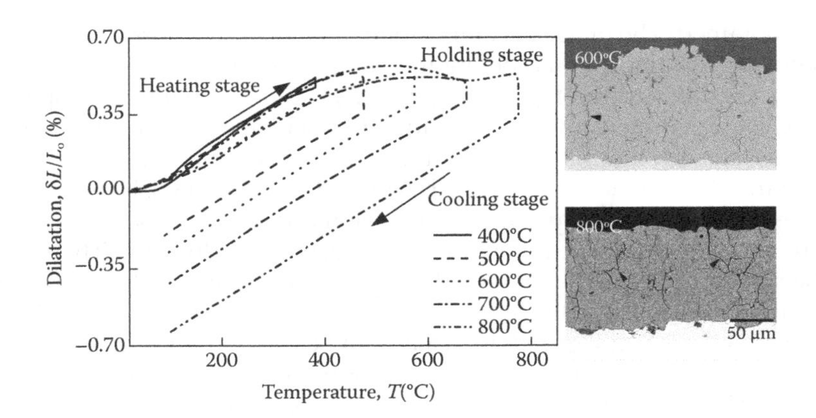

FIGURE 6.11
Dilatation curves of plasma-sprayed HACs obtained from heating, holding to cooling processes at 400°C to 800°C. (From Yang, C.W. and Lui, T.S., *Mater. Trans.*, 48(2), 211–218, 2007. With permission.)

an approximately linear thermal expansion when the heating temperature is in the range from 100°C to 400°C. The CTE of an HAC within this temperature range is also evaluated for about 15.6×10^{-6} °C^{-1}. In addition, it is worth noting that the nonlinear region of the dilatation curves represents a consequence of greater crystallization of plasma-sprayed HACs at 500°C to 800°C temperature interval. Table 6.1 lists the extent of dilatation values that are calculated from the dilatation curves cooling to about 100°C and significant crystallization-induced contraction after heat treatments have been demonstrated. This phenomenon can be recognized as a result of crystallization-induced contraction for these coatings. The CTE data of crystallized HACs at these heating temperatures are calculated from the slope of cooling stages, and the change in the CTE value also means that the effective crystallization temperature of plasma-sprayed HACs by postheat treatments should be higher than 600°C [64,120].

Compared with the as-sprayed HACs (Figure 6.6b), the cross-sectional images obtained from 600°C and 800°C crystallized HACs represent significantly cracking features, as indicated by the arrows in Figure 6.11. Figure 6.12 shows a typical SEM/SEI observation nearby these contraction-induced cracks of the heat-treated HACs in the range of 600°C to 800°C, and there is an obvious contrast within this area. Through the semiquantitative analysis of SEM/EDS, the light gray contrast denoted by "C" with a Ca/P ratio of 1.61 represents the occurrence of HA crystallization close to the contraction-induced cracks, and the dark gray

TABLE 6.1
Coefficient of Thermal Expansion (CTE, α) and Crystallization-Induced Contraction Ratio of Heat-Treated HACs

Heating Temperatures (°C)	α (×10^{-6} °C^{-1})[a]	Contraction Ratio (%)[b]
400	15.1	0.05
500	14.8	0.20
600	13.6	0.28
700	13.9	0.43
800	14.3	0.65

Source: Yang et al., *Mater. Trans.*, 48(2), 211–218, 2007. With permission.
[a] Values are measured from the slope of cooling curves to room temperature.
[b] Data obtained from total dilatation of the sample dimension after cooling.

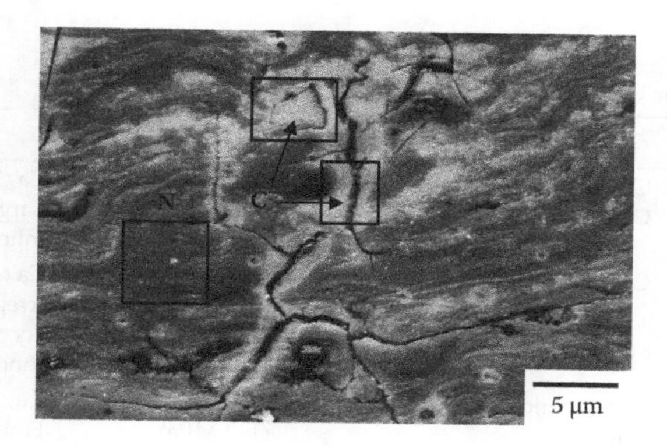

FIGURE 6.12
Enlarged cracks of heat-treated HACs, showing presence of crystallized (denoted by "C") and nonstoichiometric calcium phosphate (denoted by "N") regions that can be recognized by different contrast. (From Yang, C.W. and Lui, T.S., *Mater. Trans.*, 48(2), 211–218, 2007. With permission.)

region "N" with a low Ca/P atomic ratio of 1.35 represents a nonstoichiometric calcium phosphate region away from the "C" region. By incorporating the IOC and the thermal dilatometry results, therefore, it can be recognized that the formation and the propagation of enlarged cracks is due to the coating contraction during crystallization.

For biological applications, the dissolution rate of HA coatings is of interest because a rapidly dissolving coating may not remain on the implant for a sufficient time to allow full stabilization in bone or the desired tissue response in vivo. Ongoing development and optimization of the plasma-sprayed HACs are aimed at higher crystallinity coatings without sacrificing bonding strength. Although it is possible to evidently increase the crystallinity of plasma-sprayed HACs by postdeposition heat treatments in vacuum and in the air, heat treatments with temperatures over 600°C result in the degradation of mechanical properties with the significant formation of crystallization-induced cracks [101,120]. Therefore, it is indispensable to develop a lower-temperature treating process [58,59,63]; for example: a hydrothermal treatment with an abundant water vapor atmosphere that can simultaneously acquire higher crystallinity, good bonding strength, and biological responses without microstructural deterioration [121,122].

Hydrothermal Synthesis and Crystallization

The interest of synthesis of HA is linked with its importance as a major constituent of the inorganic component in human bones and teeth, and the characteristics of HA have significant effects on the subsequent products with HA being in the form of dense or porous structure in coatings or in composites. Since HA has been recognized as the best biocompatible ceramic material, there have been many reports on the biological aspects [6,7,15,123,124], and the fabrication processing of HA has progressed with the growing importance of the biological applications. A number of studies on the preparation of HA by various methods have been reported in the literature. Yoshimura and Suda et al. have reviewed the preparation for HA powders and grouped these methods into three categories, as listed in Table 6.2 [125–127]. Table 6.3 illustrates the chemical reactions of these processes [128]. Two

TABLE 6.2

Preparation Methods for Crystalline HA

	Starting Materials	Synthetic Conditions	Comments
Solid state reaction	$Ca_3(PO_4)_2$, CaO, $Ca_2P_2O_7$, $CaCO_3$	900–1300°C	Ca/P ~ 1.67 Large, irregular grain Inhomogeneous
Wet chemical method	$Ca(OH)_2$, H_3PO_4	RT ~100°C pH: 7–12	Ca/P < 1.67 Irregular crystals with low crystallinity Inhomogeneous
Hydrothermal method	Wet chemically prepared HA	100–200°C (1–2 MPa)	Ca/P = 1.67 Fine single crystals Homogeneous
Flux growth method	CaF_2, $CaCl_2$ as flux $Ca(OH)_2$ as flux	1325°C FA, HA	Large crystals with lattice strain

main ways for the preparation of HA powders are solid-state reactions and wet chemical methods. In the case of HA fabrication, the wet methods can be divided into precipitation, hydrothermal technique, and hydrolysis of the calcium phosphates. Depending on these techniques, materials with nanocrystalline, various morphologies of blades, rods, needles or equiaxed crystals, stoichiometry, and various levels of crystallinity can be obtained.

Solid-state reactions can usually obtain stoichiometric and well-crystallized HA products. However, they require relatively high heating temperatures and long heat-treatment time. In addition, the HA powder prepared by solid state reactions usually have irregular forms with a large grain size, and often have heterogeneity in composition due to incomplete reactions. The wet chemical method is a relatively easier way of obtaining HA powder. The reactions may occur in aqueous solutions at lower temperatures. But the lack of wet chemical methods in atmosphere means that the products are usually less crystallized, heterogeneous in composition, and irregularly formed crystals with lattice defects. The flux growth method, which is a better method since the fluxes such as CaF_2, $CaCl_2$, NaCl, KF, and $Ca(OH)_2$ mixed with starting apatite powders make lower liquid temperature, results in the production of less strained apatite crystals [129–131]. Among these methods mentioned in Table 6.2, the hydrothermal technique is a very important method

TABLE 6.3

Chemical Reactions for Various Synthesis Methods of HA

1. Solid state reaction

   $Ca_2P_2O_7 + CaCO_3 \rightarrow Ca_{10}(PO_4)_6(OH)_2$, with H_2O vapor

   $Ca_3(PO_4)_2 + CaO \rightarrow Ca_{10}(PO_4)_6(OH)_2$ (at 1000°C)

   $6CaHPO{\cdot}2H_2O + 4CaCO_3 \rightarrow Ca_{10}(PO_4)_6(OH)_2 + 4CO_2 + 14H_2O$ (at 1000°C)

2. Wet chemical method

   $10Ca(OH)_2 + 6H_3PO_4 \rightarrow Ca_{10}(PO_4)_6(OH)_2 + 18H_2O$ (at pH = 8)

   $10CaCl_2 + 6Na_2HPO_4 + 2H_2O \rightarrow Ca_{10}(PO_4)_6(OH)_2 + 12NaCl + 8HCl$ (at pH = 8)

   $10Ca(NO_3)_2 + 6(NH_4)_2HPO_4 + 2H_2O \rightarrow Ca_{10}(PO_4)_6(OH)_2 + 12NH_4NO_3 + 8HNO_3$ (at pH = 8–10)

3. Hydrothermal method

   $10CaHPO_4 + 2H_2O \rightarrow Ca_{10}(PO_4)_6(OH)_2 + 4H_3PO_4$ (at 200°C)

4. Flux method

   $CaO + P_2O_5 + B_2O_3 \rightarrow Ca_{10}(PO_4)_6(OH)_2$

in the preparation of HA. The hydrothermal technique and hydrothermal materials processing are becoming a popular field of research for scientists and technologists of various disciplines, particularly after the successful development of ceramic processing technology during the 1970s. The fabrication of HA under hydrothermal conditions usually gives well-crystallized, compositionally homogeneous, and uniform HA powders with a high degree of crystallinity, and large, perfect, single crystals of HA with a Ca/P ratio close to the stoichiometric value of 1.67 [132]. The understanding of minerals formation in nature under elevated pressure and temperature in the presence of water (hydrothermal conditions are similar to the environment of mineral formation within the earth's crust) has led to the development of the hydrothermal technique of today. In the following sections, the principles and applications of the hydrothermal technique for preparing HA are introduced. Next, the effects of hydrothermal crystallization and significantly self-healing on the microstructural homogeneity of plasma-sprayed HACs are discussed in Section 6.3.2. In addition, the kinetics, reaction rates, and activation energy of hydrothermal crystallization, which are related to the saturated steam pressure within a hermetical system, are deduced and evaluated in Section 6.3.3.

Hydrothermal Technology for the HA: Principles and Applications

Apatite is a common mineral in igneous, sedimentary, and metamorphic rocks, which has a general chemical formula of $A_{10}(BO_4)_6X_2$, where A is Ca, Sr, Ba, Fe, Pd, Cd, and rare earth elements, BO_4 can be PO_4^{3-}, VO_4^{3-}, SiO_4^{4-}, AsO_4^{3-}, CO_3^{2-} groups, and X can be OH^-, F^-, Cl^-, CO_3^{2-} groups. The inorganic phases of HA with a chemical formula $Ca_{10}(PO_4)_6(OH)_2$ present in the hard tissues contain mostly Ca, P, and H_2O, also a small amount of Na^+, Mg^{2+}, K^+, as well as F^-, Cl^-, and CO_2^{3-}. Therefore, the chemical component of the mineral constituents of teeth and bones is very important in the synthesis of HA-based biomaterials. In the present biomedical and clinical applications, HA powders, bulk implants, and surface coatings on metallic or ceramic substrates prepared under hydrothermal conditions have been effectively carried out by many research groups [133–144]. The hydrothermal method has been found to be a suitable method to prepare well-crystallized and nonagglomerated crystals that are homogeneous in size, shape, and composition that can be achieved even at low temperatures [145,146]. HA crystals with different morphologies can also be grown by hydrothermal method using various starting materials such as calcite, brushite, and monetite [135,147,148].

In the hydrothermal process, water is the most important solvent and a necessary component of the system, and indeed it is often the principal component with regard to the relative content of salts, acids, alkalis, and so forth, which may serve as mineralizers. It also exhibits unique properties, especially under supercritical conditions. In any system containing water, a certain concentration of the components occurs in the dissolved state, changing the pH of the medium, the composition of the original liquid phase, and the properties of the solution. Several previous publications have made definitions for the term "hydrothermal" [125,149–154], and a concluded definition of the hydrothermal reaction can be proposed as follows: any heterogeneous chemical reactions in the presence of a solvent (whether aqueous or nonaqueous) or mineralizers above room temperature and at pressure greater than 1 atm in a closed system to dissolve and recrystallize materials that are relatively insoluble under ordinary conditions.

During the early 1970s in the Material Research Laboratory at Pennsylvania State University, a process was developed that utilized the skeletal structure of marine invertebrates, especially reef building corals, as a template to make porous structures of other materials [155]. The calcium carbonate ($CaCO_3$) skeleton is reacted with dominium hydrogen phosphate and, by means of a hydrothermal exchange of carbonate and phosphate, is converted to HA. Moreover, the calcium carbonate can also be transformed into HA in the presence of the appropriate amounts of the dicalcium phosphate anhydrous (DCPA, $CaHPO_4$), as shown in reactions 6.11 and 6.12:

$$10CaCO_3 + 6(NH_4)_2HPO_4 + 2H_2O \rightarrow Ca_{10}(PO_4)_6(OH)_2 + 6(NH_2)CO_3 + 4H_2CO_3 \quad (6.11)$$

$$4CaCO_3 + 6CaHPO_4 \rightarrow Ca_{10}(PO_4)_6(OH)_2 + 6H_2O + 4CO_2 \quad (6.12)$$

Under stable temperature and pressure conditions, the exchange results in a nearly pure HA. The HA structure is an exact replicate of the porous marine skeleton. Ito et al. [156,157] have done the study on the single crystal growth of HA. Single crystals of carbonate-containing HA have been grown hydrothermally by gradually heating with a temperature gradient applied to the pressure vessel, using the DCPA. Reaction 6.13 also shows this hydrothermal reaction for the formation of HA single crystals.

$$10CaHPO_4 + 2H_2O \rightarrow Ca_{10}(PO_4)_6(OH)_2 + 4H_3PO_4 \quad (6.13)$$

In addition, TCP and TP can be easily converted to HA under the hydrothermal conditions [59], and the chemical reactions as shown in 6.14 and 6.15 can be carried out hydrothermally at 275°C, under a steam pressure of about 82.76 MPa [158,159].

$$3Ca_4P_2O_9 + 3H_2O \rightarrow Ca_{10}(PO_4)_6(OH)_2 + 2Ca(OH)_2 \quad (6.14)$$

$$3Ca_3(PO_4)_2 + Ca(OH)_2 \rightarrow Ca_{10}(PO_4)_6(OH)_2 + H_2O \quad (6.15)$$

Considering the biomedical applications, plasma-sprayed HACs deposited on metallic implants, which is an extensively used process in commercial products, tend to avoid the inherent mechanical property limitations of HA without any significant loss in biocompatibility. It has been generally recognized that the crystallization of hydroxyl-deficient plasma-sprayed HACs requires at least 600°C [45,64,116] for postheat treatments in vacuum or in the air. But high heating temperatures tend to cause phase decomposition (Figures 6.7 and 6.8) and undermined the microstructural integrity (Figures 6.11 and 6.12) of crystalline HA. Research results have indicated that HACs with a higher impurity content of TCP, TP, CaO, OHA, and ACP will result in a higher dissolution rate than crystalline HA in aqueous solutions or in human body fluids. The higher dissolution rate will lead to a decrease in microstructural homogeneity, poorer mechanical properties, and lack of coating adherence, which will undermine the long-term fixation between the implants and the surrounding bone tissue. To solve these problems, it has been reported that surface modifications for forming bonelike apatite can induce high bioactivity of bioinert metals in simulated body fluid [160]. Since HA is a stable phase under a partial steam pressure of 500 mmHg [70], therefore a hydrothermal crystallization process conducted with a water vapor atmosphere has been developed to minimize impurity phases and promote HA crystallization at relatively lower temperatures. Performing a hydrothermal treatment on plasma-sprayed HACs is an effective method to promote HA crystallization, increase the crystallinity, and significantly improve the extent of new bone apposition in vivo [59,63,121].

In recent years, a new hydrothermal method has been proposed that helps to prepare thin HA ceramic coatings on Ti substrates with a curved surface at low temperature. It has been demonstrated that a pure HA ceramic layer with a thickness of 50 μm could be coated to a Ti cylindrical rod at about 135°C under the confining pressure of 40 MPa [138]. However, the coating layer showed a porous microstructure with the relative density of only about 60%. Hydrothermal hot-pressing (HHP) method is also a possible route for producing a ceramic body at relatively low temperatures (generally under 300°C) [161]. The bonding of HA and Ti alloys was achieved by the HHP method through the surface modification of Ti alloys with NaOH solution at relatively low temperatures [161–163]. Because the released water can be utilized as a reaction solvent during the HHP treatment, the compression of specimens under hydrothermal conditions can help to accelerate the densification of HA and the joining of HA to metal was achieved simultaneously under hydrothermal condition following the chemical reaction 6.16 [139,164].

$$6CaHPO_4{\cdot}2H_2O + 4Ca(OH)_2 \rightarrow Ca_{10}(PO_4)_6(OH)_2 + 18H_2O \quad (6.16)$$

Hydrothermal Crystallization with Self-Healing Effect of Plasma-Sprayed HACs

Some researchers have noted that morphology-controlled HA crystals and thin HA coatings, which have high crystallinity and an enhanced interfacial adhesive strength, on a curved surface of Ti substrate can be successfully synthesized through the hydrothermal method at low temperatures [63,138,165,166]. Although the hydrothermal method has attracted great interest recently as a replacement for the high-temperature plasma-spraying process, the hydrothermal synthesis, as displayed in reaction 6.16, is more complex because the purity of the raw material (dicalcium phosphate dihydrate, $CaHPO_4{\cdot}2H_2O$, DCPD), the concentration, and the pH value of solutions must all be carefully controlled to obtain well-crystallized HA. Besides, the efficiency of forming a uniform surface coating is much lower than the plasma-spraying technique. Therefore, combining the advantages of plasma spraying and hydrothermal treatment can lead to improvements in the crystallinity, microstructural homogeneity, adhesive strength, and biological responses of HA-coated Ti-substrate implants [121,122]. The benefits of low-temperature hydrothermal crystallization of nanocrystallite HA have been clarified through x-ray photoelectron spectroscopy (XPS), transmission electron microscopy (TEM) examinations, evaluation of the crystallization rate, and the activation energy [167–171].

Figure 6.13 illustrates the schematic apparatus of the plasma-sprayed HA-coated Ti–6Al–4V specimens within the hermetical autoclave during the hydrothermal treatment. The deionized water is used as the source of steam atmosphere during the hydrothermal treatment. The specimens were isolated without immersion in the water. Figure 6.14 shows the XRD patterns of the plasma-sprayed and various hydrothermally treated HACs (HT-HACs). The sharpening of the three strongest HA main peaks and the flattening of the diffraction background (2θ at about 28° to 34°) mean that the plasma-sprayed HACs significantly crystallized and the content of ACP significantly decreased by performing the autoclaving hydrothermal treatment in an ambient saturated steam-pressure system. The quantitative results of the crystallinity (IOC) for these HT-HACs are shown in Figure 6.15. The IOC value increased with increasing the hydrothermal heating time and temperature. It is worth noting that just low heating temperatures of 150°C to 200°C are required to see a significant rise in crystallinity for the HT-HACs (the IOC is about

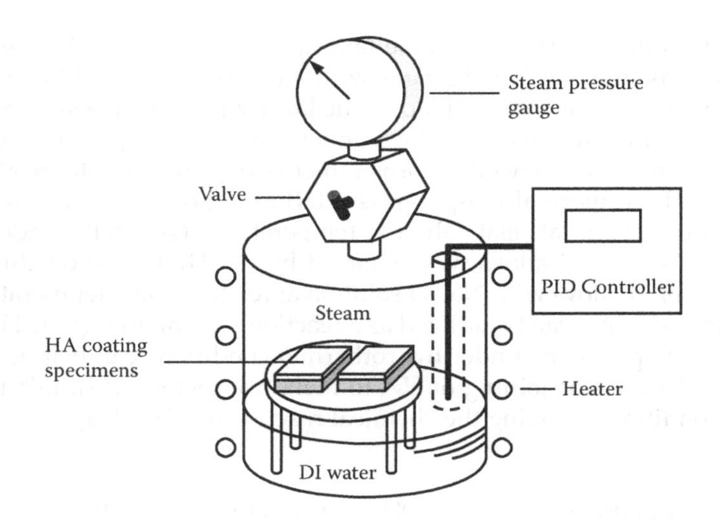

FIGURE 6.13
Schematic apparatus of HA-coated specimens within autoclave (Parr 4621) for hydrothermal treatment.

70%–85%) compared with the 600°C to 800°C heat treatments in the air or in vacuum (the IOC is about 71–80%, calculated from Figure 6.7) [120]. Since the OH^- groups can promote the reconstitution of ACP into crystalline HA [172], therefore the saturated steam-pressure atmosphere of the hydrothermal treatment can significantly improve HA crystallization and effectively eliminate ACP through the replenishment of OH^- groups.

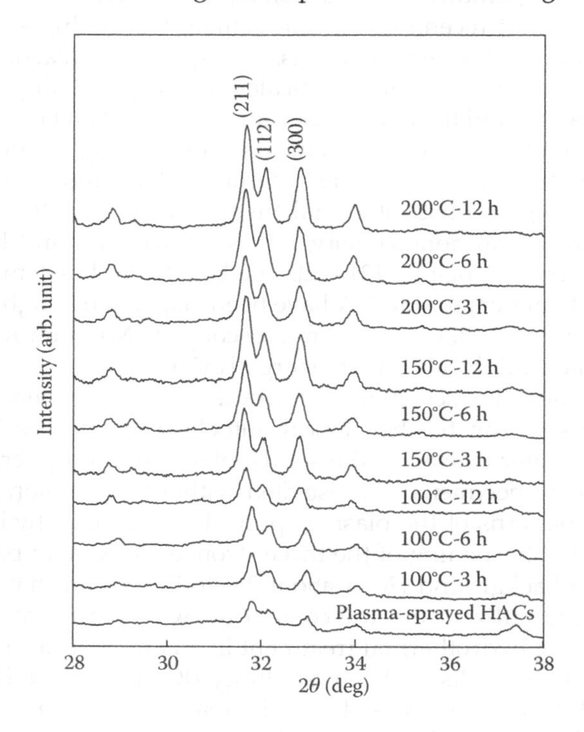

FIGURE 6.14
X-ray diffraction patterns of various hydrothermally treated HACs (HT-HACs).

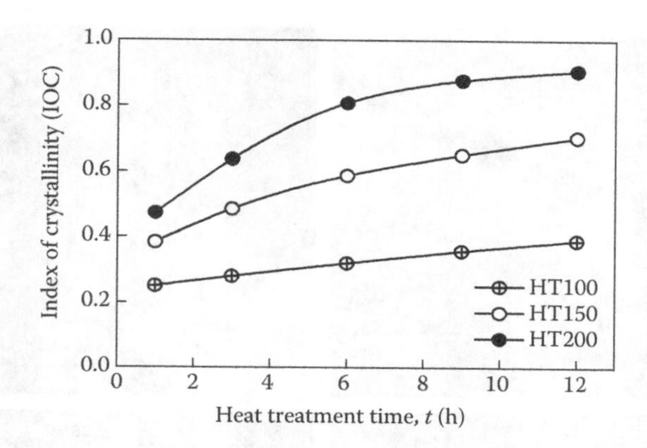

FIGURE 6.15
Index of crystallinity (IOC) for various HT-HACs.

Figure 6.16 shows typical microstructural morphologies with significant crystallization features of the HT-HACs. It provides evidence of the differences in microscopic surface features under various hydrothermal conditions, as illustrated in Figure 6.16a to e. It is worth noting that new crystalline growth, indicated by arrows in Figure 6.16a, is observed in the vicinity of the cracks and on the surface of the HT100–12h specimen. These new-growth grains can be attributed to crystalline HA, which crystallized from the hydroxyl-deficient structure of plasma-sprayed HACs through the replenishment of OH^- groups. With increasing heating temperatures and heating time of the hydrothermal treatment, the crystalline HA experiences further grain growth with a larger crystal size and a significant reduction in microcracks. Figure 6.16f shows the cross-sectional feature of the HT150–6h specimen. It can be seen that the contact between lamellar boundaries are significantly healed by the nanoscale HA crystallite after hydrothermal treatment. The microstructural homogeneity with a reduction of these defects in the HT-HACs can be recognized as the self-healing effect of the hydrothermal crystallization under an abundant saturated steam environment during hydrothermal treatment.

TEM images and select-area diffraction (SAD) patterns also reveal the crystalline microstructure of hydrothermally crystallized HA grains for different HA crystallinity. Figure 6.17a shows the TEM bright field image and the SAD patterns of the HT150 condition with partial hydrothermally crystallized grains and the ACP region within coatings. The crystalline grain can be recognized as HA crystals with a Ca/P ratio of about 1.61, and the ACP region displays a Ca/P ratio of about 1.45. It can be seen that if H_2O molecules compensated for the OH^- loss by replenishing the hydroxyl-deficient structure directly, the HACs have a Ca/P ratio of 1.67 and become pure HA [173]. Since crystalline HA can nucleate and grow from the ACP region [174], it is suggested that the crystallization of HA grains from the amorphous region is responsible for the formation of these nanocrystalline grains. Larger HA grains are observed after 200°C hydrothermal treatment (HT200), as shown in Figure 6.17b, which represents the TEM bright field image of HA polycrystals. The TEM/EDS analysis result represents an average Ca/P atomic ratio of about 1.66, which is close to the theoretical value of stoichiometric HA crystal structure.

The band observation of PO_4^{3-} and OH^- detected by the Fourier transform infrared spectrometer (FT-IR) [101,175] can provide the information concerning structural features such as the hydroxylation of HACs. In addition, the XPS analysis can further clarify the replenishment of OH^- groups and the reduction of the dehydroxylation state of hydroxyl-deficient

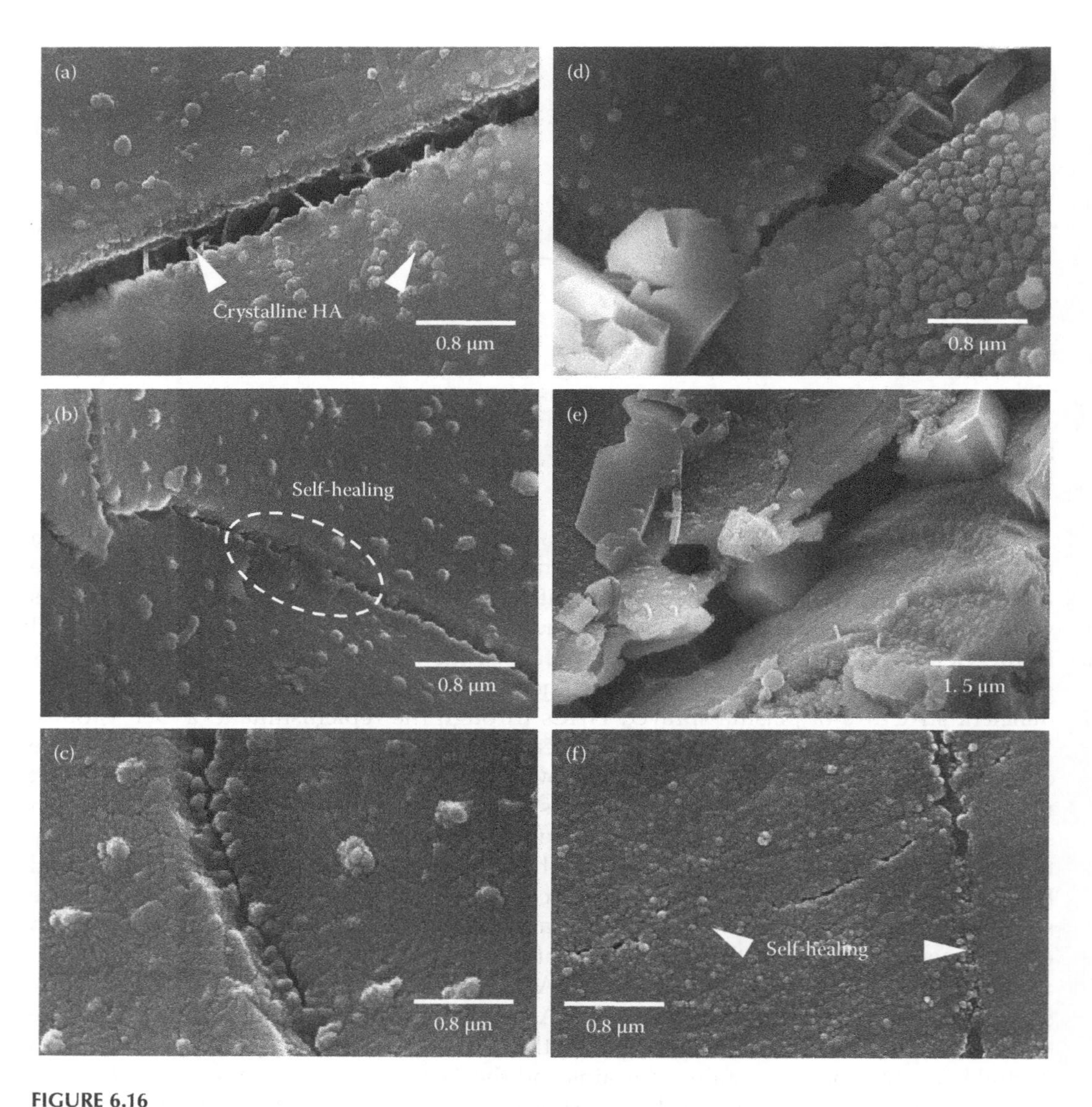

FIGURE 6.16
Surface morphologies of (a) HT100–12h, (b) HT150–6h, (c) HT150–12h, (d) HT200–6h, and (e) HT200–12h specimens. Arrows indicate HA nanocrystallite crystallized through hydrothermal crystallization. (f) A significant microstructural self-healing effect on lamellar boundaries and microcracks within HT150–6h specimen.

HACs during the hydrothermal treatment. Figure 6.18 shows the high-resolution XPS O 1*s* spectra of HT-HACs with curve fittings. The binding energy (BE) of these fit-peaks results from the Gaussian peak-fitting routine. The O 1*s* spectra presented in Figure 6.18a and b consists of two components at about BE = 531.4 and 533.4 eV, which correspond to the PO (PO_4^{3-}) and POH bonds of HA crystal [176–178]. The relatively large integration area of the POH bonding peak at HT-HACs specimens with high degree of crystallinity, as shown in Figure 6.18b, can be recognized that the hydroxyl-deficient microstructure of plasma-sprayed HACs is significantly improved with the abundant replenished OH^- groups by hydrothermal treatment. Beside the improved POH bond, previous reports indicated that the HT-HACs specimen may exhibit a substantial amount of surface adsorbed

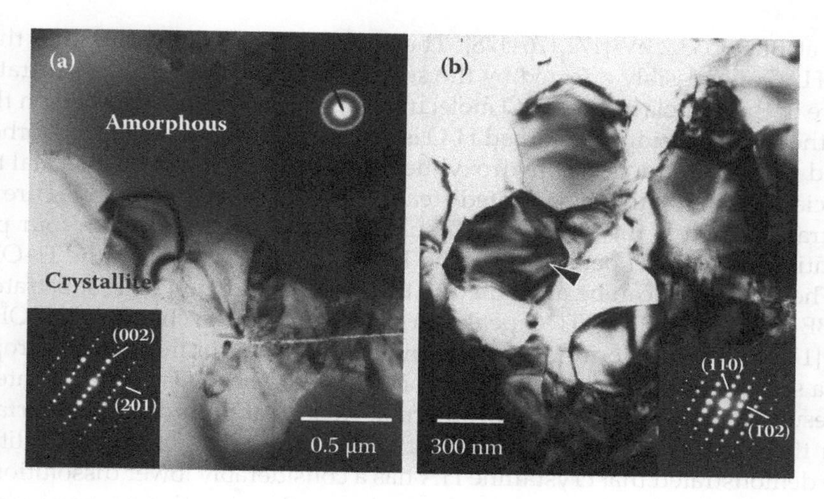

FIGURE 6.17
TEM images of hydrothermally crystallized HACs: (a) HT150 and (b) HT200.

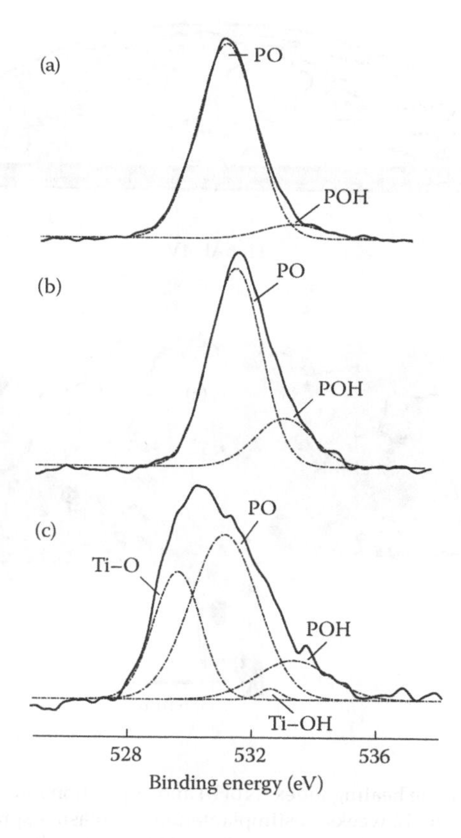

FIGURE 6.18
XPS O 1*s* spectra curve-fitting results of (a) plasma-sprayed HACs, (b) HT-HACs, and (c) surface close to HT-HACs/Ti substrate interface.

H_2O peak at BE = 533.2 eV [171,176–178]. The adsorbed H_2O represents that the surface of the HT-HACs is possibly affected by the surrounding moisture in the saturated steam atmosphere in the autoclave, and H_2O molecules can be physically adsorbed on the HACs. However, the surface residual adsorbed H_2O is absent because the surface adsorbed H_2O is diminished with the reduction of hydroxyl-deficient state during hydrothermal treatment [171], especially under a higher saturated steam-pressure atmosphere. In Figure 6.18c, the O 1s spectra obtained at the HT-HACs/Ti substrate interface are fit with four peaks: the above-mentioned PO, POH peaks of HA, the Ti–O peak at 529.6 eV, and the Ti–OH peak at 532.5 eV. The Ti–O peak can be attributed to the surface oxide ion of Ti substrate, and the peak at ΔBE about 3.0 eV from Ti–O peak can be assigned to the chemisorbed OH^- groups of Ti–OH [177–179]. Considering that the rapid solidification of molten HA droplets during plasma spraying induces the formation of ACP at the HAC/Ti substrate interface, the analysis results represent that the hydrothermal treatment promotes the interfacial crystallization through the chemical bonding of OH^- groups. The biocompatibility tests in vitro have demonstrated that crystalline HA has a considerably lower dissolution rate and the presence of Ti–OH bonding can further enhance the bioactive properties of the HA coating by promoting the osteointegration process [178,180].

In addition, Yang et al. indicated that the hydrothermally crystallized HACs also show better in vivo biological responses through examinations with the Chinese coin implant

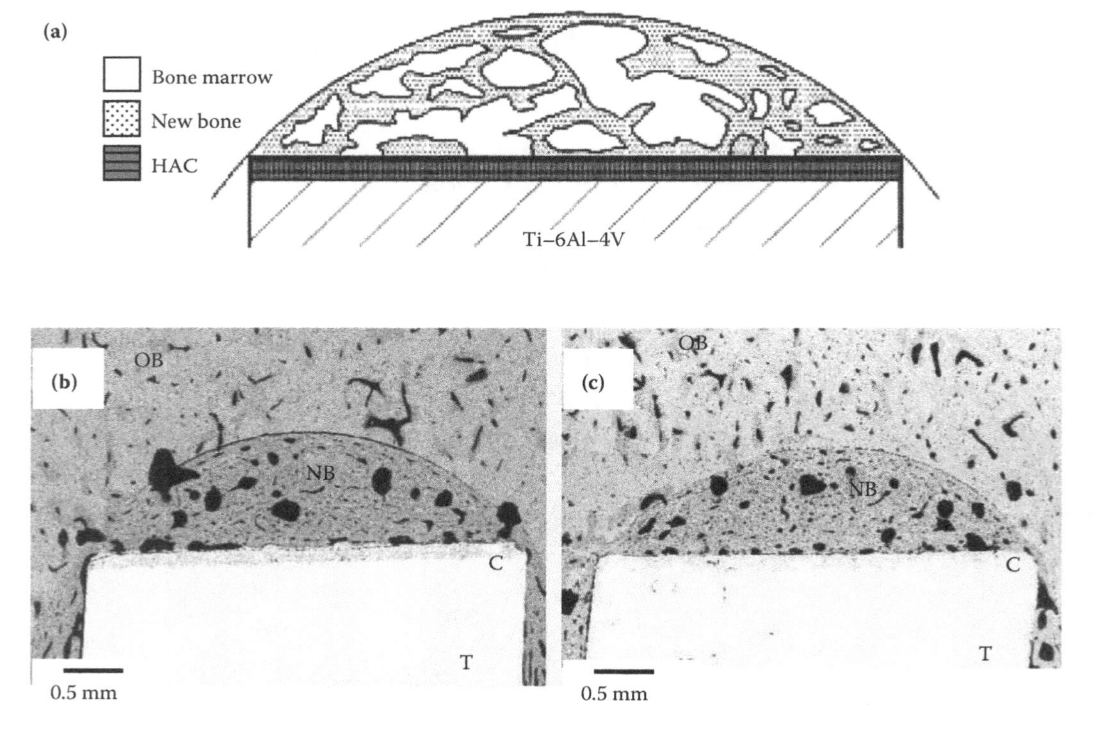

FIGURE 6.19
(a) Schematic illustration of new bone healing index (NBHI) and apposition index (AI). SEM/BEI of histological section at surgical defect region for 12 weeks postimplantation: (b) plasma-sprayed HACs and (c) HT-HACs. New bone is repaired within surgical defect regions of two HACs. Osseointegration is found at both bone/plasma-sprayed HACs and bone/HT-HACs interfaces. T, Ti–6Al–4V; C, coating; NB, new bone; OB, old bone. (From Yang et al., *J. Biomed. Mater. Res.*, 83A, 263–271, 2007. With permission.)

TABLE 6.4
NBHI and AI Values for Plasma-Sprayed HACs and HT-HACs after 12 Weeks of Implantation

	Plasma-Sprayed HACs[a]	HT-HACs[a]
NBHI (%)	75.7 ± 7.7	79.0 ± 7.5
AI (%)	68.7 ± 7.6	78.1 ± 6.4

Note: NBHI, new bone healing index; AI, apposition index.
[a] Values are given as an average ± standard deviation (SD).

model in the femoral of a goat [121]. Then the osteoconductivity of the implants is evaluated quantitatively in terms of the new bone healing index (NBHI), which is defined as the area of new bone/area of surgical defect region × 100%. The ability of osseointegration of implants is addressed as apposition index (AI), which is defined as the length of direct bone–implant contact/total length of bone–implant interface × 100%. The schematic illustrations of NBHI and AI are shown in Figure 6.19a. This method can help to determine the success or failure of an implant by evaluating the interaction occurring at the bone–biomaterial interface. Table 6.4 indicated that the HT-HACs have a statistically higher extent of new bone healing and apposition index compared to plasma-sprayed HACs after 12 weeks of implantation. The amount of new bone increased within the surgical defect regions of both coatings, as shown in Figure 6.19b and c. However, some particles dissociated from the plasma-sprayed HACs are observed at the implant–bone interface, as shown in Figure 6.20. This can be attributed to the higher content of ACP and impurity phases, and the dissolution induced the granular particles dissociated from the HACs. This result suggests that the HT-HACs can provide the firm bone/implant fixation compared to plasma-sprayed HACs. The advantage of the hydrothermal treatment performed within an abundant steam-pressure atmosphere compared with other high-temperature heating processes is that it can simultaneously acquire high crystallinity with a self-healing effect, high phase purity, and better biological responses without serious microstructural deterioration of coatings.

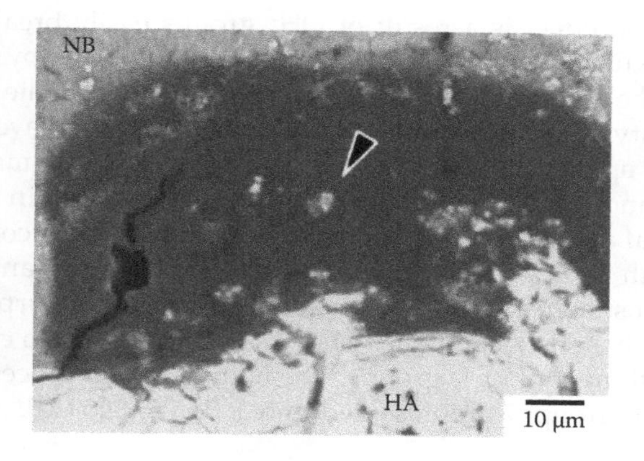

FIGURE 6.20
Histological observation at bone/plasma-sprayed HACs interface after 12 weeks implantation. Dissociated particles (indicated by arrow) from HACs are observed within remodeling canal. NB, new bone. (From Yang et al., *J. Biomed. Mater. Res.*, 83A, 263–271, 2007. With permission.)

Kinetics of Hydrothermal Crystallization under a Saturated Steam Pressure

Through XRD, XPS analysis results, and microscopical observations presented in the previous section, significant microstructural homogeneity and regeneration are achieved via autoclaving hydrothermal treatments. This is a result of the replenishment of missing OH^- groups with surrounding H_2O molecules [59,63,181]. It also demonstrates that hydrothermal treatment can actually promote significant crystallization to improve the phase purity and better crystallinity of low-crystalline plasma-sprayed HACs only at relatively lower temperatures.

Referring to the crystallization mechanism reported before, these studies have indicated that the kinetics of crystallization and chemical reactions during heat treatments are significantly related to heating temperatures, which is recognized as a main factor for promoting HA crystallization [120,167–169]. In addition, a higher crystallization rate and lower activation energy of crystallization are demonstrated for the postheat treatment in an ambient atmosphere with a partial water vapor pressure than in a vacuum environment [120]. Chen et al. [59] also reported that the crystallization of plasma-sprayed HACs can be achieved by performing postheat treatments in the nitrogen (N_2) or oxygen (O_2) atmosphere. The increase of crystallinity and the reduction of impurity phases (TCP and TP) for heat-treated HACs within these controlled atmospheres are better than that of in vacuum. There was no obvious difference in crystallinity between the HA coatings heated in dry N_2 and dry O_2. However, HACs heat-treated in humid N_2 (or humid O_2) atmosphere showed a higher degree of crystallinity than those only heat-treated in a dry atmosphere [59]. It can be seen that incorporation of water vapor can significantly promote the crystallization of HA whereas the intrinsic properties of dry atmosphere, such as N_2 and O_2, have less effect on the crystallization. Therefore, the ambient heating atmosphere with water molecules is thought to be another significant factor that should be considered to affect the reaction rate and the activation energy for the crystallization of HA [120,181]. The influence of saturated steam pressure is more notable while the reactions occurred in a hermetical atmosphere of autoclaving hydrothermal treatment. However, some previous studies did not show the steam pressure factor for the kinetics of hydrothermal HA crystallization [170,172]. Thus, this is discussed in detail with the following experimental results and the derivation to clarify the effect of saturated steam pressure on the hydrothermal crystallization kinetics.

The dehydroxylation effect is a result of OH^- groups easily breaking away from the HA crystal structure under the high temperature and high enthalpy of the plasma spraying process, while the formation of amorphous calcium phosphate with a significantly decreased crystallinity of HA occurred in the as-sprayed coating layers. When the hydrothermal treatment is applied to promote the crystallization of plasma-sprayed HACs, the water is vaporized and the ionized water vapor molecules contain H^+ and OH^- groups within the hermetical autoclave as displayed in reaction 6.17. The content of H^+ and OH^- groups increases with increasing the temperature [136]. The resultant OH^- groups within the water vapor atmosphere would be expected to react with amorphous and other low-crystalline calcium phosphate components, and convert them into crystalline HA phase through the replenishment of OH^- groups. The hydroxylation process proceeds with the replenishment of OH^- groups as represented in reaction 6.18 [59,71].

$$H_2O \rightarrow H^+ + OH^- \tag{6.17}$$

$$Ca_{10}(PO_4)_6(OH)_{2-2x}O_x{\cdot}V_x + xH_2O \rightarrow Ca_{10}(PO_4)_6(OH)_2 \tag{6.18}$$

Considering the theory of chemical reaction kinetics, the HA crystallization should follow the Arrhenius equation [167,170,182] as represented in Equation 6.19:

$$r = \frac{dx}{dt} = k(1-x)^n \tag{6.19}$$

where x represents the conversion ratio of HA from amorphous calcium phosphate to crystalline HA. This can be recognized as the IOC value for the various degrees of crystallization of the HT-HACs displayed in Figure 6.15. The symbol r is the crystallization rate and k is the rate constant. The rate constant (k) represents the reaction rate for the kinetics of Arrhenius equation, and it can be recognized as the crystallization rate during heat treatments. Next, the crystallization rate as well as the activation energy of hydrothermal crystallization can be quantitatively evaluated by the IOC data. Equation 6.20 is obtained from the natural logarithmic (ln) of 6.19, and it should be noted that the conversion ratio (i.e., the IOC) determines the overall crystallization kinetics.

$$\ln\frac{dIOC}{dt} = n\ln(1-IOC) + \ln k \tag{6.20}$$

According to the derivation in a previous study [120], the reaction order n, which is calculated from the slope by the least squares fitting method of Equation 6.20 at a maximum coefficient of determination (R^2), is approximated from 1.8 to 2.1 for the atmospheric and vacuum crystallization treatments of plasma-sprayed HACs at 500°C to 800°C. Since the total reaction order should be an integer, it can be deduced that HA crystallization should follow the second-order reaction kinetics of the Arrhenius equation, and Equation 6.19 can be converted into Equation 6.21. Table 6.5 lists the rate constant k, which can be calculated from the slope of the linear plots of $(1 - IOC)^{-1}$ versus heat-treatment time (t) from the integration of Equation 6.21 for the atmospheric and vacuum crystallization treatments. Based on the reaction kinetics of Arrhenius equation, the rate constant (k) can be thought as the reaction rate, and it represents the crystallization rate during heat treatments. Except for considering the oxidation problem of Ti–6Al–4V during high-temperature heating, the experimental results, as shown in Table 6.5, demonstrate that heat treatments in an ambient

TABLE 6.5

Results of Crystallization Kinetics of Various Heat-Treated HACs

	Rate Constant, k $k = A\exp(-E_a/RT)$			
	k_{500}	k_{600}	k_{800}	**Activation Energy, E_a (kJ/mol)[a]**
Vacuum heating[b]	0.197	0.365	0.586	24.6
Atmospheric heating[b]	0.272	0.379	0.612	19.1
	k_{100}	k_{150}	k_{200}	
Hydrothermal treatment	0.294	0.591	0.905	16.6

Source: Yang C.W. and Lui, T.S., *Mater. Trans.*, 48(2), 211–218, 120. 2007. With permission.

[a] Data calculated from the slope of ln$k$ vs. heating temperatures ($1/T$) graph.

[b] The parameters k_{500}, k_{600}, and k_{800} represent the crystallization rate constant for 500°C, 600°C, and 800°C heat treatments in the air and in vacuum, respectively.

atmosphere with water vapor or a partial steam pressure can be recognized as a better way than in vacuum under the same heating conditions [59,101,120,172].

$$r = \frac{\mathrm{dIOC}}{\mathrm{d}t} = k(1 - \mathrm{IOC})^2 \tag{6.21}$$

With regard to the hydrothermally crystallized conditions, Figure 6.21a shows the natural logarithmic plots for the relationship of ln(dIOC/dt) versus ln(1 − IOC) using the data represented in Figure 6.15. The reaction order, n value, is 1.57, 1.56, and 1.53 for the hydrothermal crystallization at 100°C, 150°C, and 200°C, respectively. On the basis of previous reports [167,170,182] and the above-mentioned results, HA crystallization should be a second-order reaction kinetics, which depends on the effects of heat-treatment time and temperatures. However, the saturated steam pressures (P_{H_2O}) in the hermetical atmosphere of the autoclaving hydrothermal treatment are 0.10 MPa (100°C), 0.48 MPa (150°C), and 1.56 MPa (200°C). Referring to the phase diagram of the CaO–P_2O_5–H_2O system as shown in Figure 6.2b [70], HA is a stable phase under an atmosphere with 500 mmHg steam pressure, and the phase stability of HA is increased with increasing steam pressure. The effect of P_{H_2O} should also be considered as another significant factor affecting the HA crystallization within a steam pressure environment.

Therefore, Equation 6.22 shows the modified form that involves a saturated steam-pressure term following the second-order reaction kinetics of Arrhenius equation. Figure 6.21b shows the $1/(1 - \mathrm{IOC})^{1/2}$ versus heat-treatment time (t, hours) plot resulting from the integration of Equation 6.12; here, P_{H_2O} can be thought of as a constant at each hydrothermal heating temperature. Since the above-mentioned saturated steam-pressure term (P_{H_2O}) is independent of time (t), the slope by the least squares fitting results in Figure 6.21b is deduced in a form of $(kP_{H_2O}^{1/2})/2$ and the hydrothermal crystallization rate constant (k) for 100°C, 150°C, and 200°C hydrothermal crystallization is obtained. According to Equation 3.13, the activation energy (E_a) for the hydrothermal crystallization of HA can be quantitatively evaluated from the Arrhenius plot of ln$k$ versus $1/T$ (heating temperatures), as shown in Figure 6.22 (where T is the heating temperature in Kelvin, R is the gas constant,

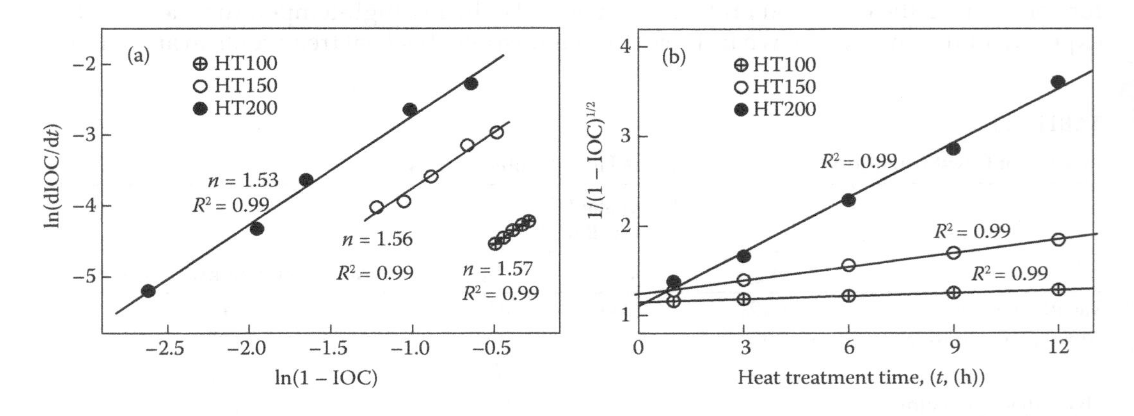

FIGURE 6.21
(a) Plots of ln(dIOC/dt) vs. ln(1 − IOC) from natural logarithm of Equation 6.19 for hydrothermal treatment, and (b) plots of $(1 - \mathrm{IOC})^{-1/2}$ vs. heat-treatment time (t, hours) from integration of Equation 6.22 for hydrothermal crystallization.

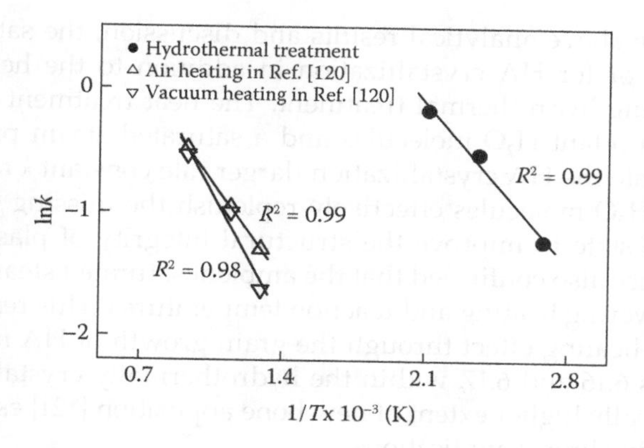

FIGURE 6.22
Arrhenius relationship plots for hydrothermal treatment in this study, and air and vacuum heat treatments according to previous analysis results [120]. Slope of plot is equal to $-E_a/R$ (where R is gas constant, 8.314 J K^{-1} mol^{-1}).

8.314 J K^{-1} mol^{-1}, and A is the Arrhenius constant). The above-calculated results are summarized in Table 6.5.

$$r = \frac{\mathrm{dIOC}}{\mathrm{d}t} = k(1 - \mathrm{IOC})^{3/2} P_{\mathrm{H_2O}}^{1/2} \tag{6.22}$$

$$k = A \exp\left(\frac{-E_a}{RT}\right) \tag{6.23}$$

Additional experiments show that the rate constant for 100°C atmospheric heat treatment (k_{100}') is about 0.011. Comparing the rate constant k_{100}' (0.011) with k_{500}, k_{600}, and k_{800} values of the atmospheric heating condition listed in Table 6.5, the heating temperature can be recognized as a factor that promotes the HA crystallization rate of the atmospheric heat treatment. Also, comparing the rate constant k_{100}' (0.011) with k_{100} (0.294), the significantly increased crystallization rate constant for 100°C hydrothermal treatment results from the effect of saturated steam pressure within the autoclave. The crystallization rate constant increased with increasing the saturated steam pressure, and the k_{200} value is larger than any other rate constant for the air heat treatment. Generally, the crystallization of hydroxyl-deficient HA requires at least 600°C in a vacuum or in the air [61,116,120,167]. However, high-temperature crystallization tends to undermine the structural integrity and cause phase decomposition of crystalline HA phase, microstructural deterioration, and degradation of mechanical properties of coating layers [64,120]. Through the analysis of Arrhenius kinetics, the hydrothermal crystallization of HA under an atmosphere of saturated steam pressure occurs only at lower temperatures with a significantly larger crystallization rate constant and lower activation energy than other heat treatments. This new reaction rate information, as displayed in Table 6.5, confirms that the ambient saturated steam pressure plays an important role in lowering crystallization temperatures.

On the basis of the above analytical results and discussion, the saturated steam pressure is a crucial factor for HA crystallization in addition to the heating temperatures during the autoclaving hydrothermal treatment. The heat treatment in a high moisture atmosphere with abundant H_2O molecules and a saturated steam pressure can further promote and accelerate the HA crystallization (larger rate constant k and lower activation energy E_a) because H_2O molecules effectively replenish the missing OH^- groups within the dehydroxylation state to improve the structural integrity of plasma-sprayed HACs. Experimental evidence also confirmed that the ambient saturated steam pressure plays an important role in lowering heating and reaction temperatures. This results in a significant microstructural self-healing effect through the grain growth of HA nanocrystallite [171], as shown in Figures 6.16 and 6.17, within the hydrothermally crystallized HACs, which also shows a statistically higher extent of new bone apposition [121] essential in the initial fixation of implants in clinical applications.

Crystallization Effect on Mechanical Properties of Plasma-Sprayed HACs

Since the use of plasma-sprayed HA-coated implants for biomedical applications is strongly influenced by the long-term stability of the coating system, the coating/substrate adhesion, which can be represented as the interfacial bonding strength, and interlamellar cohesion are of great concern. The adhesion of plasma-sprayed coatings is not only an interfacial problem of each lamella within coatings, but involves the microstructural integrity, crystallinity, residual stresses, crack propagation, defects content, and defects distribution of coatings. Therefore, the evaluation of the interfacial bonding strength between coatings and substrates is quite important to nearly all branches of the surface engineering.

According to the definition of the American Society for Testing and Materials (ASTM), adhesion is the state in which two surfaces are held together by interfacial forces that may consist of valence forces or interlocking forces or both (ASTM D907-70). To determine the adhesive bonding strength of plasma-sprayed HACs, scratch testing [183–189], in which a sharp needle under a given weight necessary to reach the underlying metallic surface is an indication of the comparative bonding strength. Push-out tests have been used to measure the ability of the implant to resist forces tending to shear the bonding between the implant surfaces and surrounding bone [190–196]. Among these methods, the most commonly used method of determining tensile strength involves the coating of a metallic disk followed by testing utilizing a variation of ASTM C633. To test the adhesive bonding strength of HA coatings to an implant such as titanium alloy, the surface of the cylindrical substrate fixtures is first prepared as the actual surface on an implant using all cleaning and grit-blasting steps. After plasma-spraying HA coatings on substrates, the loading fixtures are also grit-blasted and bonded to the surface of the HA coatings using a heat-cured adhesive glue. Then the assemblies are subjected to tensile tests after curing. It is noted that the roughness of the substrate is important in achieving high bonding strength of plasma-sprayed HACs. The bonding of the plasma-sprayed HACs to metallic substrates appears to be mostly mechanical in nature, as there is a lower degree of chemical bonding in the as-deposited coatings. In addition, the crystallization of plasma-sprayed HACs with performing postheat treatments can also help to improve the bonding strength and the effect of crystallization on bonding strength, wear resistance, and failure properties will be presented in the following sections.

Effect of Hydrothermal Crystallization on the Bonding Strength of HACs

In clinical application, a plasma-sprayed HACs failure by chipping, spalling, delamination, and dissolution is being observed on explanted endoprostheses usually close to the implant/coating interface [47,196,198]. This can be attributed to the existence of a layer of ACP formed during rapid quenching of molten or semimolten droplets of calcium phosphate with exceptionally high cooling rates at the coating/Ti interface. The ACP layer is thought to act as a fracture path [199] and owing to its comparatively high solubility will be preferentially dissolved in vitro and in vivo [76,200,201], thus further weakening the mechanical integrity of the interface [98,202]. Therefore, it is one of the challenges of coating design to reduce the ACP content and improve the adhesion of the coating to substrate by optimizing spraying parameters, modifying the precursor HA powder, or adding an intermediate coating layer [40,203–208]. In addition, applying postheat treatments for promoting the crystallization of interfacial ACP is another effective method to improve the interfacial adhesive bonding strength of plasma-sprayed HACs.

The bonding strength of the plasma-sprayed and different heat-treated HACs measured by the tensile adhesion test according to ASTM C633 is shown in Figure 6.23. For both the vacuum and atmospheric heat treatments, the bonding strength tends to increase with increasing the heating temperature up to 600°C, whereas the bonding strength markedly decreases with further increasing the heating temperature up to 800°C. For the hydrothermal treatment, the bonding strength is also significantly improved with the hydrothermal crystallization of HA, and 150°C hydrothermally treated HACs has a higher bonding strength (about 38.9 MPa for HT150) than both of the optimal conditions (at 600°C) for atmospheric and vacuum heat-treated HACs (about 37.1 MPa for AH600, and about 36.0 MPa for VH600, respectively). Considering the cross-sectional features of the HACs also shown in Figure 6.23, both the 600°C vacuum and atmospheric heat-treated specimens

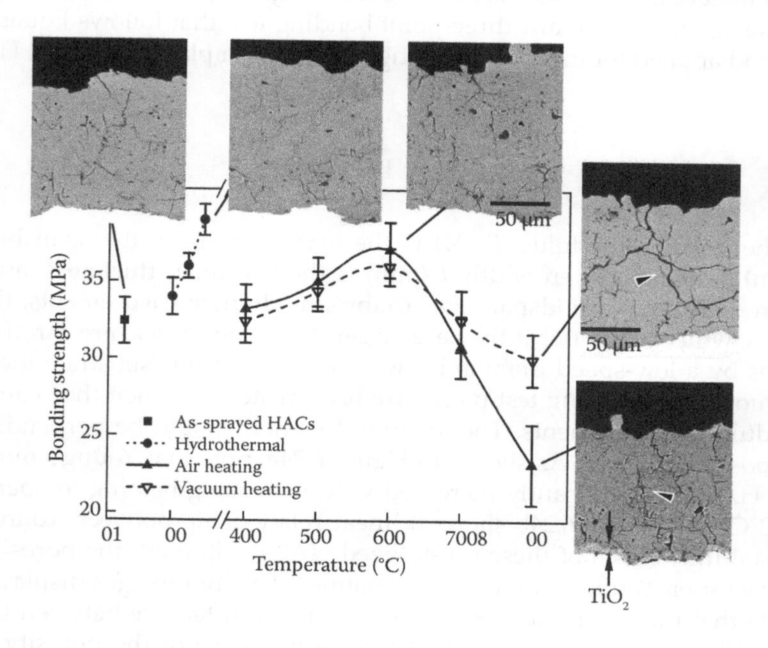

FIGURE 6.23
Variation of bonding strength correlated with microstructural features after hydrothermal treatment and atmospheric and vacuum heat treatments.

represent similar microstructures to the as-sprayed HACs, and 150°C hydrothermally treated HACs display the highest coating density of all the conditions. However, note that an obvious cracking feature (as indicated by arrows) and an interfacial TiO_2 layer can be recognized under both of the high-temperature heating processes and the formation of TiO_2 layer (characterized by XRD analysis, a rutile phase) significantly causes serious interfacial fracturing and coating debonding at elevated heating temperatures [120,209]. In addition, the deterioration of bonding strength for heat-treated HACs in vacuum and in the air should also depend on the above-mentioned detrimental crystallization-induced contraction, CTE mismatch between the coating and substrate [64,120,210] in Section 6.2.3, and the variation of residual stresses [100,210] during high-temperature heat treatments, especially in the temperature range of 600°C to 800°C. The relationship between the heating temperature and the bonding strength is found to be related to the crystallization behavior, and the affecting factors will be clarified in the following paragraphs.

According to the criterion of ASTM C633, the variation of bonding strength in situ is suggested to be governed by the cohesive strength of coatings and the adhesive strength of a coating to a metal substrate. The affecting factors of the adhesive strength of a coating and substrate interface include the surface roughness of substrate and the residual stress. As for the cohesive strength of coating, the factors include the crystallinity (IOC) and the densification of a coating that appears on Young's modulus of a coating. Since Young's modulus is a measure of the interatomic binding forces, the evolution of Young's modulus for the HACs depends on the extent of crystallization. In addition, the microstructural features such as defects, lamellar structure, and the contact between splats boundaries should also be considered as other affecting factors on Young's modulus of a coating [211,212]. Through Young's modulus measurements, it can help to clarify the effect of crystallization on the bonding strength and the failure mechanism. Several methods can measure Young's modulus of a material, including the bending test, single-edge notch test, compact tension test, and so forth, and a standard three-point bending test that follows Equation 6.24 is a suitable method applied for measuring Young's modulus of plasma-sprayed HACs [213].

$$E = \frac{PL^3}{4wt^3\delta} \tag{6.24}$$

E (GPa) is the Young's modulus, P (N) is the load, L (mm) is the span between supports, w (mm) is the specimen width, t (mm) is the specimen thickness, and δ (mm) is the specimen deflection at midspan. For Young's modulus measurements, the HA coating test pieces, which are better if they are larger than 1 mm thick, are carefully cut from the substrates by a low-speed diamond saw along the coating/substrate interface. Then substrate-removed HA coating test pieces are heat-treated and then they can be used for Young's modulus measurements. The loading direction should be perpendicular to the spraying deposition surface. As shown in Figure 6.24a, note that Young's modulus of the heat-treated HACs is significantly increased with increasing heating temperatures from 400°C to 800°C, and Figure 6.24b shows a linear relationship between Young's modulus and the crystallinity (IOC) of these crystallized HACs. Although the porosity is also an influencing factor on Young's modulus of a coating, SEM/BEI images displayed in Figure 6.24b indicate that there is no obvious microstructural difference between the HAC test pieces with different crystallinity. Except for the influence of the porosity and defects (such as pores and microcracks) distribution, therefore, it is reasonable to suggest that the crystallinity is a main controlling factor in increasing Young's modulus of crystallized

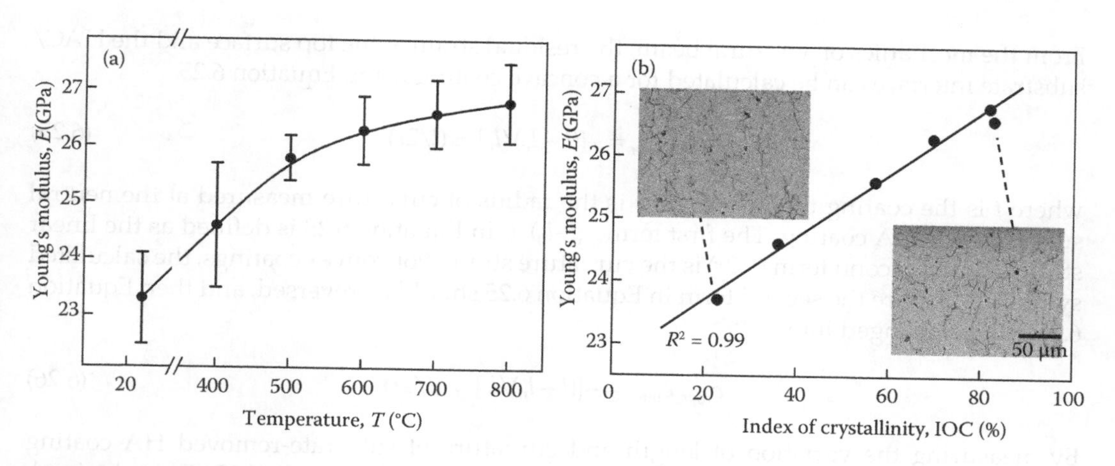

FIGURE 6.24
(a) Variation of Young's modulus as a function of heating temperatures. (b) A linear correlation between Young's modulus and crystallinity (IOC) of HACs. Images show microstructural features of Young's modulus test pieces with various IOC. (From Yang et al., *Mater. Sci. Eng.C*, 26, 1395–1400, 2006. With permission.)

HACs herein. According to the Griffith–Orowan–Irwin theory, the fracture toughness of a ceramic is correlated with the ability of impeding crack propagation (γ) and Young's modulus (E) from the relationship: $K_{IC} = \sqrt{2\gamma E}$ [214]. The relative investigations indicated that the improvement of fracture toughness can be approached to about 5% to 20% with the increase in Young's modulus for the crystallization of HACs with performing heat treatments [99,113,215]. In addition, the crystallization can also help to enhance the cohesion between splats boundaries within the coatings [211,212,215]. Therefore, the enhanced bonding strength of the heat-treated HACs can be pinpointed from the improvement of Young's modulus and fracture toughness resulting from the crystallization effect of HA coatings. Although the bonding strength is improved with the crystallization of HACs during vacuum and atmospheric heat treatments, note that detrimental effects accompanied with HA crystallization may result in the deterioration of bonding strength, as shown in Figure 6.23. These deterioration effects are the crystallization-induced contraction, CTE mismatch, interfacial oxide layers, and residual compressive stresses. Referring to the dilatation data of thermal dilatometry at 600°C to 800°C (from Figure 6.11 and Table 6.1), the enlarged cracks, as shown in Figure 6.12, induced from the crystallized-induced contraction (from 0.28% to 0.65%) of heat-treated HACs result in the deterioration of microstructural integrity as well as the bonding strength. In addition, the crystallization-induced coating contraction during high-temperature heat treatments will also significantly change the coating/substrate interfacial residual stress states.

The residual stress of plasma-sprayed HA coatings can be measured using various methods such as the $\sigma = E\varepsilon$ and $\sin^2\Psi$ methods from XRD, Raman, analytical model, and the specimen curvature method [197,202,210,216–219]. As described in the previous sections, the substrate-removed HA coating layers not only can be used for the measurements of thermal dilatations and Young's modulus, but also can be applied for measuring residual stress states through the specimen curvature method [210,220]. For measuring the residual stress, a 180 ± 20 μm thick HA coating is deposited on the substrate. After performing heat treatments, the gauge length (l) of these heat-treated HA coatings, which are separated from the substrates following the procedure detail described in [220], are measured. The curvatures of the substrate-removed HA coating strips are determined from side-view photographs.

From the mechanics of a flexural beam, the residual strain at the top surface and the HAC/substrate interface can be calculated for a concave coating using Equation 6.25:

$$\varepsilon_{top}, \varepsilon_{inter} = -[(l - l_0)/l_0] \pm (t/2r) \quad (6.25)$$

where t is the coating thickness and r is the radius of curvature measured at the neutral surface of the HA coating. The first term $-(l-l_0)/l_0$ in Equation 6.25 is defined as the linear strain and the second term $(t/2r)$ is the curvature strain. For convex coatings, the calculated symbol "±" before the second term in Equation 6.25 should be reversed, and then Equation 6.25 will be changed into:

$$\varepsilon_{top}, \varepsilon_{inter} = -[(l - l_0)/l_0] \mp (t/2r) \quad (6.26)$$

By measuring the variation of length and curvature of substrate-removed HA coating layers, the residual strain (ε) of the 400°C to 900°C vacuum heat-treated HACs is obtained, and the results are shown in Figure 6.25. The reason of performing vacuum heat treatments is to prevent the significant oxidation of metallic substrates, especially for the Ti alloy substrates. It can be seen that the plasma-sprayed HACs represents a compressive residual strain. When applying heat treatments, the crystallized-HACs displays tensile residual strains for heating temperatures performed at 400°C to 600°C. It is worth noting that the crystallized-HACs produced compressive residual strains again at heating temperatures higher than 600°C. Referring to the thermal dilatometry results represented in Figure 6.11 and Table 6.1, a significant crystallization-induced contraction is demonstrated after high-temperature heat treatments. As shown in Figure 6.24, Young's moduli of heat-treated HACs are advanced with increasing heating temperatures, and this is attributed to the crystallization effect of HACs. However, the comparison of Figures 6.23 and 6.24 showed the bonding strength of vacuum and atmospheric heat-treated HACs did not increase in accordance with increasing heating temperatures. They lowered with the temperatures after attaining the maximum value at 600°C. This results from the impact of the interfacial adhesive force between coating and substrate besides the cohesive strength of the coating layers. Figure 6.26 shows the mechanism of residual stress on the debonding of the coating [221,222]. Before debonding of a coating, interfacial and interlamellar splat cracks are assumed to exist at the coating/substrate interface, as shown in Figure 6.26a.

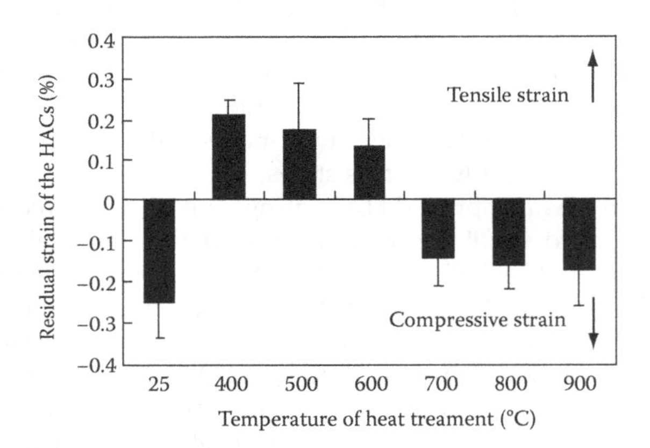

FIGURE 6.25
Measured residual strains of as-sprayed HACs and vacuum heat-treated HACs from 400°C to 900°C.

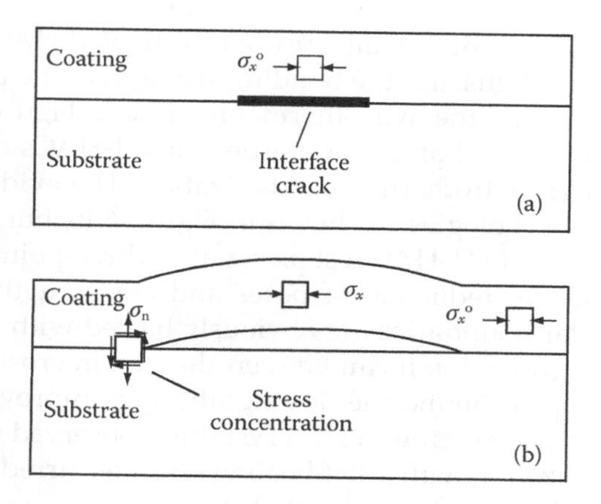

FIGURE 6.26
Effect of delamination on coating fracture driving force: (a) attached configuration and (b) delaminated configuration. σ_x^o and σ_x denote in-plane compressive stress in attached and delaminated coating, respectively. σ_n is induced through-thickness tensile stress.

The in-plane compressive residual stress, which resulted from the compressive residual strains as shown in Figure 6.25, would induce through-thickness tensile stress (the σ_n in Figure 6.26b) acting in the direction normal to the interface of the HA coating and the Ti substrate. The induced normal tensile stress will neutralize the bonding force of a coating on the substrate and weaken the interfacial adhesive bonding strength of the HA coating to substrate, especially for those HACs heat-treated under temperatures higher than 600°C. Thus, from the above demonstrations, it is difficult to simultaneously acquire high crystallinity without the microstructural deterioration and the degradation of adhesive bonding strength for plasma-sprayed HACs through the high-temperature vacuum and atmospheric heat treatments.

With regard to the hydrothermal treatment performed at relatively lower temperatures, Figure 6.27a shows a linear relationship between Young's modulus and the IOC values of

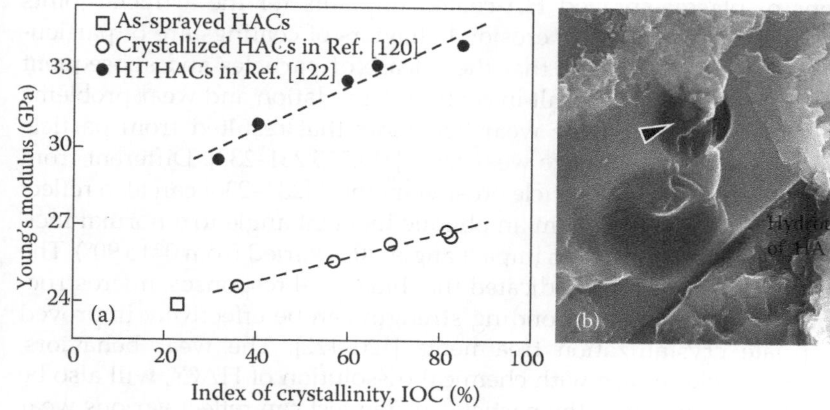

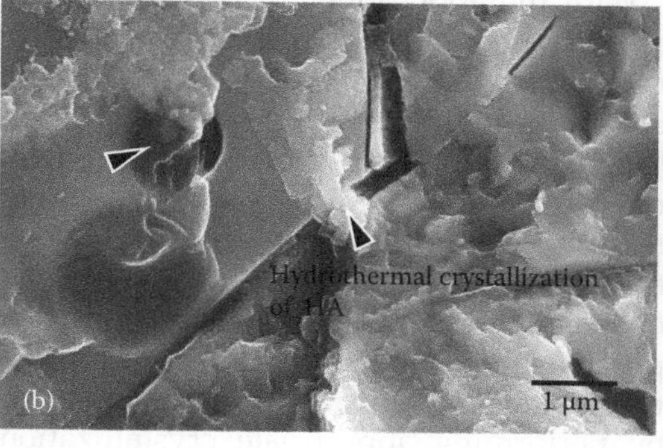

FIGURE 6.27
(a) A linear correlation between Young's modulus and crystallinity (IOC) of HACs. (b) Self-healing effect of hydrothermal crystallization (as indicated by arrows) on HT-HACs observed at coating fracture surface after three-point bending test.

HT-HACs compared with those high-temperature heat-treated HACs displayed in Figure 6.24. Since both Young's modulus and the bonding strength of the plasma-sprayed HACs are significantly improved after the hydrothermal treatment (Figure 6.23), it is worth noting that the improvement of mechanical properties for HT-HACs can be pinpointed due to the self-healing effect of hydrothermal crystallization. The evidences can not only be observed from surface morphologies as shown in Figure 6.16, but also be demonstrated from the fracture specimens of HT-HAC test pieces after three-point bending tests. Figure 6.27b represents a significant reduction of pores and cracks within the HT-HAC coatings, and the inter-lamellar boundaries are obviously healed with the nanocrystalline as indicated by arrows in Figure 6.16f. It can be seen that the microstructural homogeneity and the contact between splats boundaries are significantly improved after hydrothermal treatment. Thus, besides the new-growth HA crystallites observed on the coating surface, the hydrothermal crystallization with a self-healing effect occurred throughout the whole HA coating layers under the abundant saturated steam pressure environment. According to the above-mentioned results, it can be recognized that the overall bonding strength of plasma-sprayed HACs is effectively improved by the low-temperature hydrothermal treatment with increasing both the cohesive strength and the adhesive interfacial strength through the self-healing effect and the HAC/Ti substrate interfacial chemical bonding (Ti–OH), respectively.

Erosive Wear Behaviors

Plasma-sprayed ceramic coatings have been widely employed to provide an improved wear resistance to various industrial parts [50,223–225]. The erosion of ceramic coatings can be influenced by both coating properties and impacting particle conditions including its size and morphology, velocity, incident angle, and materials properties in a similar way to that of bulk materials. Considering the relationship between microstructural features and properties of thermal sprayed coatings, it can be recognized that the properties of thermal spraying coating will be significantly influenced by the lamellar structure inherent in the thermal spraying processes [226–229]. The difference of microstructural features of the coatings from the bulk materials makes their erosive wear behaviors in a different way.

With the applications of plasma-sprayed HA-coated implants for the artificial joints replacement, the abrasive wear and particle erosion behaviors of coatings are of particular interest. Clinical studies have indicated that the release of particles and subsequent inclusions in the surrounding bone will result in coating degradation and wear problems [49,230]. Some reports have focused on the wear behaviors that resulted from particle release of HACs by the fretting and abrasive wear tests [116,225,231–233]. Different from the fretting and abrasive wear tests, the particle erosion method [234–236] can also reflect the erosive wear behaviors of a material from an oblique incident angle to a normal incident angle through changing various erosion impact angles (θ is varied from 0° to 90°). The previously mentioned presentations have indicated that biological responses, microstructure homogeneity, Young's modulus, and bonding strength can be effectively improved by performing appropriate crystallization treatments [120–122]. The wear behaviors, which resulted from the particle release with chemical dissolution of HACs, will also be improved with HA crystallization. Since the particle erosion test can reflect various wear behaviors of ductile fracture and brittle fracture from changing the erosion impact angles, it will adequately simulate the wears of acetabular components in the human body.

The particle erosion test is generally conducted at room temperature using a sandblasting type erosion machine. The setup for the experiment is illustrated schematically in

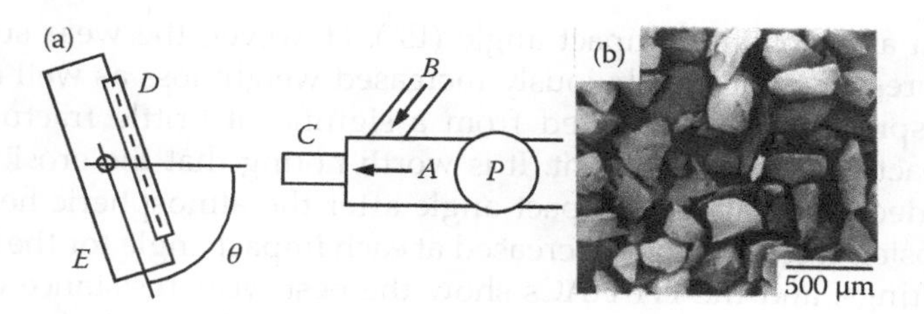

FIGURE 6.28
(a) Schematic apparatus of particle erosion test and (b) surface morphology of SiO_2 erodent. *A*, compressed air flow; *B*, erodent supplier; *C*, erodent nozzle with 6-mm inner diameter; *D*, specimen, 30 mm from the nozzle outlet; *E*, specimen holder; *θ*, impact angle; *P*, pressure gauge.

Figure 6.28a. Details of its function have been well described in the reports [234,235]. For the case of present experiments herein, the erosion test specimens are surface finished by grinding with 1200-grit SiC papers before conducting the particle erosion test. Angular SiO_2 grit with mean particle size of 295 ± 10 μm is selected as the erodent, as shown in Figure 6.28b. The pressure of compressed air flow is set at 0.3 MPa, and the average particle velocity, which is estimated from single-exposure photography, was about 73 m s^{-1}. The total erodent weight is fixed at 300 g for each run. These above-mentioned erosive wear experimental parameters can be changed with the practical situations. The impact angle can be varied from 15° (an oblique impact) to 90° (a normal impact) through rotating the specimen holder. The erosion rate, which is defined as the total weight loss per erodent weight, is taken directly as the total weight loss divided by applied total erodent weight.

Figure 6.29 shows the particle erosion test results and the representative wear surface morphologies. These data are averaged from at least two runs for each test condition (from 15° to 90°). It can be seen that the erosion rate significantly increased with increasing the erosion impact angle for plasma-sprayed HACs. Figure 6.29a shows the wear surface of plasma-sprayed HACs that displays a sliding fracture path along the erodent

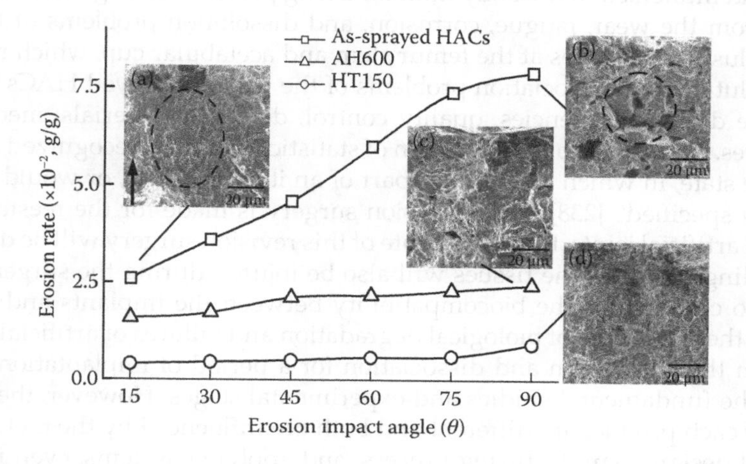

FIGURE 6.29
Variability of erosion rate with erosion impact angle for plasma-sprayed HACs, applied with atmospheric heat treatment at 600°C (AH600) and hydrothermal treatment at 150°C (HT150). Corresponding wear surface morphologies of as-sprayed HACs at impact angles of (a) 15° and (b) 90° and wear surfaces of (c) AH600 and (d) HT150 specimens at 90° normal impact angle are displayed. Arrow indicates projected impact direction of erosion test.

impact direction at an oblique impact angle (15°). However, the wear surface shown in Figure 6.29b represents that the obviously increased weight loss as well as the high erosion rate of as-sprayed HACs resulted from a significant brittle fracturing feature by the normal impact (90°) of the erodent. It is worth noting that the erosion rate of HACs is significantly decreased at each impact angle after the atmospheric heat treatment. In addition, the erosion rate is further decreased at each impact angle for the hydrothermally crystallized coatings, and the HT-HACs show the best wear resistance of all the conditions. Compared with Figure 6.29b–d, it can be seen that the brittle fracturing feature of the coating is significantly reduced with the crystallization of the HACs, especially after the hydrothermal treatment. The HT150 specimen displays a more flattened wear surface morphology than others, as shown in Figure 6.29d, and it represents that the normal impact wear resistance is improved after the hydrothermal crystallization. Since the wear fractures depend on the fracture toughness of a material, the increased fracture toughness can help to impede crack propagation [99,215] and thus the erosion resistance can be further enhanced. The reasons can be explained through the measurements of Young's modulus of the coating layers as described in the previous section. To sum up, the effects of hydrothermal crystallization with the self-healing phenomenon on the recovery of mechanical properties, such as Young's modulus, the bonding strength, and the erosion resistance, in plasma-sprayed HACs are demonstrated.

Statistical Evaluation and Reliability Engineering for Biomaterials

Unlike mechanical testing methods such as tensile, compressive, shear, and fatigue tests, under a uniaxial applied force to the experimental specimens, the artificial dental and orthopedic replacements implanted in human body are always tolerated with a complex stress field and immersed in the body fluid for a long period. The degradation and failures may occur from the wear, fatigue, corrosion, and dissolution problems of the implants. Figure 6.30 illustrates failures at the femur stem and acetabular cup, which resulted from serious dissolution and dissociation problems of the plasma-sprayed HACs [237]. Failure types include design deficiencies, quality control, defective materials, mechanical, and human failures. According to the definition of statistics, failure is recognized as "the event, or inoperable state, in which any item or part of an item does not, or would not, perform as previously specified" [238]. If the revision surgery is made for the reestablishment of implants and artificial joints, the success rate of this revision surgery will be decreased and the surrounding healthy bone tissues will also be injured during the surgery. Therefore, in addition to considering the biocompatibility between the implants and surrounding bone tissues, the evaluation of biological degradation and failures of artificial joints, which resulted from the dissolution and dissociation for a period of implantation, should also be made in the fundamental studies and experimental stages. However, the lifetime and the failure of each product are different and both are influenced by the metallurgical factors, material design, manufacturing process, and applying systems, even if they are all produced from the same manufacturing condition and equipment. Thus, the statistical analysis can help to evaluate the data distribution, statistical significance, and predict the long-term stability of biomaterials for clinical applications.

In order to prevent early failures and provide a long-term stable implantation for the plasma-sprayed HA-coated titanium implants or other biomaterials, the reliability

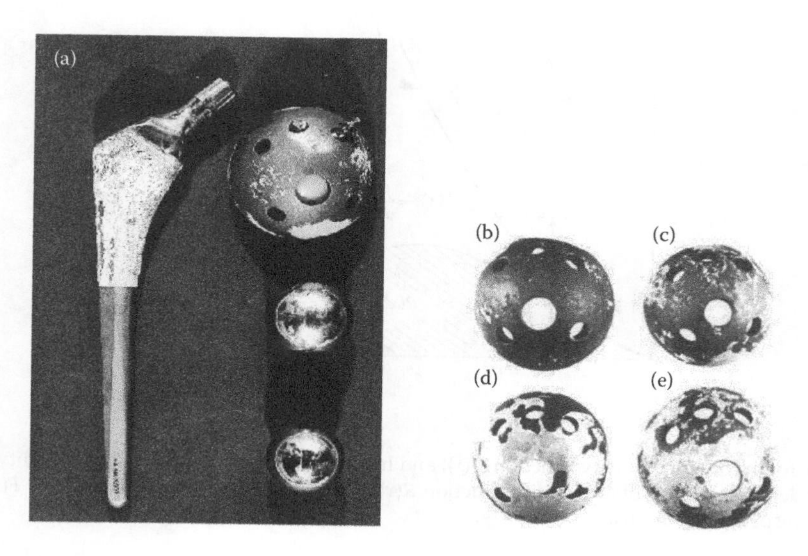

FIGURE 6.30
(a) Failure illustration of femoral stem and acetabular cup, and photographs of retrieved cups with different failure modes resulted from (b) aseptic loosening with 20.5% residual HA, (c) septic loosening with 20.3% residual HA, (d) osteolysis with 70.5% residual HA, and (e) polyethylene wear with 41.9% residual HA. Stable cups have more residual HA-coated surface than loose cups.

engineering, which is combined with the statistics and the engineering, is a commonly adopted statistical method for evaluating the most optimal design, processing, and manufacturing parameters. Reliability engineering is an engineering field that deals with the study about the ability of a system or a component to perform its required functions under stated conditions for a specified period of time. Not only it can evaluate the failure probability and failure modes of materials, but it can also predict the fracture possibility that results from the stages of material design and manufacturing processes. A basic step in many reliability engineering studies is choosing a probability density function. The relationships among the probability density function, the reliability function, and the hazard function for determining failure behaviors are deduced and described in the following section.

Statistical Significance of Data Distribution

Reliability projections are based on fitting models to life test data and both the choice of the model and the analysis methodology used can have a major influence on the result. The principal assumption underlying most statistical modeling is that a reasonably simple population model or equation will generate the smooth population curve. In addition, the larger amount of testing samples, the more closely it should resemble the population. Figure 6.31 illustrates the relationships for the probability density function and hazard function curves of the reliability engineering statistics. The model for the population curve is called the probability density function (PDF), denoted by $f(x)$. Suppose that the failure probability of a material is $P_r(x^* \leq x \leq x^* + \Delta x)$ within a limited stress increasing interval $[x^*, x^* + \Delta x]$ while the fracture occurred, and the probability of x falling between these two specified values is the integration under the probability density function from x^* to $x^* + \Delta x$, which is presented as:

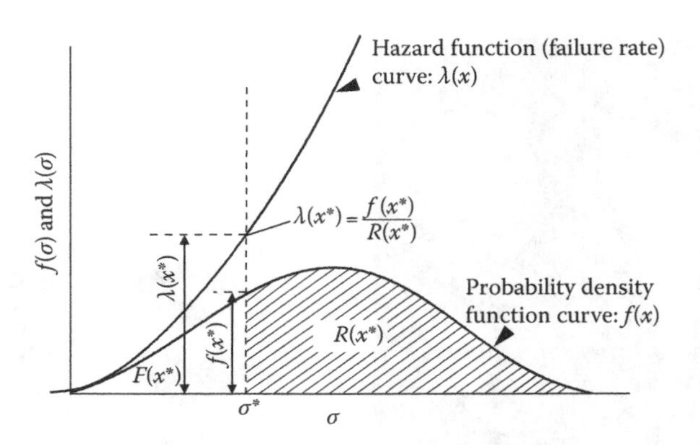

FIGURE 6.31
Relationships for probability density function ($f(x)$) and hazard function ($\lambda(x)$) curves of reliability engineering statistics. Shaded area represents reliability function $R(x^*)$, and cumulative failure probability $F(x^*)$ is defined as $1 - R(x^*)$ at a specific strength σ^*.

$$P_r\left(x^* \leq x \leq x^* + \Delta x\right) = \int_{x^*}^{x^*+\Delta x} f(x)\mathrm{d}x \tag{6.27}$$

Then the absolute value for the probability density function of failure at x^* ($f(x^*)$) can be presented as follows:

$$f(x^*) = \lim_{\Delta x \to 0} \frac{P_r\left(x^* \leq x \leq x^* + \Delta x\right)}{\Delta x} \tag{6.28}$$

As shown in Figure 6.31, the area under curve of $f(x)$ is called the cumulative distribution function (CDF), which is denoted by $F(x)$. Note that $f(x)$ is just the derivative of $F(x)$. $F(x)$ describes where the population failures lie. When the fracture occurred at a certain value x^*, Equation 6.29 displays the cumulative failure probability $F(x^*)$, which is the integrated area under the PDF curve to the right of a specific value x^*, as the value is varied from 0 to x^*. The cumulative failure probability $F(x^*)$ can also be recognized as the unreliability function.

$$F(x^*) = P(x^*) - P(0) = \int_{x=0}^{x=x^*} f(x)\mathrm{d}x \tag{6.29}$$

Suppose that the total sample space is 1.0, therefore, the complementary event of the cumulative failure probability is defined as the survival probability, which is also recognized as the survivor function and denoted by $R(x)$ [239]. Therefore, the reliability of a material larger than $x^*(R(x^*))$ with a relation of $R(x^*) = 1 - F(x^*)$ can be shown in Equation 6.30.

$$R(x^*) = 1 - F(x^*) = \int_{x=x^*}^{x=\infty} f(x)\mathrm{d}x \tag{6.30}$$

Another important statistical function for the reliability engineering and failure analysis is failure rate. Failure rate is the frequency with which an engineered system or component fails. It is often denoted by the Greek letter λ and is important in reliability theory. By calculating the failure rate for smaller and smaller intervals of Δx, the interval becomes infinitely small. This results in the hazard function, which is the instantaneous failure rate at any point for the continuous sense, as shown in Figure 6.31. The mathematical formulas are shown in Equations 6.31 and 6.32.

$$\lambda(x) = \lim_{\Delta x \to 0} \frac{R(x) - R(x + \Delta x)}{\Delta x \cdot R(x)} \tag{6.31}$$

$$\lambda(x^*) = \frac{f(x^*)}{R(x^*)} = -\ln\left[1 - F(x^*)\right] \tag{6.32}$$

Unlike the above-mentioned probability density function $f(x)$, the statistical significance of the hazard function means the failure probability of a specimen, which is failed at the infinitely small interval of Δx.

The Weibull Distribution Function

Statisticians always prefer large samples of data, but engineers and clinicians are forced to do statistical analysis with very small samples, even as few as three to five failures. When the result of a failure involves safety or extreme costs, it is inappropriate to request more failures. The Student's *t* test and the analysis of variance (ANOVA) analysis [100,120,218] are the most used statistical analysis methods for biological application. These two analysis methods can simply decide the statistical significance between several groups with different experimental variables and parameters. In addition, to characterize the strength data fluctuation, reliability, failure probability, and failure mechanism of materials, Equation 6.33 represents a powerful statistical distribution function. This function is the Weibull distribution function, invented by Waloddi Weibull in 1937 and delivered in his hallmark American paper in 1951 [240]. He claimed that this model can be applied to a wide range of problems, and the Weibull models have been used in many different applications for solving a variety of problems from many different disciplines [240–247].

$$F(x_i) = 1 - \exp\left[-\left(\frac{x_i - x_o}{\eta}\right)^m\right] \tag{6.33}$$

A powerful theoretical argument explains why the Weibull distribution function works so well for many failure mechanisms. The Weibull model can be derived theoretically as a form of extreme value distribution, governing the time to occurrence of the "weakest link" of many competing failure processes. This argument provides the theoretical basis for choosing a Weibull life distribution model for a particular mechanism. The Weibull distribution function has been successfully modeling failures for several diverse applications such as capacitor, gate oxide, ball bearing, relay, and material strength failure mechanisms. The Weibull distribution most frequently provides the best fit of life data. The primary advantage of Weibull statistical analysis is the ability to provide reasonable accurate failure analysis and failure forecasts with extremely small amounts of testing samples. Solutions are possible at the earliest indications of a problem without having to crash a few more. If all the bearings are tested to failure, the cost and time required is much greater. Therefore, a small amount of testing samples also allow cost-effective component testing. Another advantage of the Weibull statistical analysis is that it provides a sample and useful graphical plot. The data plot is extremely important to engineering clinicians and managers.

With regard to clinical applications, plasma-sprayed HA-coated implants with a sufficient, reliable strength and reliability are indispensable due to their long-term stability. However, many metallurgical variables affect the coating strength, including variables associated with materials manufacturing, and result in a certain extent of data fluctuation. To solve these problems and determine the reliability and failure modes of the coatings, this statistical method of survival analysis has been accepted as an engineering design method for such materials [239,248]. In the present subject, the variable x in Equation 6.33 can be defined as a certain mechanical strength (denoted by σ), such as the adhesive bonding strength, shear strength, fracture strength, toughness, and so forth, resulting from a mechanical testing. In order to evaluate the statistical significance for the data fluctuation of the measured bonding strength as shown in Figure 6.23, therefore, the Weibull model is applied to clarify the metallurgical effects on the failure mechanism of plasma-sprayed HACs. Equation 6.34 shows the general form of the Weibull distribution function, where σ represents the bonding strength, and at least 20 specimens (n = 20) are tested for the purpose of statistical significance of the Weibull analysis.

$$F(\sigma_i) = \int_{\sigma=0}^{\sigma=\sigma_i} f(\sigma)\mathrm{d}\sigma = 1-\exp\left[-\left(\frac{\sigma_i-\sigma_\mathrm{o}}{\sigma_\mathrm{c}}\right)^m\right] \tag{6.34}$$

$F(\sigma_i)$ is the cumulative failure probability corresponding to a measured bonding strength σ_i (i is the ranking of specimens from the lowest value to the highest one, i = 1–20). According to the definition of the Weibull statistics, the failure behavior of materials is determined by three parameters: m, σ_c, and σ_o. The Weibull modulus (m), which controls the shape of function curves, is a measure of the variability of the data. In addition, it should be worth noting that the failure behaviors can also be determined by the value distribution of the Weibull modulus (m) as shown in Figure 6.32, and can be interpreted as follows:

- A value of $m < 1$ indicates that the failure is an "early failure" mode. The failure probability and the failure rate are very high as shown in Figure 6.32a. However, the decreasing of the failure rate (DFR) occurred over time when the significant infant mortality or those defective items failing early are weeded out of the population. This situation is mostly resulted from the error of design and preexisted defects in materials or systems during the manufacturing processes.
- A value of $m = 1$ indicates that the failure probability or the failure rate is constant over time as shown in Figure 6.32b (constant failure rate, CFR), that is, a random failure. This might suggest that random external events result in the mortality and failures.

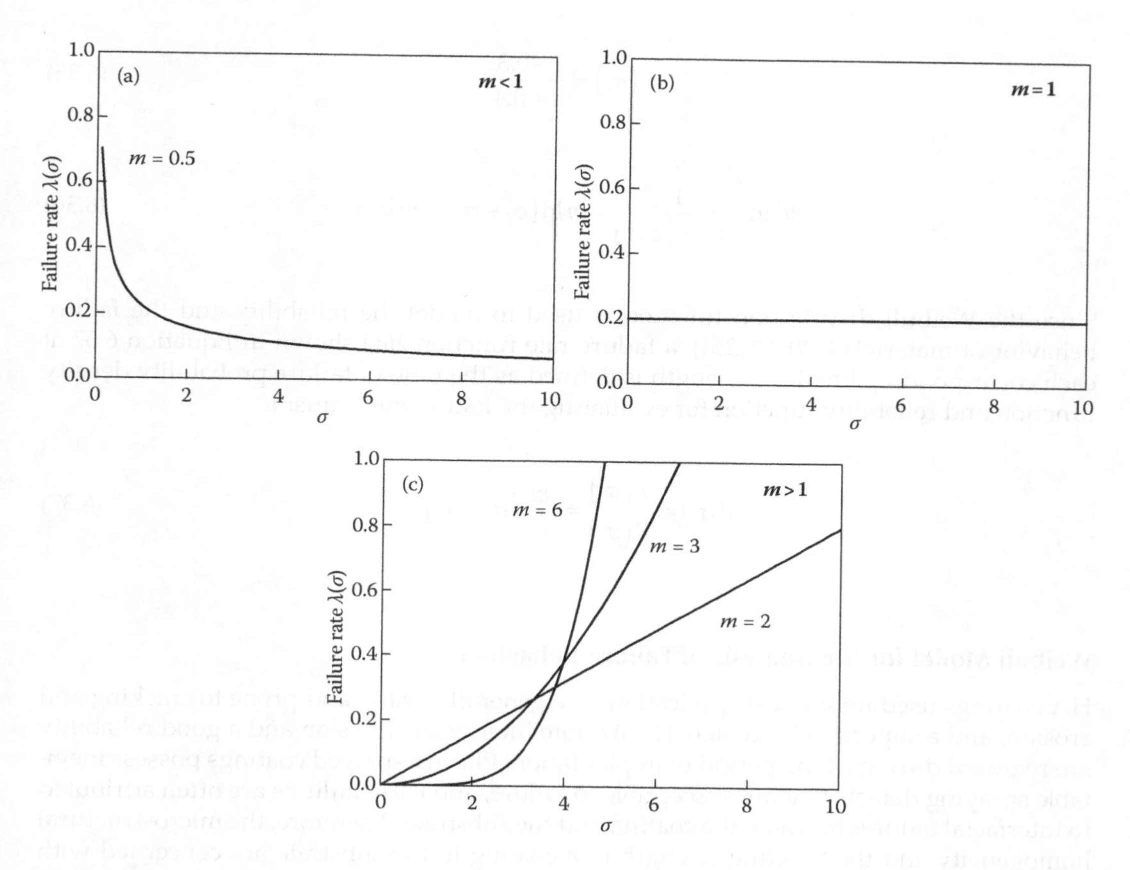

FIGURE 6.32
Three failure modes of materials (other parameters are $\eta = 5$, $\sigma_o = 0$): (a) decreasing failure rate (DFR) of an early failure with $m < 1$; (b) constant failure rate (CFR) of random failure with $m = 1$; and (c) increasing failure rate (IFR) of a wearout failure with $m > 1$.

- A value of $m > 1$ indicates that the system belongs to a wearout failure model and the failure rate increases with time (IFR). In addition, the slope of failure rate function curve increased with increasing the Weibull modulus, as shown in Figure 6.32c. This situation occurs if there is an aging process, or parts that are more likely to fail as time go on.

The characteristic strength σ_c corresponds to the strength at which the cumulative failure probability is 63.2%. The minimum strength σ_o means that the failure probability of HACs lower than this strength is zero. The Weibull model is a very flexible life distribution model with two defining parameters, which are the Weibull modulus (m) and the characteristic strength (σ_c).

The cumulative failure probability $F(\sigma_i)$ is estimated using the Benard's median rank in Equation 6.35 [249], which is a very close approximated solution of a statistical function [248,250], and the reliability function $R(\sigma_i)$ with a relation of $R(\sigma_i) = 1 - F(\sigma_i)$ is defined as the survival probability [239]. Through the natural logarithmic (ln) graphs for the cumulative failure probability at each corresponding bonding strength σ_i (i = 1–20) of the specimens, it can graphically evaluate the Weibull modulus (m) from the slope of a least-squares fitting method of Equation 6.36.

$$F(\sigma_i) = \frac{i - 0.3}{n + 0.4} \tag{6.35}$$

$$\ln \ln \left(\frac{1}{1 - F(\sigma_i)} \right) = m \ln(\sigma_i - \sigma_o) - m \ln \sigma_c \tag{6.36}$$

Since the Weibull distribution function is used to model the reliability and the failure behavior of materials [120,239,251], a failure rate function $\lambda(\sigma_i)$ shown in Equation 6.37 at each corresponding bonding strength is defined as the ratio of failure probability density function and reliability function for evaluating the failure mechanism.

$$\lambda(\sigma_i) = \frac{f(\sigma_i)}{R(\sigma_i)} = \frac{m}{\sigma_c^m} (\sigma_i - \sigma_o)^{m-1} \tag{6.37}$$

Weibull Model for the Analysis of Failure Behaviors

HA coatings used for clinical applications are generally brittle and prone to cracking and erosion, and a superior HA-coated Ti substrate interfacial adhesion and a good reliability are required during a long period of implantation. Plasma-sprayed coatings possess inevitable spraying defects that are susceptible to failure, and early failures are often attributed to interfacial failures between the coating and the substrate. Therefore, the microstructural homogeneity and the bonding strength of a coating to the substrate are concerned with determining the performance and reliability of HACs. The plasma-sprayed HACs and the HT-HACs, which are hydrothermally treated at 125°C for 12 h (HT125) and at 150°C for 6 h (HT150), are selected for evaluating the coating reliability and failure behaviors through the Weibull statistics. Fitting the measured bonding strength data into the Weibull distribution function, the failure probability density function $f(\sigma)$ curves of the plasma-sprayed HACs, HT125, and HT150 conditions are plotted in Figure 6.33a. Figure 6.33b shows the natural logarithmic (ln) graphs for the cumulative failure probability at each corresponding bonding strength σ_i (i = 1–20), so as to graphically evaluate the Weibull modulus (m) from the slope of a least-squares fitting, and the results of Weibull statistical analysis are listed in Table 6.6.

Since the Weibull distribution function can be used to model the reliability and the failure behavior of materials [120,239,251], a failure rate function $\lambda(\sigma_i)$ shown in Equation 6.37 at each corresponding bonding strength is further applied for evaluating the failure mechanism of coatings. Figure 6.34 shows the failure rate function ($\lambda(\sigma)$) and reliability function ($R(\sigma)$) curves of the plasma-sprayed and HT-HACs. These curves start from the minimum strength (σ_o), which implies the failure probability of HACs less than this strength is zero and the reliability of HACs is 1.0. The minimum strength can be recognized as safety strength. Meanwhile, knowledge of the Weibull modulus (m) can provide further explanation for the self-healing effect of hydrothermal crystallization on the bonding strength of HACs, and it can be used to determine which coating has higher uniformity and reliability. The examination of the Weibull modulus listed in Table 6.6 represents that the plasma-sprayed HACs (m = 3.8) is a reliable surface coating with a wearout failure model

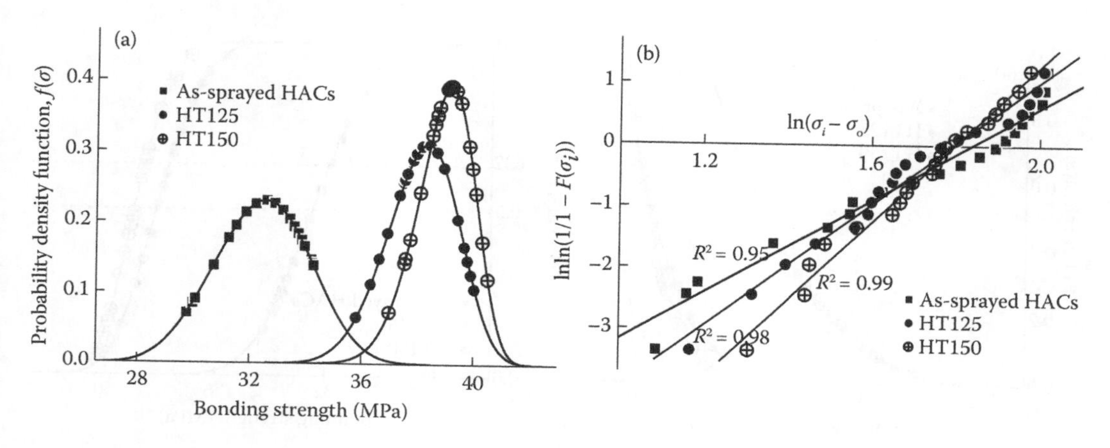

FIGURE 6.33
(a) Failure probability density function $f(\sigma)$ curves and (b) Weibull distribution plots of plasma-sprayed and HT-HACs. $F(\sigma_i)$ is cumulative failure probability at corresponding bonding strength (σ_i), and slope represents Weibull modulus (m), which calculated by least-squares fitting method of Equation 6.36 at a maximum coefficient of determination (R^2).

($m > 1$) of increasing failure rate (IFR) [249,251]. The HT-HACs also show a wearout failure model with a higher Weibull modulus ($m = 5.0$ and 6.4 for HT125 and HT150, respectively), which represents the microstructural self-healing and homogeneity resulted from hydrothermal crystallization has evident benefits to effectively enhance the bonding strength of plasma-sprayed HACs. A material with a higher Weibull modulus is selected as it may be an indicator for clinical use or lesser technique sensitivity. The Weibull modulus can be also a measure of the variability of the data, which gets larger as the degree of bonding strength fluctuation decreases. Evident benefits of the failure probability density function (Figure 6.33a) and failure rate (Figure 6.34a) curves shift to a higher bonding strength with a concentrated data distribution are achieved for HT150 specimens. The hydrothermal treatment not only effectively enhances the bonding strength of plasma-sprayed HACs, but helps to acquire more stable HACs with less reliability decrease (Figure 6.34b) while the loading exceeds the minimum strength.

The representative failure morphologies of these coatings are shown in Figure 6.35. It can be seen that the failure morphology represents a combination of the cohesive failure region (co) and the adhesive failure region (ad). The cohesive failure is dominated by microstructural features such as crystallinity, defects, lamellar texture, and a large area fraction of cohesive failure can be commonly observed at high strength coatings [63,99]. Compared with the failures of plasma-sprayed HACs shown in Figure 6.35a, since strengthening

TABLE 6.6

Results of Bonding Strength Measurements and Weibull Statistical Analysis of Plasma-Sprayed HACs and HT-HACs

	Bonding Strength (MPa), σ [a]	Minimum Strength (MPa), σ_o [b]	Characteristics Strength (MPa), η [b]	Weibull Modulus, m [b]
Plasma-sprayed HACs	32.4 ± 1.5	26.8	33.1	3.8
HT125 (12 h)	38.1 ± 1.2	32.6	38.7	5.0
HT150 (6 h)	38.9 ± 1.0	33.3	39.4	6.4

[a] Each value is the average of 20 tests ($n = 20$).
[b] Data obtained from $\ln\ln(1/1 - F(\sigma_i))$ vs. $\ln(\sigma_i - \sigma_o)$ plots (Figure 6.32b) using Equation 6.36.

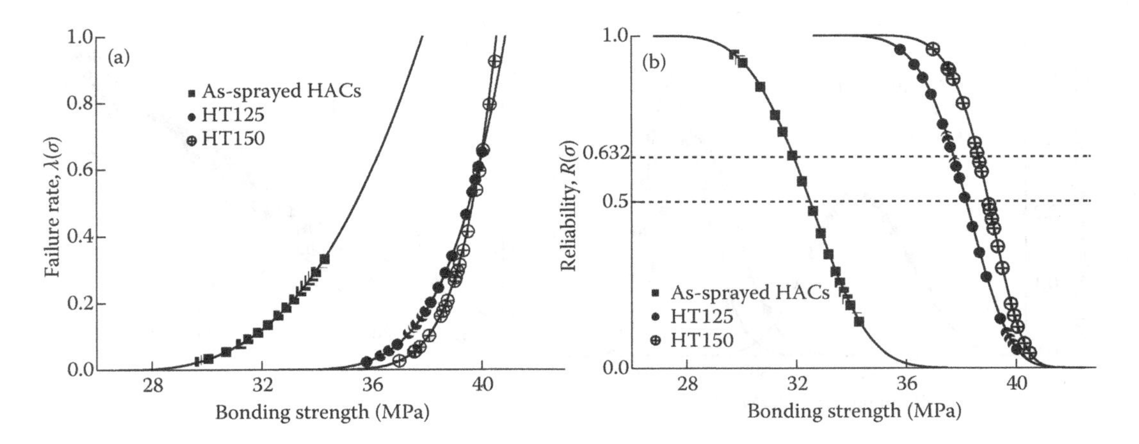

FIGURE 6.34
(a) Failure rate function $\lambda(\sigma)$ curves, and (b) reliability function $R(\sigma)$ curves of plasma-sprayed and various HT-HACs. These curves start from minimum strength (σ_o), which is the safety strength for biological application of HACs.

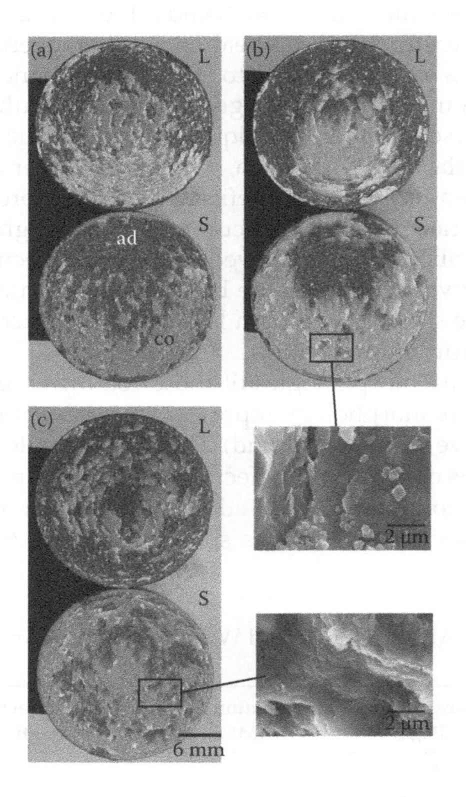

FIGURE 6.35
Failure morphologies of (a) plasma-sprayed HACs, (b) HT150, and (c) HT125 specimens after tensile adhesion tests. Bonding strength of coatings measured is a manifestation of cohesive (co) and adhesive (ad) strength. L, loading fixture; S, substrate fixture.

coatings resulted from the microstructural self-healing effect of hydrothermal crystallization, the failure morphologies of HT-HACs represent crystallized, homogeneity, and display a larger area fraction of cohesive failure as displayed in Figure 6.35b and c. In contrast, the decreased area fraction of adhesive failure represents that the adhesion of HT-HACs to the Ti–6Al–4V substrate is significantly improved, especially for the HT125 condition. Referring to the evidences demonstrated from the XPS analysis as shown in Figure 6.18, the hydrothermal treatment effectively helps to promote the interfacial crystallization through the replenished and the chemisorbed OH^- groups, which results in a significant chemical bonding of the HA coating to Ti substrate interface. It can be summarized from the above-mentioned results that performing low-temperature hydrothermal treatments is an available process and will allow plasma-sprayed HA-coated implants to have desirable mechanical fixation and reliability for long-term applications without dissociation problems.

Summary

HA is today a conventional applied bioactive ceramic material, which is considered an excellent hard tissue substitute in dentistry and orthopedics due to its favorable osteoconductivity and osseointegration properties. Plasma-sprayed HAs on metallic substrate exhibits enhanced interfacial strength and tends to avoid the inherent mechanical property limitations of HA without significant loss in biocompatibility. As has been represented in this chapter, plasma-sprayed HACs have advantages and disadvantages as far as their properties (i.e., microstructural, mechanical, biological, and material reliability), and applications are concerned with the realization of chemical stability in solution and thermal stability of HA.

Since the phase stability of crystalline HA is reduced during plasma spraying, a good understanding of phase decomposition products, such as ACP, TCP, TP, CaO, and other nonstoichiometric calcium phosphate, would contribute to the knowledge on dissolution mechanism and stability of HACs. The identification of these phases can be achieved by XRD and Raman spectroscopy techniques. The quantification of the crystallinity and phase content of plasma-sprayed HACs can be obtained by the internal standard method and the quantitative phase analysis (QPA) of Rietveld method by x-ray or neutron diffraction.

Postspray heat treatment is required and is an effective way to improve the crystallization state and the dissolution problems of plasma-sprayed HACs. Compared with different heat treatments, hydrothermal treatment is more favorable to eliminate the impurity phases and ACP than high temperature heat treatments in vacuum or in the air. The derivation from Arrhenius kinetics demonstrates that heating temperature is a controlling factor for HA crystallization. A higher crystallization rate and lower activation energy of HA crystallization for the hermetically hydrothermal treatment can be recognized as the effect of ambient heating atmosphere with a saturated steam pressure.

Hydrothermal crystallization obviously improves the microstructural homogeneity of plasma-sprayed HACs through the self-healing effect. The enhanced bonding strength and erosion resistance are resulted from the increased cohesive strength of dense coatings and the increased adhesive strength with a significant chemical interlocking between the hydrothermally treated HACs and substrate interface. Relative low-temperature hydrothermal treatment can help to avoid the detrimental oxidation layer and compressive residual strain, which resulted from high-temperature heat treatments, at the coating/substrate interface.

In addition, the failure behaviors of plasma-sprayed HACs is also an important task review, and the statistics can help to evaluate the data distribution, statistical significance, and predict the long-term stability of biomaterials for the further clinical applications. Reliability engineering via a powerful statistical function of the Weibull model can not only evaluate the failure probability and failure modes of materials, but predict the fracture possibility, which resulted from the stages of material design and manufacturing processes. Biological coatings with a higher Weibull modulus and a wearout failure with IFR are adopted as it is an indicator for clinical use or lesser technique sensitivity. According to the results of Weibull model analysis, an increased Weibull modulus represents that the bonding strength and the reliability of plasma-sprayed HACs are further improved by the hydrothermal crystallization.

References

1. Holmes, R. E., Bucholz, R. W., and V. Mooney. 1986. Porous hydroxyapatite as a bone-graft substitute in metaphyseal defects. *J. Bone Jt. Surg.* 68A:904–911.
2. Bucholz, R. W., Carlton, A., and R. E. Holmes. 1989. Interporous hydroxyapatite as a bone graft substitute in tibial plateau fractures. *Clin. Orthop.* 240:53–62.
3. Munting, E., Verhelpen, M., Li, F., and A. Vincent. 1990. Contribution of hydroxy-apatite coatings to implant fixation. In *CRC Handbook of Bioactive Ceramics, Vol. II*, T. Yamamuro, L. L. Hench, and J. Wilson (eds.), 143–148. Boca Raton, FL: CRC Press Inc., Taylor & Francis.
4. Jansen, J. A., van de Waerden, J. P. C. M., Wolke, J. G. C., and K. de Groot. 1991. Histologic evaluation of the osseous adaptation to titanium and hydroxy-apatite-coated titanium implants. *J. Biomed. Mater. Res.* 25:973–989.
5. Yuan, H., Yang, Z., de Bruijn, J. D., de Groot, K., and X. Zhang. 2001. Material-dependent bone induction by calcium phosphate ceramics: A 2.5-year study in dog. *Biomaterials* 22:2617–2623.
6. Hench, L. L. 1991. Bioceramics: From concept to clinic. *J. Am. Ceram. Soc.* 74[7]:1487–1510.
7. Schreurs, B. W., Huiskes, R., Buma, P., and T. J. J. H. Slooff. 1996. Biomechanical and histological evaluation of a hydroxyapatite-coated titanium femoral stem fixed with an intramedullary morsellized bone grafting technique: An animal experiment on goats. *Biomaterials* 17:1177–1186.
8. de Groot, K. 1983. Ceramic of calcium phosphates: Preparation and properties. In *Bioceramics of Calcium Phosphate*, K. de Groot (ed.), 100–114. Boca Raton, FL: CRC Press Inc., Taylor & Francis.
9. Denissen, H., Mangano, C., and G. Cenini. 1985. *Hydroxylapatite Implants*. India: Piccin Nuova Libraria, S.P.A.
10. Hench, L. L. 1998. Bioceramics. *J. Am. Ceram. Soc.* 81[7]:1705–1728.
11. van Audekercke, R., and M. Martens. 1984. Mechanical properties of cancellous bone. In *Natural and Living Biomaterials*, G. W. Hastings and P. Ducheyne (eds.), 89–98. Boca Raton, FL: CRC Press Inc., Taylor & Francis.
12. de Groot, K., Klein, C. P. A. T., Wolke, J. G. C., and J. M. A. de Bliek-Hogervost. 1990. Chemistry of calcium phosphate bioceramics. In *Handbook of Bioactive Ceramics, Vol. II*, T. Yamamuro, L. L. Hench, and J. Wilson (eds.), 3–16. Boca Raton, FL: CRC Press Inc., Taylor & Francis.
13. van Audekercke, R., and M. Martens. 1984. Mechanical properties of cancellous bone. In *Natural and Living Biomaterials*, G. W. Hastings, and P. Ducheyne (eds.), 89–98. Boca Raton, FL: CRC Press Inc., Taylor & Francis.

14. Choi, J. W., Kong, Y. M., and H. E. Kim. 1998. Reinforcement of hydroxyapatite bioceramic by addition of Ni_3Al and Al_2O_3. *J. Am. Ceram. Soc.* 81:1743–1748.
15. Ducheyne, P., Hench, L. L., Kagan, A., Martens, M., Bursens, A., and J. C. Mulier. 1980. Effect of hydroxyapatite impregnation on skeletal bonding of porous coated implants. *J. Biomed. Mater. Res.* 14:225–237.
16. Wolke, J. G. C., Klein, C. P. A. T., and K. de Groot. 1991. Bioceramics for maxillofacial applications. In *Bioceramics and the Human Body*, A. Ravaglioli and A. Krajewski (eds.), 166–180. England: Elsevier Science Publishers Ltd.
17. Geesink, R. G. T., de Groot, K., and C. P. A. T. Klein. 1988. Bonding of bone to apatite-coated implants. *J. Bone Jt. Surg. [Br]* 70B:17–22.
18. Cook, S. D., Thomas, K. A., Delton, J. E., Volkman, T. K., Whitecloud, T. S., and J. F. Key. 1992. Hydroxyapatite coating of porous implants improves bone ingrowth and interface attachment strength. *J. Biomed. Mater. Res.* 26:989–101.
19. Wang, B. C., Chang, E., Yang, C. Y., and D. Tu. 1993. A histomorphometric study on osteoconduction and osseointegration of titanium alloy with and without plasma-sprayed hydroxyapatite coating using back-scattered electron images. *J. Mater. Sci.: Mater. Med.* 4:394–403.
20. Bauer, T. W., Geesink, R. C. T., Zimmerman, R., and J. T. McMahon. 1991. Hydroxyapatite-coated femoral stems: Histological analysis of components retrieved at autopsy. *J. Bone Jt. Surg. [Am]* 73A:1439–1452.
21. Lintner, F., Böhm, G., Huber, M., and R. Scholz. 1994. Histology of tissue adjacent to an HAC-coated femoral prostheses: A case report. *J. Bone Jt. Surg. [Br]* 76B:824–830.
22. Jarcho, M. 1981. Calcium Phosphate Ceramics as Hard Tissue Prosthetics. *Clin. Orthop.* 157:259–278.
23. Geesink, R. G. T., de Groot, K., and C. P. A. T. Klein. 1987. Chemical implant fixation using hydroxyapatite coatings. *Clin. Orthop.* 225:147–170.
24. Cook, S. D., Thomas, K., Kay, J. F., and M. Jarcho. 1988. Hydroxylapatite coated titanium for orthopaedic implant applications. *Clin. Orthop. Rel. Res.* 232:225–243.
25. Wei, M., Uchida, M., Kim, H. M., Kokubo, T., and T. Nakamura. 2002. Apatite-forming ability of CaO-containing titania. *Biomaterials* 23:167–172.
26. Wei, M., Ruys, A. J., Milthorpe, B. K., and C. C. Sorrell. 2005. Precipitation of hydroxyapatite nano-particles: Effects of precipitation method on electrophoretic deposition. *J. Mater. Sci.: Mater. Med.* 16:319–324.
27. Ong, J. L., Appleford, M., and S. Oh et al. 2006. The characterization and development of bioactive hydroxyapatite coatings. *JOM* 58:67–69.
28. Peng, P., Kumar, S., Voelcker, N. H., Szili, E., Smart, R. S. C., and H. J. Griesser. 2006. Thin calcium phosphate coatings on titanium by electrochemical deposition in modified simulated body fluid. *J. Biomed. Mater. Res.* 76A:347–355.
29. Ozeki, K., Aoki, H., and Y. Fukui. 2006. Dissolution behavior and in vitro evaluation of sputtered hydroxyapatite films subject to a low temperature hydrothermal treatment. *J. Biomed. Mater. Res.* 76A:605–613.
30. Ben-Nissan, B., and A. H. Choi. 2006. Sol–gel production of bioactive nano-coatings for medical applications: Part 1. An introduction. *Nanomedicine* 1:311–319.
31. Liu, X., Chu, P. K., and C. Ding. 2007. Formation of apatite on hydrogenated amorphous silicon (a-Si:H) film deposited by plasma-enhanced chemical vapor deposition. *Mater. Chem. Phys.* 101:124–128.
32. Kokubo, T., Hayashi, T., Sakka, S., Kitsugi, T., and T. Yamamuro. 1987. Bonding between bioactive glasses, glass-ceramics or ceramics in a simulated body fluid. *J. Ceram. Soc. Jpn.* 95:785–791.
33. Oonishi, H., Yamamoto, M., and H. Ishimaru et al. 1989. The effect of hydroxyapatite coating on bone growth into porous titanium alloy implants. *J. Bone Jt. Surg.* 71B:213–216.
34. Hardy, D. C. R., Frayssinet. P., and P. E. Delince. 1999. Osteointegration of hydroxyapatite-coated stems of femoral prostheses. *Eur. J. Orthop. Surg. Traumatol.* 9:75–81.

35. Hayashi, K., Inadome, T., Mashima, T., and Y. Sugioka. 1993. Comparison of bone–implant interface shear strength of solid hydroxyapatite and hydroxyapatite-coated titanium implants. *J. Biomed. Mater. Res.* 27:557–563.
36. Burr, D. B., Mori, S., and R. D. Boyd et al. 1993. Histomorphometric assessment of the mechanisms for rapid ingrowth of bone to HA/TCP coated implants. *J. Biomed. Mater. Res.* 27:645–653.
37. Jaffe, W. L., and D. F. Scott. 1996. Current concepts review: Total hip arthroplasty with hydroxyapatite-coated prostheses. *J. Bone Jt. Surg. [Am]* 78A:1918–1934.
38. Block, M. S., Kent, J. N., and J. F. Kay. 1987. Evaluation of hydroxyapatite-coated titanium dental implants in dogs. *J. Oral Maxillofac. Surg.* 45:601–607.
39. Kitsugi, T., Yamamuro, T., Takeuchi, H., and M. Ono. 1988. Bonding behavior of 3 types of hydroxyapatite with different sintering temperatures implanted in bone. *Clin. Orthop.* 234:280–290.
40. Filiaggi, M. J., Coombs, N. A., and R. M. Pilliar. 1991. Characterization of the interface in the plasma sprayed HA coating/Ti–6Al–4V implant system. *J. Biomed. Mater. Res.* 25:1211–1229.
41. Chen, J., Zhou, J., Zhang, X., and D. Wan. 1991. A study on Ha-coated titanium dental implants part: II. Coating properties in vivo, implant design and clinical evaluation. In *Bioceramics and the Human Body*, A. Ravaglioli and A. Krajewski (eds.), 89–100. England: Elsevier Science Publishers Ltd.
42. Galante, J., Rostoker, W., Lueck, R., and R. D. Ray. 1971. Sintered fiber metal composites as a basis for attachment of implants to bone. *J. Bone Jt. Surg.* 53A:101–114.
43. Albrektsson, T., Branemark, P. I., and H. A. Hansson et al. 1983. The interface zone of inorganic implants in vivo: Titanium implants in bone. *Ann. Biomed. Eng.* 11:1–27.
44. Ravaglioli, A., and A. Krajewski. 1992. *Bioceramics: Materials, Properties, Applications.* London: Chapman and Hall Press.
45. Wang, B. C., Chang, E., Lee, T. M., and C. Y. Yang. 1995. Changes in phases and crystallinity of plasma-sprayed hydroxyapatite coatings under heat treatment: A quantitative study. *J. Biomed. Mater. Res.* 29:1483–1492.
46. Gross, K. A., and C. C. Berndt. 1998. Thermal processing of hydroxyapatite for coating production. *J. Biomed. Mater. Res.* 39:580–587.
47. Yang, C. Y., Wang, B. C., Chang, E., and B. C. Wu. 1995. Bond degradation at the plasma-sprayed HA coating/Ti–6Al–4V alloy interface: An in vitro study. *J. Mater. Sci.: Mater. Med.* 6:258–265.
48. Yang, C. Y., Lin, R. M., and B. C. Wang et al. 1997. In vitro and in vivo mechanical evaluations of plasma-sprayed hydroxyapatite coatings on titanium implants: The effect of coating characteristics. *J. Biomed. Mater. Res.* 37:335–345.
49. Bauer, T. W., Taylor, S. K., Jiang, M., and S. V. Medendorp. 1994. An indirect comparison of 3-rd body wear in retrieved hydroxyapatite-coated porous and cemented femoral components. *Clin. Orthop.* 298:11–18.
50. Fu, Y. Q., Batchelor, A. W., Wang, Y., and K. A. Khor. 1998. Fretting wear behaviors of thermal sprayed hydroxyapatite (HA) coating under unlubricated conditions. *Wear* 217:132–198.
51. Gross, K. A., and M. Babovic. 2002. Influence of abrasion on the surface characteristics of thermally sprayed hydroxyapatite coatings. *Biomaterials* 23:4731–4737.
52. Ji, H., and P. M. Marquis. 1993. Effect of heat treatment on the microstructure of plasma-sprayed hydroxyapatite coating. *Biomaterials* 14:64–68.
53. Zyman, Z., Weng J., Liu X., and X. Zhang. 1994. Phase and structural changes in hydroxyapatite coatings under heat treatment. *Biomaterials* 15:151–155.
54. Weng, J., Liu X., Zhang X., and K. de Groot. 1996. Integrity and thermal decomposition of apatite in coatings influenced by underlying titanium during plasma spraying and post-heat-treatment. *J. Biomed. Mater. Res.* 30:5–11.
55. Lu, Y. P., Li S. T., Zhu R. F., Li M. S., and T. Q. Lei. 2003. Formation of ultrafine particles in heat treated plasma-sprayed hydroxyapatite coatings. *Surf. Coat. Technol.* 165:65–70.
56. Lu, Y. P., Song Y. Z., Zhu R. F., Li M. S., and T. Q. Lei. 2003. Factors influencing phase compositions and structure of plasma sprayed hydroxyapatite coatings during heat treatment. *Appl. Surf. Sci.* 206:345–354.

57. Yang, Y., Kim K. H., Agrawal C. M., and J. L. Ong. 2004. Interaction of hydroxyapatite-titanium at elevated temperature in vacuum environment. *Biomaterials* 25:2927–2932.
58. Cao, Y., Weng, J., Chen, J., Feng, J., Yang, Z., and X. Zhang. 1996. Water vapor-treated hydroxyapatite coatings after plasma spraying and their characteristics. *Biomaterials* 17:419–424.
59. Chen, J., Tong, W., Cao, Y., Feng, J., and X. Zhang. 1997. Effect of atmosphere on phase transformation in plasma-sprayed hydroxyapatite coatings during heat treatment. *J. Biomed. Mater. Res.* 34:15–20.
60. Kumar, R., Cheang, P., and K. A. Khor. 2004. Phase composition and heat of crystallization of amorphous calcium phosphate in ultra-fine radio frequency suspension plasma sprayed hydroxyapatite powders. *Acta Mater.* 52:1171–1181.
61. Feng, C. F., Khor, K. A., Liu, E. J, and P. Cheang. 2000. Phase transformations in plasma sprayed hydroxyapatite coatings. *Scr. Mater.* 42:103–109.
62. Lee, Y. P., Wang, C. K., Huang, T. H., Chen, C. C., Kao, C. T., and S. J. Ding. 2005. *In vitro* characterization of post heat-treated plasma-sprayed hydroxyapatite coatings. *Surf. Coat. Technol.* 197:367–374.
63. Yang, C. W., Lui, T. S., Lee, T. M., and E. Chang. 2004. Effect of hydrothermal treatment on microstructural feature and bonding strength of plasma-sprayed hydroxyapatite on Ti–6Al–4V. *Mater. Trans.* 45[9]:2922–2929.
64. Yang, C. W., Lee, T. M., Lui, T. S., and E. Chang. 2006. Effect of post vacuum heating on the microstructural feature and bonding strength of plasma-sprayed hydroxyapatite coatings. *Mater. Sci. Eng. C.* 26:1395–1400.
65. Yu, L. G., Khor, K. A., Li, H., and P. Cheang. 2003. Effect of spark plasma sintering on the microstructure and in vitro behavior of plasma sprayed HA coatings. *Biomaterials* 24:2695–2705.
66. Li, H., Khor, K. A., and P. Cheang. 2006. Effect of steam treatment during plasma spraying on the microstructure of hydroxyapatite splats and coatings. *J. Thermal Spray Technol.* 15[4]:610–616.
67. Driessens, F. C. M. 1983. Formation and stability of calcium phosphates in relation to the phase composition of the mineral in calcified tissue. In *Bioceramic of Calcium Phosphate*, K. de Groot (ed.), 1–32. Boca Raton, FL: CRC Press Inc., Taylor & Francis.
68. Adam, P., Nebelung, A., and M. Vogt. 1988. Verhalten von mit Tricalciumphosphat beschichteten Titanimplantaten bei der Behandlung mit Wasser von 80°C (Behavior of titanium implants coated with tricalcium phosphate during treatment with water at 80°C). *Sprechsaal.* 121[10]:941–944.
69. Newesely, H. 1997. High temperature behavior of hydroxy- and fluorapatite. *J. Oral Rehab.* 4:97.
70. Moreno, E. C., Kresak, M., and R. T. Zahradnik. 1977. Physicochemical aspects of fluoride-apatite systems relevant to the study of dental caries. *Caries Res.* 11: 142–177.
71. LeGeros, R. Z., and M. S. Tung. 1983. Chemical stability of carbonate and fluoride-containing apatites. *Caries Res.* 17:419–429.
72. Christofferssen, J., and M. R. Christofferssen. 1982. Kinetics of dissolution of calcium hydroxyapatite: V. The acidity constant for the hydrogen phosphate surface complex. *J. Cryst. Growth* 57:21–26.
73. Hench, L. L., Splinter, R. J., Allen, W. C., and T. K. Greenlee. 1971. Bonding mechanisms at the interface of ceramic prosthetic materials. *J. Biomed. Mater. Res.* 2:117–141.
74. Margoils, H. C., and E. C. Moreno. 1992. Kinetics of hydroxyapatite dissolution in acetic, lactic and phosphoric acid solutions. *Calcif. Tissue. Int.* 50:137–143.
75. Kent, J. N., Quinn, J. H., Zide, M. F., Guerra, L. R., and P. J. Boyne. 1983. Augmentation of deficient alveolar ridge with non-resorbable hydroxyapatite alone or with autogenous cancellous bone. *J. Oral Maxillofac. Surg.* 41:429–435.
76. Ducheyne, P., Radin, S., and L. King. 1993. The effect of calcium phosphate ceramic composition and structure on in vitro behavior: I. Dissolution. *J. Biomed. Mater. Res.* 27:25–34.
77. Radin, S. R., and P. Ducheyne. 1993. Effect of calcium phosphate ceramic composition and structure on *in vitro* behavior: II. Precipitation. *J. Biomed. Mater. Res.* 27:35–45.

78. Garcia, R., and R. H. Doremus. 1992. Electron microscopy of the bone–hydroxyapatite interface from a human dental implant. *J. Mater. Sci.: Mater. Med.* 3:154–156.
79. Gregory, T. M., Moreno, E. C., Patel, J. M., and W. E. Brown. 1974. Solubility of β-$Ca_3(PO_4)_2$ in the system $Ca(OH)_2$-H_3PO_4-H_2O at 5, 15, 25 and 37°C. *J. Res. Natl. Bur. Stand.* 78A:667–674.
80. McDowell, H., Gregory, T. M., and W. E. Brown. 1977. Solubility of $Ca_5(PO_4)_3OH$ in the system $Ca(OH)_2$-H_3PO_4-H_2O at 5, 15, 25 and 37°C. *J. Res. Natl. Bur. Stand. A Phys. Sci.* 81A:273–281.
81. Roth, R. S., Negas, T., and L. P. Cook. 1983. *Phase Diagrams for Ceramists*, Vol. 5, (pp. 321–322). Washington, DC: American Ceramic Society.
82. Zhou, J., Zhang, X., Chen, J., Zeng, S., and K. de Groot. 1993. High temperature characteristics of synthetic hydroxyapatite. *J. Mater. Sci.: Mater.* Med. 4:83–85.
83. Vogel, J., Russel, C., Gunther, G., Hartmann, P., Vizethum, F., and N. Bergner. 1996. Characterization of plasma-sprayed hydroxyapatite by ^{31}P-MAS-NMR and the effect of subsequent annealing. *J. Mater. Sci.: Mater.* 7:495–499.
84. Locardi, B., and U. E. Pazzaglia. 1993. Thermal behaviour of hydroxyapatite intended for medical applications. *Biomaterials* 14:437–441.
85. Tucker, R. C. 1994. Advanced thermal spray deposition techniques. In *Handbook of Deposition Technologies for Films and Coatings*, R. F. Bunshah (ed.), 591–642. Park Ridge, NJ: Noyes.
86. de Groot, K., Geesink, R., Klein, C. P. A. T., and P. Serekian. 1987. Plasma sprayed coatings of hydroxyapatite. *J. Biomed. Mater. Res.* 21:1375–1381.
87. Bourdin, E., Fauchais, P., and M. Boulos. 1983. Transient heat conduction under plasma conditions. *Int. J. Heat Mass Transfer*. 26:567–582.
88. Fauchias, P., Coudert, J. F., Vardelle, M., Vardelle, A., and A. Denoirjean. 1992. Diagnostics of thermal spray plasma jets. *J. Thermal Spray Technol.* 1:117–128.
89. Pfender, E. 1994. Plasma jet behavior and modeling associated with the plasma spray process. *Thin Solid Films* 238:228–241.
90. Wang, M. 2004. Bioactive materials and processing. In *Biomaterials and Tissue Engineering*, D. Shi (ed.), 40–45. Berlin: Springer Verlag.
91. Grabmann, O., and R. B. Heimann. 2000. Compositional and microstructural changes of engineered plasma-sprayed hydroxyapatite coatings on Ti6Al4V substrates during incubation in protein-free simulated body fluid. *J. Biomed. Mater. Mater. B* 53[6]:685–693.
92. Carayon, M. T., and J. L. Lacout. 2003. Study of the Ca/P atomic ratio of the amorphous phase in plasma-sprayed hydroxyapatite coatings. *J. Solid State Chem.* 172:339–350.
93. Montel, G., Bonel, G., Trombe, J. C., Heughebaert, J. C., and C. Rey. 1980. Progress in the area of chemistry of solid phosphorus-compounds with apatite structure—Application to biology and processing of minerals. *Pure Appl. Chem.* 52:973–987.
94. Heimann, R. B. 2006. Thermal spraying of biomaterials. *Surf. Coat. Technol.* 201:2012–2019.
95. Riboud, P. V. 1973. Composition and stability of apatites in system CaO-P_2O_5-iron oxide H_2O at high-temperature. *Ann. Chim.* 8:381–390.
96. Dyshlovenko, S., Pateyton, B., Pawlowski, L., and D. Murano. 2004. Numerical simulation of hydroxyapatite powder behaviour in plasma jet. *Surf. Coat. Technol.* 179:110–117.
97. Dyshlovenko, S., Pateyton, B., Pawlowski, L., and D. Murano. 2004. Erratum: Numerical simulation of hydroxyapatite powder behaviour in plasma jet. *Surf. Coat. Technol.* 187:408–409.
98. LeGeros, R. Z. 1993. Biodegradation and bioresorption of calcium phosphate ceramics. *Clin. Mater.* 14:65–88.
99. Kweh, S. W. K., Khor, K. A., and P. Cheang. 2000. Plasma-sprayed hydroxyapatite (HA) coatings with flame-spheroidized feedstock: Microstructure and mechanical properties. *Biomaterials* 21:1223–1234.
100. Yang, Y. C., and E. Chang. 2003. The bonding of plasma-sprayed hydroxyapatite coatings to titanium: Effect of processing, porosity and residual stress. *Thin Solid Films* 444:260–275.
101. Yang, C. W., Lee, T. M., Lui, T. S., and E. Chang. 2005. A comparison of the microstructural feature and bonding strength of plasma-sprayed hydroxyapatite coatings with hydrothermal and vacuum post-heat treatment. *Mater. Trans.* 46[3]:709–715.

102. Gross, K. A., Berndt, C. C., and H. Herman. 1998. Amorphous phase formation in plasma-sprayed hydroxyapatite coatings. *J. Biomed. Mater. Res.* 39:407–414.
103. Zyman, Z., Weng, J., Liu, X., Zhang, X., and Z. Ma. 1993. Amorphous phase and morphological structure of hydroxyapatite plasma coatings. *Biomaterials* 14:225–228.
104. Li, H., Ng, B. S., Khor, K. A., Cheang, P., and T. W. Clyne. 2004. Raman spectroscopy determination of phases within thermal sprayed hydroxyapatite splats and subsequent in vitro dissolution examination. *Acta Mater.* 52:445–453.
105. Darimont, G. L., Gilbert, B., and R. Cloots. 2004. Non-destructive evaluation of crystallinity and chemical composition by Raman spectroscopy in hydroxyapatite-coated implants. *Mater. Lett.* 58:71–73.
106. Young, R. A. 1988. Pressing the limits of Rietveld refinement. *Aust. J. Phys.* 41:297–310.
107. Young, R. A. 1993. *The Rietveld Method*, International Union of Crystallography. New York: Oxford University Press.
108. Kumar, R., Cheang, P., Khor, K. A., and T. White. 2001. XRD and Rietveld quantitative phase analysis of radio frequency suspension plasma sprayed nano-hydroxyapatite powders. In *Proceedings of the International Thermal Spray Conference*, 93–98. ASM International.
109. Kumar, R., Cheang, P., and K. A. Khor. 2003. Radio frequency (RF) suspension plasma sprayed ultra-fine hydroxyapatite (HA)/zirconia composite powders. *Biomaterials* 24:2611–2621.
110. Keller, L. 1995. X-ray powder diffraction patterns of calcium phosphate analyzed by the Rietveld method. *J. Biomed. Mater. Res.* 29:1403–1413.
111. Keller, L., and W. A. Dollase. 2000. X-ray determination of crystalline hydroxyapatite to amorphous calcium-phosphate ratio in plasma sprayed coatings. *J. Biomed. Mater. Res.* 49:244–249.
112. Wang, B. C., Chang, E., Yang, C. Y., Tu, D., and C. H. Tsai. 1993. Characteristics and osteoconductivity of three different plasma-sprayed hydroxyapatite coatings. *Surf. Coat. Technol.* 58:107–117.
113. Li, H., Khor, K. A., and P. Cheang. 2002. Properties of heat-treated calcium phosphate coatings deposited by high-velocity oxy-fuel (HVOF) spray. *Biomaterials* 23:2105–2112.
114. Khor, K. A., Gu, Y. W., Pan, D., and P. Cheang. 2004. Microstructure and mechanical properties of plasma sprayed HA/YSZ/Ti-6Al-4V composite coatings. *Biomaterials* 25:4009–4017.
115. Espanol, M., Guipont, V., Khor, K. A., Jeandin, M., and N. Ilorca-Isern. 2002. Effect of heat treatment on high pressure plasma sprayed hydroxyapatite coatings. *Surf. Eng.* 18[3]:213–218.
116. Gross, K. A., Gross, V., and C. C. Berndt. 1998. Thermal analysis of amorphous phases in hydroxyapatite coatings. *J. Am. Ceram. Soc.* 81:106–112.
117. Chou, B. Y., and E. Chang. 2002. Phase transformation during plasma spraying of hydroxyapatite–10-wt%-zirconia composite coating. *J. Am. Ceram. Soc.* 85:661–669.
118. Cullity, B. D. 1978. *Elements of X-ray Diffraction*. Philippines: Addison-Wesley.
119. Yang, C. W., and T. S. Lui. 2008. Crystallization effect on bonding strength and failure mechanism of plasma-sprayed hydroxyapatite coatings. In *Biomimetic and Supramolecular Systems Research*, Arturo H. Lima (ed.), Hauppauge, NY: Nova Science Publishers Inc.
120. Yang, C. W., and T. S. Lui. 2007. Effect of crystallization on the bonding strength and failures of plasma-sprayed hydroxyapatite. *Mater. Trans.* 48[2]:211–218.
121. Yang, C. Y., Lee, T. M., and C. W. Yang et al. 2007. The in vitro and in vivo biological responses of plasma-sprayed hydroxyapatite coatings with post-hydrothermal treatment. *J. Biomed. Mater. Res.* 83A:263–271.
122. Yang, C. W., and T. S. Lui. 2008. The self-healing effect of hydrothermal crystallization on the mechanical and failure properties of hydroxyapatite coatings. *J. Eur. Ceram. Soc.* 28:2151–2159.
123. Aoki, H. 1991. *Science and Medical Applications of Hydroxyapatite*. Takayama Press System Center Co., Tokyo: Japanese Association of Apatite Science, JAAS.
124. Ducheyne, P., Kokubo, T., and C. A. van Blitterswijk (eds.) 1992. *Bone-Bonding Biomaterials*. London: Reed Healthcare Communications.

125. Yoshimura, M., and H. Suda. 1994. Hydrothermal processing of HAp: Past, present and future. In *Hydroxyapatite and Related Compounds*, P. W. Brown and B. Constantz (eds.), 45–72. Cleveland, OH: CRC Press Inc., Taylor & Francis.
126. Yamashita, K., and T. Kanazawa. 1989. Hydroxyapatite. In *Inorganic Phosphate Materials*, T. Kanazawa (ed.), 15. *Materials Science Monograph* 52. Tokyo: Kodansha and Elsevier.
127. Ioku, K., Yoshimura, M., and S. Somiya. 1989. Microstructure-designed HAp ceramics from fine single crystals synthesized hydrothermally. In *Bioceramics, Proc. 1st Int. Bioceram. Symp.*, H. Oonishi, H. Aoki, and K. Sawai (eds.), 62–67. Tokyo: Ishiyaku Euro-America Inc.
128. Shi, D. 2004. *Biomaterials and Tissue Engineering*. Berlin: Springer.
129. Prener, J. S. 1967. The growth and crystallographic properties of calcium fluor- and chlorapatite crystals. *J. Electrochem. Soc.* 114:77–83.
130. Oishi, S., and T. Kamiya. 1994. Flux growth of fluorapatite crystals. *J. Chem. Soc. Jpn*. 9:800–804.
131. Oishi, S., and I. Sugiura. 1997. Growth of chlorapatite crystals from a sodium chloride flux. *Bull. Chem. Soc. Jpn*. 70:2483–2487.
132. Aoki, H. 1994. *Medical Applications of Hydroxyapatite*. Tokyo: Ishiyaku EuroAmerica.
133. Suchanek, W., and M. Yoshimura. 1998. Processing and properties of hydroxyapatite-based biomaterials for use as hard tissue replacement implant. *J. Mater. Res.* 13:1–24.
134. Hsu, Y. S., Chang, E., and H. S. Liu. 1998. Growth of phosphate coating on titanium substrate by hydrothermal process. *Ceram. Int.* 24:7–12.
135. Han, Y., Xu, K., and J. Lu. 1999. Morphology and composition of hydroxyapatite coatings prepared by hydrothermal treatment on electrodeposited brushite coatings. *J. Mater. Sci.: Mater. Med.* 10:243–248.
136. Zhang, H., Li, S., and Y. Yan. 2001. Dissolution behavior of hydroxyapatite powder in hydrothermal solution. *Ceram. Int.* 27:451–454.
137. Suchanek, W. L., Byrappa, K., Shuk, P., Riman, R. E., Janas, V. F., and K. S. TenHuisen. 2004. Preparation of magnesium-substituted hydroxyapatite powders by the mechanochemical–hydrothermal method. *Biomaterials* 25:4647–4657.
138. Oniki, T., and T. Hashida. 2006. New method for hydroxyapatite coating of titanium by the hydrothermal hot isostatic pressing technique. *Surf. Coat. Technol.* 200:6801–6807.
139. Hosoi, K., Hashida, T., Takahashi, H., Yamasaki, N., and T. Korenaga. 1996. New processing technique for hydroxyapatite ceramics by the hydrothermal hot-pressing method. *J. Am. Ceram. Soc.* 79[10]:2771–2774.
140. Jinawath, S., Polchai, D., and M. Yoshimura. 2002. Low-temperature hydrothermal transformation of aragonite to hydroxyapatite. *Mater. Sci. Eng. C* 22:35–39.
141. Zhang, X., and K. S. Vecchio. 2007. Hydrothermal synthesis of hydroxyapatite rods. *J. Cryst. Growth* 308:133–140.
142. Ashok, M., Kalkura, S. N., Sundaram, N. M., and D. Arivuoli. 2007. Growth and characterization of hydroxyapatite crystals by hydrothermal method. *J. Mater. Sci.: Mater. Med.* 18:895–898.
143. Zhu, R., Yu, R., Yao, J., Wang, D., and J. Ke. 2008. Morphology control of hydroxyapatite through hydrothermal process. *J. Alloys Compd.* 457:555–559.
144. Zhang, H.-B., Zhou, K.-C., Li, Z.-Y., and S.-P. Huang. 2009. Plate-like hydroxyapatite nanoparticles synthesized by the hydrothermal methods. *J. Phys. Chem. Solids* 70:243–248.
145. Yoshimura, M., Sujaridworakun, P., Koh, F., Fujiwara, T., Pongkao, D., and A. Ahniyaz. 2004. Hydrothermal conversion of calcite crystals to hydroxyapatite. *Mater. Sci. Eng. C* 24:521–525.
146. Riman, R. E., Suchanek, W. L., Byrappa, K., Chen, C. W., Shuk, P., and C. S. Oakes. 2002. Solution synthesis of hydroxyapatite designer particulates. *Solid State Ionic* 151:393–402.
147. Ishikawa, K., and E. D. Eanes. 1993. The hydrolysis of anhydrous dicalcium phosphate into hydroxyapatite. *J. Dent. Res.* 72:474–480.
148. Zhu, K., Yanagisawa, K., Onda, A., and K. Kajiyoshi. 2004. Hydrothermal synthesis and morphology variation of cadmium hydroxyapatite. *J. Solid State Chem.* 177:4379–4385.
149. Morey, G. W., and P. Niggli. 1913. The hydrothermal formation of silicates, a review. *J. Am. Chem. Soc.* 35:1086–1130.

150. Laudise, R. A. 1970. *The Growth of Single Crystals*, 278–281. Englewood Cliffs, NJ: Prentice-Hall.
151. Rabenau, A. 1985. The role of hydrothermal synthesis in preparative chemistry. *Angew. Chem. (Engl. Ed.)* 24:1026–1040.
152. Lobachev, A. N. 1973. *Crystallization Process under Hydrothermal Conditions*, 1–255. New York, NY: Consultants Bureau.
153. Roy, R. 1994. Acceleration the kinetics of low-temperature inorganic syntheses. *J. Solid State Chem.* 111:11–17.
154. Byrappa, K. 1992. *Hydrothermal Growth of Crystals*, 1–365. Oxford, UK: Pergamon Press.
155. Roy, D. M., and S. K. Linnehan. 1974. Hydroxyapatite formed from coral skeletal carbonate by hydrothermal exchange. *Nature* 247:220–222.
156. Ito, A., Nakamura, S., and H. Aoki, et al. 1996. Hydrothermal growth of carbonate-containing hydroxyapatite single crystals. *J. Cryst. Growth* 163:311–317.
157. Ito, A., Teraoka, K., Tsutsumi, S., and T. Tateishi. 1996. Single crystal hydroxyapatite: Preparation, composition and mechanical properties. *Bioceramics* 9:189–192.
158. LeGeros, R. Z. 1991. *Calcium Phosphates in Oral Biology and Medicine Vol. 15*. Basel: S. Karger.
159. LeGeros, R. Z. 1967. Crystallographic studies of the carbonate substitution in the apatite structure. PhD thesis, New York University.
160. Kokubo, T., Kim, H. M., and M. Kawashita. 2003. Novel bioactive materials with different mechanical properties. *Biomaterials* 24:2161–2175.
161. Yamasaki, N., Yanagisawa, K., Nishioka, M., and S. Kanahara. 1986. Hydrothermal hot-pressing method: Apparatus and application. *J. Mater. Sci. Lett.* 5:355–356.
162. Onoki, T., Hosoi, K., and T. Hashida. 2003. Joining hydroxyapatite ceramics and titanium alloys by hydrothermal method. *Key Eng. Mater.* 240–242:571–574.
163. Onoki, T. Higashi, T., and X. Wang et al. 2009. Interface structure between Ti-based bulk metallic glasses and hydroxyapatite ceramics jointed by hydrothermal techniques. *Mater. Trans.* 50[6]:1308–1312.
164. Monma, H., and T. Kamiya. 1987. Preparation of hydroxyapatite by the hydrolysis of brushite. *J. Mater. Sci.* 22:4247–4250.
165. Li, J., and T. Hashida. 2007. Preparation of hydroxyapatite ceramics by hydrothermal hot-pressing method at 300°C. *J. Mater. Sci.* 42:5013–5019.
166. Onoki, T., Hosoi, K., and T. Hashida et al. 2008. Effects of titanium surface modifications on bonding behavior of hydroxyapatite ceramics and titanium by hydrothermal hot-pressing. *Mater. Sci. Eng. C* 28:207–212.
167. Chang, C., Huang, J., Xia, J., and C. Ding. 1999. Study on crystallization kinetics of plasma sprayed hydroxyapatite coating. *Ceram. Int.* 25:479–483.
168. Roeder, R. K., Converse, G. L., Leng, H., and W. Yue. 2006. Kinetics effects on hydroxyapatite whiskers synthesized by the chelate decomposition method. *J. Am. Ceram. Soc.* 89[7]:2096–2104.
169. Campos, A. L., Silva, N. T., Melo, F. C. L., Oliverira, M. A. S., and G. P. Thim. 2002. Crystallization kinetics of orthorhombic mullite from diphasic. *J. Non-Cryst. Solids* 304:19–24.
170. Huang, L. Y., Xu, K. W., and J. Lu. 2000. A study of the process and kinetics of electrochemical deposition and the hydrothermal synthesis of hydroxyapatite coatings. *J. Mater. Sci.: Mater. Med.* 11:667–673.
171. Yang, C. W., and T. S. Lui. 2009. Kinetics of hydrothermal crystallization under saturated steam pressure and the self-healing effect by nanocrystallite for hydroxyapatite coatings. *Acta Biomater.* 5:2728–2737.
172. Tong, W., Chen, J., Cao, Y., Lu, L., Feng, J., and X. Zhang. 1997. Effect of water vapor pressure and temperature on the amorphous-to-crystalline HA conversion during heat treatment of HA coatings. *J. Biomed. Mater. Res.* 36:242–245.
173. Zeng, H., and W. R. Lacefield. 2001. XPS, EDX and FTIR analysis of pulsed laser deposited calcium phosphate bioceramic coatings: The effects of various process parameters. *Biomaterials* 21:23–30.

174. Dong, Z. L., Khor, K. A., Quek, C. H., White, T. J., and P. Cheang. 2003. TEM and STEM analysis on heat-treated and *in vitro* plasma-sprayed hydroxyapatite/Ti-6Al-4V composite coatings. *Biomaterials* 24:97–105.
175. Arias, J. L., Garcia-Sanz, F. J., and M. B. Mayor, et al. 1998. Physicochemical properties of calcium phosphate coatings produced by pulsed laser deposition at different water vapour pressures. *Biomaterials* 19:883–888.
176. Boyd, A., Akay, M., and B. J. Meenan. 2003. Influence of target surface degradation on the properties of RF magnetron-sputtered calcium phosphate coatings. *Surf. Interface. Anal.* 35:188–198.
177. Takadama, H., Kim, H. M., Kokubo, T., and T. Nakamura. 2001. An X-ray photoelectron spectroscopy study of the process of apatite formation on bioactive titanium metal. *J. Biomed. Mater. Res.* 55:185–193.
178. Massaro, C., Baker, M. A., Cosentino, F., Ramires, P. A., Klose, S., and E. Milella. 2001. Surface and biological evaluation of hydroxyapatite-based coatings on titanium deposited by different techniques. *J. Biomed. Mater. Res.* 58B:651–657.
179. Healy, K. E., and P. Ducheyne P. 1992. The mechanisms of passive dissolution of titanium in a model physiological environment. *J. Biomed. Mater. Res.* 26:319–338.
180. Ramires, P. A., Romito, A. M., Cosentino, F., and E. Milella. 2001. The influence of titania/hydroxyapatite composite coatings on in vitro osteoblasts behavior. *Biomaterials* 22:1467–1474.
181. Yang, Y., Kim, K. H., Agrawal, C. M., and J. L. Ong. 2003. Influence of post-deposition heating time and the presence of water vapor on sputter-coated calcium phosphate crystallinity. *J. Dent. Res.* 82:833–837.
182. Liu, C., Huang, Y., Shen, W., and J. Cui. 2001. Kinetics of hydroxyapatite precipitation at pH 10 to 11. *Biomaterials* 22:301–306.
183. Ueda, M., Imai, Y., Motoe, A., Uchida, K., and N. Aso. 2000. Adhesion of hydroxyapatite layer prepared by thermal plasma spraying to titanium or titanium (IV) oxide substrate. *J. Ceram. Soc. Jpn.* 108:865–868.
184. Fernández-Pradas, J. M., García-Cuenca, M. V., Clèries, L., Sardin, G., and J. L. Morenza. 2002. Influence of the interface layer on the adhesion of pulsed laser deposited hydroxyapatite coatings on titanium alloy. *Appl. Surf. Sci.* 195:31–37.
185. Cheng, K., Zhang, S., Weng, W., Khor, K. A., Miao, S., and Y. Wang. 2008. The adhesion strength and residual stress of colloidal-sol gel derived β-tricalcium phosphate/fluoridated-hydroxyapatite biphasic coatings. *Thin Solid Films* 516:3251–3255.
186. Ievlev, V. M., Domashevskaya, E. P., and V. I. Putlyaev et al. 2008. Structure, elemental composition, and mechanical properties of films prepared by radio-frequency magnetron sputtering of hydroxyapatite. *Glass Phys. Chem.* 34:608–616.
187. Cheng, K., Ren, C., and W. Wang et al. 2009. Bonding strength of fluoridated hydroxyapatite coatings: A comparative study on pull-out and scratch analysis. *Thin Solid Films* 517:5361–5364.
188. Heleno, R. A., Wagner, N. S., and J. R. T. Branco. 2009. Performance evaluation of hydroxyapatite coatings thermally sprayed on surgical fixation pins. *Key Eng. Mater.* 396–398:69–75.
189. Xiong, X.-B., Zeng, X.-R., Zou, C.-L., Li, P., and Y.-B. Fan. 2009. Influence of hydrothermal temperature on hydroxyapatite coating transformed from monetite on HT-C/C composites by induction heating method. *Surf. Coat. Technol.* 204:115–119.
190. Wang, B. C., Lee, T. M., Chang, E., and C. Y. Yang. 1992. Effect of coating thickness on the shear strength and failure mode of plasma sprayed hydroxyapatite coatings to bone. *Biomed. Eng.* 4:605–609.
191. Hayashi, K., Inadome, T., Mashima, T., and Y. Sugioka. 1993. Comparison of bone-implant interface shear strength of solid hydroxyapatite and hydroxyapatite-coated titanium implants. *J. Biomed. Mater. Res.* 27:557–563.
192. Moroni, A., Caja, V. L., Sabato, C., Egger, E. L., Gottsauner-Wolf, F., and E. Y. S. Chao. 1994. Bone ingrowth analysis and interface evaluation of hydroxyapatite coated versus uncoated titanium porous bone implants. *J. Mater. Sci.: Mater. Med.* 5:411–416.
193. Wang, S., Lacefield, W. R., and J. E. Lemons. 1996. Interfacial shear strength and histology of plasma sprayed and sintered hydroxyapatite implants in vivo. *Biomaterials* 17:1965–1970.

194. Thompson, J. I., Greqson, P. J., and P. A. Revell. 1999. Analysis of push-out test data based on interfacial fracture energy. *J. Mater. Sci.: Mater. Med.* 10:863–868.
195. Lopes, M. A., Santos, J. D., and F. J. Monteiro, et al. 2001. Push-out testing and histological evaluation of glass reinforced hydroxyapatite composites implanted in the tibia of rabbits. *J. Biomed. Mater. Res.* 54:463–469.
196. Lee, T. M., Yang, C. Y., Chang, E., and R. S. Tsai. 2004. Comparison of plasma-sprayed hydroxyapatite coatings and zirconia-reinforced hydroxyapatite composite coatings: In vivo study. *J. Biomed. Mater. Res. A* 71:652–660.
197. Sergo, V., Sbaizero, O., and D. R. Clarke. 1997. Mechanical and chemical consequences of the residual stresses in plasma sprayed hydroxyapatite coatings. *Biomaterials* 18:477–482.
198. Spivak, J. M., Ricci, J. L., Blumenthal, N. C., and H. Alexander. 1990. A new canine model to evaluate the biological response of intramedullary bone to implant materials and surfaces. *J. Biomed. Mater. Res.* 24:1121–1149.
199. Park, E., Condrate, R. A., Hoelzer, D. T., and G. S. Fischman. 1998. Interfacial characterization of plasma-spray coated calcium phosphate on Ti-6Al-4V. *J. Mater. Sci.: Mater. Med.* 9:643–649.
200. Wen, J., Leng, Y., Chen, J., and C. Zhang. 2000. Chemical gradient in plasma-sprayed HA coatings. *Biomaterials* 21:1339–1343.
201. DeBruijn, J. D., Bovell, Y., and C. van Blitterswijk. 1994. Structural arrangements at the interface between plasma sprayed calcium phosphates and bone. *Biomaterials* 15:543–550.
202. Tsui, Y. C., Doyle, C., and T. W. Clyne. 1998. Plasma sprayed hydroxyapatite coatings on titanium substrates: Part 1. Mechanical properties and residual stress levels. *Biomaterials* 19:2015–2029.
203. Ji, H., Ponton, C. B., and P. M. Marquis. 1992. Microstructural characterization of hydroxyapatite coating on titanium. *J. Mater. Sci.: Mater. Med.* 3:283–287.
204. Kurzweg, H., Heimann, R. B., and T. Troczynski. 1998. Adhesion of thermally sprayed hydroxyapatite-bond-coat systems measured by a novel peel test. *J. Mater. Sci.: Mater. Med.* 9:9–16.
205. Heimann, R. B., Kurzweg, H., Ivey, D. G., and M. L. Wayman. 1998. Microstructural and *in vitro* chemical investigations into plasma-sprayed bioceramic coatings. *J. Biomed. Mater. Res. B* 43[4]:441–450.
206. Heimann, R. B. 1999. Design of novel plasma sprayed hydroxyapatite-bond coat bioceramic systems. *J. Therm. Spray Technol.* 8[4]:597–604.
207. Heimann, R. B., Schürmann, N., and R. T. Müller. 2004. In vitro and in vivo performance of Ti6Al4V implants with plasma-sprayed osteoconductive hydroxylapatite-bioinert titania bond coat "duplex" systems: An experimental study in sheep. *J. Mater. Sci.: Mater. Med.* 15:1045–1052.
208. Heimann, R. B., and R. Wirth. 2006. Formation and transformation of amorphous calcium phosphates on titanium alloy surfaces during atmospheric plasma spraying and their subsequent in vitro performance. *Biomaterials* 27:823–831.
209. Lo, T. N., Chang, E., and T. S. Lui. 2004. Interfacial characterization of porcelain veneered on the pure titanium under vacuum firing. *Mater. Trans.* 45:3065–3070.
210. Yang, Y. C. 2007. Influence of residual stress on bonding strength of plasma-sprayed hydroxyapatite coating after the vacuum heat treatment. *Surf. Coat. Technol.* 201:7187–7193.
211. Li, C.-J., Ohmori, A., and R. McPherson. 1997. The relationship between microstructure and Young's modulus of thermally sprayed ceramic coatings. *J. Mater. Sci.* 32:997–1004.
212. Kim, H. J., and Y. G. Kweon. 1999. Elastic modulus of plasma-sprayed coatings determined by indentation and bend tests. *Thin Solid Films* 342:201–206.
213. Yang, Y. C., Chang, E., and S. Y. Lee. 2003. Mechanical properties and Young's modulus of plasma-sprayed hydroxyapatite coating on Ti substrate in simulated body fluid. *J. Biomed. Mater. Res. A* 67:886–899.
214. Chiang, Y. M., Birnie, D. P., and W. D. Kingery. 1997. *Physical Ceramics: Principles for Ceramics Science and Engineering*, 478–484. New York: John Wiley & Sons, Inc.
215. Beshish, G. K., Florey, C. W., Worzala, F. J., and W. J. Lenling. 1993. Fracture toughness of thermal spray ceramic coatings determined by the indentation technique. *J. Thermal Spray Technol.* 2:35–38.

216. Brown, S. R., Turner, I. G., and H. Reiter. 1994. Residual stress measurement in thermal sprayed hydroxyapatite coatings. *J. Mater. Sci.: Mater. Med.* 5:756–759.
217. Yang, Y. C., Chang, E., Hwang, B. H., and S. Y. Lee. 2000. Biaxial residual stress states of plasma-sprayed hydroxyapatite coatings on titanium alloy substrate. *Biomaterials* 21:1327–1337.
218. Yang, Y. C., and E. Chang. 2001. Influence of residual stress on bonding strength and fracture of plasma-sprayed hydroxyapatite coatings on Ti-6Al-4V substrate. *Biomaterials* 22:1827–1836.
219. Yang, Y. C., and C. Y. Yang. 2008. The influence of residual stress on the shear strength between the bone and plasma-sprayed hydroxyapatite coating. *J. Mater. Sci.: Mater. Med.* 19:1051–1060.
220. Yang, Y. C., and E. Chang. 2004. Measurements of residual stresses in plasma-sprayed coatings on titanium alloy. *Surf. Coat. Technol.* 190:122–131.
221. Evans, A. G., Crumley, G. B., and R. E. Demaray. 1983. On the mechanical behavior of brittle coatings and layers. *Oxidat. Met.* 20:196–216.
222. Mevrel, R. 1987. Cyclic oxidation of high-temperature alloys. *Mater. Sci. Technol.* 3:531–535.
223. Tucker, R. C. 2002. Thermal spray coatings: Broad and growing applications. *Int. J. Powder Metall.* 38:45–53.
224. Toma, D., Brandl, W., and G. Marginean. 2001. Wear and corrosion resistance of thermally sprayed cermet coatings. *Surf. Coat. Technol.* 138:149–158.
225. Liao, H., Normand, B., and C. Coddet. 2000. Influence of coating microstructure on the abrasive wear resistance of WC/Co cermet coatings. *Surf. Coat. Technol.* 124:235–242.
226. Li, C.-J., and A. Ohmori. 2002. Relationship between the structure and properties of thermally sprayed coatings. *J. Thermal Spray Technol.* 11:365–374.
227. McPherson, R., and B. V. Shafer. 1982. Interlamellar contact within plasma-sprayed coatings. *Thin Solid Films* 97:201–214.
228. Ohmori, A., and C.-J. Li. 1991. Quantitative characterization of the structure of plasma sprayed Al_2O_3 coating by using copper electroplating. *Thin Solid Films* 201:241–252.
229. Ohmori, A., Li, C.-J., and Y. Arata. 1990. Influence of plasma spray conditions on the structure of Al_2O_3 coatings. *Trans. Jpn. Weld. Res. Inst.* 19:259–270.
230. Lintner, F., Bohm, G., Huber, M., and R. Scholz. 1994. Histology of tissue adjacent to an HAC-coated femoral prosthesis—a case report. *J. Bone Jt. Surg.* 76B:824–830.
231. Fu, Y. Q., Batchelor, A. W., and K. A. Khor. 1999. Fretting wear behavior of thermal sprayed hydroxyapatite coating lubricated with bovine albumin. *Wear* 230:98–102.
232. Coathup, M. J., Blackburn, J., Goodship, A. E., Cunninghum, J. L., Smith, T., and G. W. Blunn. 2005. Role of hydroxyapatite coating in resisting wear particle migration and osteolysis around acetabular components. *Biomaterials* 26:4161–4169.
233. Morks, M. F. 2008. Fabrication and characterization of plasma-sprayed HA/SiO_2 coatings for biomedical application. *J. Mech. Behav. Biomed. Mater.* 1:105–111.
234. Liou, J. W., Chen, L. H., and T. S. Lui. 1995. The concept of effective hardness in the abrasion of coarse 2-phase materials with hard 2nd-phase particles. *J. Mater. Sci.* 30:258–262.
235. Liou, J. W., Lui, T. S., and L. H. Chen. 1997. SiO_2 particle erosion of A356.2 aluminum alloy and the related microstructural changes. *Wear* 211:169–176.
236. Yang, C. W., Lui, T. S., and L. H. Chen. 2009. Hydrothermal crystallization effect on the improvement of erosion resistance and reliability of plasma-sprayed hydroxyapatite coatings. *Thin Solid Films* 517:5380–5385.
237. Lai, K. A., Shen, W. J., Chen, C. H., Yang, C. Y., Hu, W. P., and G. L. Chang. 2002. Failure of hydroxyapatite-coated acetabular cups: Ten-year follow-up of 85 Landos Atoll arthroplasties. *J. Bone Jt. Surg. [Br]* 84B:641–646.
238. Dodson, B., and D. Nolan. 2002. *Reliability Engineering Handbook*. Boca Raton, FL: CRC Press Inc., Taylor & Francis.
239. Burrow, M. F., Thomas, D., Swain, M. V., and M. J. Tyas. 2004. Analysis of tensile strengths using Weibull statistics. *Biomaterials* 25:5031–5035.
240. Weibull, W. 1951. A statistical distribution function of wide applicability. *J. Appl. Mech.* 18:293–297.

241. Keshevan, K., Sargent, G., and H. Conrad. 1980. Statistical analysis of the Hertzian fracture of Pyrex glass using the Weibull distribution function, *J. Mater. Sci.* 15:839–844.
242. Phani, K. K. 1987. A new modified Weibull distribution function. *Commun. Am. Ceram. Soc.* 70:182–184.
243. Yang, L., English, J. R., and T. L. Landers. 1995. Modeling latent and patent failures of electronic products. *Microelectron. Reliab.* 35:1501–1505.
244. Quereshi, F. S., and A. K. Sheikh. 1997. Probabilistic characterization of adhesive wear in metals. *IEEE Trans. Reliab.* 46:38–44.
245. Almeida, J. B. 1999. Application of Weibull statistics to the failure of coatings. *J. Mater. Process. Technol.* 93:257–263.
246. Talker, P., and R. O. Weber. 2000. Power spectrum and detrended fluctuation analysis: Application to daily temperatures. *Phys. Rev. E* 62:150–160.
247. Fok, S. L., Mitchell, B. C., Smart, J., and B. J. Marsden. 2001. A numerical study on the application of the Weibull theory to brittle materials. *Eng. Fract. Mech.* 68:1171–1179.
248. Villora, J. M., Callejas, P., Barba, M. F., and C. Baudin. 2004. Statistical analysis of the fracture behaviour of porous ceramic Raschig rings. *J. Eur. Ceram. Soc.* 24:589–594.
249. Abernethy, R. B. 2000. *The New Weibull Handbook: Reliability and Statistical Analysis for Predicting Life, Safety, Survivability, Risk, Cost and Warranty Claims*, 4th edition. North Palm Beach, FL: Robert B. Abernathy.
250. Faucher, B., and W. R. Tyson. 1988. On the determination of Weibull parameters. *J. Mater. Sci. Lett.* 7:1199–1203.
251. Lima, R. S., and B. R. Marple. 2003. High Weibull modulus HVOF titania coatings. *J. Thermal Spray Technol.* 12:240–249.

7

Bioceramic Coating on Titanium by Physical and Chemical Vapor Deposition

Takashi Goto, Takayuki Narushima, and Kyosuke Ueda

CONTENTS

Introduction

Metals, typically titanium (Ti) and its alloys, are reliable for use as biomaterials due to their strength, ductility, and durability in the human body. However, the tissue compatibility of such specific metals (metallic biomaterials) is insufficient for biomedical applications. Since the microstructure and phase of metallic materials are generally well-controlled by thermomechanical treatment in order to satisfy the mechanical properties required for biomedical applications, tissue compatibility should be improved while maintaining the microstructure and mechanical properties of these materials. Surface modification, in particular bioceramic coating, is a promising way to improve the tissue compatibility of biomaterials.

In this chapter, the preparation of bioceramic coatings on metallic biomaterials, mainly Ti and its alloys, by vapor deposition and their properties are discussed. Calcium phosphate coatings such as apatite with bone compatibility are commonly used as coating phases, and the Ti and its alloys are the metallic biomaterials mainly used as substrates. Since these metals can be directly connected to living bone at an optical microscopic level (i.e., osseointegration),[1,2] they have been used as substitutes for hard tissues such as in stems of artificial hip joints and dental implants for long-term implantation in bones.[3,4] Metallic biomaterials should usually be fixed in the human body without being moved for more than 3 months. A coating of bioactive calcium phosphate on Ti is applied for the stems of artificial hip joints and dental implants to obtain a strong bonding with bones and to shorten the fixation period.

Surface Modification of Metallic Biomaterials

The surface modification processes for improving the bone compatibility of metallic biomaterials are summarized in Figure 7.1.[5] They can be classified as dry and wet processes. Morphology and/or phase/composition of the surface layer of metallic biomaterials are modified in dry and wet processes by using ions/gases and solutions, respectively. The phase/composition is controlled by applying an apatite coating or by modifying the surface characteristics with nonapatite coating.

Vapor deposition can be used to apply apatite and other bioactive layers on metallic biomaterials. Apatite coating on metallic biomaterials has been developed since the 1970s, and plasma spraying has been clinically applied to apatite coating on Ti–6Al–4V implants since the mid-1980s after FDA approval in 1981.[6–8] Although plasma spraying has a long history of clinical applications in apatite coating due to the advantages of high deposition rates with sufficiently low cost, more reliable coatings have been sought to improve the bonding strength between the implants and the coatings while controlling the microstructure.

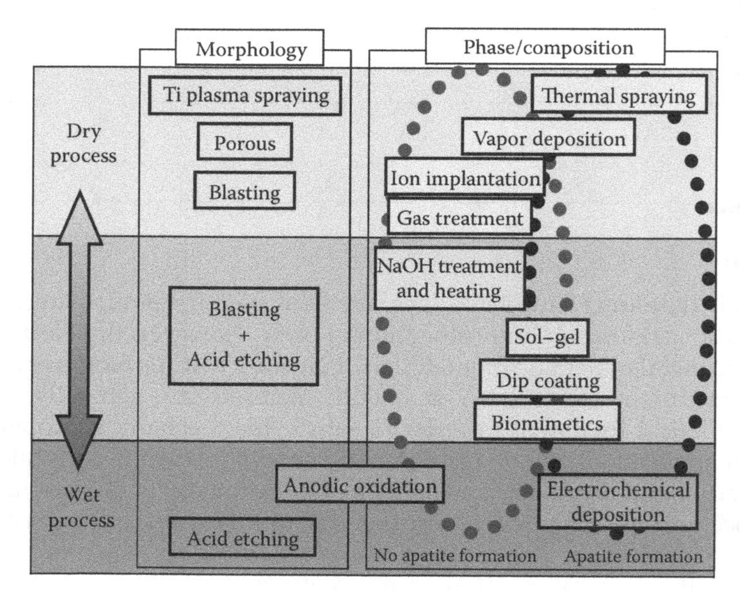

FIGURE 7.1
Surface modification processes of metallic biomaterials.

In order to develop more advanced bioceramic coatings on metallic biomaterials, many calcium phosphate coating processes including vapor deposition, biomimetics, and electrochemical deposition have been investigated.[9] These coating processes are shown in Figure 7.2, where they are categorized by processing temperature and thickness of coating, and also as to adherence and coating area.[5] Vapor deposition can be advantageous for the preparation of uniform and dense coatings of calcium phosphate with a well-controlled phase, composition, film thickness, and high bonding strength to metallic biomaterials. Vapor deposition is generally classified into physical vapor deposition (PVD) and chemical vapor deposition (CVD). Both PVD and CVD are used to prepare solid films or powders from a gas phase. Although hybrid processes such as activated reactive evaporation[10] have been reported, chemical reactions in the gas phase are basically involved in the CVD methods but not in the PVD methods. Ceramics are generally fabricated by powder sintering with various additives due to their high melting points, covalent nature, low self-diffusivities, and so forth. Vapor deposition techniques are suitable for the fabrication of highly pure and dense ceramics at relatively lower temperature without additives. Typical methods of PVD and CVD are summarized in Figure 7.3. The details of each method are described in the next section. All the vapor deposition methods require energy for the activation of source gases. The interaction between the particles (atoms/ions/clusters) and solid surface changes depending on their kinetic energy as shown in Figure 7.4: deposition, sputtering, and ion implantation.[11] Sputtering as a PVD method utilizes the above-mentioned phenomena of the kinetic energy of particles less than 10^3 eV for vaporization of target materials and of the kinetic energy of particles less than 10 eV for deposition from the gas phase.

PVD and CVD Methods

In PVD, a solid source material is physically vaporized by energy such as heat, plasma, or laser, and then thin films are deposited on a substrate. Consequently, the composition of

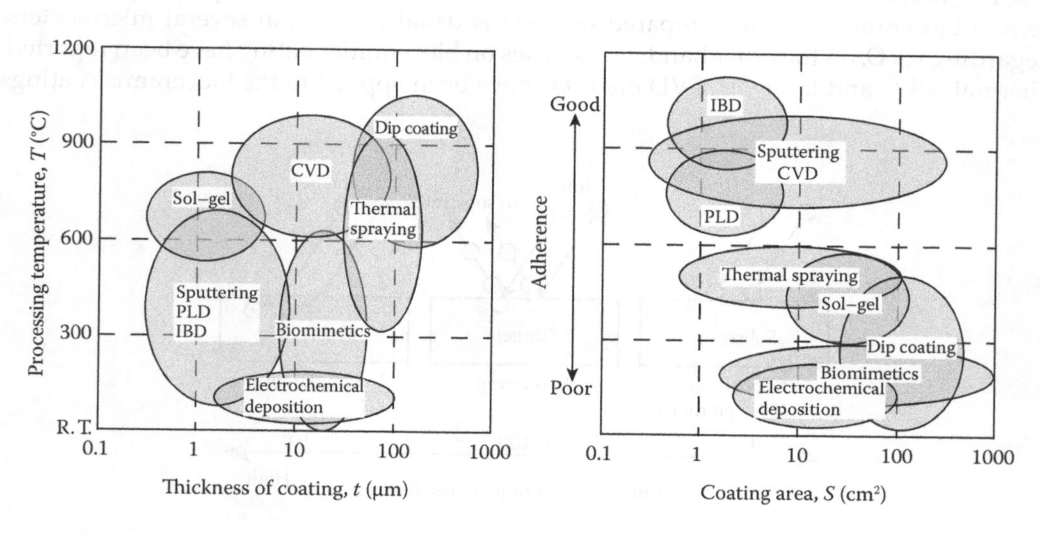

FIGURE 7.2
Processes for coating calcium–phosphate film on Ti substrate.

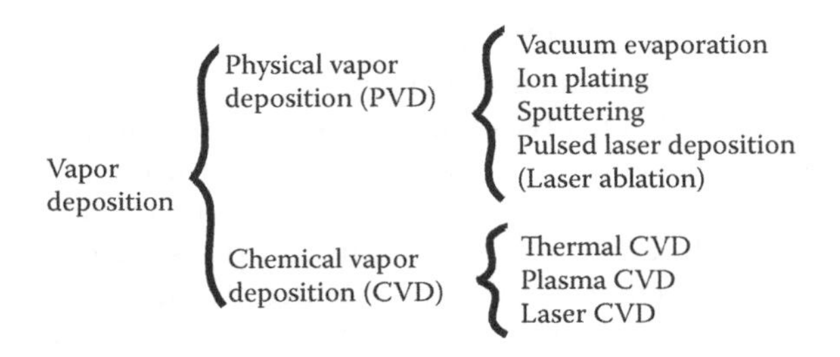

FIGURE 7.3
Typical methods of PVD and CVD.

thin films does not change significantly from that of the source materials. PVD methods such as vacuum deposition, sputtering, ion plating, pulsed laser deposition (PLD), and ion beam deposition (IBD) have been applied to bioceramic coating of metallic biomaterials. Figure 7.5 shows schematics of vacuum deposition, sputtering, ion plating, and PLD methods. In CVD, on the other hand, thin films or powders via chemical reactions such as thermal decomposition or hydrogen reduction of source gases are synthesized, and therefore the composition of films are often significantly different from that of the source gases. A schematic of the CVD method is depicted in Figure 7.6. Since CVD has generally more process parameters (deposition temperature, total pressure, partial pressure of each source gas, etc.) than PVD, the morphology and crystallographic orientation of coatings are more widely controllable. Therefore, pure, dense, and highly oriented films can be synthesized by CVD. In order to activate the chemical reactions, various energy sources such as heat, plasma, and laser are utilized in CVD.

Tables 7.1 and 7.2 summarize studies[12–23] of bioceramic coatings on Ti by PVD and CVD, respectively. Some characteristics and advantages of each PVD and CVD methods are included in these tables. As the target or source materials for PVD, hydroxyapatite ($Ca_{10}(PO_4)_6(OH)_2$, HAp)[12–14,18,19], β-type tricalcium phosphate ($Ca_3P_2O_8$, β-TCP),[15] HAp + β-TCP[17], and $CaO–P_2O_5$ glasses[24] have been fabricated by sintering or spraying. The thickness of bioceramic coatings prepared by PVD is usually less than several micrometers. Regarding CVD, on the other hand, few studies on bioceramic coating have been reported. Thermal[22,25–27] and laser[23,28] CVD methods have been applied to the bioceramic coatings

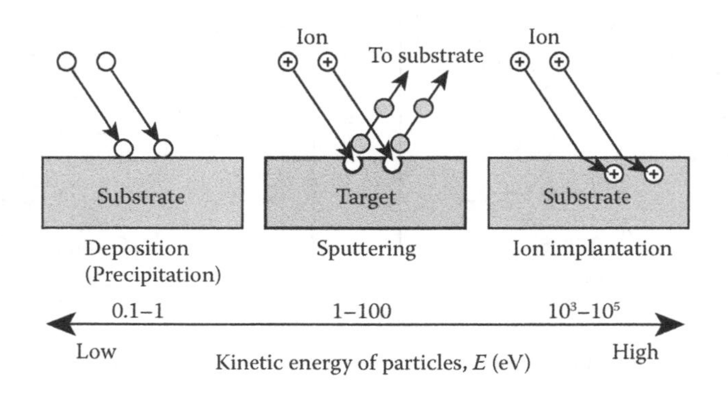

FIGURE 7.4
Interaction between particles and the solid surface.

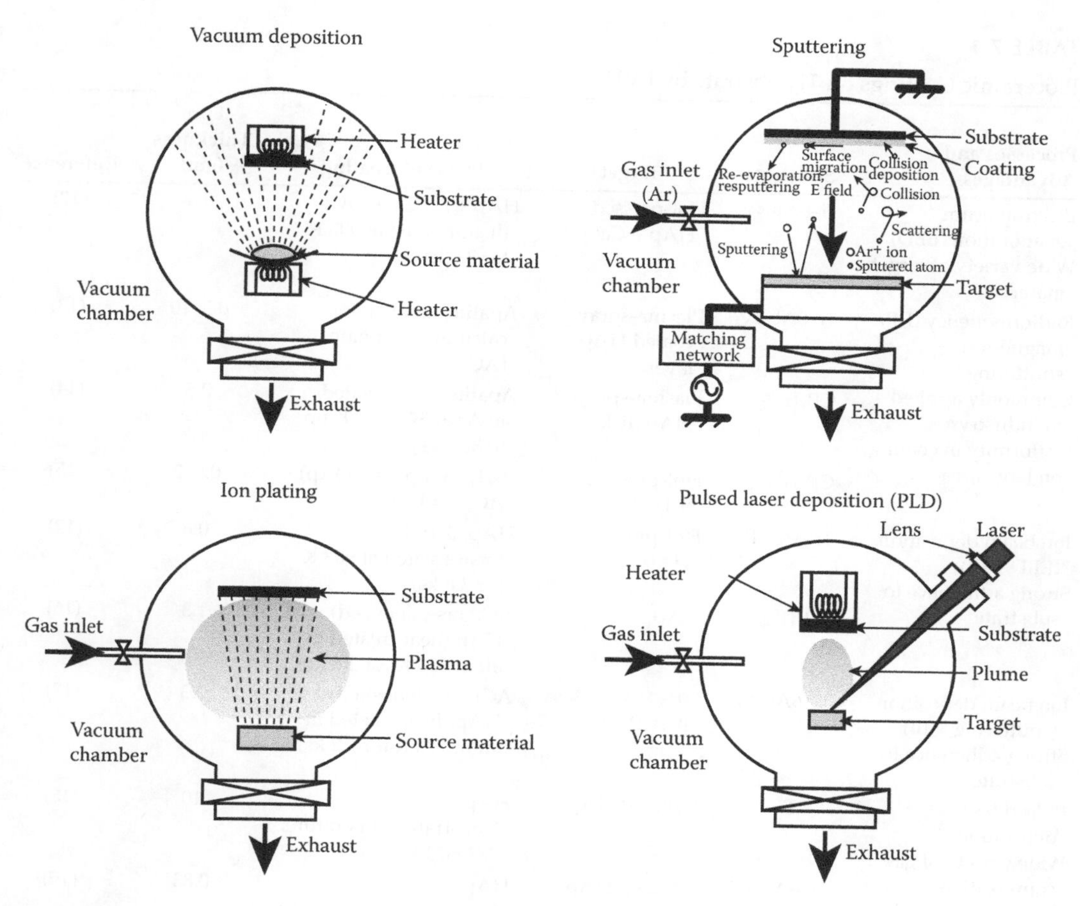

FIGURE 7.5
Schematic of vacuum deposition, sputtering, ion plating, and pulsed laser deposition methods.

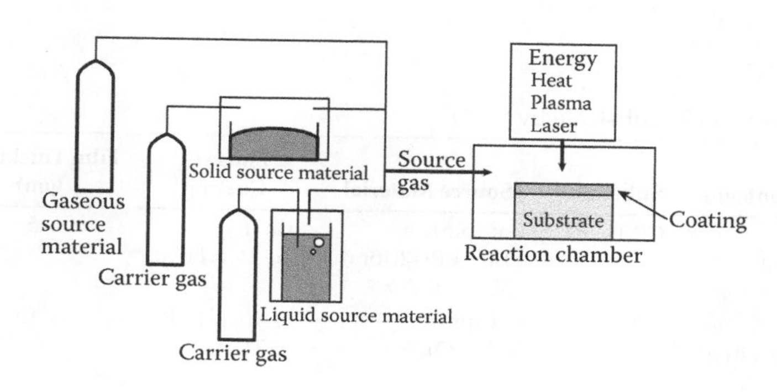

FIGURE 7.6
Schematic of CVD method.

TABLE 7.1

Bioceramic Coatings on Ti Substrate by PVD

Processes and Advantages	Substrate	Target	Phase of Coating	Film Thickness (μm)	Reference
Electron beam evaporation (EBD) Wide variety of target materials	Ti–6Al–4V	Hot-pressed HAp + CaO	HAp + β-TCP +CaO (heat-treated at 903 K for 3.6 ks)	0.6	(12)
Radiofrequency (RF) magnetron sputtering Commonly applied in industry Uniformity in coating on large area	Ti–6Al–4V	Plasma-spray coated HAp layer	Apatite, amorphous calcium phosphate (ACP)	0.5–10	(13)
	CP Ti	Plasma-sprayed HAp disk	Apatite (heat-treated in Ar at 573–973 K up to 86.4 ks)	2.5	(14)
	CP Ti	Hot-pressed β-TCP	ACP, oxyapatite (OAp), ACP + OAp	0.5–2	(15)
Ion beam deposition (EBD + IB) Strong adherence to substrate	Ti–6Al–4V	Hot-pressed HAp	HAp, β-TCP (heat-treated at 903 K for 3.6 ks)	0.6	(12)
	CP Ti	HAp	ACP (as-deposited) HAp (heat-treated in air at 873 K for 3.6 ks)	1.3	(16)
Ion beam deposition (sputtering + IB) Strong adherence to substrate	Ti–6Al–4V	70% HAp + 30% β-TCP	ACP (as-deposited) HAp (heat-treated in air at 773 K for 7.2 ks)	0.3	(17)
Pulsed laser deposition Wide variety of gas composition Coating composition close to target	CP Ti	Sintered HAp	HAp (substrate temperature: 773–873 K)	10	(18)
	Ti–6Al–4V	Sintered HAp	HAp (substrate temperature: 758 K)	0.83	(19)
	Ti–6Al–4V	Compressed HAp	HAp + α-TCP + TTCP (substrate temperature: 848 K)	<5	(20)
Ion plating High deposition rate	Ti–6Al–4V	HAp	HAp (heat-treated in air at 773 K for 14.4 ks)	1–5	(21)

TABLE 7.2

Bioceramic Coatings on Ti Substrate by CVD

Processes and Advantages	Substrate	Source Material	Phase of Coating	Film Thickness (μm)	Reference
Thermal CVD High deposition rate	CP Ti	$Ca(dpm)_2$, $Ti(O\text{-}i\text{-}Pr)_2(dpm)_2$, $(C_6H_5O)_3PO$	$CaTiO_3$, α-TCP, HAp	<5	(22)
Laser CVD Extremely high deposition rate Relatively low deposition temperature	CP Ti	$Ca(dpm)_2$, $(C_6H_5O)_3PO$	HAp, β-TCP, TTCP	< 10	(23)

such as Ca–Ti–O and Ca–P–O system films on Ti. Although the deposition temperature of CVD is generally higher than that of PVD and resulting in the mechanical degradation of Ti, lowering of the deposition temperature in CVD has been attempted by adopting metal organic (MO) precursors combined with auxiliary energy by laser.

Bioceramic Coating by PVD

Sputtering

Sputtering is most widely and commonly employed to manufacture thin films in many industries. In sputtering, highly accelerated ions, typically Ar^+, are emitted to a source material (target), and then sputtered atoms or clusters are deposited on a substrate to form thin films.

Radio-frequency (RF) magnetron sputtering is the process in which the Ar^+ ions forming plasma by the radiofrequency radiation sputter the target and then deposit the target material on the substrate. Figure 7.7 shows a schematic illustration of the RF magnetron sputtering apparatus. The sputtering chamber is evacuated to a total pressure of less than 10^{-4} Pa, and then sputtering gas such as Ar or a mixture of Ar-O_2 is introduced into the chamber where it reaches a total pressure of several pascals. As shown in Figure 7.8, a permanent magnet is located behind a target, and the magnetic field forms a closed-loop annular path. Since the secondary electrons ejected from the target take a cycloidal path, the probability of ionization of the sputtering gas within the confinement zone increases greatly.[29]

The RF magnetron sputtering process has many advantages:[30]

- High deposition rate
- Ease of sputtering any metal, alloy, or compound
- High-purity films
- High adhesion of films
- Excellent coverage of steps and small features
- Ability to coat low refractory substrates
- Ease of automation
- Uniformity in thickness and roughness on large-area substrates

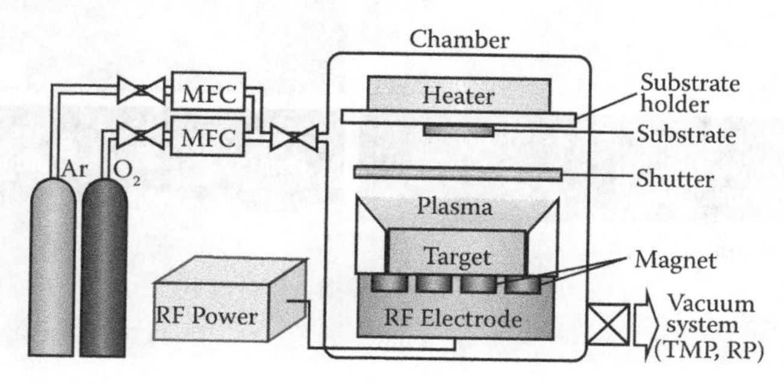

FIGURE 7.7
Schematic illustration of RF magnetron sputtering.

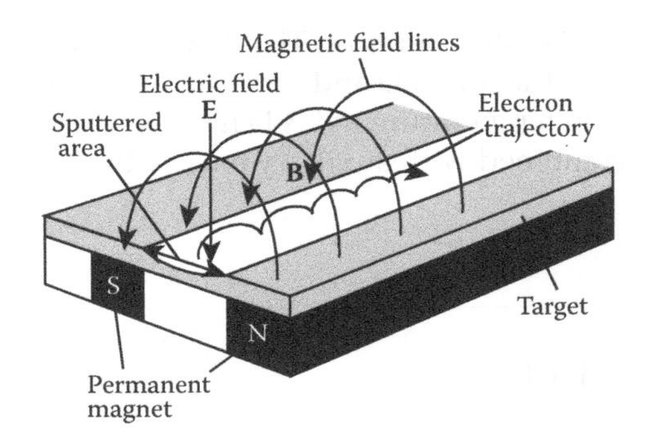

FIGURE 7.8
Schematic illustration of magnetron and target.

RF magnetron sputtering is promising for bioceramic coating of metallic biomaterials because highly adhered Ca–P–O coatings can be prepared uniformly at low temperature.

Figure 7.9 shows the appearance of amorphous calcium phosphate (ACP) coatings on mirror-polished commercially pure (CP) Ti and blasted Ti–6Al–4V alloy substrates prepared by RF magnetron sputtering. The surface feature of the coating well preserved the original roughness of the blasted Ti–6Al–4V alloy substrate, proving good step-coverage even on a complicated rough surface. Thermal spraying would not usually maintain the surface roughness of the original substrate after application of a thick calcium phosphate coating, while RF magnetron sputtering can achieve thin coatings with good adherence and coverage. Some studies on calcium phosphate coating on metallic biomaterials prepared by RF magnetron sputtering have been reported.[13–15,31–38] The crystallinity of calcium phosphate coating prepared by RF magnetron sputtering changed depending on process parameters such as RF power, gas pressure in the sputtering chamber, and oxygen gas concentration. Figure 7.10 depicts the effects of RF power and total gas pressure in the chamber on the phase of calcium phosphate coating prepared at room temperature without the addition of

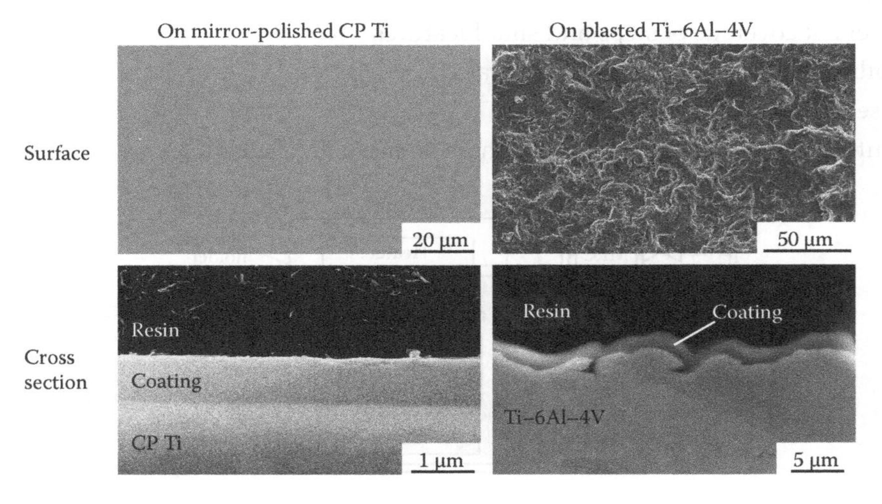

FIGURE 7.9
SEM images of surface and cross section of ACP coatings prepared by RF magnetron sputtering.

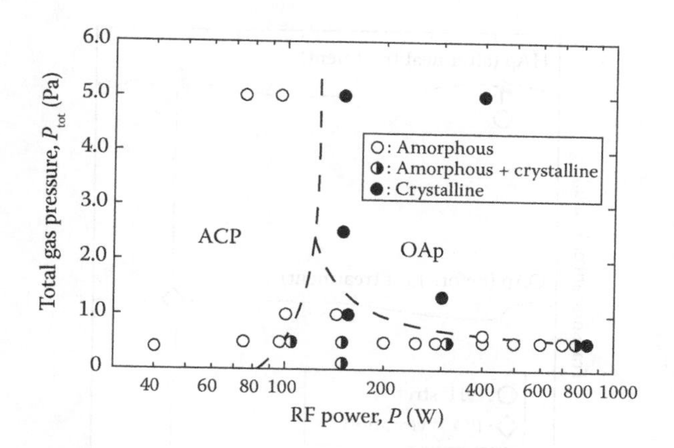

FIGURE 7.10
Effects of total gas pressure and RF power on phase of calcium phosphate coating prepared at room temperature without addition of oxygen gas.

oxygen gas. Figure 7.11 shows the effects of oxygen gas concentration in the sputtering gas and RF power on the phase of coatings.[15] The crystallinity of calcium phosphate coating depends on the degrees of RF power, oxygen gas concentration in the sputtering gas, and total pressure. Sputtering is advantageous for low-temperature coating; however, calcium phosphate coatings may be crystallized by an increase in substrate temperature[31–33] or by heat treatment of ACP coatings.[14,34,38] Figure 7.12 shows the FTIR spectra of the oxyapatite ($Ca_{10}(PO_4)_6O$, OAp) coatings prepared by RF magnetron sputtering on mirror-polished CP Ti substrates before and after heat treatment at 873 K for 7.2 ks in air. A hydroxyl stretching band was observed at 3570 cm^{-1} in the coating after the heat treatment. Hydroxyl group is not usually introduced into the calcium phosphates by sputtering methods because sputtering is conducted under low total gas pressure conditions. The heat treatment in air or

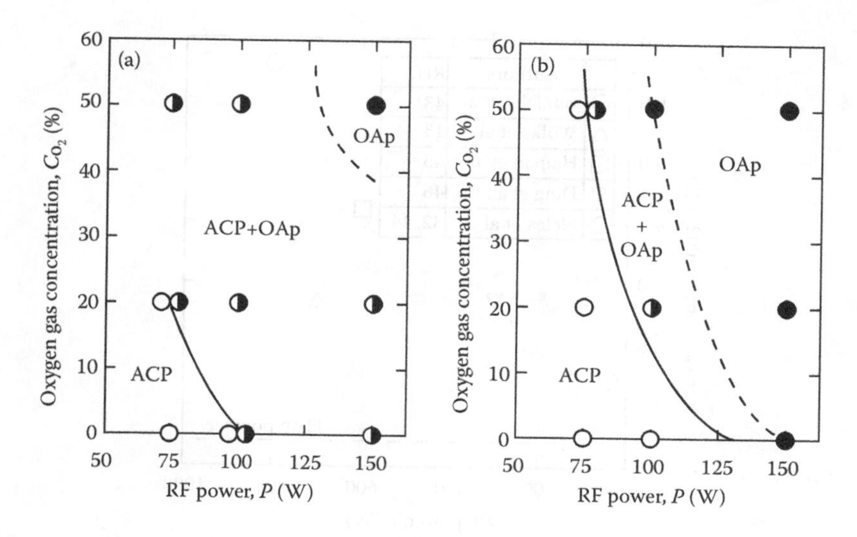

FIGURE 7.11
Effects of oxygen gas concentration in sputtering gas (C_{O2}) and RF power on phase in coatings at total pressures of (a) 0.5 Pa and (b) 5 Pa. (Deposition time = 18 ks.)

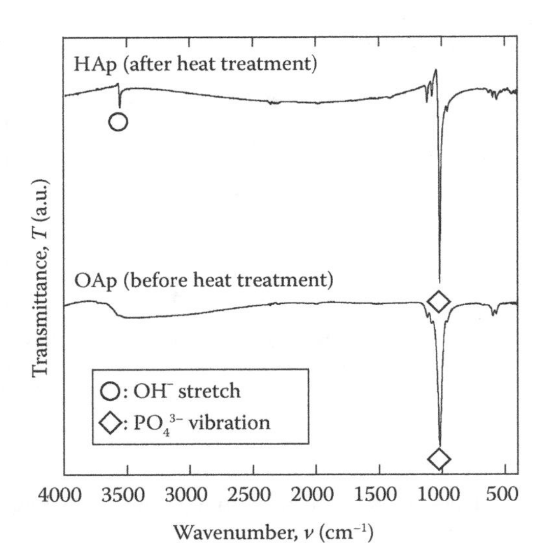

FIGURE 7.12
FTIR spectra of OAp coatings prepared using RF magnetron sputtering on mirror-polished CP Ti substrates before and after heat treatment at 873 K for 7.2 ks in air.

in a water-vapor containing atmosphere is required in order to obtain HAp coating, which contains hydroxyl group.

HAp has a hexagonal structure and it is known that HAp exhibits anisotropic reactivity with human saliva[(39)] and also anisotropic mechanical properties.[(40–42)] There are some reports that the preferentially oriented HAp can be obtained using RF magnetron sputtering. Figure 7.13 indicates the reported results of the peak intensity ratio of (002) and (211) of HAp coating prepared using RF magnetron sputtering.[(13,32,43–46)] The preferential

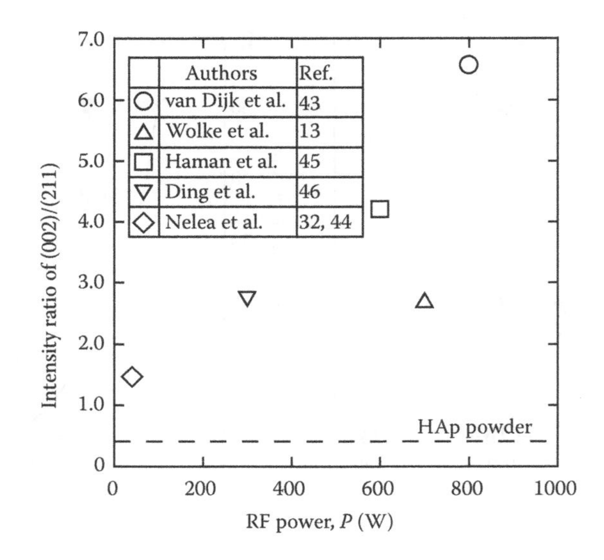

FIGURE 7.13
Effect of RF power on intensity ratio of (002)/(211) of HAp coating prepared using RF magnetron sputtering.

orientation to the *c*-axis of HAp increased with increasing RF power during the sputtering. Since the biological apatite crystallites were reported to exhibit preferential orientation of the *c*-axis (⟨002⟩ direction),[42] control of the orientation in calcium phosphate coatings on metallic biomaterials will be effective for implant applications.

Ion Beam Deposition

IBD has been widely used for surface modification by combining ion impregnation and various PVD techniques. IBD also includes dynamic mixing (DM), ion beam enhanced deposition (IBED), and ion beam assisted deposition (IBAD). Ions are able to impregnate the surface of solids by kinetic acceleration and the modified surface layer very strongly. Calcium phosphate coating on a Ti substrate has been conducted by IBD by combinations such as electron beam (EB) deposition/Ar^+ ion impregnation,[12] EB deposition/Ca^{2+} ion impregnation,[16] and sputtering/Ar^+ ion impregnation.[17] Figure 7.14 shows the apparatus of IBD for the preparation of HAp coating on a Ti substrate.[47] During implantation of the Ca^{2+} ions into the Ti substrate, an HAp source material is evaporated using the EB gun and deposited in the Ti substrate in an atmosphere containing water vapor. Figure 7.15 shows a schematic illustration of a graded coating prepared by the IBD method. The graded coating can be prepared by controlling the amount of the current of Ca^{2+} ions and the amount of HAp evaporation. Ca^{2+} ions are implanted into the Ti substrate, and a mixing layer containing Ca^{2+} ions and HAp is formed on the substrate. The top surface of the coating is the HAp layer. Since the composition of the coating gradually changes from Ti to Ti–Ca and Ca–P–O, the graded coating shows significantly strong adherence to the Ti substrate. As-deposited coatings by these methods are usually amorphous and then crystallize to HAp and β-TCP coatings by heat treatment.[12,16]

Pulsed Laser Deposition

PLD is a common technique to prepare thin films by high-power pulsed laser ablation of a solid target and subsequent deposition of the ablated species on a substrate. Therefore, this method is often called laser ablation. A target can be instantly melted and directly evaporated or be formed into atom/molecular clusters, and therefore the composition of such thin films is usually very close to that of the target. Even complicated multicomponent thin films can be prepared by PLD. A laser is emitted from outside the PLD chamber and forms a plasma plume around the deposition zone without sensitive control of the deposition conditions such as total pressure and gas species. Therefore, PLD has a wide

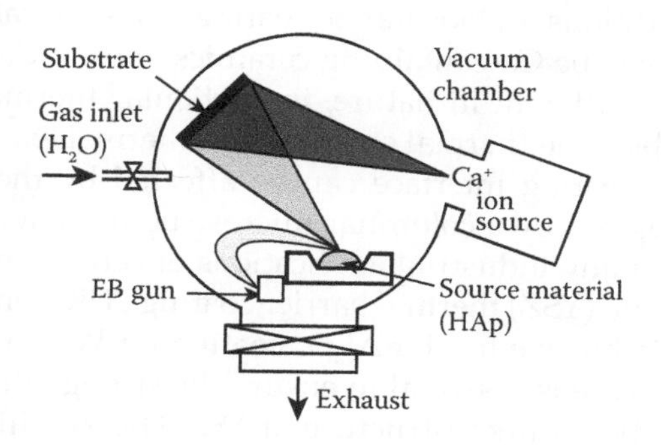

FIGURE 7.14
Schematic illustration of IBD apparatus.

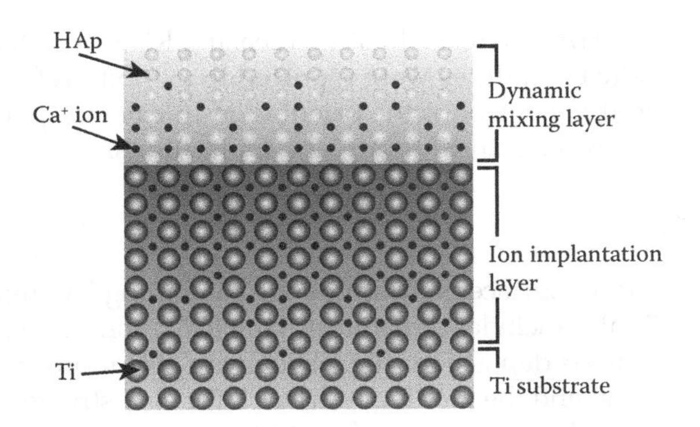

FIGURE 7.15
Schematic illustration of modified surface layer prepared by IBD.

range of degrees of freedom with regard to gas composition.[48] PLD can be used to prepare apatite coatings containing OH groups by introducing water vapor into the PLD chamber at a substrate temperature of 873 K by using an HAp target.[18,19,48] The Ca/P ratio and OH content in calcium phosphate coatings can be controlled in PLD by changing the water vapor pressure in a gas atmosphere.[19] Without water vapor, on the other hand, single-phase HAp cannot be obtained; instead α-TCP and/or TTCP are formed. Water vapor plays a significant role in the crystal phase of calcium phosphate in PLD.[20]

Bioceramic Coating by CVD

CVD is a versatile process to prepare a wide range of materials in various forms and with various microstructures, mainly because CVD has many deposition parameters such as gas concentration, deposition temperature, geometric configuration of CVD chamber, and so forth.[49] The morphology of deposits can be controlled by these parameters, in particular deposition temperature and supersaturation of precursor gases as depicted in Figure 7.16. Supersaturation can be defined as the ratio of an input source gas pressure to an equilibrium gas pressure. A powdery deposit may form at low temperature and under high supersaturation conditions, while platelike or epitaxial films form at high temperature and low supersaturation conditions. In bioceramic coating, the substrate is commonly Ti or its alloys, and the coating may be Ca-containing ceramics, mostly Ca–P–O films. Obviously, metals and ceramics are different in nature, in particular thermal expansion, and they may often be incompatible. The thermal stress due to thermal expansion mismatch at the metal substrate/ceramic coating interface can be affected by the microstructure of the coating, and it can be relaxed by a columnar microstructure having small gaps between each column. There are many industrial applications of ceramic coatings on metals such as yttria-stabilized zirconia (YSZ) thermal barrier coating (TBC) on Ni-base superalloy gas turbine blade[50] and antiabrasive hard α-Al_2O_3 coating on WC-Co cutting tools,[51] where the columnar microstructure is essential to ensure the strong adherence of ceramic coatings. A typical cross-sectional microstructure of YSZ TBC coating by CVD is presented in Figure 7.17.[52] The columnar grains are well grown, and small gaps can be seen at the columnar grain boundary.

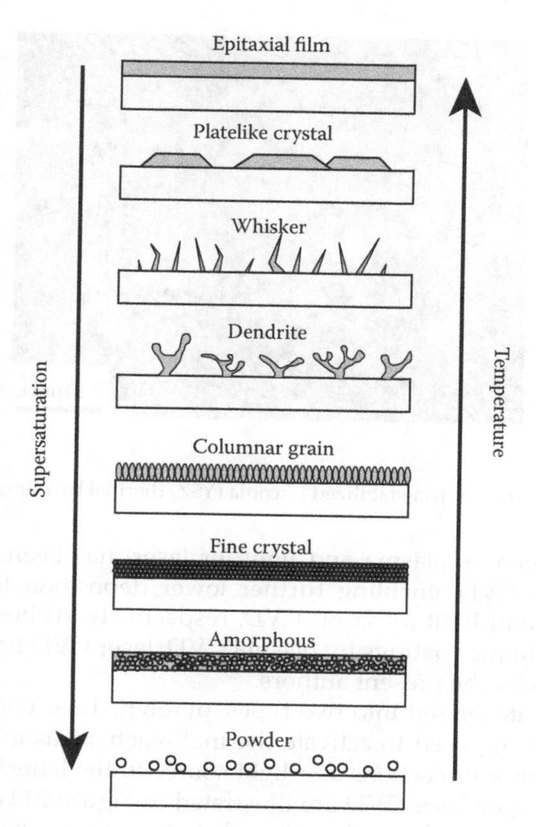

FIGURE 7.16
Effects of temperature and supersaturation on morphology of deposits in CVD.

Conventional CVD is often termed thermal CVD because CVD is a sequential thermally activated process including many chemical reactions and mass-transfer steps as illustrated in Figure 7.18.(53) Therefore, CVD commonly requires a higher deposition temperature than PVD; this may be a disadvantage of CVD. This disadvantage relates to the microstructural change in Ti substrates during CVD processes. Ti transforms from α to β type around 1170 K. When α type and α + β type Ti materials are held over β transus temperature in the single β phase region, very rapid β grain growth occurs and their microstructure is coarsened. The resultant transformed microstructure is unable to be refined by postheat treatment. In bioceramic coatings, therefore, the deposition temperature should be lowered. Precursor (source gas) can be a key factor to determine the deposition temperature in CVD. In many industrial applications, a halide precursor, particularly chloride and bromide compounds, has been employed in CVD; this is termed halide CVD. Since halides are usually thermally stable, halide CVD commonly requires a high deposition temperature, typically more than 1300 K. On the other hand, many kinds of metal-organic compounds (MO) have been developed these days, and MOs are more chemically reactive than halide compounds. CVD using MO precursors (termed MOCVD) often enables deposition temperature lower than halide CVD. However, the lower deposition temperature of MOCVD often results in lower crystallinity and remaining of impurity hydrocarbons in deposited films. This may be a drawback of MOCVD.

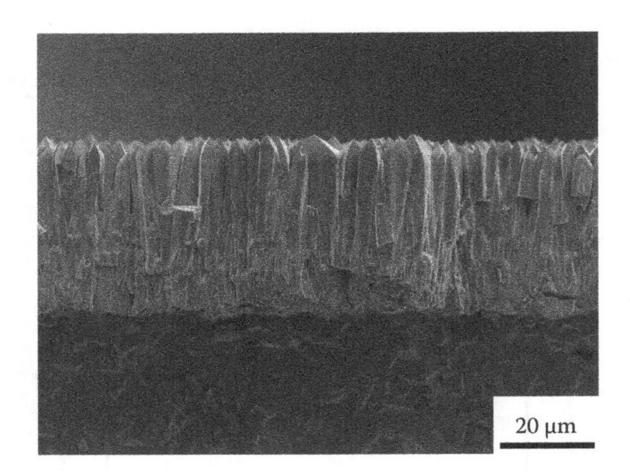

FIGURE 7.17
Cross-sectional microstructure of yttria-stabilized zirconia (YSZ) thermal barrier coating (TBC).

Auxiliary energy such as plasma and light (or laser) has been employed to enhance chemical reactions in CVD, enabling further lower deposition temperature. They are termed plasma CVD and light (or laser) CVD, respectively. Although there has been no report so far on bioceramic coatings by plasma CVD, laser CVD has been applied to prepare Ca–P–O coatings by the present authors.

Laser CVD can be categorized into two types: pyrolytic laser CVD and photolytic laser CVD, with the laser being used to activate thermal reactions as a heat source in the first type and for photochemical reactions as a light source in the latter.[54] Schematic diagrams of pyrolytic and photolytic laser CVD are illustrated in Figure 7.19a and b, respectively. In pyrolytic laser CVD, a laser is focused on the substrate surface, where the spot size may be commonly less than several tens of micrometers. Nanodots/nanowires and patterned deposits have been prepared without etching by pyrolytic laser CVD. In photolytic laser CVD, a laser passes through source gas often parallel to the substrate. Without heating the substrate,

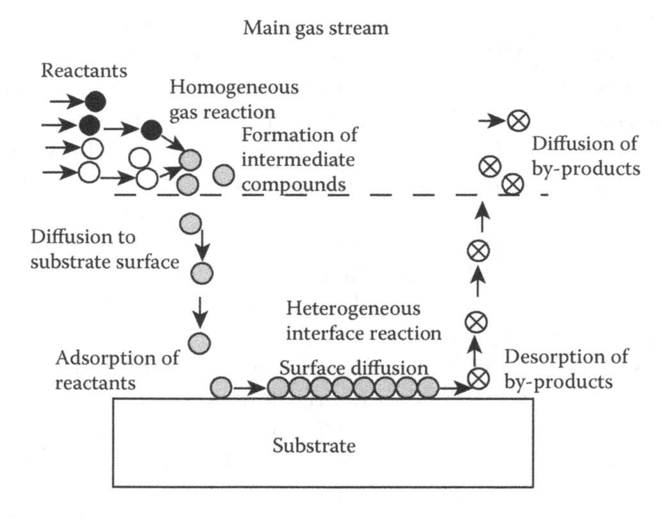

FIGURE 7.18
Schematic representation of various chemical reactions and mass-transfer steps in CVD.

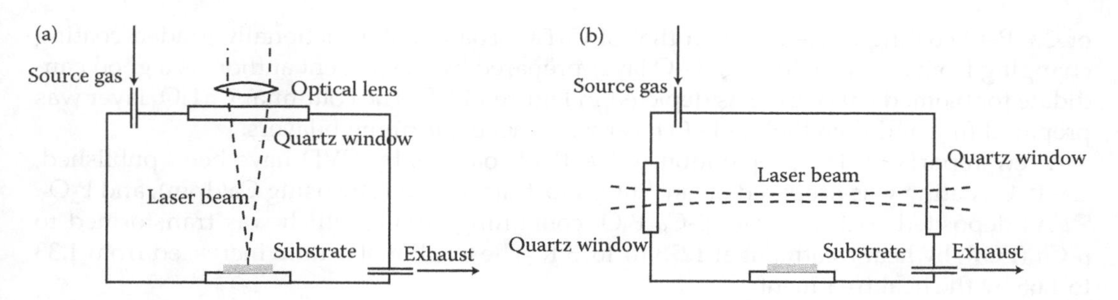

FIGURE 7.19
Schematic diagrams of (a) pyrolytic laser CVD and (b) photolytic laser CVD.

precursor gases react to form a film by a high-energy laser. In conventional pyrolytic and photolytic laser CVD, however, deposits are limited to nanosized or thin-film forms. For thick and wide-area coatings for engineering applications such as thermal barriers, antiabrasive and bioceramic coatings by laser CVD have been thought to be impossible.

The present authors have developed a large spot size (~20 mm) laser CVD enabling a high deposition rate of several hundreds μm/h to several tens mm/h for various ceramic coatings. This laser CVD is different from the conventional pyrolytic or photolytic laser CVD; a laser can ionize precursor gases forming plasma (plasma laser CVD), where the precursor gases can be highly activated as illustrated in Figure 7.20, enabling significant high-speed and low-temperature deposition of films. YSZ and SiO_2 coatings several hundreds μm in thickness have been prepared by this laser CVD at 660[55] and 27.5 mm/h[56], respectively.

Thermal CVD

PVD, mainly plasma spray, and sol–gel have been widely applied for bioceramic coatings. CVD has not been applied for such applications, the lack of appropriate precursors being one of the reasons. $CaTiO_3$ bioceramic coating by thermal CVD was first prepared by the present authors at 950 to 1050 K using Ca(dpm) (dpm: dipivaloylmethanate) and $Ti(OiPr)_2dpm_2$ (OiPr: orso-iso-propoxide).[25] $CaTiO_3$ coating with a well-developed columnar microstructure exhibited good adherence and compatibility with a Ti substrate. Although $CaTiO_3$ coating is bioactive and well compatible with a Ti substrate, the osteoconductivity

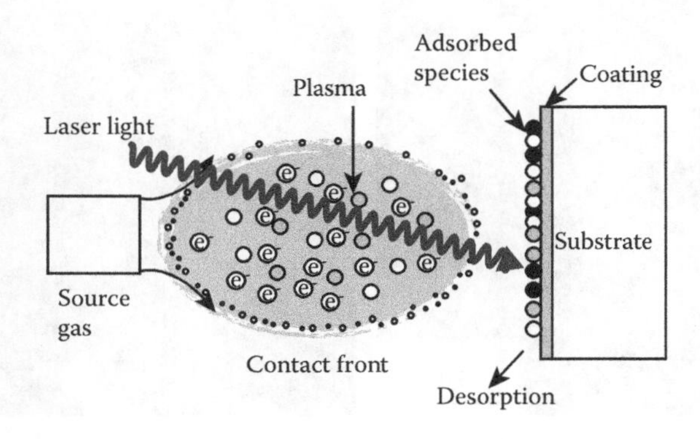

FIGURE 7.20
Schematic diagram of plasma laser CVD.

of Ca–P–O coating is greater than that of $CaTiO_3$ coating. A functionally graded coating changing from a $CaTiO_3$ to a Ca–P–O layer prepared by the present authors is a good candidate for biomedical coating as depicted in Figure 7.21.(57) The columnar $CaTiO_3$ layer was prepared first and then the Ca–P–O layer was stacked, forming bilayers.

A few reports on the preparation of Ca–P–O coatings by CVD have been published. Ca–P–O coating was prepared on an Al_2O_3 substrate at 1123 K by using $Ca(dpm)_2$ and P_2O_5.(58) As-deposited coatings were β-$Ca_2P_2O_7$ containing $AlPO_4$, which was transformed to β-$Ca_3(PO_4)_2$ by heat treatment at 1273 to 1623 K. The Ca/P molar ratio increased from 1.33 to 1.66 by the heat treatment.

A fluorine-containing carbonated HAp coating was conducted on Ti–6Al–4V substrate by using $Ca(hfpd)_2$ (hfpd: hexafluro-pentadione) and tributylphosphate at 873 K.(59) The as-deposited coating had a cauliflower-like nodule microstructure with a Ca/P molar ratio of 1.3 close to OCP containing impurity C–H. This coating was heat-treated at 1073 K, and then the Ca/P molar ratio changed from 1.3 to 1.71 close to that of HAp, whereas the crystal structure was not investigated. No biomedical properties of this coating were reported.

The present authors have prepared Ca–P–O coatings on Ti substrate by using $Ca(dpm)_2$ and $(C_6H_5O)_3PO$ precursors by changing the deposition temperature from 873 to 1073 K and the Ca/P molar ratio from 0.1 to 2.5.(22,26,27) Single phase HAp and α-TCP were first prepared in as-deposited forms at 950 to 1000 K. The crystal phase of Ca–P–O coatings changed widely with deposition temperature and Ca/P molar ratio in source gases as illustrated in Figure 7.22. Mixed phases of CaO and $CaCO_3$ formed below 900 K, whereas HAp and α-TCP formed over 900 K. Single-phase HAp and α-TCP coatings were prepared at 973 to 1073 K and at a Ca/P molar ratio below 1.0.

CVD is in general advantageous for controlling the preferred orientations by controlling deposition conditions, and (002) preferred orientation, which is often observed in bone, can be achieved in HAp coating on Ti substrate. The typical surface morphology of (002)-oriented HAp along with that of (510)-oriented α-TCP coating by thermal CVD is presented in Figure 7.23. Both have a grainlike surface microstructure and columnar cross section. The deposition rates of these Ca–P–O coatings are 10 to 20 μm/h, which are 10 to 100 times higher than that of common sputtering.

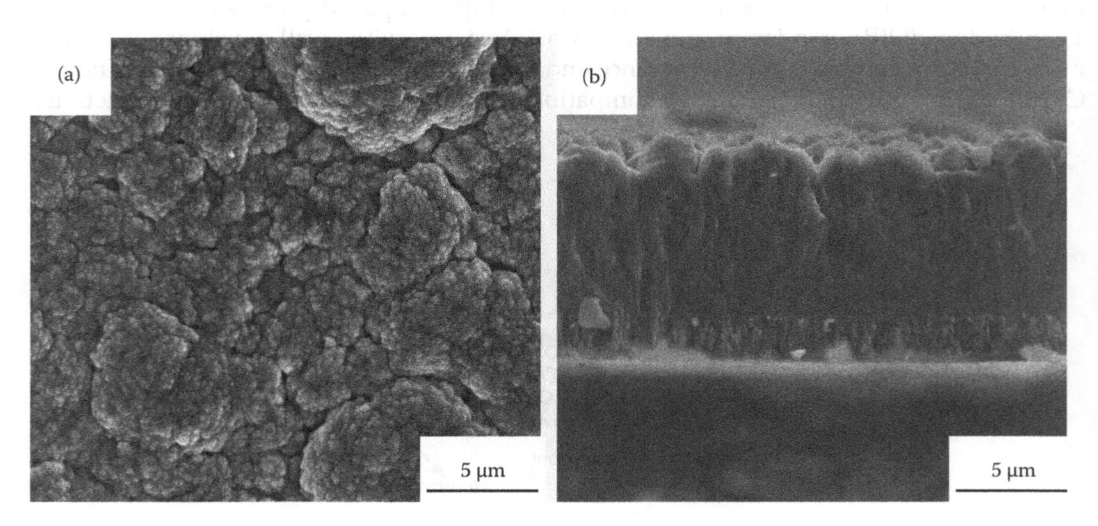

FIGURE 7.21
Microstructure of functionally graded $CaTiO_3$/Ca–P–O coating. (a) Surface, (b) cross section.

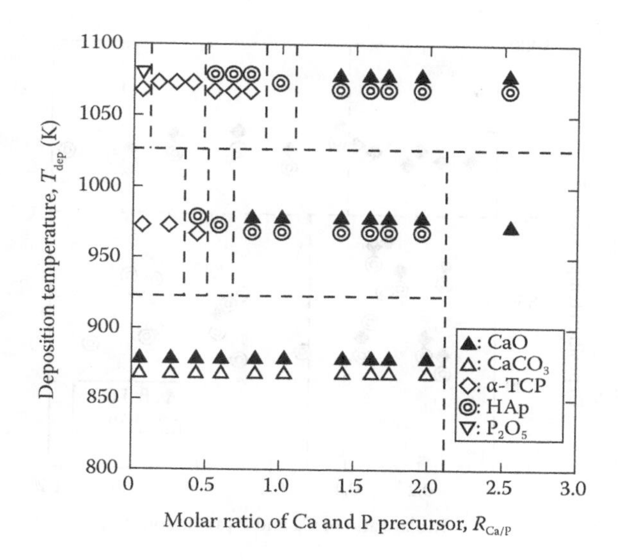

FIGURE 7.22
$T_{dep} - R_{Ca/P}$ phase formation diagram of Ca–P–O coatings at P_{O2} = 0.32 kPa and P_{tot} = 0.8 kPa.

Laser CVD

Laser CVD has been commonly applied to prepare small-scale materials such as thin films, nanotubes and nanodots, mainly for semiconductor devices. Since the use of a laser can significantly accelerate chemical reactions, laser CVD can achieve tremendously high deposition rates at relatively low deposition temperature, which is advantageous for bioceramic coatings on Ti substrates. The present authors first applied laser CVD for bioceramic coatings.

The effects of deposition temperature and Ca/P molar ratio on the crystal phase of Ca–P–O coatings at a laser power of 50W are illustrated in Figure 7.24.[28] Single-phase

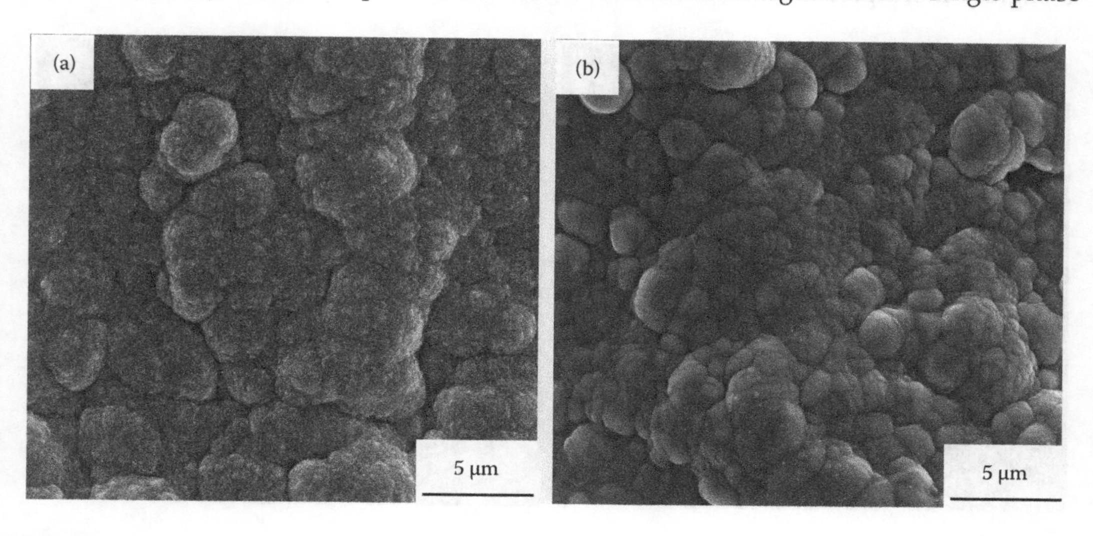

FIGURE 7.23
Surface morphology of (a) HAp and (b) α-TCP coatings prepared at T_{dep} = 1073 K and P_{tot} = 0.8 kPa.

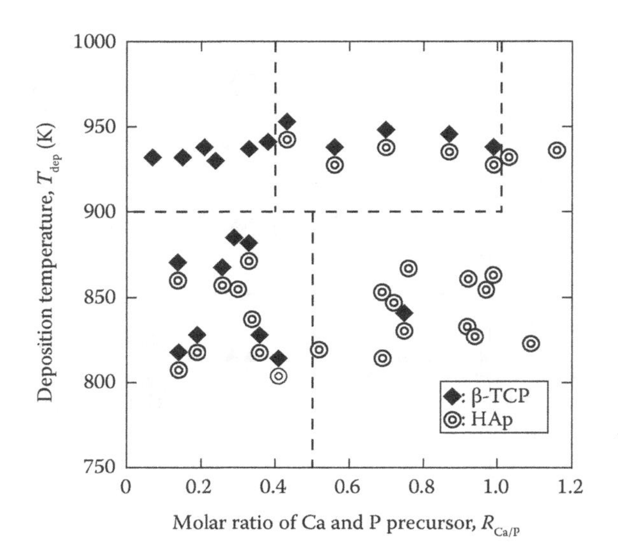

FIGURE 7.24
CVD phase diagram of Ca–P–O coatings prepared at P_L = 50 W and P_{tot} = 0.6 kPa.

HAp coatings were obtained at 800 to 900 K and Ca/P molar ratios more than 0.4, while single-phase β-TCP coatings were obtained around 950 K and at Ca/P molar ratios less than 0.4. The deposition temperature for HAp by laser CVD was about 200 K lower than that by thermal CVD. The preferred orientation was controlled mainly by the changing Ca/P molar ratio. Typical surface morphologies of (002)- and (300)-oriented HAp coatings, respectively, are presented in Figure 7.25a and b. β-TCP coating prepared at a laser power of 100 to 200 W also showed preferred orientations of (290) and (400). The surface morphology of β-TCP coatings prepared at Ca/P molar ratios of 0.4 and 0.7 about 1320 to 1330 K, respectively, is presented in Figure 7.26a and b, where the (290) orientation of Figure 7.26a is slightly more prominent than that of Figure 7.26b. The deposition rate for Ca–P–O

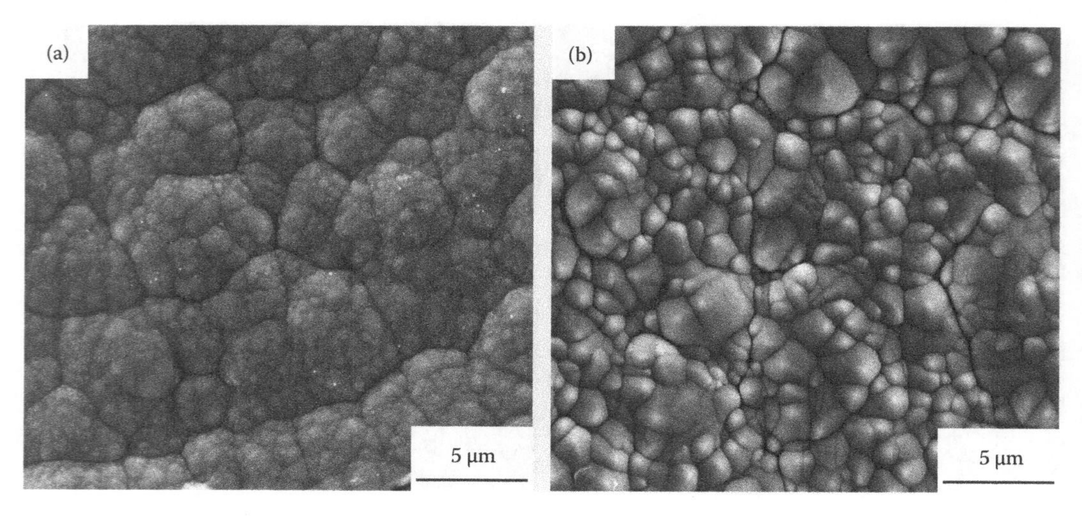

FIGURE 7.25
Surface morphology of (a) (002)-oriented and (b) (300)-oriented HAp coatings prepared by laser CVD.

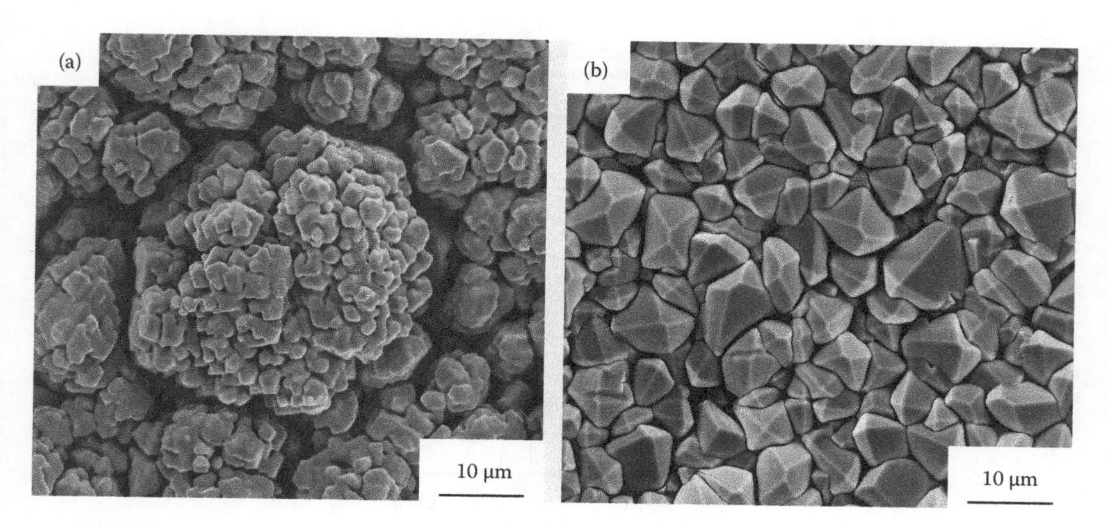

FIGURE 7.26
Surface morphology of (290)- and (400)-oriented β-TCP (290). Orientation of (a) is more prominent than that of (b).

coatings by laser CVD is about 1000 μm/h at most; that is, 10 to 100 times faster than that of thermal CVD and more than 1000 times of sputtering.

Performance of Bioceramic Coating Prepared by Vapor Deposition

In this section, the properties of bioceramic coatings prepared by vapor deposition are discussed with a focus on bonding strength to substrates, apatite formation in simulated body fluid (SBF), and biological response.

Bonding Strength

High bonding strength of bioceramic coatings to substrates is essential for implant applications because of the possible delayed failures associated with inflammatory diseases.

Figure 7.27 shows the values of bonding strength of ACP and OAp coatings with a thickness of 0.5 μm, which were prepared using RF magnetron sputtering, to mirror-polished CP Ti and blasted Ti–6Al–4V alloy substrates. The values were calculated from the maximum load in a pulling test using aluminum studs. It appears that the bonding strength of the coatings were 60 to 70 MPa independent of the crystallinity of the coatings and the surface roughness of the substrates. Table 7.3 summarizes the bonding strengths between Ti substrates and calcium phosphate coatings prepared by PVD[12,18,33,35–38] as compared with those by plasma spraying.[60–64] The bonding strengths listed in Table 7.3 were obtained by pulling tests using aluminum studs attached to the surface of the coating on Ti substrates using epoxy glue. The bonding strength exceeded 60 MPa for the calcium phosphate coatings prepared by RF magnetron sputtering and IBD, which is much higher than that prepared by plasma spraying. The higher bonding strength in coatings prepared by PVD is perhaps caused by (1) the thin thickness of the coatings as compared with that prepared

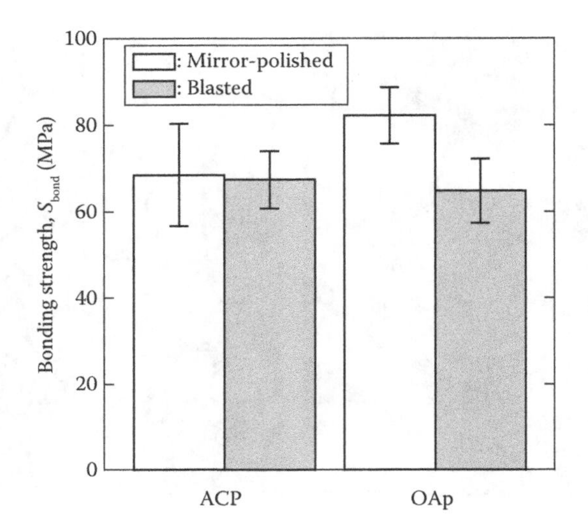

FIGURE 7.27
Bonding strengths of the ACP and OAp coatings fabricated on mirror-polished CP Ti and blasted Ti–6Al–4V alloy substrates.

by plasma spraying, and (2) the removal of adsorbed gases on the substrate surface in RF magnetron sputtering and the formation of a functionally graded layer in IBD. Table 7.3 suggests that the bonding strength is affected by heat treatment and immersion in aqueous solution such as SBF. The thermal expansion coefficient difference between a calcium phosphate coating and a Ti substrate together with preferential and partial dissolution of the coating would decrease the bonding strength. The bonding strength of coatings, around 60 MPa, is close to that of the epoxy glue used in the pulling tests. As shown in Figure 7.28,[(65)] the calcium phosphate coating prepared on a Ti substrate by RF magnetron sputtering remained even after the pulling tests.[(33)] The actual bonding strength of the coating would be more than 60 MPa. The bonding strength of the thin films to metal substrates should be more precisely evaluated theoretically and experimentally.

The bonding strengths between α-TCP and HAp coatings prepared by thermal CVD and Ti substrates are 48 and 42 MPa, respectively. These values are slightly smaller than those of calcium phosphate coatings prepared by sputtering and IBD, but they are higher than those reported in the coatings prepared by sol–gel and plasma spraying.

Apatite Formation in SBF

Apatite formation on a bioactive glass surface in SBF can be an indicator of *in vivo* bone formation.[(66,67)] The apatite formation in SBF would be affected by the physical/chemical properties and roughness of the substrate surface.

CVD can be used to prepare bioceramic coatings such as calcium phosphate and calcium titanate with a wide variety of surface morphology and crystallographic orientation, and apatite formation on these coatings in SBF has been reported. Table 7.4 shows the time required for apatite formation in Hanks' solution over the whole surface of Ca–Ti–O and Ca–P–O coatings prepared by CVD[(27,28,68)] and other coating methods[(69,70)] on Ti substrates. Figure 7.29a and b show the surface morphology of the HAp coatings prepared by thermal CVD after immersion in Hanks' solution for 3.6 and 21.6 ks, respectively. Apatite was identified on the HAp coating after 3.6 ks, and the whole surface of the HAp coating was

TABLE 7.3
Bonding Strength Between Calcium Phosphate Coating and Ti Substrate

Coating Method	Substrate	Thickness of Coating (μm)	As-Coated (MPa)	Heat-Treated (MPa)	Immersed in SBF (MPa)	Reference
RF magnetron sputtering	Mirror-polished Ti–6Al–4V	3	60	-	45	(35)
RF magnetron sputtering	Mirror-polished Ti–6Al–4V	3–4	42–56	-	-	(36)
RF magnetron sputtering	Mirror-polished Ti–6Al–4V	3–4	27	23	-	(37)
RF magnetron sputtering	Mirror-polished CP Ti	0.5	60–80	-	30–60	(33)
RF magnetron sputtering	Blasted Ti–6Al–4V	0.5	60–80	50–60	-	(38)
IBD	Mirror-polished Ti–6Al–4V	0.6	64.8	-	-	(12)
PLD	Mirror-polished CP Ti	10	30–40	-	-	(18)
Plasma spraying	Blasted CP Ti	80–100	45	-	39.1	(60)
Plasma spraying	Blasted Ti–6Al–4V	200	30	-	20	(61)
Plasma spraying	Blasted Ti–6Al–4V	150	23	26	4.6	(62)
Plasma spraying	Blasted Ti–6Al–4V	50	35	-	-	(63)
Plasma spraying	Blasted CP Ti	135	6.7	-	-	(64)

covered with apatite with a needlelike texture after 21.6 ks.[27] The surface texture of the HAp coating on which the apatite phase formed in a short period had a cauliflower-like structure, and the formation of an apatite phase was preferential at hollow places of the cauliflower-like texture.[27] Apatite formation is perhaps closely related to the elution of calcium and phosphate ions from bioceramics into SBF.[67] The concentration of these eluted ions increased at the hollow places in the film, which must have caused the formation of the apatite phase in a short period by increasing the supersaturation of apatite in the solution. The spatial gap on the surface of thermally oxidized Ti substrates induced apatite

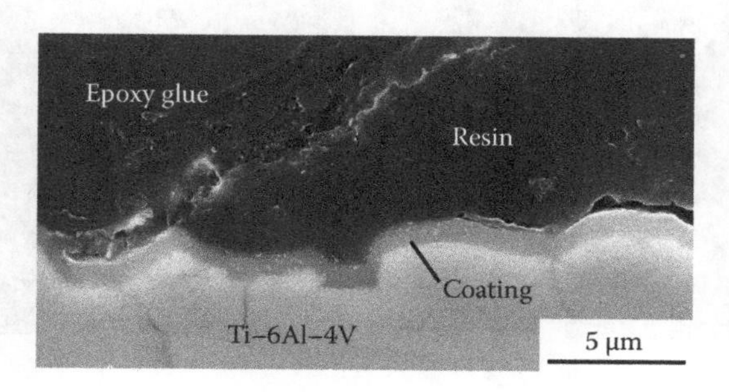

FIGURE 7.28
SEM image of cross section of OAp-coated Ti–6Al–4V plate with blasted surface after adherence test.

TABLE 7.4

Apatite Formation Time on Bioceramic Coatings in SBFs

Coating Method	Phase of Coating	SBF	Apatite Formation (ks)	Reference
Thermal CVD	HAp	Hanks' solution	21.6	(27)
Thermal CVD	α-TCP	Hanks' solution	1209.6	(27)
Thermal CVD	$CaTiO_3$ complicated surface	Hanks' solution	259.2	(68)
Thermal CVD	$CaTiO_3$ smooth surface	Hanks' solution	3628.8	(68)
Laser CVD	HAp, β-TCP	Hanks' solution	259.2	(28)
Plasma spraying	HAp	Kokubo solution	86.4	(69)
Sol–gel	HAp + TiO_2	Kokubo solution	691.2	(70)

formation in Kokubo solution.[71] In CVD, a spatial gap suitable to apatite formation can be introduced by controlling the surface morphology of the bioceramic coatings.

The relationship between the crystallographic orientation of HAp coatings prepared by CVD and apatite formation in SBF has been studied. Apatite formation on an HAp coating oriented to the *c*-axis (i.e., the ⟨002⟩ direction) in Hanks' solution was faster than that oriented to other directions. Preferential apatite formation on the *c*-face of HAp has been reported in the immersion test of a highly oriented HAp sintered body in Kokubo solution.[72] Figure 7.30a and b show the surface morphology of HAp coatings prepared by laser CVD oriented to the *a*-axis (i.e., the ⟨300⟩ direction) after immersion in Hanks' solution for 259.2 and 604.8 ks, respectively. Although the apatite formation rate on the (300)-oriented HAp coating was not high, apatite formation was observed at hollow places 259.2 ks after immersion and the whole surface was covered with needlelike apatite crystallites 604.8 ks after immersion. These results suggest that the hollow places and (002) preferred orientation in bioceramic coatings enhance the apatite formation in SBF.

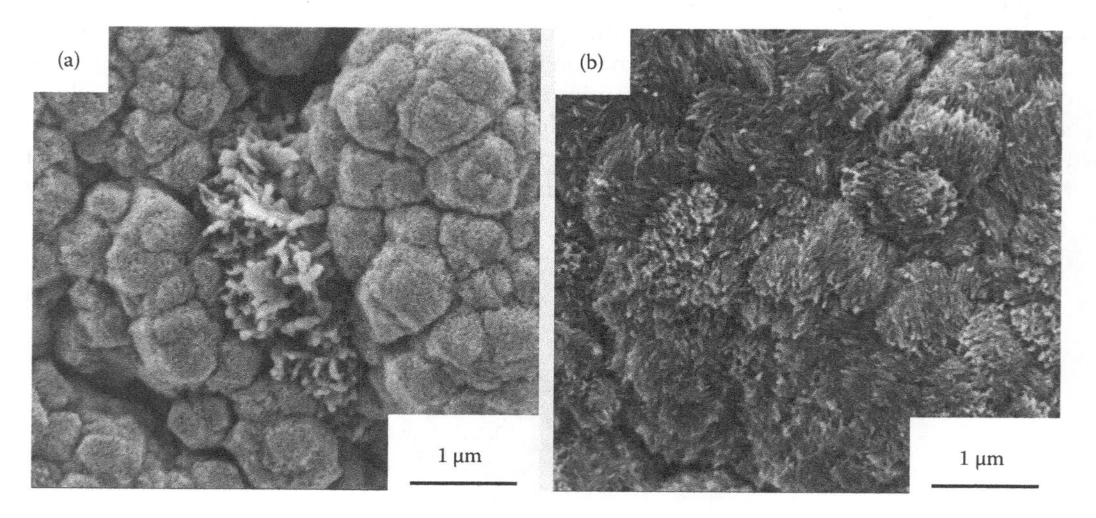

FIGURE 7.29
Surface morphology of HAp coatings prepared by thermal CVD after immersion in Hanks' solution for (a) 3.6 ks and (b) 21.6 ks.

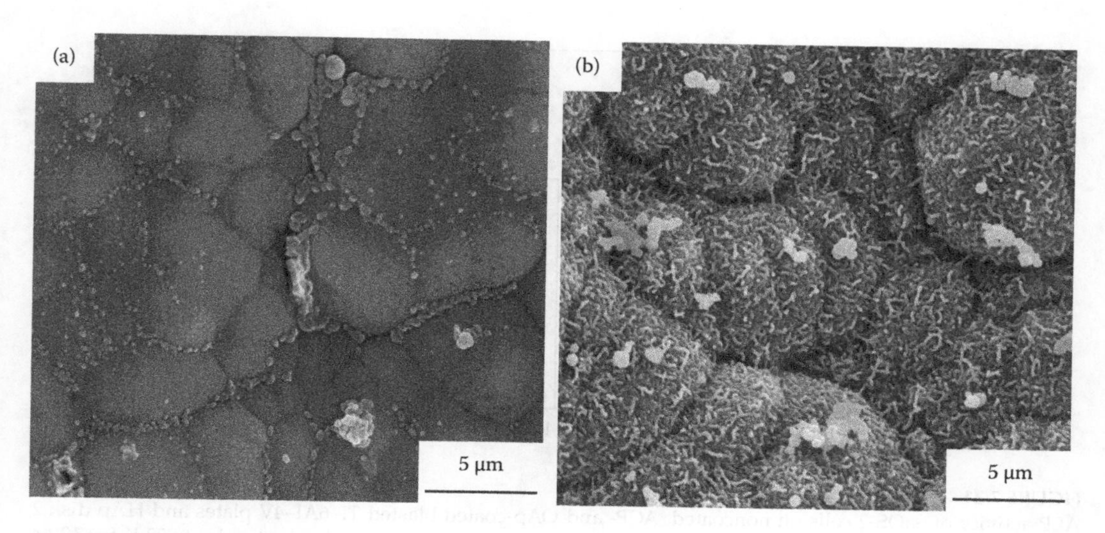

FIGURE 7.30
Surface morphology of HAp coatings prepared by laser CVD after immersion in Hanks' solution for (a) 259.2 ks and (b) 604.8 ks.

The degradation of bioceramic coatings prepared by PVD in SBF has been investigated. ACP coating exhibited higher bioresorbability as compared with crystalline coating.[73–75] The elution from an ACP coating accelerated apatite formation in SBF,[74] which would be advantageous in bone formation *in vivo*. In the immersion of thick calcium phosphate coatings in Kokubo solution prepared by plasma spraying, the nucleation and growth of bonelike apatite might be closely associated with the ACP phase suitably dissolving and releasing calcium and phosphate ions.[76] On the contrary, apatite formation was observed on the crystalline calcium phosphate coating but not on the ACP coating.[73] The surface morphology and the mass of the eluted ions from the coatings might be also associated with the apatite formation.

Biological Response

In vitro and *in vivo* evaluations using cells and animals have been carried out for bioceramic coatings prepared by PVD, focusing on the improvement of bone compatibility of metallic biomaterials.

Alkaline phosphatase (ALP) activity can be an osteoblastic phenotypic marker and an indicator of the first stage of osteoblastic differentiation.[77] Figure 7.31 shows ALP production per DNA production of SaOS-2 cells on the coatings of ACP and OAp heat-treated in a silica ampoule at 873 K for 7.2 ks prepared by RF magnetron sputtering on blasted Ti–6Al–4V alloy substrates, compared with a noncoated blasted Ti–6Al–4V alloy substrate and HAp disks.[38] The thickness of the coatings was 0.5 μm. The ALP activity of the SaOS–2 cells on the calcium phosphate coatings on Ti substrates was significantly greater than that on noncoated Ti substrates after culturing.[33,38] The calcium phosphate coating enhances the osteogenic differentiation of osteoblasts on the surface of the Ti implant. The interaction between calcium phosphate coatings and cells such as fibroblasts[78] and rat bone marrow cells[79] has been investigated, and the calcium phosphate coating would improve the soft tissue compatibility due to the increase in cell spreading area and collagen I formation.[78]

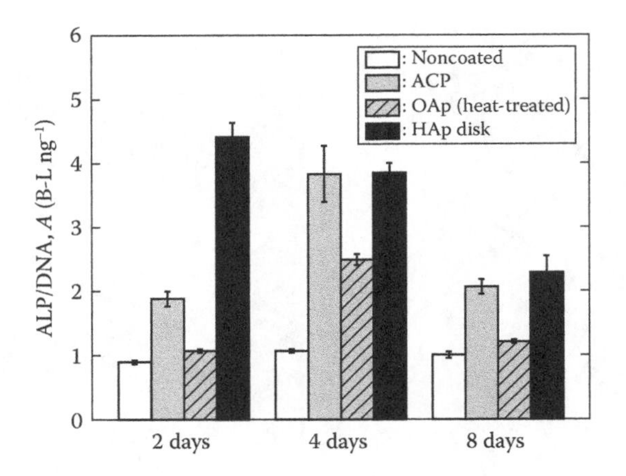

FIGURE 7.31
ALP activity of SaOS-2 cells on noncoated, ACP- and OAp-coated blasted Ti–6Al–4V plates and HAp disk 2, 4, and 8 days after they were cultured. OAp coatings were heat-treated in a silica ampoule at 873 K for 7.2 ks. (B-L × 16.7 = U/l, 310 K).

Many studies on in vivo evaluation of Ti implants with calcium phosphate coatings by PVD have been reported.(33,38,80–85) The improvement in the bone compatibility of the Ti implants has been demonstrated by evaluating the removal torque,(38,80) ultimate interfacial strength(81) and bone–implant contact (BIC)(33,48,80–82) in animals. The values of removal torque of noncoated and ACP-coated blasted Ti–6Al–4V alloy implants from the femurs of Japanese white rabbits are shown in Figure 7.32.(38) The removal torque increased with the duration of implantation, and the values for the ACP-coated implants were greater than those of noncoated implants. It was statistically improved by the ACP coating 2 weeks

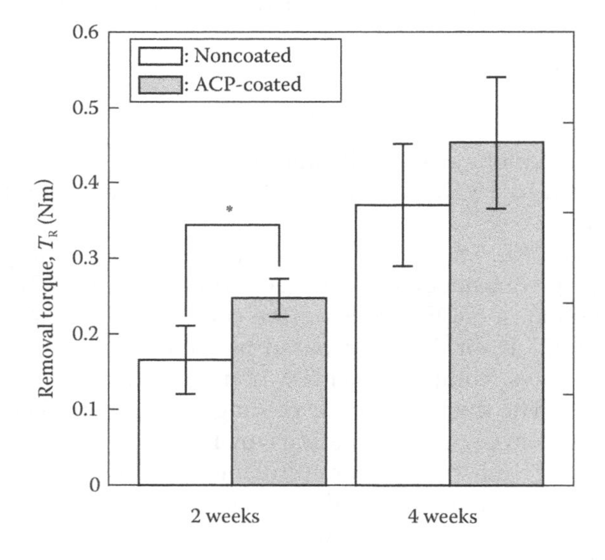

FIGURE 7.32
Removal torque values of noncoated and ACP-coated blasted Ti–6Al–4V alloy implants 2 and 4 weeks after implantation in femurs of Japanese white rabbits (*$p < 0.05$).

after the implantation ($p < 0.05$). For the applications of calcium phosphate coating to dental implants, implantation tests of coated Ti have been reported. Figure 7.33 shows optical micrographs of the interface between the ACP-coated and noncoated (control) CP Ti cylinders and bones 2, 4, 8, and 12 weeks after implantation in mandibles of beagle dogs.(86) BIC, which is the ratio of the surface area of the implant in direct contact with bone to total surface area, is shown in Figure 7.34. The percentage of BIC for the ACP-coated CP Ti cylinders was greater than that for the noncoated cylinders 8 to 12 weeks after implantation.(86)

In the evaluation of calcium phosphate coatings, both the amorphous and crystalline phases have been employed. Crystalline calcium phosphate coating with a thickness of 1 μm on Ti substrates implanted into the backs of New Zealand white rabbits was still detected 12 weeks after implantation, while ACP coating with a thickness of 4 μm disappeared and then a crystalline carbonate apatite layer was precipitated.(83) A crystalline calcium phosphate coating with a thickness of 0.1 μm remained 3 weeks after implantation in the femur of goats, owing to the high stability of crystalline calcium phosphate thin film under biological conditions.(84)

Cross sections of Ti implants with amorphous and crystalline calcium phosphate coatings after implantation in the femurs of Japanese white rabbits for 4 weeks are shown in Figure 7.35a and b, respectively. The ACP coating was prepared by RF magnetron sputtering and the crystalline phase was obtained by the postheat treatment of as-sputtered OAp in air for 7.2 ks. Direct contact between implants and new bones was microscopically observed for both types of implants. The crystalline calcium phosphate coating still existed at the interface between Ti and new bone 4 weeks after implantation, while no layer was detected on the ACP-coated Ti implant. The high bioresorbability of ACP coating can be confirmed in bones similar to that in SBF. The elution of calcium and phosphate ions from bioceramic coatings might have affected the bone forming ability. Vapor deposition methods are suitable to control the composition and phase of the bioceramic coatings. The effect of eluted ions, not only calcium and phosphate ions but also other ions such as silicon or zinc, should be studied using calcium phosphate coatings prepared by vapor deposition.

The bone forming ability of implants may be closely related to the initial interaction with biomolecules. The immobilization of biomolecules such as bisphosphonates(47,85,87) and fibronectin(88) on the surface of calcium phosphate-coated Ti by PVD has been studied.

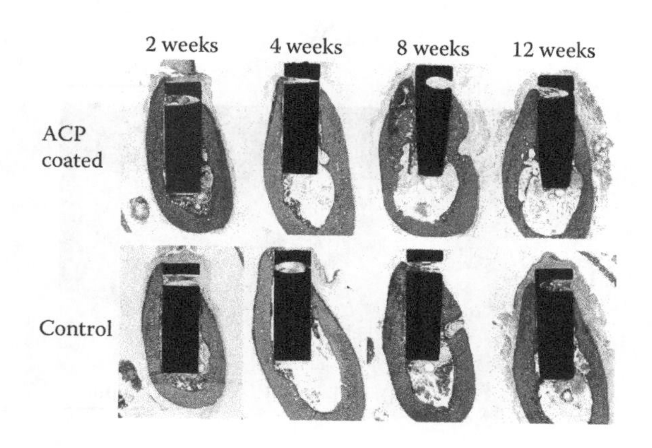

FIGURE 7.33
Optical micrographs of interface between ACP-coated and noncoated (control) CP Ti cylinders and bones 2, 4, 8, and 12 weeks after implantation in mandibles in beagle dogs.

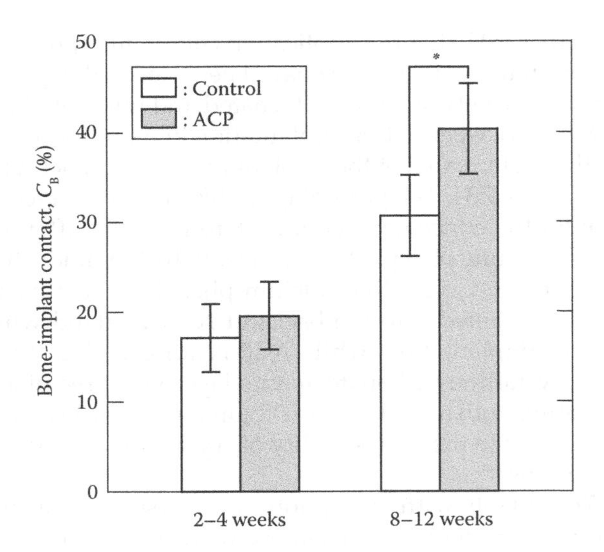

FIGURE 7.34
Percentage of bone-implant contact of ACP-coated and noncoated (control) CP Ti cylinders ($*p < 0.05$).

Yoshinari et al.[47] immobilized bisphosphonates on calcium phosphate coatings on Ti substrates prepared by IBD and showed that the initial adherence of bacteria[87] was suppressed and the BIC values in the mandibles of beagle dogs were increased.[85] Coatings by vapor deposition can be applied to surface modification of metallic biomaterials in combination with the immobilization of biomolecules.

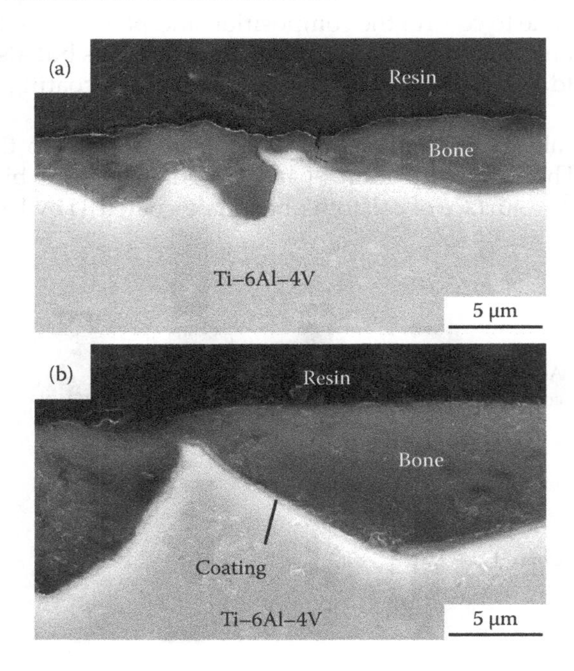

FIGURE 7.35
SEM images of cross section of (a) ACP- and (b) OAp-coated Ti implants after implantation in femurs of Japanese white rabbits for 4 weeks.

Improvement in Wear and Corrosion Resistance

Metallic biomaterials are mainly applied to the load-bearing parts in the human body. Wear debris generated from biomaterials by a tribological reaction are thought to be an important factor related to implant loosening and bone resorption.[89] The surface of metallic biomaterials are usually covered with spontaneously formed thin oxides (i.e., passive films, which cause high corrosion resistance in metallic biomaterials). In the case that the protective passive films on metallic biomaterials are destroyed by the tribological reaction of wear debris, elusion of metal ions from the metallic biomaterials would be accelerated. Therefore, the wear and corrosion properties of metallic biomaterials are closely related to their biocompatibility.

Improving wear and corrosion resistance of metallic biomaterials by surface coating using PVD methods has been conducted. TiN[90–92] and diamondlike carbon (DLC)[93] coatings have been prepared on metallic biomaterials using sputtering and ion plating methods because of their high hardness and low friction coefficients. TiN coating on type 316L stainless steel and Ti alloys such as Ti–6Al–4V and Ti–6Al–7Nb showed improvements in their tribological properties against ultrahigh molecular weight polyethylene (UHMWPE[90] and corrosion resistance.[90,92]

TiO_2 coating by PVD methods is another approach to improving corrosion resistance of stainless steels and Ti and its alloys. An ion beam sputtering technique has been used to deposit thick and dense TiO_2 coating on Ti and type 316L stainless steel surface.[94] The TiO_2 coating with the low defect concentration and a slow mass transport process across the coating will improve the corrosion resistance and are also expected to improve the blood compatibility of the implants such as artificial heart valves and stents.[95,96]

Factors Considered in Biomedical Coating on Metallic Biomaterials

Many factors should be considered when applying bioceramic coating on metallic biomaterials (Figure 7.36).[97] Tissue compatibility is the first priority of the bioceramic coatings and is affected by surface morphology, phase, composition, and orientation of the coatings. The high bonding strength between a coating and metallic biomaterial, which is affected by physical and chemical properties and surface morphology of substrates, is also crucial.

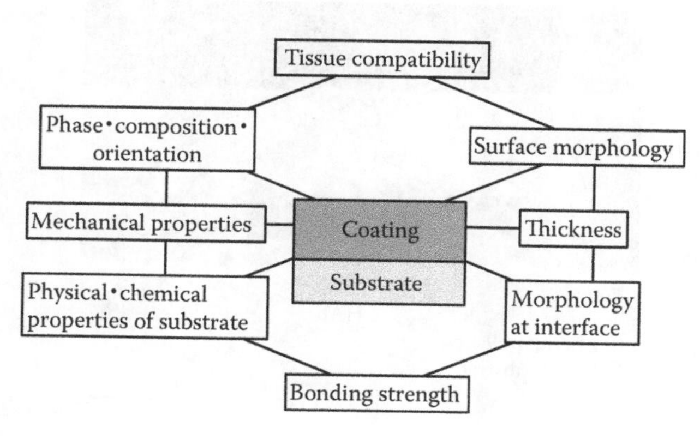

FIGURE 7.36
Factors in biomedical coating on metallic biomaterials by vapor deposition.

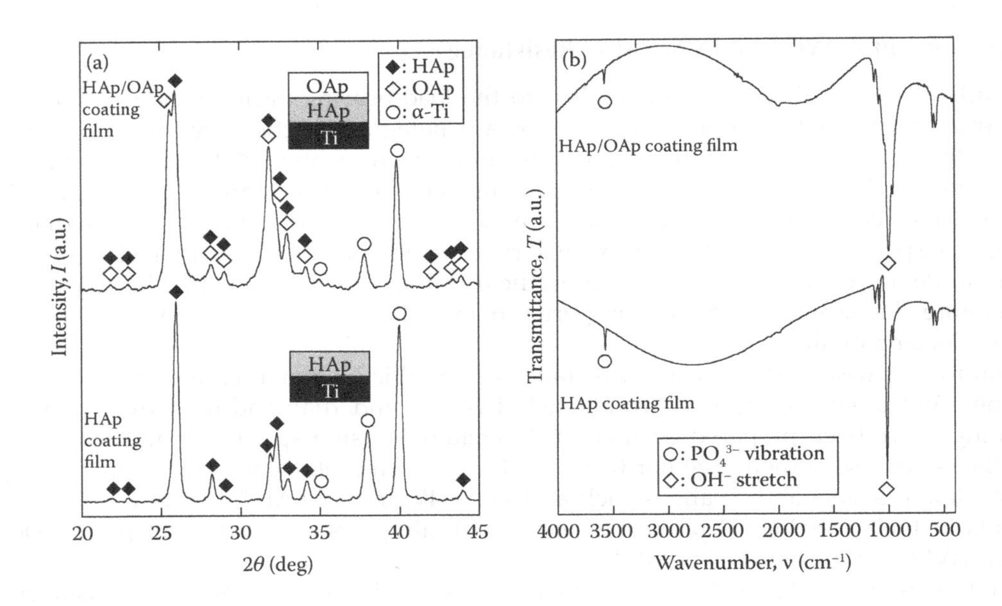

FIGURE 7.37
(a) XRD patterns and (b) FTIR spectra of HAp and HAp/OAp coatings prepared on mirror-polished CP Ti substrates.

Comprehensive understanding of the coating, substrate, and vapor deposition process is needed to develop practical biomedical coatings.

In order to control the coating/substrate and human body/coating interfaces independently, multilayered coating by vapor deposition may be useful. The preparation of double-layered calcium phosphate coatings consisting of films with different crystallinities on CP Ti substrates by RF magnetron sputtering has been reported.[98] The first layer of the double-layered coating (i.e., the inner layer) was high-crystalline calcium phosphate, and the second layer (i.e., the outer layer) was low-crystalline calcium phosphate

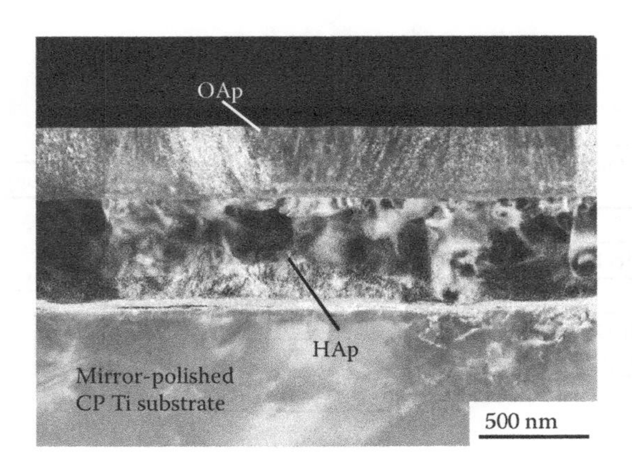

FIGURE 7.38
TEM image of cross section of HAp/OAp coating prepared on a mirror-polished CP Ti substrate.

because calcium phosphate coatings with high and low crystallinity are expected to have high bonding strength and biocompatibility, respectively. Preparation of double-layered HAp/OAp and OAp/ACP coatings was carried out. In the preparation of double-layered HAp/OAp coating, an HAp film was first prepared on a substrate by heat treating an as-sputtered OAp film in air at 873 K for 7.2 ks; this HAp film was considered to be the inner layer, which was then covered with an as-sputtered OAp film. In the case of double-layered OAp/ACP coating, inner-layer OAp and outer-layer ACP films were coated on the CP Ti substrate under different sputtering conditions. The thickness of each layer was controlled to be 0.5 μm, and the total thickness of the double-layered coatings was around 1 μm. The XRD patterns and FTIR spectra of the HAp (inner) layer and HAp/OAp double layer are demonstrated in Figure 7.37a and b, respectively. Figure 7.38 shows a cross section of the double-layered HAp/OAp coating prepared on the mirror-polished CP Ti substrate. Both layers of the coating were dense, uniform, and firmly in contact with each other.

TABLE 7.5

Phase, Structure, and Properties of Coatings Prepared by RF Magnetron Sputtering and Thermal and Laser CVD

Processes	Parameters		Phase and Structure	Remarks
RF magnetron sputtering	Heat treatment (>773 K)	In air (water–vapor containing atmosphere)	HAp (crystalline)	Bioactive
		In vacuum	OAp (crystalline)	Bioactive
	RF power (as-sputtered)	High (>150 W)	OAp (low crystalline)	Bioresorbable Bioactive Possible (002) orientation
		Low (<150 W)	ACP (amorphous)	Highly bioresorbable Bioactive
Thermal CVD	Temperature	Over 900 K (Ca/P molar ratio < 1)	HAp	Bioactive Highly (002) orientation
			α-TCP	Bioresorbable Highly (510) orientation: grainlike
Laser CVD	Temperature (laser power: 30 W)	750–950 K (Ca/P molar ratio > 0.5)	HAp + TTCP	Bioactive Non-orientation
		800–900 K (Ca/P molar ratio = 0.5)	HAp	Bioactive Non-orientation
		850–950 K (Ca/P molar ratio < 0.4)	β-TCP + HAp	Bioresorbable Non-orientation
	Temperature (laser power: 50 W)	800–900 K (Ca/P molar ratio > 0.4)	HAp	Bioactive (300) orientation
		950 K (Ca/P molar ratio < 0.4)	β-TCP	Bioresorbable (220) orientation

Summary

Bioceramic coating by PVD and CVD on metallic biomaterials has been discussed, focusing on improving the bone compatibility of metallic biomaterials. Finally, the relationship between process parameters and phase, structure, and properties of coatings prepared by RF magnetron sputtering and thermal and laser CVD, which have been the main processes discussed in this chapter, are shown in Table 7.5. The vapor deposition can be promising processes for preparation of bioceramic coatings because it can provide well-defined coatings by adjusting many process parameters.

Research and development of bioceramic coatings for applications to hard tissue replacements will continue. Bioceramic coating by vapor deposition is a promising surface modification method accommodating mechanical, chemical, and biomedical properties.

References

1. Brånemark, P.-I., Hansson, B.O., and Adell, R., et al. 1977. Osseointegrated implants in the treatment of the edentulous jaw, experience from a 10-year period. *Scand J Plast Reconstr Surg* 11 Suppl 16: 1–132.
2. Brånemark, P.-I. 1983. Osseointegration and its experimental background. *J Prosthet Dent* 50: 399–410.
3. Williams, D.F. 2001. Titanium for medical applications. In Brunette, D.M., Tengvall, P., Textor, M., and Thomsen, P. (eds.), *Titanium in Medicine*, pp. 13–24, Berlin: Springer.
4. Niinomi, M. 2003. Recent research and development in titanium alloys for biomedical applications and healthcare goods. *Sci Technol Adv Mat* 4: 445–454.
5. Narushima, T. 2008. Surface modification for improving biocompatibility of titanium materials with bone. *J Jpn Inst Light Metals* 58: 577–582.
6. LeGeros, R.Z. 1988. Calcium phosphate materials in restorative dentistry: a review. *Adv Dent Res* 2: 164–180.
7. Yankee, S.J., Pletka, B.J., Salsbury, R.L., and Johnson, W.A. 1991. Historical development of plasma sprayed hydroxylapatite biomedical coatings. In Sudarshan, T.S., Bhat, D.G., and Jeandin, M. (eds.), *Surface Modification Technologies IV*, pp. 261–270, Warrendale, PA: TMS.
8. de Groot, K., Geesink, R., Klein, C.P.A.T., and Serekian, P. 1987. Plasma sprayed coatings of hydroxylapatite. *J Biomed Mater Res* 21: 1375–1381.
9. Yang, Y., Kim, K.H., and Ong, J.L. 2005. A review on calcium phosphate coatings produced using a sputtering process—An alternative to plasma spraying. *Biomaterials* 26: 327–337.
10. Nimmagadda, R. and Bunshah, R.F. 1971. Temperature and thickness distribution on substrate during high-rate physical vapor-deposition of materials. *J Vac Sci Technol* 8: VM85–VM94.
11. Narushima, T. 2007. Surface morphology and composition/phase control in metallic biomaterials. *J Jpn Soc Biomater* 25: 252–260.
12. Lee, I.-S., Whang, C.-N., Kim, H.-E., Park, J.-C., Song, J.H., and Kim, S.-R. 2002. Various Ca/P ratios of thin calcium phosphate films. *Mater Sci Eng C* 22: 15–20.
13. Wolke, J.C.G., van Dijk, K., Schaeken, H.G., de Groot, K., and Jansen, J.A. 1994. Study of the surface characteristics of magnetron-sputter calcium phosphate coatings. *J Biomed Mater Res* 28: 1477–1484.
14. Yoshinari, M., Hayakawa, T., Wolke, J.G.C., Nemoto, K., and Jansen, J.A. 1997. Influence of rapid heating with infrared radiation on RF magnetron-sputtered calcium phosphate coatings. *J Biomed Mater Res* 37: 60–67.

15. Narushima, T., Ueda, K., Goto, T., et al. 2005. Preparation of calcium phosphate films by radio-frequency magnetron sputtering. *Mater Trans* 46: 2246–2252.
16. Yoshinari, M., Ohtsuka, Y., and Dérand, T. 1994. Thin hydroxyapatite coating produced by the ion beam dynamic mixing method. *Biomaterials* 15: 529–535.
17. Cui, F.Z., Luo, Z.S., and Feng, Q.L. 1997. Highly adhesive hydroxyapatite coatings on titanium alloy formed by ion beam assisted deposition. *J Mater Sci Mater Med* 8: 403–405.
18. Wang, C.K., Chern Lin, J.H., Ju, C.P., Ong, H.C., and Chang, R.P.H. 1997. Structural characterization of pulsed laser-deposited hydroxyapatite film on titanium substrate. *Biomaterials* 18: 1331–1338.
19. Arias, J.L., García-Sanz, F.J., Mayor, M.B., et al. 1998. Physicochemical properties of calcium phosphate coatings produced by pulsed laser deposition at different water vapour pressures. *Biomaterials* 19: 883–888.
20. Fernández-Pradas, J.M., Clèries, L., Sardin, G., and Morenza, J.L. 2002. Characterization of calcium phosphate coatings deposited by Nd:YAG laser ablation at 355 nm: Influence of thickness. *Biomaterials*, 23: 1989–1994.
21. Yoshinari, M., Ozeki, K., and Sumii, T. 1991. Properties of hydroxyapatite-coated Ti-6Al-4V alloy produced by the ion-plating method. *Bull Tokyo Dent Coll* 32: 147–156.
22. Sato, M., Tu, R., Goto, T., Ueda, K., and Narushima, T. 2008. Apatite formation behavior on bioceramic films prepared by MOCVD. *J Ceram Soc Jpn* 117: 461–465.
23. Sato, M., Tu, R., Goto, T., Ueda, K., and Narushima, T. 2009. Preparation behavior in a Hanks' solution on Ca-P-O films prepared by laser CVD. *Mater Trans* 50: 2455–2459.
24. Yamashita, K., Matsuda, M., Arashi, T., and Umegaki, T. 1998. Crystallization, fluoridation and some properties of apatite thin films prepared through RF-sputtering from $CaO-P_2O_5$ glasses. *Biomaterials* 19: 1239–1244.
25. Sato, M., Tu, R., and Goto, T. 2006. Preparation conditions of $CaTiO_3$ film by metal-organic chemical vapor deposition. *Mater Trans* 47: 1386–1390.
26. Sato, M., Tu, R., and Goto, T. 2007. Preparation of hydroxyapatite and calcium phosphate films by MOCVD. *Mater Trans* 48: 3149–3153.
27. Sato, M., Tu, R., Goto, T., Ueda, K., and Narushima, T. 2008. Hydroxyapatite formation on Ca–P–O coating prepared by MOCVD. *Mater Trans* 49: 1848–1852.
28. Sato, M., Tu, R., Goto, T., Ueda, K., and Narushima, T. 2009. Precipitation behavior in a Hanks' solution on Ca–P–O films prepared by laser CVD. *Mater Trans* 50: 2455–2459.
29. Kelly, P.J. and Arnell, R.D. 2000. Magnetron sputtering: a review of recent developments and applications. *Vacuum* 56: 159–172.
30. Swann, S. 1988. Magnetron sputtering. *Phys Technol* 19: 67–75.
31. Wolke, J.G.C., van der Waerden, J.P.C.M., de Groot, K., and Jansen, J.A. 1997. Stability of radiofrequency magnetron sputtered calcium phosphate coatings under cyclically loaded conditions. *Biomaterials* 18: 483–488.
32. Nelea, V., Morosanu, C., Iliescu, M., and Mihailescu, I.N. 2004. Hydroxyapatite thin films grown by pulsed laser deposition and radio-frequency magnetron sputtering: comparative study. *Appl Surf Sci* 228: 346–356.
33. Ueda, K., Narushima, T., Goto, T., Taira, M., and Katsube, T. 2007. Fabrication of calcium phosphate films for coating on titanium substrates heated up to 773 K by RF magnetron sputtering and their evaluations. *Biomed Mater* 2: S160–S166.
34. Yang, Y., Kim, K.H., Agrawal, C.M., and Ong, J.L. 2003. Effect of post-deposition heating temperature and the presence of water vapor during heat treatment on crystallinity of calcium phosphate coatings. *Biomaterials* 24: 5131–5137.
35. Ding, S.-J., Ju, C.-P., and Lin, J.-H.C. 1999. Immersion behavior of RF magnetron-assisted sputtered hydroxyapatite/titanium coatings in simulated body fluid. *J Biomed Mater Res* 47: 551–563.
36. Zhao, Y.T., Zhang, Z., Dai, Q.X., Lin, D.Y., and Li, S.M. 2006. Microstructure and bond strength of HA($+ZrO_2+Y_2O_3$)/Ti6Al4V composite coatings fabricated by RF magnetron sputtering. *Surf Coat Technol* 200: 5354–5363.

37. Chen, M., Liu, D., You, C., Yang, X., and Cui, Z. 2007. Interfacial characteristic of graded hydroxyapatite and titanium thin film by magnetron sputtering. *Surf Coat Technol* 201: 5688–5691.
38. Ueda, K., Kawasaki, Y., Narushima, T., et al. 2009. Calcium phosphate films with/without heat treatments fabricated using RF magnetron sputtering. *J Biomech Sci Eng* 4: 392–403.
39. Aoki, H. 1989. Surface design and functions of hydroxyapatite. *J Surf Sci Soc Jpn* 10: 96–101.
40. Nakano, T., Fujitani, W., and Umakoshi, Y. 2004. Synthesis of apatite ceramics with preferential crystal orientation. *Mater Sci Forum* 449–452: 1289–1292.
41. Hoepfner, T.P. and Case, E.D. 2004. An estimate of the critical grain size for microcracks induced in hydroxyapatite by thermal expansion anisotropy. *Mater Lett* 58: 489–492.
42. Nakano, T., Kaibara, K., Tabata, Y., et al. 2002. Unique alignment and texture of biological apatite crystallites in typical calcified tissues analyzed by microbeam X-ray diffractometer system. *Bone* 31: 479–487.
43. van Dijk, K., Schaeken, H.G., and Wolke, J.C.G., et al. 1995. Influence of discharge power level on the properties of hydroxyapatite films deposited on Ti6Al4V with RF magnetron sputtering. *J Biomed Mater Res* 29: 269–276.
44. Nelea, V., Morosanu, C., Iliescu, M., and Mihailescu, I.N. 2003. Microstructure and mechanical properties of hydroxyapatite thin films grown by RF magnetron sputtering. *Surf Coat Technol* 173: 315–322.
45. Haman, J.D., Scripa, R.N., Rigsbee, J.M., and Lucas, L.C. 2002. Production of thin calcium phosphate coatings from glass source materials. *J Mater Sci Mater Med* 13: 175–184.
46. Ding, S.-J., Ju, C.-P., and Chern Lin, J.-H. 1999. Characterization of hydroxyapatite and titanium coatings sputtered on Ti–6Al–4V substrate. *J Biomed Mater Res* 44: 266–274.
47. Yoshinari, M., Oda, Y., Inoue, T., and Shimono, M. 2002. Dry-process surface modification for titanium dental implants. *Metall Mater Trans A* 33A: 511–519.
48. Zeng, H., Lacefield, W.R., and Mirov, S. 2000. Structural and morphological study of pulsed laser deposited calcium phosphate bioceramic coatings: Influence of deposition conditions, laser parameters, and target properties. *J Biomed Mater Res*, 50: 248–258.
49. Bryant, W.A. 1977. Review: The fundamentals of chemical vapor deposition. *J Mater Sci* 12: 1285–1306.
50. Clarke, D.R. and Levi, C.G., 2003. Materials design for the next generation thermal barrier coatings. *Annu Rev Mater Res* 33: 383–417.
51. Kadokura, H., Itoh, A., Kimura, T., and Goto, T. 2010. Moderate temperature and high-speed synthesis of α-Al_2O_3 films by laser chemical vapor deposition using Nd:YAG laser. *Surf Coat Technol* 204: 2302–2306.
52. Tu, R. and Goto, T. 2005. Thermal cycle resistance of yttria stabilized zirconia films prepared by MOCVD. *Mater Trans* 46: 1318–1323.
53. Pattanaik, A.K. and Sarin, V.K. 2001. Basic principles of CVD thermodynamics and kinetics. In Park, J.-H. (ed.), *Chemical Vapor Deposition, Surface Engineering Series* Vol. 2, pp. 23–43. Materials Park, OH: ASM International.
54. Duty, C., Jean, D., and Lackey, W.J. 2001. Laser chemical vapor deposition: Materials, modeling, and process control. *Inter Mater Rev* 46: 271–287.
55. Kimura, T. and Goto, T. 2003. Rapid synthesis of yttria-stabilized zirconia films by laser chemical vapor deposition. *Mater Trans* 44: 421–424.
56. Endo, J., Itoh, A., Kimura, T., and Goto, T. 2010. High-speed deposition of dense, dendritic and porous SiO_2 films by Nd: YAG laser chemical vapor deposition. *Mater Sci Eng B* 166: 225–229.
57. Sato, M., Tu, R., Goto, T., Ueda, K., and Narushima, T. 2008. Preparation of Ca–Ti–O/Ca–P–O functionally graded bio-ceramic film by MOCVD. *J Jpn Soc Powder Powder Metallurgy* 55: 325–330.
58. Allen, G.C., Ciliberto, E., Fragalà, I., and Spoto, G. 1996. Surface and bulk study of calcium phosphate bioceramics obtained by metal organic chemical vapor deposition. *Nucl Instrum Meth B* 116: 457–460.

59. Darr, J.A., Guo, Z.X., Raman, V., Bououdina, M., and Rehman, I.U. 2004. Metal organic chemical vapour deposition (MOCVD) of bone mineral like carbonated hydroxyapatite coatings. *Chem Commun* 6: 696–697.
60. Cao, Y., Weng, J., Chen, J., Feng, J., Yang, Z., and Zhang, X. 1996. Water vapour-treated hydroxyapatite coatings after plasma spraying and their characteristics. *Biomaterials* 17: 419–424.
61. Yang, C.Y., Lin, R.M., Wang, B.C., et al. 1997. In vitro and in vivo mechanical evaluations of plasma-sprayed hydroxyapatite coatings on titanium implants: The effect of coating characteristics. *J Biomed Mater Res* 37: 335–345.
62. Kweh, S.W.K., Khor, K.A., and Cheang, P. 2002. An in vitro investigation of plasma sprayed hydroxyapatite (HA) coatings produced with flame-spheroidized feedstock. *Biomaterials* 23: 775–785.
63. Silva, P.L., Santos, J.D., Monteiro, F.J., and Knowles, J.C. 1998. Adhesion and microstructural characterization of plasma-sprayed hydroxyapatite/glass ceramic coatings onto Ti–6Al–4V substrates. *Surf Coat Technol* 102: 191–196.
64. Filiaggi, M.J., Coombs, N.A., and Pilliar, R.M. 1991. Characterization of the interface in the plasma-sprayed HA coating/Ti–6Al–4V implant system. *J Biomed Mater Res* 25: 1211–1229.
65. Narushima, T., Ueda, K., Goto, T., et al. 2008. Fabrication and evaluation of calcium phosphate coating films on blast-treated Ti–6Al–4V alloy substrate. *J Jpn Soc Powder Powder Metall* 55: 318–324.
66. Ducheyne, P. and Qiu, Q. 1999. Bioactive ceramics: The effect of surface reactivity on bone formation and bone cell function. *Biomaterials* 20: 2287–2303.
67. Kokubo, T., and Takadama, H. 2006. How useful is SBF in predicting in vivo bone bioactivity? *Biomaterials* 27: 2907–2915.
68. Sato, M., Tu, R., Goto, T., Ueda, K., and Narushima, T. 2007. Hydroxyapatite formation on MOCVD-$CaTiO_3$ coated Ti. *Key Eng Mater* 352: 301–304.
69. Weng, J., Liu, Q., Wolke, J.G.C., Zhang, X., and de Groot, K. 1997. Formation and characteristics of the apatite layer on plasma-sprayed hydroxyapatite coatings in simulated body fluid. *Biomaterials* 18: 1027–1035.
70. Wen, C.E., Xu, W., Hu, W.Y., and Hodgson, P.D. 2007. Hydroxyapatite/titania sol–gel coatings on titanium–zirconium alloy for biomedical applications. *Acta Biomater* 3: 403–410.
71. Sugino, A., Tsuru, K., Hayakawa, S., et al. 2009. Induced deposition of bone-like hydroxyapatite on thermally oxidized titanium substrates using a spatial gap in a solution that mimics a body fluid. *J Ceram Soc Jpn* 117: 515–520.
72. Tanase, T., Akiyama, J., Iwai, K., and Asai, S. 2007. Characterization of surface biocompatibility of crystallographically aligned hydroxyapatite fabricated using magnetic field. *Mater Trans* 48: 2855–2860.
73. Wolke, J.G.C., de Groot, K., and Jansen, J.A. 1998. Dissolution and adhesion behavior of radiofrequency magnetron-sputtered Ca-P coatings. *J Mater Sci* 33: 3371–3376.
74. Verestiuc, L., Morosanu, C., Bercu, M., Pasuk, I., and Mihailescu, I.N. 2004. Chemical growth of calcium phosphate layers on magnetron sputtered HA films. *J Cryst Growth* 264: 483–491.
75. van der Wal, E., Wolke, J.G.C., Jansen, J.A., and Vredenberg, A.M. 2005. Initial reactivity of rf magnetron sputtered calcium phosphate thin films in simulated body fluids. *Appl Surf Sci* 246: 183–192.
76. Weng, J., Liu, Q., Wolke, J.G.C., Zhang, D., and de Groot, K. 1997. The role of amorphous phase in nucleating bone-like apatite on plasma-sprayed hydroxyapatite coatings in simulated body fluid. *J Mater Sci Lett* 16: 335–337.
77. Ogata, K., Imazato, S., Ehara, A., et al. 2005. Comparison of osteoblast responses to hydroxyapatite and hydroxyapatite/soluble calcium phosphate composites. *J Biomed Mater Res* 72A: 127–135.
78. Zhao, B.H., Lee, I.-S., Bai, W., Cui, F.Z., and Feng, H.L. 2005. Improvement of fibroblast adherence to titanium surface by calcium phosphate coating formed with IBAD. *Surf Coat Technol* 193: 366–371.

79. Hulshoff, J.E.G., van Dijk, K., van der Waerden, J.P.C.M., Wolke, J.G.C., Ginsel, L.A., and Jansen, J.A. 1995. Biological evaluation of the effect of magnetron sputtered Ca/P coatings on osteoblast-like cells in vitro. *J Biomed Mater Res* 29: 967–975.
80. Lee, I.-S., Kim, D.-H., Kim, H.-E., Jung, Y.-C., and Han, C.-H. 2002. Biological performance of calcium phosphate films formed on commercially pure Ti by electron-beam evaporation. *Biomaterials* 23: 609–615.
81. Ong, J.L., Bessho, K., Cavin, R., and Carnes, D.L. 2002. Bone response to radio frequency sputtered calcium phosphate implants and titanium implants in vivo. *J Biomed Mater Res* 59: 184–190.
82. Hayakawa, T., Yoshinari, M., Kiba, H., Yamamoto, H., Nemoto, K., and Jansen, J.A. 2002. Trabecular bone response to surface roughened and calcium phosphate (Ca–P) coated titanium implants. *Biomaterials* 23: 1025–1031.
83. Wolke, J.G.C., van der Waerden, J.P.C.M., Schaeken, H.G., and Jansen, J.A. 2003. In vivo dissolution behavior of various RF magnetron-sputtered Ca–P coatings on roughened titanium implants. *Biomaterials* 24: 2623–2629.
84. Wolke, J.G.C., de Groot, K., and Jansen, J.A. 1998. Subperiosteal implantation of various RF magnetron sputtered Ca-P coatings in goats. *J Biomed Mater Res* 43: 270–276.
85. Yoshinari, M., Oda, Y., Inoue, T., Matsuzaka, K., and Shimono, M. 2002. Bone response to calcium phosphate-coated and bisphosphonate-immobilized titanium implants. *Biomaterials* 23: 2879–2885.
86. Ueda, K., Narushima, T., Goto, T., et al. 2007. Evaluation of calcium phosphate coating films on titanium fabricated using RF magnetron sputtering. *Mater Trans* 48: 307–312.
87. Yoshinari, M., Oda, Y., Ueki, H., and Yokose, S. 2001. Immobilization of bisphosphonates on surface modified titanium. *Biomaterials* 22: 709–715.
88. Chen, C., Lee, I.-S., Zhang, S.-M., and Yang, H.C. 2010. Biomimetic apatite formation on calcium phosphate coated titanium in Dulbecco's phosphate buffered saline solution containing $CaCl_2$ with and without fibronectin. *Acta Biomater* 6: 2274–2281.
89. Akisue, T., Kurosaka, M., Matsui, N., et al. 2001. Paratibial cyst associated with wear debris after total knee arthroplasty. *J Arthroplasty* 16: 389–393.
90. Streicher, R.M., Weber, H., Schön, R., and Semlitsch, M. 1991. New surface modification for Ti–6Al–7Nb alloy: Oxygen diffusion hardening (ODH). *Biomaterials* 12: 125–129.
91. Kola, P.V., Daniels, S., Cameron, D.C., and Hashmi, M.S.J. 1996. Magnetron sputtering of TiN protective coatings for medical applications. *J Mater Proc Technol* 56: 422–430.
92. Paschoal, A.L., Vanâncio, E.C., de Campos Franceschini Canale, L., da Silva, O.L., Huerta-Vilca, D., and de Jesus Motheo, A. 2003. Metallic biomaterials TiN-coated: Corrosion analysis and biocompatibility. *Artif Organs* 27: 461–464.
93. Li, D.J. and Gu, H.Q. 2002. Cell attachment on diamond-like carbon coating. *Bull Mater Sci* 25: 7–13.
94. Pan, J., Leygraf, C., Thierry, D., and Ektessabi, A.M. 1997. Corrosion resistance for biomaterial applications of TiO_2 films deposited on titanium and stainless steel by ion-beam-assisted sputtering. *J Biomed Mater Res* 35: 309–318.
95. Huang, N., Yang, P., Leng, Y.X., et al. 2003. Hemocompatibility of titanium oxide films. *Biomaterials* 24: 2177–2187.
96. Leng, Y.X., Chen, J.Y., Wang, J., et al. 2006. Comparative properties of titanium oxide biomaterials grown by pulsed vacuum arc plasma deposition and by unbalanced magnetron sputtering. *Surf Coat Technol* 201: 157–163.
97. Narushima, T. 2010. Calcium phosphate coating on titanium using dry process. *Mater Sci Forum* 654–659: 2162–2167.
98. Ueda, K., Kawasaki, Y., Goto, T., Kurihara, J., Kawamura, H., and Narushima, T. 2010. Fabrication and evaluation of multi-layered calcium phosphate coating film on titanium. *J Jpn Soc Powder Powder Metall* 57: 314–320.

8

Coating of Material Surfaces with Layer-by-Layer Assembled Polyelectrolyte Films

Thomas Crouzier, Thomas Boudou, Kefeng Ren, and Catherine Picart

CONTENTS

Introduction

In the field of implantable biomaterials and tissue engineered constructs, the bulk properties of materials are usually recognized as being important for the overall properties, such as mechanical strength, of the materials. Surface properties, however, are of utmost importance because they have an impact on subsequent tissue and cellular events, including protein adsorption, cell adhesion, and inflammatory response (Thevenot et al. 2008), all of which are necessary for tissue remodeling. Considerable efforts are thus currently devoted toward the functionalization of biomaterial surfaces commonly used in biomedical applications (typically metals, polymers, ceramics) in order to provide them with new functional biological properties and to render them more biomimetic. In this work, biomimetic indicates an attempt to reproduce the self-organization of natural matrices. In particular, one of the major aims is to recreate the complex cell structure and environment at various length scales: from the cell membrane structure and pericellular coat (also called glycocalyx), which are important for signal transduction and the mechanical and chemical sensing of the cell (Zaidel-Bar et al. 2004), to the extracellular matrix composed of an entangled and hydrated network of proteins and glycosaminoglycans (Alberts et al. 1994). To this end, thin film coatings deposited on the "bulk" materials offer great potentialities. Designing thin films with nanometer-scale control over their internal structures while preserving the bioactivity of embedded molecules and adjusting their delivery is thus a great challenge, in particular when the delivery must be performed under physiological conditions (limited pH range, fixed ionic strength, presence of physiological fluids and cells). Not only are thin films of utmost importance for the biomedical field, but also in many other fields such as electronics, optical devices, sensors, and catalysis. Several techniques have thus been developed to design thin films at the molecular level, including Langmuir–Blodgett (LB) and self-assembled monolayers (SAMs). As already indicated by Tang et al. (2006) in their review, both present a certain number of limitations and disadvantages. The most problematic are probably the limited amounts of biological molecules incorporated into LB films because of their limited stability, their monolayer nature, and the need for the presence of thiols on the substrate (e.g., for only noble metals or silane) in order to deposit SAMs. For biological applications, there is thus a need for easier and more versatile deposition methods.

The layer-by-layer (LbL) method initially introduced by Moehwald, Decher, and Lvov 15 years ago consists of alternately depositing polyelectrolytes that self-assemble and self-organize on the material's surface, leading to the formation of polyelectrolyte multilayer (PEM) Films (Decher et al. 1992; Lvov et al. 1994). The procedure is simple and in principle applicable to many different kinds of substrate. In the first 10 years of the development of this technique for biomedical applications, the proofs of concept were given and different types of films containing charged species were successfully prepared, including biological molecules (polypeptides, polysaccharides, DNA, proteins, and viruses) and various kinds of nanoparticles (clay platelets, carbon nanotubes, etc.) (Ai et al. 2003; Decher and Schlenoff 2003). In a second phase of the technical development, the behavior of the cells deposited on films began to be explored in 2001 (Chluba et al. 2001). At the same period, a different mechanism for film growth—exponential growth—was discovered, which opened up new opportunities for the design of thick films with reservoir capacities (Picart et al. 2002). Within the past 5 years, possibilities for the spatiotemporal control of cell growth have emerged and the first in vivo studies have been performed. It is only recently that more complex cell processes such as cell differentiation have begun to be explored and controlled via PEM films. Overall, the possibilities for using a wide range of polyelectrolytes and nano-objects combined with the advantages offered by PEM coatings, such as spatial confinement and localized delivery, as well as protective effects on exposure to physiological media and external stresses, considerably enrich the biological applications for PEM films. Several reviews that include the biological field have been published in the past 3 years. They concern either the internal structure of the films (Jaber and Schlenoff 2006; Schönhoff et al. 2007; Sukhishvili et al. 2006; von Klitzing 2006) or the applications of PEM films at the nanoscale (Hammond 2004). These applications can be for controlled erosion (Lynn 2007), protein inspired nanofilms (Zhang et al. 2007), polyelectrolyte blends (Quinn et al. 2007), and biomedical applications including drug delivery, biosensors, biomimetism, and tissue engineering (Tang et al. 2006). In this chapter, we focus our attention on the design of PEM films for biomaterial surface coatings and tissue engineering. We provide a global view of the biological applications for PEM films as a template for tissue mimetism and as biomaterial coatings that have been achieved within the past 5 years. This includes a survey of the physical and chemical properties that have emerged as key points for controlling film nanostructure in relation to biological processes. We also include the different possibilities for controlling cell behavior via film composition, bioactivity, mechanical properties, and spatiotemporal or three-dimensional organization (Figure 8.1). We focus on supported LbL films, although other forms, such as membranes and capsules, also show great promise for biomedical applications. In particular, PEM-based films are widely explored and have already been the subject of several reviews (De Geest et al. 2007; Sukhorukov et al. 2005; Sukhorukov et al. 2007). However, the field of biosensors, which is very wide, will not be evoked because of space constraints.

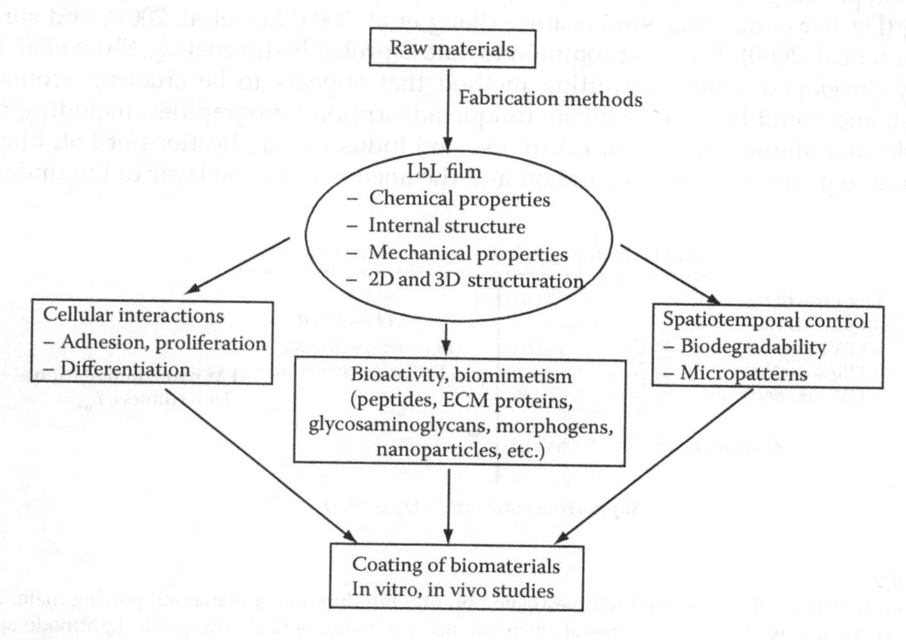

FIGURE 8.1
Scheme of different levels of controls that can lead to LbL films (also called polyelectrolyte multilayer films) with defined functionalities. One of their numerous potential applications is in the field of biomaterials and tissue engineering. (Reproduced with permission from Boudou et al., *Adv. Mater.*, 21, 1–27, 2009. Copyright Wiley-VCH Verlag GmbH & Co. KGaA 2010.)

Processing Parameters Influencing Film Growth and Structure

Driving Forces for Film Buildup

Figure 8.2 presents a schematic of all the techniques that can be employed to characterize film growth for films deposited on a supporting material. The growth of linearly and exponentially growing films can indeed be followed by quartz crystal microbalance with dissipation monitoring (QCM-D). The driving forces behind polyelectrolyte deposition using the LbL technique in order to form PEM have been already widely described and reviewed (von Klitzing 2006). These include electrostatic interactions as well as nonelectrostatic interactions, including short-range interactions such as hydrophobicity (Guyomard et al. 2005), hydrogen bonds (Sukhishvili and Granick 2002), van der Waals forces, charge transfer halogen interactions (Wang, Ma 2007), and possibly covalent bonds formed by click chemistry (Kinnane, Wark 2009). Thus, both the intrinsic properties of the polyelectrolytes themselves (structure of the polyelectrolyte, charge density, chain stiffness) and the physical and chemical properties of the suspending medium (presence and type of salt, pH) are key parameters. Importantly, it is now acknowledged that the driving force behind multilayer formation is not only of electrostatic origin, but also the gain in entropy due to the release of counterions (Dubas and Schlenoff 1999; von Klitzing 2006), very similar to what is observed in the formation of polyelectrolyte complexes (Sukhishvili et al. 2006).

Different Deposition Methods: Dip Coating, Spraying, Spin Coating

Various depositing methods have already been proposed for LbL buildup, including dip coating (Decher et al. 1992), spin coating (Jiang et al. 2004; Lee et al. 2001), and spraying (Schlenoff et al. 2000). The most common to date is probably dip coating. Shim et al. (2007) recently developed a new dewetting method that appears to be efficient, economical, and fast, and could be used to create unique adsorption topographies, including fractal networks and aligned fibers. For future use and industrial applications of LbL films, the total time required for film preparation and the anchorage of the layer to the underlying

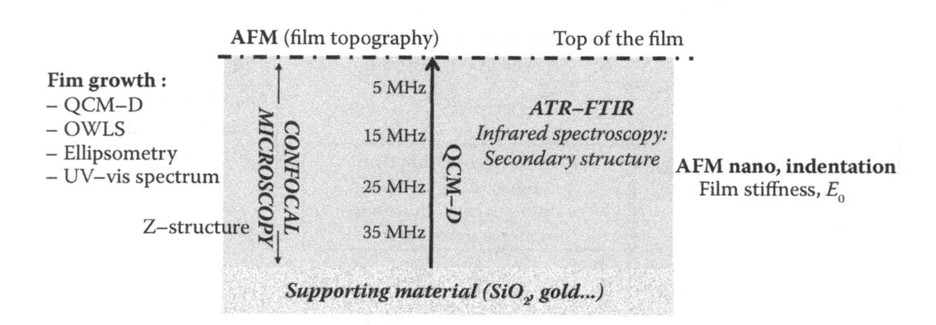

FIGURE 8.2
Scheme of different techniques used to investigate LbL film buildup onto a planar supporting material. Film growth can be followed by quartz crystal microbalance (QCM-D), optical waveguide lightmode spectroscopy (OWLS), UV–visible spectrometry, and ellipsometry. Film chemical structure can be probed by Fourier-transform infrared spectroscopy, and z-structure can be imaged by confocal laser scanning microscopy (CLSM) for films thicker than ~800 nm. AFM can be used both in topography mode to image film surface and in force mode to perform nanoindentations (AFM nanoindentation) to determine film Young's modulus, E_0. E_0 is a parameter characterizing film's mechanical properties.

substrate are probably important constraints. Therefore, particularly rapid methods such as spraying are being further developed (Izquierdo et al. 2005). Spray depositing was found to be effective even under conditions for which dipping failed to produce homogeneous films (e.g., extremely short contact times). Moreover, it was found that the rinsing step could be skipped, making it possible to speed up the whole buildup process.

Regarding anchorage to the underlying substrate, a recent development reported by Lee et al. (2008) paves the way to better anchoring of the film and could be applied in the case of particularly hydrophobic surfaces such as poly(tetrafluoroethylene) (PTFE) and poly(ethylene) (PE), which often require priming methods. These authors showed that mussel adhesive-inspired polymers containing catechol and amine functional groups, such as dopamine, can be grafted to various polyelectrolytes that allow the adsorption of polyelectrolytes and LbL buildup on various polymeric surfaces such as PTFE, polyethyleneterephthalate, and polycarbonate. These catecholamine polymers could thus be used as universal surface primers for facilitating LbL assembly on metal, oxide, and polymer substrates.

Overall, the numerous possibilities for depositing methods and the recent development of reinforced polyelectrolyte/surface anchoring strengthen the notion that films can be efficiently and reproducibly coated onto any kind of substrate.

Growth Mode: Linear versus Exponential

The first investigated polyelectrolyte systems were described by Decher et al. (1992). These systems showed linear growth of both mass and film thickness with the number of layers deposited. Poly(styrene sulfonate)/poly(allylamine hydrochloride) (PSS/PAH) films are one of the most prominent examples of linearly growing systems (Caruso et al. 1997; Picart et al. 2001a). These films have a stratified structure, each polyelectrolyte layer interpenetrating only its neighboring layers.

Films that grow exponentially have been described more recently by Elbert et al. (1999) and Picart et al. (2001b) for poly(L-lysine)/alginate (PLL/ALG) and PLL/hyaluronan (PLL/HA) films. Initially, this type of growth was mostly observed in films based on polyamino-acids and polysaccharides (Lavalle et al. 2002; Richert et al. 2004c; Tezcaner et al. 2006) before being found to be much more commonly encountered. Either film roughness (McAloney et al. 2001) or polyelectrolyte diffusion in and out of the film of one of the polyelectrolytes (Picart et al. 2002) was found to be at the origin of this growth, with the latter mechanism being increasingly recognized as a key feature in film growth. Even films made of synthetic polyelectrolytes such as polyacrylic acid (PAA) can exhibit an exponential growth (Sun et al. 2007; Zacharia et al. 2007). Exponential growth can be evidenced by QCM-D (Figure 8.3a). In addition, polyelectrolyte diffusion can be easily visualized via confocal laser scanning microscopy (CLSM) when the films are thick enough (at least 1 μm) (Figure 8.3b). This was shown by observing PLL^{FITC} (Picart et al. 2002), chitosan $(CHI)^{FITC}$ (Richert et al. 2004c), and end-labeled PAA (Sun et al. 2007) diffusion. A mechanism for this diffusion has also been proposed (Lavalle et al. 2004). According to a theoretical model by Salomaki and Kankare (2007), PLL/HA and CHI/HA films should always grow exponentially. Recently, the exponential growth mechanism has seen some significant developments. Films containing inorganic sheets can thus also show exponential growth (Podsiadlo et al. 2008). In addition, growth can be amplified by pH leading to even thicker films obtained in a very limited number of depositing cycles (Ji et al. 2006). Better understanding of the different growth mechanisms is also emerging (von Klitzing 2006). For instance, Porcel et al. (2006) showed that a transition from exponential to linear growth occurs at a certain level in film buildup. It also appears that even for synthetic polyelectrolyte films, exponential

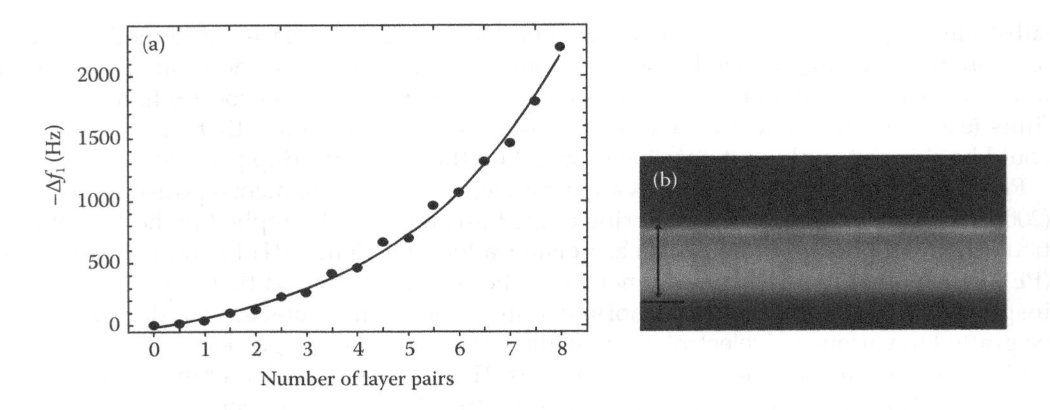

FIGURE 8.3
(a) QCM frequency shifts $-\Delta f/\nu$ for each layer as a function of number of layer pair n deposited on SiO_2 substrate. Data are given for fundamental frequency at 5 MHz. Black line corresponds to fit of data by an exponential law. (b) Z observation of a $(PLL/HA)_{19}$-PLL_{20} multilayer film by CLSM. Vertical section through film containing two labeled PLL_{19}^{FITC} (green) and $HA_{19}TR$ layers. Image size is 26.2 × 8.4 μm. Supporting glass slide is indicated with a white line. Green fluorescence (corresponding to PLL^{FITC}) is visible over a total thickness of about 4 μm (white arrow). (Adapted from Picart et al., *Proc. Natl. Acad. Sci. U S A*, 99, 12531–12535, 2002.)

growth becomes dominant when NaCl concentrations increase (McAloney et al. 2001) or when temperature is increased (Salomaki et al. 2005). Interestingly, isothermal titration microcalorimetry investigations indicate that the linear growth regime is associated with exothermic complexation, whereas the exponential growth regime relates to endothermic complexation (Laugel et al. 2006).

Film Hydration and Swellability: Sensitivity to External Parameters Such as pH and Ionic Strength

Film hydration can be estimated by measuring the film refractive index using techniques such as optical waveguide lightmode spectroscopy (Picart et al. 2001) or ellipsometry (by measuring respectively dry and hydrated film thickness) (Burke and Barrett 2003). Refractive index of synthetic PEM films, such as (PSS/PAH) films, was measured in situ by OWLS to be approximately 1.5 under physiological conditions (Picart et al. 2001). This indicates that these films are relatively dense and contain only about 25% of water (a simple approximation of the water content is based on the following formula: $n_{PEM} = 1.3340 \times a + (1 - a) \times 1.56$, where 1.334 is the refractive index of a 0.15 M NaCl solution, 1.56 is the refractive index of a pure polymer film (Burke and Barrett 2003), and a being the fraction of water). Similar measurements have been done using PLL, poly(D-lysine) (PDL), or even chitosan as polycation in combination with polyanions such as gelatin (Ai et al. 2003), poly(L-glutamic) acid (PGA) (Tryoen-Toth et al. 2002), or hyaluronan (Richert et al. 2004c). In general, films made of polypeptides and polysaccharides in comparable ionic strength conditions are more hydrated than films made of synthetic polyelectrolytes such as (PSS/PAH). This observation is based on refractive indices that are ≈1.36–1.38 for polysaccharide films (Picart et al. 2001; Richert et al. 2004c) and ≈1.42 for (PGA/PLL) films (Lavalle et al. 2002), which would correspond to water contents ranging respectively from 95% to 60%. Of note, the majority of synthetic polyelectrolytes have hydrophobic chain backbones, which determine film properties before complex formation. On the other hand, natural polyelectrolytes have hydrophilic groups on the backbone. This refractive index for (PLL/HA) films is of the same order of magnitude of that found via ellipsometry (Burke and Barrett 2003) for wet films (1.35), and has to be compared to the refractive index for dried films (1.56). This indicates that the film swells by about 830% (initial conditions for film assembly were pH 9 and 0.1 M NaCl). The high swelling capacities of polysaccharides, and in particular for hyaluronan (Lapcik et al. 1998) renders the buildup of much thicker films possible—up to several hundred nanometers (Richert et al. 2004c) or even several micrometers after deposition of 20 to 30 layer pairs (Picart et al. 2002). Because water content is an important parameter in film structure, the temperature of film buildup or of posttreatment storage can also play a role in the internal secondary structure of the film. This was nicely demonstrated by Boulmedais et al. (2003) for (PLL/PGA) films heated up to 89°C.

These polysaccharide-based films were often, if not always, found to inhibit cell attachment (Elbert et al. 1999; Richert et al. 2004a; Richert et al. 2004c), except when films were stiffened by covalent cross-linking (Richert et al. 2004). Therefore, a trend that seems to emerge from all these cell lines and primary cell studies is that nanometer-thin and dense films formed by few layer pairs, which are also very stiff, are more favorable for cellular adhesion than thick and highly hydrated films that are much softer (Picart et al. 2007).

A detailed study of the hydration and swelling properties of (PLL/HA) films indicates that the most important parameters are (1) the assembly pH (that can be varied from 5 to 9 for these particular films) and ionic strength and (2) the swelling medium (Burke and Barrett 2003). Thus, depending on the combination of these parameters, very different film properties can be achieved. Polysaccharides such as HA have a random coil conformation but can form hydrogen bonds with water (Hammond 1999). They can also exhibit hydrophobic interactions (Laurent 1998), which are influenced by ionic strength. Very interestingly, the pK_a of polyelectrolytes in the film demonstrates that both PLL and HA experience a significant shift in their $pK_{a(apparent)}$ values upon adsorption, compared to the accepted values (in dilute solution) of 9.36 ± 0.08 and 3.08 ± 0.03, respectively, in the presence of 1.0 mM NaCl. The $pK_{a(apparent)}$ values of both PLL and HA remained relatively constant after the first three to four deposited layers (at pH = 7, it is 4.8 for HA and 6.8 for PLL). This decrease in the acid strength of HA and base strength of PLL is similar to that reported for other polyelectrolyte pairs (Boulmedais et al. 2002). It has been previously speculated and experimentally shown that the charge on the multilayer film surface strongly influences the acid–base equilibria of adsorbing polyelectrolyte chains (Shiratori and Rubner 2000). According to Barret et al., for (PLL/HA) multilayer films, the overall trends in the $pK_{a(apparent)}$ shifts upon adsorption are influenced by the ability of both of these polymers to adopt some degree of secondary conformational order with changes in the local pH and ionic strength environment (Burke and Barrett 2003, 2005; Turner et al. 1988; Yasui and Keigerling 1986). In the intermediate pH range, HA is known to have some degree of chain stiffening in solution due to local hydrogen bonded regions, whereas PLL chains are reported to experience a random coil to α-helix transition at pH = 10.5 (Yasui and Keigerling 1986). The same authors also investigated the swelling of (PAH/HA) films and found that these films exhibit a high dependence of swelling on the assembly solution pH. The swelling ratio varied between 2 at physiological pH = 7 to more than 8 at very acidic pH = 2 and was more pronounced than that at basic pH = 10 (swelling ratio of about 5).

Influence of Molecular Weight on Film Buildup

Few studies have systematically investigated the influence of polymer molecular weight on the physical properties of PEM, either for synthetic polyelectrolytes (Sui et al. 2003) or for natural polyelectrolytes. One of the reasons is the difficulty in obtaining monodispersed polymers, especially for natural polyelectrolytes that have very diverse production methods and are subjected to natural variation. Kujawa et al. (2005) found that CHI/HA film thickness increased when the M_W of these polysaccharides was higher. However, this effect was only attributed to a difference in film growth onset and not to actual differences in mass deposited per layer. Sun et al. (2007) used the (PAH/PAA) synthetic film model to underline the importance of molecular weight in the buildup process. With lower molecular weight PAA, they observed that growth approached that of exponentially growing systems. The use of low-molecular-weight PAA instead of a higher MW (the one commonly used and commercially available) made it possible to diffuse it within these films, resulting in thicker and exponentially growing films. Such differences in diffusion were also observed by Porcel et al. (2007), who studied MW changes in the PLL/HA system. Changes in PLL and HA molecular weight did not significantly affect the mass deposited per layer, but the use of high MW PLL did restrain PLL diffusion within the upper part of the film. Most of the investigations that focused on the influence of polymer length essentially studied the influence on the film growth curve and thickness, with other properties (e.g., mechanical) rarely investigated (Lingstrom and Wagberg 2008). Overall, both the nature of diffusing species and its length are important.

Mechanical Properties

In recent years, designing PEM with adjustable mechanical properties has become a major challenge for applications in chemistry, physics, and biology. The characterization of their viscoelastic properties is thus crucial, and several methods that are specific to thin films have been employed. A common one is to perform nanoindentation experiments via atomic force microscopy (AFM), possibly using a colloidal probe as indenter (Dimitriadis et al. 2002; Richert et al. 2004b). Several other methods, relying on different physical principles, are well suited to characterizing thin films, some of them in a liquid state. These include quartz crystal microbalance (Salomaki et al. 2004; Salomaki and Kankare 2007), piezorheometry (Collin et al. 2004), or bulging tests (Lin et al. 2007). The stiffness of PEM can be modulated from a few kPa to several GPa depending on the structural properties of the polyelectrolytes, and also on the degree of cross-linking inside the film. In fact, both ionic cross-links, affected mostly by pH and ionic strength, and covalent cross-links induced by chemicals or photoactivation will impact film stiffness. It can also be observed that the stiffness of a native multilayer film is also related to the buildup regime in the LBL process. Films that grow exponentially are generally considered to be softer than those with a linear buildup (Collin et al. 2004). For instance, PLL/HA native films are rather viscous and Young's modulus (E_0) for cross-linked films reaches a maximum of 500 kPa, whereas PSS/PAH microcapsules in water are 300 MPa (Picart et al. 2007).

A first means of modulation consists in modifying the film's internal structure by using polyelectrolytes with different conformations such as carrageenans. Schoeler et al. (2006) thus characterized the stiffness of PEM containing PAH as the polycation and two different anionic sulfated polysaccharides: ι-carrageenan, which forms helical structures, and λ-carrageenan, which has a random coil conformation. Using AFM indentation, they found that films prepared with ι-carrageenan were about three times stiffer than those with λ-carrageenan, highlighting the strong influence of polyelectrolyte structures on the film's rigidity (Schoeler et al. 2006; Schönhoff et al. 2007). In a similar manner, grafting phospholipid (Kujawa et al. 2007) or sugar molecules, such as lactose or mannose

(Schneider et al. 2006), onto one of the polyelectrolytes can significantly influence the film's stiffness.

A second strategy for adjusting the mechanical properties of PEM films is to incorporate nanoparticles into the films. Inspired by the inorganic–organic composite material of seashells and lamellar bone, Kotov et al. studied the buildup of composite multilayer films containing cationic polyelectrolytes and anionic nanoparticles, such as carbon nanotubes (Tang et al. 2003; Gheith et al. 2005), montmorrillonite (Podsiadlo et al. 2007; Tang et al. 2003), or metallic nanoparticles (Jiang et al. 2004; Koktysh et al. 2002; Ostrander et al. 2001; Park et al. 2005). Evaluation of the mechanical properties of these composite films displayed up to 2 orders of magnitude more on Young's modulus when compared with the pure polyelectrolyte (Srivastava and Kotov 2008).

Another method of stiffening "soft" PEM films consists in inserting "stronger" polyelectrolytes. Caruso et al. and Schaaf et al. groups thus tailored PEM rigidity by mixing polyanions, whose behavior usually differed considerably when considered individually as film constituents (Ball et al. 2009; Cho et al. 2004; Hubsch et al. 2004). Although the rigidity in these studies was not measured directly, in many cases, the growth regime could be changed from exponential to linear by suitable blending, showing that most likely the mechanical properties had also changed. Considerable stiffening of the film was thus observed, for instance, by inserting "stiff" PSS/PAH layers on top of a "soft" PLL/HA film (Francius et al. 2007) or between layers of CHI/HA (Salomaki and Kankare 2009).

One of the many attractive features of PEM is the extent to which their mechanical properties can be tailored by varying the conditions used to assemble the films. Because of the pH-dependent dissociation of the weak acidic and alkaline functional groups on the chains, films prepared from weak polyelectrolytes (only partially charged at moderate pH near their p*K*) are strongly modulated by the pH and ionic strength environment. Mermut et al. (2003) thus showed that Young's modulus of films made of PAH and an azobenzene-containing polyelectrolyte was reduced from 6.5 to about 0.1 MPa when the assembly pH increased from 5 to 9. Several other groups, in particular Rubner et al., investigated the remarkable nanoscale control that can be exercised over the properties of (PAH/PAA) films (i.e., stiffness, thickness, roughness, wettability, and swelling behavior), by varying the pH conditions used to assemble the films (Mendelsohn et al. 2003; Pavoor et al. 2004; Thompson et al. 2005). In brief, PAH/PAA films assembled at a relatively neutral pH are significantly thinner and about 2 orders of magnitude stiffer than those assembled in acidic conditions.

It is also possible to adjust the mechanical properties of PEMs by chemical means, for instance, by creating covalent cross-links within the films. As an example, it is already known that high temperature (130°C) can induce the formation of amide or imide bonds within films (Dai et al. 2001). A protocol based on the carbodiimide chemistry for cross-linking carboxyl groups with amine groups in "mild" conditions (room temperature, salt-containing medium), thereby forming covalent amide bonds (also called peptide bonds), was proposed by Richert et al. (2004a) and Schuetz and Caruso (2003). Of note, the carbodiimide used (1-ethyl-3-(3-dimethylaminopropyl) carbodiimide [EDC]) was a zero-length cross-linker, which means that no additional molecule was inserted into the film. The cross-linking results in the selective transformation of ionic (ammonium and carboxylate) cross-links into covalent amide bonds (Figure 8.4). This versatile protocol can be applied to many different types of polyelectrolyte films, provided that they possess carboxylic and amine groups.

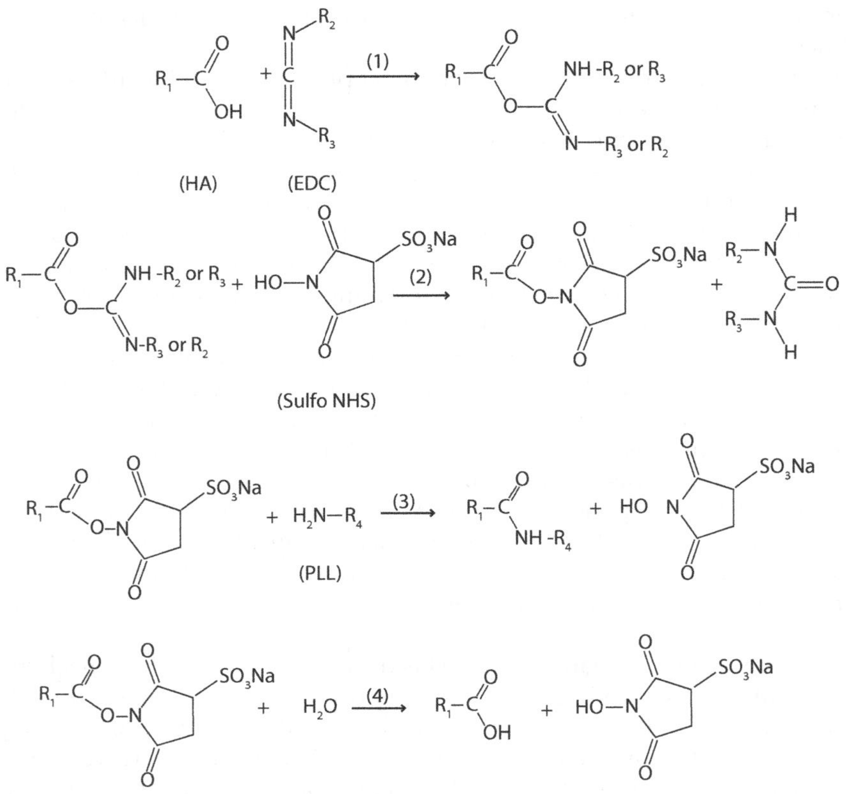

FIGURE 8.4
EDC and sulfo-NHS coupling scheme. EDC reacts with a carboxylic group and activates it (1). Activated complex is conversed into an active ester with sulfo-NHS (2). Active ester reacts with primary amine to form an amide bound (3). Unreacted sites are hydrolyzed to give a regeneration of carboxyls (4). (Reproduced with permission from Richert et al., *Biomacromolecules*, 5, 284–294, 2004. Copyright American Chemical Society 2004.)

Cross-linking has major consequences on film structure and mechanical properties. Using AFM nanoindentation, considerable stiffening of both PLL/HA and CHI/HA films was evidenced and Young's modulus was much higher when compared to the native (uncross-linked) films (Francius et al. 2006; Richert et al. 2004b; Schneider et al. 2007b). Moreover, another consequence of cross-linking is to significantly improve their resistance to the biodegradation of CHI/HA films, both in vitro and in vivo (Etienne et al. 2005b; Picart et al. 2005b). Tuning the EDC cross-linker concentration allows us to vary the Young's modulus of (PLL/HA) films over 2 orders of magnitude (Figure 8.5) (Francius et al. 2006). Of note, the percentage of decrease in the carboxylic peak, which can be precisely quantified by FTIR spectroscopy (Crouzier and Picart 2009), is found to be related to the film Young's modulus E_0 (Figure 8.6).

Using a different strategy, Li and Haynie (2004) investigated cross-linking and stabilization of polypeptide PEMs by formation of disulfide bonds, which are reversible. Disulfide bonds are involved in the structural stabilization of proteins. More recently, Such et al. (2007) reported a new method for covalent cross-linking via click chemistry to facilitate the LbL assembly of thin films.

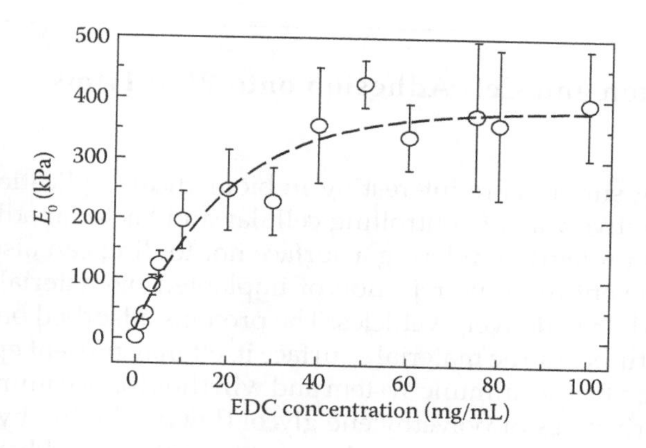

FIGURE 8.5
Surface Young's modulus E_0 determined by AFM nanoindentation technique for various EDC concentrations up to 100 mg/mL. An exponential asymptotic fit to data is also represented (thick line). Error bars represent standard deviation of 6 to 16 measurements of E_0 corresponding to various approach velocities. (Reproduced with permission from Francius et al., *Microsc. Res. Tech.*, 69, 84–92, 2006. Copyright Wiley-VCH Verlag GmbH & Co. KGaA.)

A few recent approaches to adjusting the mechanical properties of PEMs are based on photo-cross-linking. One major advantage to photo-cross-linking is that it offers the possibility of patterning PEMs. Yang and Rubner (2002) extensively demonstrated the proofs of concept for this type of cross-linking.

Pozos-Vásquez et al. (2009) also reported on the preparation of polyelectrolyte films based on PLL and HA derivatives modified by photoreactive vinylbenzyl (VB) groups. The VB-modified HA incorporated into the films was cross-linked on UV irradiation, and the force measurements taken by AFM proved that the rigidity of the cross-linked films was increased up to fourfold.

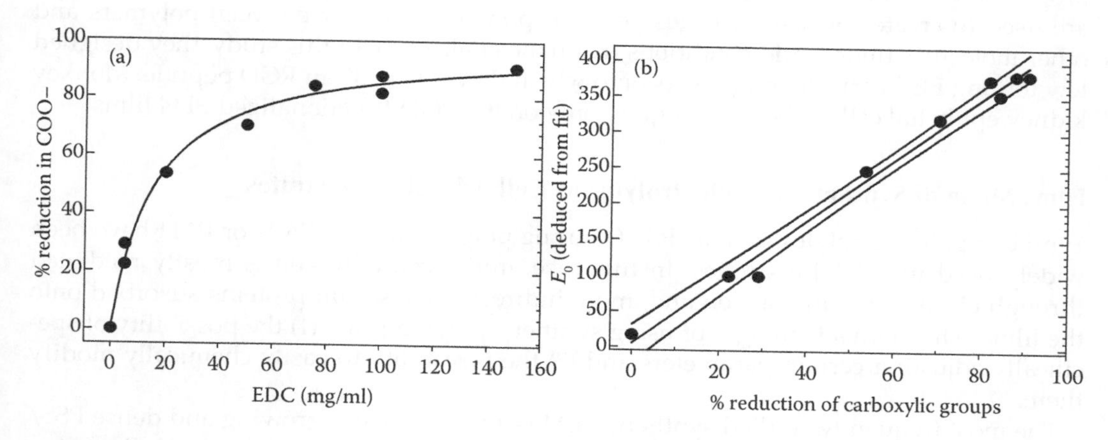

FIGURE 8.6
(a) Percentage of carboxylic groups remaining in film after cross-linking procedure, as a function of initial EDC concentration. (b) Film Young's modulus E_0 plotted as a function of percentage of reduction of carboxylic groups (band at 1610 cm^{-1}). Also shown is a regression line with the error interval (95%, dashed lines).

Protein Adsorption and Cell Adhesion onto PEM Films

Nonfouling Films

Non- or low-fouling surfaces are interesting in biomedical applications for two reasons. They can be an effective way of controlling cellular and bacterial adhesion by enhanced resistance to serum proteins. Rendering a surface nonfouling can also serve as immuno-"camouflage" to prevent immune rejection of implanted biomaterials or to enhance the efficiency of injected drug delivery vehicles. The proteins adsorbed on a material's surface may in fact be denatured, or the material's surface itself may present epitopes that could be recognized as foreign by the immune system and will thus induce immune reactions (Chen and Scott 2001). Derivatives of polyethylene glycol (PEG), a highly hydrated polymer, are very effective in rendering surfaces nonadsorbent to proteins and have been widely used since the 1990s to modify various substrates (Wagner et al. 2004). Compared to the standard chemical grafting techniques used for PEG surface functionalization, multilayer film depositing has the advantage of being rather independent of the nature or topology of the material. Thus, PEM films have been constructed using PEG-grafted polymers (Boulmedais et al. 2004) or by depositing a PEG layer on top of the films (Kidambi et al. 2008), yielding a nonfouling multilayer film. In a more biomimetic approach, phosphorylcholine (PC) and ethylene oxide $(EO)_3$ groups, which are naturally nonfouling components of erythrocyte membranes, have been grafted onto a (PSS/PAH) film, thereby lowering protein adsoption (Reisch et al. 2009). The nonfouling properties were attributed to the zwiterionic properties of the molecules. Films containing natural polysaccharides are often nonfouling and nonadhesive for cells because of their high water content and softness.

One of the advantages of nonfouling PEM is their ability to create a so-called "blank slate" (Croll et al. 2006) (e.g., a nonadhesive surface that can be subsequently modified by covalently grafting adhesion peptides). Croll et al. (2006) presented cytophobic PEM made from high-molecular-weight hyaluronanic acid and chitosan that was resistant to serum protein adsorption. Upon covalent grafting of collagen IV on top of the films, the films switched to cytophilic. A similar strategy based on "click" chemistry was recently proposed by Kinnane et al. (2009). Alkyne or azide groups incorporated into the polymer are used to create covalent linkages between polymer layers or between polymers and other molecules under mild conditions (Kinnane et al. 2009). In this study, they designed low fouling PEG acrylate multilayers onto which they "clicked" an RGD peptide. Monkey kidney epithelial cells adhered and grew only on the RGD-functionalized PEG films.

Films Made of Synthetic Polyelectrolytes as Cell Adhesive Substrates

Synthetic polyelectrolytes such as PSS (a strong polyelectrolyte), PAA, or PAH have been widely used in cell/film studies. In this case, initial cell adhesion is mostly mediated through electrostatic interaction and, more indirectly, via serum proteins adsorbed onto the films. The main advantages of using synthetic polymers are: (1) the possibility of specifically adjusting certain parameters and (2) the possibility to easily chemically modify them.

The most frequently studied synthetic PEM is, by far, linearly growing and dense PSS/PAH films. Cell types such as endothelial cells (Boura et al. 2003), fibroblasts (Brunot et al. 2008; Mhamdi et al. 2006), osteoblastic cells (Tryoen-Toth et al. 2002), and hepatocytes (Wittmer et al. 2008) have been cultured on these films. As a general rule, adhesion and proliferation on these films are very good, which may be attributed partly to the presence of sulfonate groups. The importance of such groups was evidenced in hepatocytes by using films made from PDDA and PSS (Kidambi et al. 2004). The hepatocytes adhered only on the films terminated with a PSS layer and not on PDDA ending films. However, other cells lines, such as fibroblasts, were less sensitive and adhered on both the PDDA and PSS. Of note, certain serum proteins present in the cell culture medium, such as bovine serum albumin (BSA), adsorb onto the PSS-ending films, although only weakly (Ladam et al. 2000). PAH/PAA films are also widely studied. PAA-ending films were found to be resistant to the adsorption of BSA, fibrinogen or even to lysozyme, which is oppositely charged to PAA (Salloum and Schlenoff 2004). This was explained not only by the low charge density of PAA, but also by its strong hydration that creates an exclusion volume above the PAA layer.

Usually, proteins adsorb preferentially onto films of opposite charge (Gergely et al. 2004; Ladam et al. 2001; Salloum and Schlenoff 2004). However, it now seems to be accepted that protein adsorption cannot account for the significant differences in cell adhesion (Mendelsohn et al. 2003; Olenych et al. 2005). For PAH/PAA films, the nonadhesiveness of the films built at pH 2 and the high adhesion observed for films built at pH 6.5 were instead attributed to the ability of the former to swell (Mendelsohn et al. 2003).

Synthetic polymers were also employed by Salloum et al. (2005) to investigate the combined effects of increasing surface charge and hydrophobicity on vascular smooth muscle cell (SMCs) adhesion. On the most hydrophobic surfaces, the A7R75 SMCs spread and were not very motile, whereas on the most hydrophilic surfaces, these cells adhered poorly and displayed characteristics of being highly motile.

If synthetic polymers are to be used for in vivo implantations, their possible toxicity must also be evaluated. The biocompatibility of a single PEI layer was tested on both fibroblastic and osteoblastic cells. Pure titanium (Ti) and nickel–titanium (NiTi) alloy were coated with PEI and morphology, adhesion and viability were assessed for up to 7 days after seeding. The results show that the cells were less viable and proliferated less on PEI-coated titanium than on the control, suggesting that PEI is potentially cytotoxic (Brunot et al. 2007). On the other hand, PSS/PAH films deposited on human umbilical arteries showed good grafting behavior and no inflammation in a rabbit model after 12 weeks of implantation (Kerdjoudj et al. 2008). Systematic studies for each specific case are thus required.

Film as Mimics of Extracellular Matrix for Specific Cell Cultures

A step closer to recreating the original matrix into which cells develop in vivo is to use ECM components as building blocks for the films. One advantage of these natural components is their bioavailability and their possible biodegradability, as specific enzymes are present in tissue and biological fluids. Thus, besides being used as natural mimics, they can be potentially employed as biodegradable delivery systems.

PEM made of ECM proteins such as collagen (COL) (Gong et al. 2007; Sinani et al. 2003; Zhang et al. 2005) or gelatin (GEL) (Zhu et al. 2003) and of glycoaminoglycans such as HA (Picart et al. 2001b), CS (Liu et al. 2005c; Tezcaner et al. 2006), and HEP (Mao et al. 2005; Tan et al. 2003; Wood et al. 2005) have been reported. Other polysaccharides, which are not present in the human body but can be found in algae, crustacean shells, or fungi, are also used. This is the case for ALG (Elbert et al. 1999; Yuan et al. 2007), dextran sulfate (DEXS) (Nakahara et al. 2007), and CHI (Richert et al. 2004c; Serizawa et al. 2002; Yuan et al. 2007), which are already being used in tissue engineering (Kumar 2000; Coviello et al. 2006) and have also been the subject of several studies. However, it is difficult to find a general rule concerning cell behavior for such films, as this depends both on the properties of the film (thickness, hydration, mechanical properties) and cell type. For instance, PEM made from highly hydrated polysaccharides from a combination of polysaccharides and polyamino-acids often yield gel-like films. Some cells are known to adhere poorly to hydrated surfaces and materials that are too soft (Discher et al. 2005). This was indeed observed for chondrosarcoma cells, chondrocytes, and osteoblast adhesion onto films such as PLL/HA (Richert et al. 2004a; Richert et al. 2004b), CHI/HA (Croll et al. 2006; Schneider et al. 2007b), PLL/ALG (Elbert et al. 1999), or PLL/PGA (Picart et al. 2005a). However, for certain cell types, softness is preferred. For instance, neuronal cells were found to adhere to COL/HA films (Wu et al. 2007). The outer layer chemistry has been found to be important in some cases as COL ending films showed improved adhesion, but COL was not necessary for adhesion. Cortical neurons and hippocampal neurons were sensitive to a different surface chemistry. Similarly, Tezcaner et al. (2006) showed that photoreceptor cells exhibit good viability on PLL/HA and PLL/CSA films. Gong et al. (2007) also reported that cartilage-mimetic PEM films made of COL and CSA have a beneficial effect on cell attachment, proliferation and also on glycosaminoglycan secretion. (CHI/PGA) films promoted the attachment and growth of C2C12 myoblast cells (Song et al. 2009).

So far, it appears that there is limited understanding of the detailed molecular mechanisms of cell adhesion onto these biomimetic films. In particular, there is only a study that aimed to characterize the types of integrins involved in cell adhesion, PSS/PAH films being taken as substrate (Boura et al. 2005).

ECM Protein and Peptide Coatings on PEM Films

Several studies have tried to increase cell adhesion on PEM films by coating the final layer with adhesion-promoting molecules such as fibronectin (FN), vitronectin (VN), or COL that are known to engage specific cell receptors (Alberts et al. 1994). In this paragraph, we discuss studies that deal with cell interactions onto the ECM protein modified films. The first step of these studies is to characterize and quantify protein adsorption on the films. The underlying idea is to give an additional functionality to the films by enhancing cell interactions while preserving the "bulk" properties (biodegradability, mechanical properties, etc.). Wittmer et al. (2007) added a final fibronectin layer to PLL/DEXS films and found that higher amounts of fibronectin were adsorbed on positively charged PLL ending films. Human umbilical vein endothelial cells spread to a greater extent and more symmetrically on FN-coated films. They also concluded that the presence of FN is a more important factor than film charge or layer number in controlling the interactions between multilayer films and living cells. Kreke et al. (2005) quantified FN adsorption onto PAH/HEP films at various pH solutions and found the highest FN adsorption at pH 8.4, which they attributed to a charge effect. However, adsorbed amount of FN was not the sole factor explaining the differences observed in cell adhesion strength. Semenov et al. (2009) showed recently that FN adsorbed onto cross-linked PLL/HA films promoted focal adhesion formation and was critical for maintaining densely grown mesenchymal stromal cell cultures over weeks for their differentiation.

A similar study was conducted on PAH/PSS films by Li et al. (2005). After coating the films with FN or GEL, they observed a general increase in the adhesion and proliferation of SMCs. However, they also noted that these properties depend on the number of layers in the PEM, meaning that not only outer layer chemistry but also film bulk nanostructure control cellular adhesion.

Another strategy for selectively improving cell adhesion on PEM films is to graft peptides that are known to interact with specific cell adhesion receptors. Basically, the idea underlying this strategy is similar to the previous one except that the method is different: here, only short sequences of the ECM proteins are considered and have to be covalently grafted to one of the polyelectrolyte. This requires first a synthetic chemistry step. The most prominent example is that of the RGD sequence. Hersel et al. reviewed the considerable number of strategies that have been developed to immobilize RGD on polymers, RGD being a central integrin-binding region in FN and COL. Using PEM, a new strategy consisted of grafting the peptide to one of the polyelectrolytes and then adsorbing the modified polyelectrolyte as a regular layer. PEM films exhibiting a poor adhesion are excellent candidates for such functionalization, which was applied using PAH-RGD and PGA-RGD for cell attachment (Berg et al. 2004; Picart et al. 2005a). Thus, the grafting of a 15–amino acid peptide containing the RGD motif (Figure 8.7) increased significantly the initial adhesion of primary osteoblasts onto PLL/PGA films. Interestingly, both film cross-linking and peptide grafting had an effect on the adhesion that could be potentialized when combined together (Picart et al. 2005a). Recently, in an elegant work by Werner et al. (2009), it was shown that a laminin-5–derived peptide grafted to PGA could induce specific cell adhesive structures in epithelial cells called hemidesmosomes and activate β_4 integrins. Using a different strategy, HA/CHI films onto which cells adhered poorly were rendered adherent by functionalization with an RGD containing peptide using carbodiimide chemistry (Chua et al. 2008). The immobilized RGD was shown to have a beneficial influence on osteoblast adhesion and proliferation. Other peptides, such

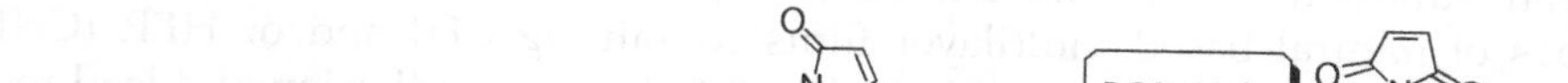

FIGURE 8.7
Scheme of synthesis of 15–amino acid peptide that contained a –RGD– sequence (PGA-RGD15m). In a first step, PGA was conjugated to maleimide groups (PGA-Mal). Then, conjugated PGA-Mal was mixed with PGD15m peptide. Mercaptopropionic acid was used to neutralize unreacted maleimide groups. Final product contains thus both RGD function and carboxylic sites that have a polyelectrolyte character. Grafting ratio was 10%. (Reproduced with permission from Picart et al., *Adv. Funct. Mater.*, 15, 83–94, 2005a. Copyright Wiley-VCH Verlag GmbH & Co. KGaA 2005.)

as alpha-melanocyte-stimulating hormone (α-MSH), with anti-inflammatory properties, have also successfully been integrated into multilayer films. Initially coupled with PLL, α-MSH was effective toward melanoma cells that were induced to produce melanocortin (Chluba et al. 2001.) Then, coupled with PGA and introduced into PLL/PGA films, it was efficient in annihilating the effect of a bacterial endotoxin that stimulated an inflammatory response in human monocytic cells (Jessel et al. 2004). The morphology of the monocytes was also affected by α-MSH as the cells formed many "fiber like" protrusions not visible on standard PLL/PGA films.

Importantly, however, the question has been raised as to whether these chemical modifications in the polyelectrolytes alter other physical chemical properties such as protein adsorption or mechanical properties, in turn influencing cell adhesion and proliferation. This is supported by recent findings by Thompson et al. (2006) and Schneider et al. (2006b), who measured the mechanical properties of the films with or without modified polyelectrolytes.

Antibacterial Coatings

The use of CHI in antibacterial dressings has received considerable attention in the past decade (Kumar 2000). The exact antibacterial mechanism of CHI is still unknown. One mechanism proposed is based on the interaction between positively charged chitosan molecules and negatively charged microbial membranes causing leakage of intracellular constituents.

Bacterial adhesion (*Escherichia coli* Gram-negative strain) was investigated on certain types of natural based multilayer films containing CHI and/or HEP. $(CHI/HA)_{10}$ films (built in 0.15 M NaCl) are highly resistant to bacterial adhesion and lead to a ≈80% decrease in bacterial adhesion as compared to bare glass (Richert et al. 2004c). On the other hand, $(CHI/HA)_{20}$ films built in 10^{-2} M NaCl were less resistant to bacterial adhesion (40% less than control on the CHI ending films and 20% less on the HA-ending films). The differences observed were explained by the lower thickness of the (CHI/HA) films built in 10^{-2} M NaCl (120 nm as compared to 300 nm for those built in 0.15 M NaCl). CHI/κ-carrageenan films were found to have a greater effect in decreasing initial bacterial adhesion than a thinner CHI coating, which was explained by the greater hydration of the multilayer films (Bratskaya et al. 2007). Adhesion of negatively charged enterococci was slightly enhanced on CHI-terminated multilayers, but the antibacterial effect was absent on κ-carregan–terminated multilayers.

Heparin, with its antithrombogenicity and strong hydrophilicity, also prevented adhesion of bacteria. The antibacterial properties of films containing both polysaccharides have thus been explored. CHI/HEP multilayer films were found to kill the bacteria that had adhered to the surface. Initial *E. coli* adhesion was also greatly decreased on the multilayer films (Fu et al. 2005). The assembly pH was found to be an important parameter in the design of efficient antiadhesive and antibacterial films.

To enhance the antibacterial effect of multilayer films, the same authors prepared films containing silver nanoparticles and coated a polyethylene terephthalate graft with alternating layers of CHI/HEP, chitosan being complexed with silver nanoparticles of 10–40 nm in size (Fu et al. 2006). The multilayer films containing nanosilver not only had effective antibacterial properties but also anticoagulant properties, while remaining nontoxic for the cells. Other types of film, such as PGA/lysozyme, were also found to inhibit bacterial adhesion (Rudra et al. 2006).

Other strategies rely on the use of antifungal peptides embedded in films (Etienne et al. 2005a), possibly incorporated by means of an amphiphilic polyelectrolyte precomplex with an hydrophobic peptide (Guyomard et al. 2008) or on Ag^+ ions as bactericides. In a first approach, Lee et al. (2005) prepared hydrogen-bonded multilayers containing Ag nanoparticles synthesized in situ and that were deposited on both planar surfaces and magnetic colloidal particles. The duration of the sustained release of antibacterial Ag ions from these coatings was prolonged by increasing the total supply of zero valent silver in the films via multiple loading and reduction cycles. Later, Li et al. (2006) constructed thin films with two distinct layered functional regions: a reservoir for the loading and release of bactericidal chemicals and a nanoparticle surface cap with immobilized bactericides. This resulted in dual-functional bactericidal coatings with both a chemical-releasing bacteria-killing capacity and a contact bacteria-killing capacity. These dual-functional coatings showed very high initial bacteria-killing efficiency due to the release of the Ag ions and retained significant antibacterial activity after the depletion of the embedded Ag because of the immobilized quaternary ammonium salts. Another strategy consists in loading silver ions into liposomes and subsequently embedding liposome aggregates into PLL/HA films (Malcher et al. 2008). The strong bactericidal effect observed was attributed to the diffusion of the silver ions out of the $AgNO_3$ coatings, leading to a significant bactericidal concentration close to the membrane of the bacteria.

Film Biodegradability

Although, in principle, multilayer films can be built under extremely different conditions in terms of pH and ionic strength, the final suspending medium may depend on the foreseen application. In particular, when cell culture studies or deposition on biomaterial surfaces are foreseen, it is then necessary that the films are stable in culture medium and in physiological conditions. These requirements may greatly limit the range of possible buildup conditions due to stability constraints. On the other hand, if the films are to be used for a subsequent release of a film component itself or of a bioactive molecule (see below), then stability is not a matter of importance, or at least is not as important as in the first case.

It stems from the aforementioned properties of the natural-based multilayer films (weak electrostatic charge, high hydration and swellability, secondary interactions) that these softer films are also more fragile than synthetic ones. This is particularly true when the films are built in a medium that has a different pH and/or ionic strength from a physiological medium (ionic strength of about 0.15 M NaCl, neutral pH). Next, the films are subjected to stresses upon medium change and can potentially be disrupted due to very high internal stresses. Typical cases are films built at acidic pH such as COL/HA films or CHI/HA films, for which COL and CHI are polycationic at acidic pH (4 for COL and less than ~5.5 for CHI). Johansson et al. (2005) found that COL/HA films are not stable when the pH is raised from 4 to 7. This could be explained by the protonation/deprotonation process for the polyelectrolytes involved in the interaction. At pH 4.0, most acid functionalities are protonated, whereas they are deprotonated at pH 7. Regarding collagen, the number of negatively charged acids on collagen approaches the number of protonated amines or the isoelectric point. The protonation/deprotonation processes induces the changes in the three-dimensional structure of the polyelectrolytes, which affects the electrostatic forces that existed between the polyelectrolyte layers. This dissolution was found to be irreversible.

However, and importantly, the film stability can be tuned depending on the nature of the film components and on the film's posttreatment. Regarding CHI/HA films, we found that the stability depends on the molecular weight of the chitosan: whereas films built with high-molecular-weight chitosan are stable in physiological medium (Richert et al. 2004c), films built with chitosan oligosaccharides (M_W = 5000 g/mol) are exhibiting a change in structure when introduced into the culture medium (Picart et al. 2005b). We evidenced that this change in structure was mostly due to the presence of divalent ions (Ca^{2+}, Mg^{2+} in the culture medium) and not to the change in pH. In fact, divalent ions are known to complex chitosan (Rhazi et al. 2002) and also alginate (Amsden and Turner 1999). Interestingly, the films can be degraded by enzymes present in body fluids such as hyaluronidase (Figure 8.8) or lysozyme, a biodegradation that depends on the extent of film cross-linking (the more cross-linked the films are, the more resistant they are).

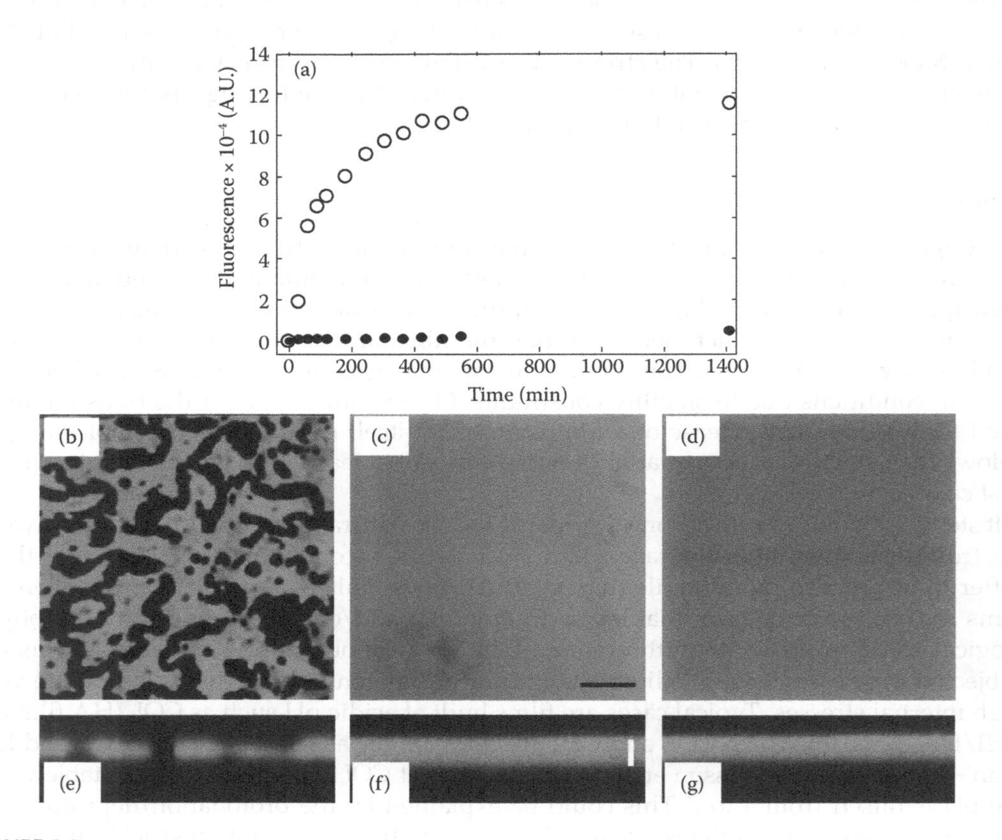

FIGURE 8.8
Degradation of a $(CHI/HA)_{24}$-CHI^{FITC} film after contact with hyaluronidase (type IV, 500U/mL) (same polyelectrolytes as in Figure 8.4): (a) followed by fluorimetry versus time for a native film (open symbols) and for a cross-linked film (closed symbols). (b, c, e, f) observed by CLSM after 4 h of contact for native (b, e) and cross-linked films (c, f) films. Cross-linking was achieved at 200 mM EDC concentration. Top views (56 × 56 μm²) of the films (b, c) (scale bar, 10 μm) and vertical sections are shown (e, f). Control images of film before contact with enzyme are also given (d and g). Vertical section scales are respectively 18.5 μm for image e and 19.5 μm for images f and g (film thickness is about 6 μm, white line). (Reproduced with permission from Picart et al., *Adv. Funct. Mater.*, 15, 1771–1780, 2005b. Copyright Wiley-VCH Verlag GmbH & Co. KGaA 2005.)

Even when films are not built in acidic or basic conditions, they may be subjected to dissolution in physiological medium. This was observed for films containing PEI as polyanion and a mixture of heparin and acid fibroblast growth factors whose degradation could be observed in PBS at 37°C (Mao et al. 2005). In contrast, films built with basic fibroblast growth factor and chondroitin sulfate (Ma et al. 2007) were stable in PBS. However, it is difficult to establish a common rule and each type of film needs to be tested. It also has to be noted that the presence of cells, which are able to exert strong stress on their matrix (Discher et al. 2005), can also affect the film stability.

It is important to stress that different strategies have been proposed to increase the mechanical resistance of the most fragile films (i.e., polypeptide or polysaccharide-based ones), in particular by cross-linking them using various strategies for increasing their mechanical properties (see Section 8.2.6).

Besides spatial control of film organization, a great amount of work deals with the temporal control of film durability and, in particular, controlled degradability. This has become of utmost importance in the field of drug delivery, in which PEMs have found many applications. The different stimulus pathways used to trigger deconstruction or dissolution have already been detailed by Tang et al. (2006) and Lynn (2007) for PEM films and De Geest et al. (2007) for PEM capsules.

A new strategy relies on the preparation of films with adjustable biodegradability, depending on the D- over L-lysine enantiomer ratio in the polyelectrolyte solution (Benkirane-Jessel et al. 2005). THP-1 macrophages produced TNF-α when they came into contact with protein A embedded in the film. The production of TNF-α started after a varying induction time and displayed a transition from no-production to full-production, which took place over a period that depended on both the film's composition and the embedding depth. The same type of macrophages degraded cross-linked CHI/HA films in an adjustable manner that depended on the extent of film cross-linking (Picart et al. 2005b). Of note, the initial adhesion of these macrophages was also related to the degree of cross-linking.

A development of the widely explored hydrolytically degradable polymers was recently presented by Liu et al. (2005c). It consists in synthesizing "charge-shifting" cationic polymers. Liu et al. demonstrated that the addition of citraconic anhydride to PAH yields an anionic, carboxylate-functionalized polymer (called polymer 2) that can be converted readily back to cationic PAH in acidic environments. The incorporation of polymer 2 into PEMs thus provides an approach to the manufacture of films that are stable at neutral pH but that erode over a period of several days in acidic media (e.g., a pH of 5).

As proof of concept, they demonstrated that ultrathin films roughly 100 nm thick manufactured using polymer 2 sustained the release of fluorescently labeled PAH for up to 4 days when incubated at pH 5.0. Furthermore, the synthetic approach was more recently applied to the release of DNA (Liu et al. 2008) using two different degradable polymers.

Delivery of Bioactive Molecules to Cells via PEM Films

Small Molecules or Drugs

Delivery of bioactive molecules (ions, drugs, proteins) often relies on diffusive processes that will depend on the film's internal structure and nanometer scale porosity. Such processes are also extremely present in real tissues for the delivery of nutrients (Thorne et al. 2008).

For instance, in the case of PEM capsules, diffusion is a method for loading molecules within the capsule's interior and investigating their permeability using fluorescent dextrans (Tong et al. 2005). The diffusion of small model molecules, such as dyes, in planar LbL films is often investigated. Kharlampieva and Sukhisvili (2004) found for hydrogen-bonded multilayers that dye loading capacity was largely affected by the nature of the polyelectrolyte on top of the film (of opposite charge to that of the dye). An extraction of the dye through the film by polymers in solution contributed significantly to dye release in the case of electrostatically assembled films. Control of entrapment and the diffusion of silver (Ag) ions have attracted great interest due to the antibacterial properties of these ions (see Section 8.3.5).

Thick films that are hydrated and/or porous are particularly suitable for being used as reservoirs for active compounds. Using PLL/HA film as a matrix, Vodouhê et al. (2006) observed, using CLSM, that paclitaxel Green 488 molecules diffused throughout the whole $(PLL/HA)_{60}$ film section and that the fluorescence was homogeneously distributed over the whole thickness of the film (12 μm). A similar strategy was employed by Schneider et al. (2007c), who loaded cross-linked PLL/HA films with the anti-inflammatory drug sodium diclofenac and with paclitaxel. The amount of drug loaded could be adjusted by varying the film's thickness (Schneider et al. 2007a). Paclitaxel-loaded films were efficient in killing cells, as less than 10% of the cells were still alive after 3 days of culture (Figure 8.9) (Schneider et al. 2007c). Control of film porosity at the micrometer and nanometer scales is an important step toward controlling diffusion. Berg et al. (2006) showed that it is possible to adjust the amount of ketoprofen and cytochalasin D released from films by varying the number of layers in the porous regions of films, and the release rate depended on film pore size.

Larger molecules, such as proteins, can diffuse within or at the surface of films, depending on the film's structural properties. Thus, albumin was found to diffuse in and on PSS/PAH films (Szyk et al. 2001). Recently, the diffusion of staphylococcal nuclease (SNase) was investigated by neutron reflectometry (Jackler et al. 2005). It was shown that the SNase is

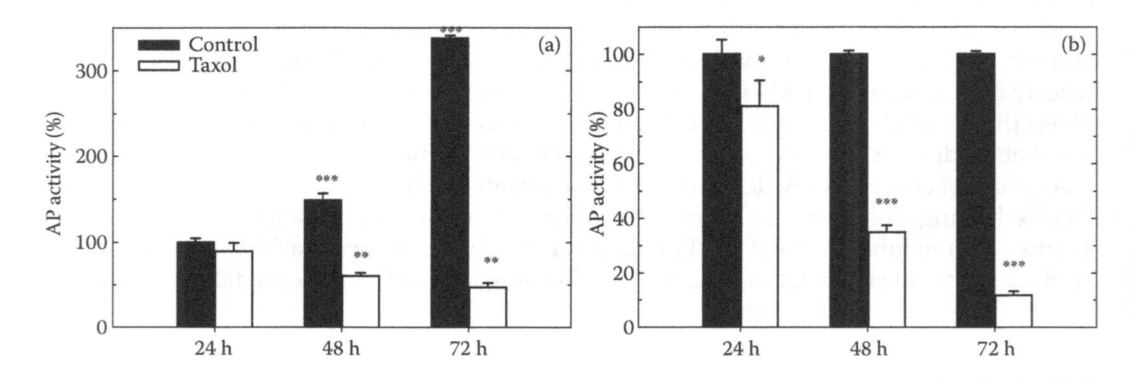

FIGURE 8.9
Acid phosphatase (AP) activity for HT29 cells cultured on cross-linked $(PLL/HA)_{12}$ films loaded or not with paclitaxel, after different time periods of 24, 48, and 72 h in culture. Error bars represent standard deviation. Two different representations are shown: (a) value of 100% has been arbitrarily attributed to CL films at 24 h ($^{**}p < 0.01$; $^{***}p < 0.001$ versus control at 24 h for control films or versus paclitaxel at 24 h for paclitaxel loaded films). (b) Value of 100% has been arbitrarily set at 100% for CL films at each time period ($^{*}p < 0.05$; $^{**}p < 0.01$; $^{***}p < 0.001$ versus controls, which are CL films at time 24, 48, and 72 h, respectively. (Reproduced with permission from Schneider et al., *Biomacromolecules*, 8, 139–145, 2007c. Copyright ACS 2007.)

partially penetrating (or diffusing) into a PSS terminating PEM upon adsorption. This penetration is preferred when the positive charge of the protein is high.

Release of bioactive molecules or of film components can be triggered by a wide variety of stimuli, such as ionic strength, light, temperature, and sensitivity to hydrolysis. The various methods developed for controlling each of these parameters have been reviewed in detail by De Geest et al. (2007) in their recent review on polyelectrolyte capsules and by Tang et al. (2006). It appears that film porosity, a certain level of hydration, and diffusion are important to allow for molecule mobility.

Surface Mediated Transfection

The controlled delivery of DNA complexes from PEMs offers the potential to enhance gene transfer by maintaining an elevated concentration of DNA within the cellular microenvironment with an appropriate polyelectrolyte film carrier that will facilitate DNA introduction. There are already several very interesting reviews about gene delivery through LbL method (Jewell and Lynn 2008; Lynn 2007). In this chapter, we will highlight recent studies that present new advances in this field.

Jessel et al. (2006) reported the fabrication of substrates containing β-cyclodextrin–DNA (CD-DNA) complexes embedded in a PEM film in which specific expression of nuclear or cytoplasmic proteins is selectively and sequentially produced. These CD-DNA complexes adsorbed on PEM films acted as an efficient gene delivery tool to transfect cells. Synthesis of new cationic polymers is one of the important developments in the field of PEMs for gene delivery. Lu et al. (2008) reported a biodegradable polycation poly(2-aminoethyl propylene phosphate), which could form multilayers with plasmid DNA (pDNA) and lead to prolonged pDNA delivery up to 2 months. Reducible polycations such as those containing disulfide bonds are also of interest for triggering gene release from PEM films under reductive conditions in the presence of DTT for instance (Blacklock et al. 2007; Blacklock et al. 2009; Chen et al. 2007). Cai et al. (2008) reported multilayers of galactosylated CHI and pDNA. Because the galactose group is a specific ligand for the asialoglycoprotein receptor (ASGP-R) of hepatocytes, these films have a specific higher transfection rate on hepatoma G2 cells. An elegant strategy for bifunctionalization of PEM films was developed by Meyer et al. (2008). These authors show that it is possible to functionalize PEM films both for cell transfection and for activation via a peptide signaling pathway. Toward this end, they prepared films containing pDNA precomplexed with PEI and a peptide molecule NBPMSH. This peptide, grafted to PGA was used as a signal molecule for melanoma cells B16-F1 and for its ability to enhance gene delivery in a receptor-independent manner.

Another development relies on the incorporation and functionality of other gene materials, such as viral vectors and silencing (Dimitrova et al. 2007; Dimitrova et al. 2008; Jia et al. 2007). Recently, Dimitrova et al. (2008) demonstrated, using hepatitis C virus infection (HCV) as a model, that siRNAs targeting the viral genome were efficiently delivered by PEM films. This delivery method resulted in a marked, dose-dependent, specific, and sustained inhibition of HCV replication and infection in hepatocyte-derived cells. Comparative analysis demonstrated that delivery of siRNAs by the films was more sustained and durable than siRNAs delivery by standard methods, including electroporation or liposomes. The antiviral effect of siRNAs films was reversed by a hyaluronidase inhibitor, suggesting that active degradation of films by cellular enzymes is required for siRNA delivery.

Bioactive Proteins and Growth Factors

Since PEM films were first developed, proteins have been employed as building blocks in LbL films. Thus, multicomponent LbL films containing proteins have been assembled via electrostatic interactions (Lvov et al. 1995; Onda et al. 1996; Lvov et al. 1998). One of the first pieces of evidence that protein embedded in PEM films retain their bioactivity came from Jessel et al. (2003). In their study, protein A was embedded at different levels in (PLL/PGA) films and was found to induce a time-dependent expression of TNF-α in THP-1 phagocytic cells. Interestingly, the cells were shown to come into contact with the protein by local degradation of the films. Notably, the cells were able to degrade the PLL but not poly(D-lysine), which forms a barrier between the cells and protein A. In this case, TNF-α production was significantly reduced.

Nonphagocytic cells such as neurons have also been shown to respond to protein embedded in a multilayer architecture. In the study by Vodouhe et al. (2005), multilayer films (mostly ending by PSS) were functionalized with a growth factor, brain derived neurotrophic factor (BDNF) or a chemorepulsive protein, semaphorin 3A (Sema3A). The quantitative amount of protein adsorbed was estimated by optical waveguide lightmode spectroscopy. The authors showed that the embedded proteins were stable in the multilayer architecture and that the protein was not released in the culture medium after 2 days in culture (or at least, the release level was below the detection level). Very interestingly, BDNF induced an increased neuronal activity and an increased neurite length, whereas Sema3A induced a decreased activity and neurite length. Thus, the structure of the films could be correlated to their effective biological activity.

Ma et al. introduced a new class of bioactive films using directly growth factors (acidic or basic fibroblasts growth factors, aFGF or bFGF, respectively) as building blocks, either mixed with heparin and deposited alternately with PEI, or directly used as polycation and deposited with chondroitin sulfate A (Ma et al. 2007; Mao et al. 2005). An enhanced secretion of collagen type I and interleukin 6 (IL-6) by fibroblasts seeded on the five layer pairs of (aFGF/HEP)/PEI was also observed by immunohistochemistry. When bFGF was directly built in multilayer films with CSA, the films containing bFGF had an improved bioactivity. In vitro incubation of the CSA/bFGF multilayers in PBS showed that about 30% of the incorporated bFGF was released within 8 days. The fact that growth factors retained their biological activity is extremely interesting for biomedical applications.

Using films made of (PLL/CSA), Tezcaner et al. (2006) prepared functionalized multilayers by adsorbing bFGF or the insoluble fraction of the intercellular photoreceptor matrix (IPM) on or within the PLL/CSA PEMs. They showed that bFGF and IPM adsorption on top of the $(PLL/CSA)_{10}/PLL$ polyelectrolyte films increased the number of photoreceptor cells attached, and in particular bFGF adsorbed on the top led to a statistically significant increase in photoreceptor cell survival at day 7. Recent developments include the use of films containing growth factors, such as bone morphogenetic protein 2 (BMP2) and transforming growth factor 1 (TGFβ1) for inducing the specific differentiation of embryonic stem cells to form bone tissue (Dierich et al. 2007). The authors used monocarboxylic β-cyclodextrins to favor the insertion of both growth factors and showed that both were required for inducing an effective differentiation. However, little is known about the exact amount of protein adsorbed or about the interaction mechanism of the growth factors and the embryonic-like bodies.

Recently, the vascular endothelial growth factor was adsorbed onto (PLL/PGA) and (PSS/PAH) films deposited on porous titanium implants (Muller et al. 2008). The $(PAH/PSS)_4$ architecture was selected to functionalize porous titanium, both for its high efficiency to adsorb VEGF and for its biocompatibility toward endothelial cells. The authors demonstrated that the VEGF adsorbed on $(PAH/PSS)_4$ maintained its bioactivity in vitro and stimulated endothelial cells proliferation. A specific activation of the intracellular pathway (VEGF receptor and MAP ERK1/2 kinase) was also evidenced.

Cell and Stem Cell Differentiation

Cells with capacities to differentiate, and stem cells in particular, are currently the subject of several studies thanks to their potential applications in tissue repair in situ and tissue engineering. Stem cells in vitro or in vivo are in "niches," a term that refers to the stem cell microenvironment (Scadden 2006). These niches are found during embryonic development (embryonic stem cells) but also in the human body (adult stem cells), where the stem cells can be activated by several signals to either promote self-renewal or differentiation to form new tissues. Important characteristics within the niche are cell–cell interactions between stem cells, as well as interactions between stem cells and neighboring differentiated cells, interactions between stem cells and adhesion molecules, extracellular matrix components, growth factors, cytokines, and physiochemical nature of the environment.

Scientists are studying the various components of the niche and trying to replicate the in vivo niche conditions in vitro. This is because for regenerative therapies, cell proliferation and differentiation must be controlled in flasks, so that a sufficient quantity of the proper cell type is produced before being introduced back into the patient for therapy. Other cells, such as skeletal muscle cells are called pluripotent in that they can differentiate in to different cell types depending on the signals received (Darabi and Perlingeiro 2008).

Studies concerning stem cell adhesion, proliferation, and differentiation on PEM films are just emerging. Given the possibilities for spatially controlling film topography, providing cell cocultures, loading films with chemical factors such as morphogens and modulating film mechanical properties, PEM films appear to have great potential for applications in stem cell-based tissue engineering.

Dierich et al. (2007) were the first to show the use of PEM films for the differentiation of embryonic bodies (EBs) into cartilage and bone. A poly(L-lysine succinylated)/PGA film, into which BMP2 and TGFβ1 had been embedded, was chosen for this purpose. They found that both BMP2 and TGFβ1 needed to be present simultaneously in the film to trigger proteoglycan production and drive the EBs to cartilage and bone formation. This constituted the first example of a multilayer whose biological activity was based on a synergy effect between two active compounds.

The same authors subsequently investigated the effect of a growth factor, BMP4, and its antagonist, Noggin, embedded in a PLL/PGA film on tooth development (Nadiri et al. 2007). They showed that these films can induce or inhibit cell death in tooth development and that the biological effects of the active molecules are conserved. The functionalized PEMs could thus act as efficient delivery tools for activating cells. This approach shows promise because it can be used to finely reproduce architectures with cell inclusions as well as to provide tissue organization.

A recent study by Crouzier et al. (2009) gave the proof that controlled amounts of a morphogen such as BMP2 can be trapped in a thick film made of (PLL/HA) and retain their activity. The amount of BMP2 trapped could be adjusted by varying both the number of layers in the film and the initial BMP2 concentration in solution. Interestingly, myoblast cells grown on unloaded films differentiated into myotubes in a manner that depended on the stiffness of the PLL/HA film (Ren et al. 2008). The same cells grown on BMP2-loaded films differentiated into osteoblasts, the expression of alkaline phosphatase (a marker for

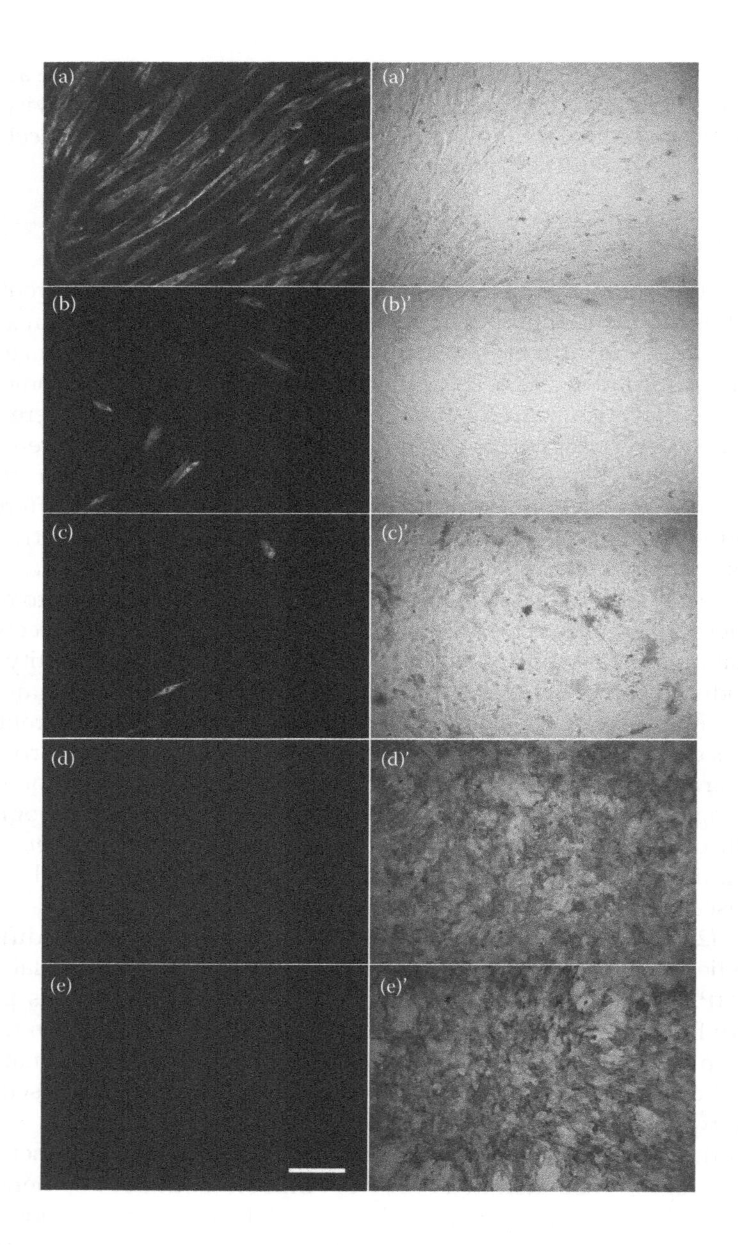

FIGURE 8.10
Immunochemical and histochemical staining of troponin T (a marker for myotube) (a–e) and alkaline phosphatase (a marker for osteoblasts) (a′–e′) of C2C12 on BMP2 loaded films for increasing BMP-2 initial concentrations: (a) 0; (b) 0.5 μg/mL; (c) 1 μg/mL; (d) 10 μg/mL, (e) 50 μg/mL (scale bar: 150 μm). (Reproduced with permission from Crouzier et al., *Small*, 5, 598–608, 2009. Copyright Wiley-VCH Verlag GmbH & Co. KGaA, 2009.)

osteoblastic activity) depending on the amount of BMP2 loaded in the films (Figure 8.10) (Crouzier et al. 2009).

A first step in the development of nanomaterials for neural interfaces was provided by Jan and Kotov (2007), who demonstrated the differentiation of environment-sensitive neuronal stem cells (NSCs), both as neurospheres and single cells, on a (PEI/single-wall carbon nanotube) multilayer film. NSCs behaved similarly to those cultured on the standard and widely used poly(L-ornithine) substratum in terms of cell viability, development of neural processes, and appearance and progression of neural markers.

In the vascular field, an application of PEM in the endothelialization of vascular grafts has been investigated. Berthelemy and coworkers (2008) found that endothelial progenitors differentiated much faster on PSS/PAH multilayer films than on any other extracellular matrix that had been used up until then, including a layer of jugular venous endothelial cells. The differentiation occurred in 2 weeks as compared to 2 months for classical coatings, and the cells formed an endothelium-like confluent cellular monolayer. This system is, of course, extremely relevant for future therapeutic approaches, but it could also provide a very interesting template for further studies on the mechanisms of endothelial cell differentiation.

In a recent study describing further efforts for providing stem cells with a biomimetic niche environment, Nichols et al. (2009) built an elegant scaffold with an inverted colloidal crystal topography reminiscent of bone marrow architecture, which was further coated with albumin/PDDA films. Bone marrow stromal cells were first allowed to attach to the scaffold. Subsequently, CD34+ hematopoietic stem cells were seeded in the scaffold to create a three-dimensional coculture. By allowing CD34+ stem cells to self-organize within this scaffold in the presence of stromal cells, the authors could recreate ex vivo part of the complexity occurring in vivo. The authors demonstrated that the scaffold supports CD34+ cell expansion and B lymphocyte differentiation with production of antigen specific IgG antibodies. Finally, implantation of these bone marrow constructs onto the backs of severe combined immunodeficiency mice proved successful and led to the generation of human immune cells. In addition to providing a structure that could be used for amplifying a large part of hematopoietic tissue, this three-dimensional matrix may also be useful for investigating the complex interactions occurring in bone marrow.

Cell Encapsulation

PEM films can potentially be employed for cell encapsulation as they can coat various cell types or even be used to build multilayered cell architectures.

One of the first examples was presented by Ai et al. (2002), who reported that platelets can be coated with LbL films and modified with antibodies as a means of investigating targeted-delivery mechanisms within the walls of blood vessel substitutes. Krol et al. (2004) later reported that single yeast cells encased within PSS/PAH polyelectrolyte shells were able to maintain their viability, functionality, and normal exchange of nutrients and waste. LbL assembly has also been used for encapsulation of *E. coli* cells (Hillberg and Tabrizian 2006). Later on, Veerabadran et al. coated mesenchymal stem cells with PLL/HA layers and showed that the cells maintained their shape and viability for up to 1 week (Veerabadran et al. 2007; Veerabadran et al. 2009). Using platelets as model cells, Fatisson et al. (2008) detected cytoskeletal changes in blood platelets coated with CHI/HA multilayers by QCM-D.

Applications for cell coatings in pancreas tissue engineering have also emerged recently. Krol et al. (2006) applied a nanometer-thick PAH/PSS/PAH coating to cover and protect human pancreatic islets. Macroscopically, no significant changes in the morphology of the islets were observed and their functionality was proved by insulin release. In contrast, however, Wilson et al. (2008) found that these films were cytotoxic to human pancreatic islets. As an alternative coating, they employed PLL-g-PEG in combination with biotin and proved cell viability in a coating composed of eight layer pairs.

Toward Biomedical Applications

PEM-Coated Implantable Biomaterials

For applications in the fields of implantable biomaterials and tissue engineering, films are used as surface coatings with the aim of providing an additional functionality for the original materials or engineered tissue. Several aspects therefore appear particularly important, as discussed in the following paragraphs.

For coating the surfaces of biomaterials (metals, synthetic or natural polymers, ceramics), it is first important to characterize the coating of the film on the materials and then to investigate the behavior of specific cell types, depending on the planned application. Very interestingly, several type of materials have been modified by LbL films (Figure 8.11 and Table 8.1). Table 8.1 summarizes all the studies performed in vitro on various materials as initial substrates. They are classified according to the type of application: bone, vascular tissue, dental tissue, neuronal tissue, pancreas, tracheal prostheses, and general engineering applications. It appears that bone and vascular tissue engineering are the fields that have attracted the greatest number of studies. This is not surprising as these two fields represent the largest markets of implantable biomaterials.

For applications in the field of orthopedics, osteoblasts are usually investigated. One of the most studied materials is titanium because of its large application for orthopedic implants (Geetha et al. 2009). New types of nano- and microporous scaffolds as future tissue engineered constructs are also currently being investigated, including electrospun fibers (Li et al. 2008) and polymer-based scaffolds (Liu et al. 2005b). As first step, cell adhesion, proliferation, and viability are quantified. The film coating has to allow cells to adhere.

In the vascular engineering field, the most used materials are stainless steels (standard material for stents) and synthetic polymers such as polyethylene terephtalate (PET), polycaprolactone, and polytetrafluoroethylene (or PTFE, Teflon®). These later ones are currently employed as vascular grafts. As the film-coated materials are going to be in contact with blood and with the vascular wall, studies often concern endothelial cells, platelets, or inflammatory cells such as macrophages. In this context, natural polyelectrolytes can potentially be used in multilayer films because of their intrinsic bioactivity. DEX and HEP can be used for their antithrombogenicity. HA can be used for its high water retention capacity. CHI/DEX films were found to exhibit anticoagulant properties only when dextran was the outermost layer of the film and when the films were built in 0.5 M NaCl or 1 M NaCl (Serizawa et al. 2002). On the other hand, CHI/HEP films built in 1 M NaCl also exhibited strong anticoagulant activity regardless of the outermost surface of the film (Serizawa et al. 2002). This type of multilayer film thus has good potential for the surface modification of medical implants in contact with blood. The thromboresistance of a $(CHI/HA)_4$-coated NiTi substrate was also demonstrated by Thierry et al. (2003). These films were found to significantly reduce platelet adhesion by 38% after 1 h of exposure to platelet-rich plasma. On the contrary, the adhesion of polymorphonuclear neutrophils onto the coated surface increased slightly, compared to bare metal.

Applications in the field of dentistry are also foreseen, with titanium being again one of the materials of choice due to its biocompatibility.

The design of the surfaces with a targeted functionality is a considerable challenge for future applications in tissue engineering and biomaterials. It is possible that adhesive peptides or ECM proteins may enhance specific cell adhesion (see Section 8.3.4). The growth factors embedded in films can provide both a new functionality and a way to adjust cell differentiation. The first studies concerning the beneficial effect of various proteins and growth factors have been presented (Section 8.4.3). Very interestingly, in all the works reported above, the bioactivity of the proteins or growth factors was always preserved. This indicates that the films are a good nano- and microenvironment for allowing an adequate preservation of the protein bioactivity, which is often a major concern when the bioactive moiety is grafted onto an underlying substrate. Thus, the very simple strategy of bioactive protein adsorption (physisorption) proves to be efficient when applied to PEM films.

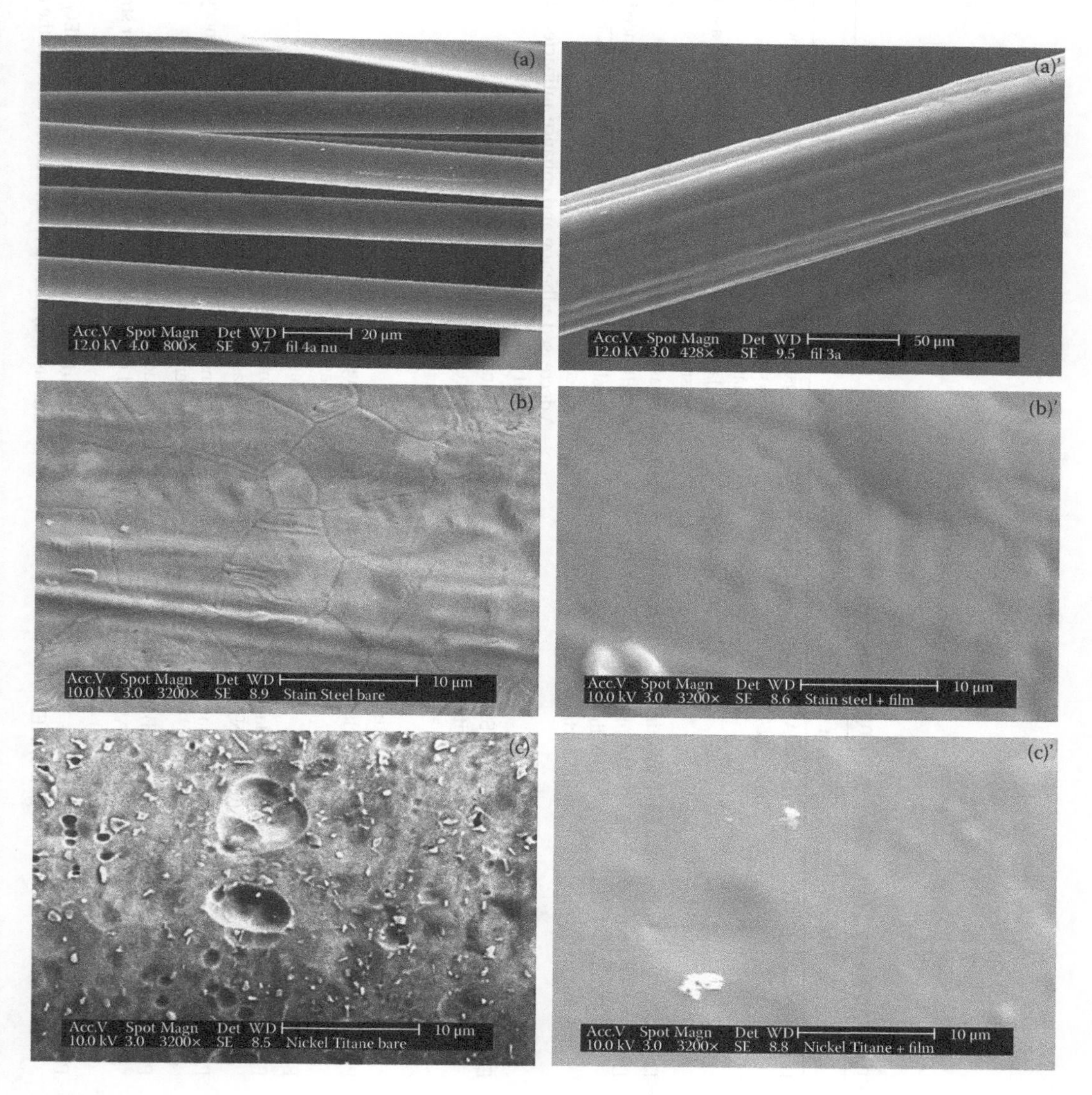

FIGURE 8.11
Coating of materials used in vascular engineering by LbL films made of PLL and HA. Scanning electron microscope images of bare materials (a, b, c) and of cross-linked $(PLL/HA)_{24}$ film coated materials (a′, b′, c′): (a, a′) polyethylene terephtalate; (b, b′) stainless steel; (c, c′) nickel–titanium alloy. (Scale bar: 20 μm (a), 50 μm (a′), and 10 μm for all other images.)

TABLE 8.1

PEM Coatings on Materials for Different Tissue Engineering Applications

Application	Substrate	Film	Cells	Main Findings	Reference
Bone	Ti	(PLL/DNA) (PAH/DNA)	Osteoblasts	– Deposition of calcium phosphate was enhanced on DNA coatings – Formation of carbonate apatite – Simulated body fluids pretreated films increased the deposition of osteocalcin	van den Beucken et al. 2007a, 2007b
	Ti	CHI/gelatine	Osteoblasts	– Increased viability and proliferation	Cai et al. 2005
	Ti	CHI/HA films + RGD X-linked at the surface	Osteoblasts *Staphylococcus aureus*	– No adhesion for native CHI/HA film, enhanced adhesion in the presence of the peptide for CHI ending surface only – A decreased adhesion and enhance antibacterial activity of CHI/HA films (w or w/o RGD)	Chua et al. 2008
	Electrospun PCL fibers	Gelatin/PSS coated with bonelike calcium phosphate	Osteoblasts	– Enhancement of cytocompatibility – Increased proliferation	Li et al. 2008
	PLA nanofibrous scaffold	PDDA/gelatine	Osteoprogenitors	– Change in surface wettability – Increase adhesion and proliferation	Liu et al. 2005b
Bone Marrow	PLA scaffold	PEI/GEL	Chondrocytes	– Increased adhesion and growth	Zhu et al. 2004
	PDMS (μfluidic channels)	(PDDA/clay)/(COL/FN)	Murine bone marrow cells	– Automated microfluidic perfusion system – Increased cell attachment and spreading	Mehta et al. 2007
	PA hydrogel ICC scaffolds	PDDA/Clay platelets	Hematopoietic stem cells	– Expansion of CD34+ stem cells and B-lymphocyte differentiation	Nichols et al. 2009
Vascular engineering	PET filaments, thread and prostheses	(PSS/PAH) (PLL/PGA) (PLL/HA)	–	– Characterization of film deposition – Good mechanical stability of the films under stretching	Rinckenbach et al. 2007
	PCL	–CHI-CL–gPEG/HEP	Platelets	– New derivative of CHI: chitosan-g-PCL-b-PEG – Increased in plasma recalcification time for the coating	Liu et al. 2007

	PTFE	PSS/PAH	Endothelial cells	– Enhanced adhesion and spreading on the films	Moby et al. 2007
	Vascular artery	CHI/HA	–	– Film coated in situ in the artery in physiological conditions – Prevention of platelet adhesion	Thierry et al. 2003
	Cryopreserved artery	PAH/PSS	Endothelial cells	– Adhesion and spreading of endothelial cells – Increased expression of von Willebrand factor	Kerdjoudj et al. 2007
	NiTi	Photo X-linked ALG/HEP/*p*-diazonium diphenylamine polymer	–	– Chemical—enhanced wettability, antifouling, and anticoagulation properties	Liu et al. 2007
	Stainless steel	CHI/HEP HA/HEP		– Longer blood clotting time than pure steel substrates – Control of releasing rate of Sirolimus by the number of layers – Suppression of smooth muscle cells growth	Huang and Yang 2008 Huang and Yang 2006
	Polyethersulfone	HEP/ALB	Leucocytes	– Reduced activation of coagulation – Reduction of the blood level of complement fragment C5a	Sperling et al. 2006
	Polyethyleneterephtalate	CHI/HEP	Platelets	– Decrease in the number of viable bacteria	Fu et al. 2005
Neuronal tissue	HYAFF 11	(PDDA/PSS)-(PDL/anti-TGFβ1)	–	– Immunological activity of anti-TGFβ1 preserved	Pastorino et al. 2006
	Free standing membrane	SWNT/PAA	Neuroblastoma and glyoma	– Good attachment and neuronal differentiation – Guidance of neurites outgrowth	Gheith et al. 2005
Pancreas	Islets of Langerhans	PVA-SH/PVA-Pyridyl disulfide Biotin-BSA/streptavidin	–	– Efficient encapsulation of islets in thin films while preserving cell viability and insulin release function	Teramura et al. 2007 Teramura et al. 2008

(continued)

TABLE 8.1 (Continued)

PEM Coatings on Materials for Different Tissue Engineering Applications

Application	Substrate	Film	Cells	Main Findings	Reference
Dental applications	Ti and SiO_2	(PLL/PGA)-PGA- EMD	–	– Immobilization of enamel matrix derivate (EMD) both on top and within PEM films	Halthur et al. 2006
	Porous Ti	(PLL/PGA) and laminin derived peptide	Epithelial cells	– In vitro, the films enhance epithelial cell colonization and proliferation – Specific formation of adhesive structures (hemidesmosomes) in the presence of the peptide	Werner et al. 2009
	PMMA disks	(CHI/HA)	–	– Enhanced resistance to enzymatic degradation of X-linked films	Etienne et al. 2005b
	Ti	(PAH/PSS) (PLL/HA)	Fibroblasts	– Enhanced adhesion and proliferation on (PAH/PSS) films	Brunot et al. 2008
Tracheal prostheses	Ti	(PLL/PGA-αMSH)	–	– In vivo study (see Table 8.2)	Schultz et al. 2005
	3D porous Ti	(PSS/PAH) (PLL/PGA)	Chondrosarcomas	– More stable adhesion (focal contacts) on negatively charged or uncoated surfaces	Vautier et al. 2003
	3D porous Ti	(PAH/PSS) (PLL/PGA)	Endothelial cells	– Enhanced spreading and proliferation of endothelial cells via activation of VEGFR2 receptors and downstream kinases	Muller et al. 2008

Source: Boudou et al., *Adv. Mater.*, 21, 1–27, 2009. Copyright Wiley-VCH Verlag GmbH & Co. KGaA 2010. With permission.

TABLE 8.2

Summary of Studies Investigating Properties of LbL Films in Vivo

Film Type and Experimental Model	Main Findings	Reference
(PLL/PGA) αMSH films deposited on tracheal prostheses	– Fibroblastic colonization of the peripharic site and respiratory epithelium on the internal side – More regular layer on PGA ending films – IL-10 production only when MSH is present	Schultz et al. 2005
(CHI/HA) native and X-linked films in a rat mouth model	– Much slower degradation of X-linked films – 60% of the film retained on PMMA disks	Etienne et al. 2005
(CHI/HA) native and X-linked in a mouse peritoneal cavity	– Partial degradation of CL films – Control of degradation by MW and extent of film X-linking	Picart et al. 2005b
(PLL/ALG)-PC coated alginate microcapsules	– Adherent cells at the periphery of the capsule – macl positive cells, no type B and T lymphocytes	Wilson et al. 2007
PAH/DNA or poly(D-lysine)/DNA in rats	– Uniform tissue response – Induction of fibrous tissue capsules for all the conditions	van den Beucken et al. 2007b
(PLL/PGA)-laminin 5 derived peptide or CL films on porous titanium	– Focal contact formation on CL films – Colonization of the implant by cells of soft tissue	Werner et al. 2009
(PDDA/clay platelet) films In inverted colloidal crystals	– High vascularization around the construct – Production of CD34+ cells – Presence of both mature and immature precursor cells	Nichols et al. 2009
Bis-ureio-surfactant and DNA coating in rats	– Increase of bone to implant contact after 1 week – Simulated body fluid DNA based coating was found to increase both early and late peri-implant bone respone	Schouten et al. 2009
(CHI/HEP) film on stainless steel coronary stents in pigs	– Promotion of reendothelialization on the film – Improved anticoagulation properties	Meng et al. 2009

Source: Boudou et al., *Adv. Mater.*, 21, 1–27, 2009. Copyright Wiley-VCH Verlag GmbH & Co. KGaA 2010. With permission.

An important aspect toward the development of future bioactive materials coated with LbL films is the stability of the anchoring of the films to the materials. If physisorption does not lead to sufficiently strong interactions, other strategies such as covalent attachment of the first layer or grafting of mussel adhesive–inspired polymers can be envisioned (see Section 8.2.2). Future tests will have to evaluate these aspects of film resistance toward mechanical stresses in the framework of specific applications (vascular tissue engineering, bone tissue engineering, etc.).

In Vivo Studies on PEM-Coated Materials

In vitro studies must be followed by in vivo studies to investigate the effects of the coatings in a more complex biological environment and for a specific purpose. As the studies on PEM films and animal and human cells started only about 8 years ago, the in vivo studies on PEM films began to emerge only 4 years ago. The number of in vivo studies has grown rapidly over the past years (four articles published in 2009). Table 8.2 shows all the in vivo studies to date.

The first studies have been published in 2005 for films deposited on tracheal prostheses (Schultz et al. 2005) or deposited on model surfaces and implanted in the rat mouth (Etienne et al. 2005b) or in the mouse peritoneal cavity (Picart et al. 2005b). Films containing polysaccharides such as chitosan and hyaluronan were found to be biodegradable, which can probably be attributed to the presence of enzyme in body fluids (hyaluronidase, lyzozyme, etc.). Recently, a porous titanium implant coated with a film containing a specific peptide (laminin-5 derived peptide) proved to induce the formation of specific adhesive structures called hemidesmosomes. In addition, the implant was colonized by the cells of the soft surrounding tissue. Nichols et al. (2009) explored the possibility to create an artificial bone marrow construct by using inverted colloidal crystals coated with a PDDA/platelet film. A high vascularization was observed around the construct and the presence of both mature and immature precursor cells was also evidenced.

Acknowledgments

The authors are grateful to the following funding agencies for their support over the past years through research and equipment grants as well as a postdoctoral (KR) and a PhD fellowship (TC): "Association Française contre les Myopathies" (AFM), "Association pour la Recherche sur la Cancer" (ARC), CNRS, "Fondation Recherche Médicale" (FRM), "Agence Nationale pour la Recherche" (ANR PNANO program), and by the NIH (R21 grant).

List of Abbreviations

ALG: alginate
BDNF: brain-derived neurotrophic factor
BMP: bone morphogenetic protein
BSA: bovine serum albumin (BSA)

CHI: chitosan
CS: chondroitin sulfate
CLSM: confocal laser scanning microscopy
CMP: carboxymethylpullulan
COL: collagen
DEX(S): dextran (sulfate)
aFGF: acidic fibroblast growth factor (resp. bFGF for basic)
EDC: 1-ethyl-3-(3-dimethylaminopropyl) carbodiimide
ECM: extracellular matrix
FN: fibronectin
GEL: gelatin
HA: hyaluronan
HEP: heparin
PAA: polyacrylic acid (PAA)
PAH: poly(allylamine) hydrochloride
PEG: polyethylene glycol
PEI: poly(ethylene)imine
PGA: poly(L-glutamic) acid
PLL: poly(L-lysine)
PEM: polyelectrolyte multilayer
PSS: poly(styrene) sulfonate
PLGA: poly(lactic-*co*-glycolic) acid
VB: vinylbenzyl
VEGF: vascular endothelial growth factor
VN: vitronectin

References

Ai, H., M. Fang, S.A. Jones, and Y.M. Lvov. 2002. Electrostatic layer-by-layer nanoassembly on biological microtemplates: Platelets. *Biomacromolecules* 3: 560–564.

Ai, H., S.A. Jones, and Y.M. Lvov. 2003. Biomedical applications of electrostatic layer-by-layer nanoassembly of polymers, enzymes, and nanoparticles. *Cell Biochem Biophys* 39: 23–43.

Ai, H., Y. Lvov, D. Mills, et al. 2003. Coating and selective deposition of nanofilm on silicone rubber for cell adhesion and growth. *Cell Biochem Biophys* 38: 103–114.

Alberts, B., D. Bray, J. Lewis, et al. 1994. *Molecular biology of the cell*. New York, NY: Garland Publishing Inc.

Amsden, B., and N. Turner. 1999. Diffusion characteristics of calcium alginate gels. *Biotechnol Bioeng* 65: 605–610.

Balkundi, S.S., N.G. Veerabadran, D.M. Eby, G.R. Johnson, and Y.M. Lvov. 2009. Encapsulation of bacterial spores in nanoorganized polyelectrolyte shells (dagger). *Langmuir* 25: 14011–14016.

Ball, V., F. Bernsmann, C. Betscha, et al. 2009. Polyelectrolyte multilayer films built from poly(L-lysine) and a two-component anionic polysaccharide blend. *Langmuir* 25: 3593–3600.

Benkirane-Jessel, N., P. Lavalle, E. Hubsch, et al. 2005. Short-time timing of the biological activity of functionalized polyelectrolyte multilayers. *Adv Funct Mater* 15: 648–654.

Berg, M.C., S.Y. Yang, P.T. Hammond, and M.F. Rubner. 2004. Controlling mammalian cell interactions on patterned polyelectrolyte multilayer surfaces. *Langmuir* 20: 1362–1368.

Berg, M.C., L. Zhai, R.E. Cohen, and M.F. Rubner. 2006. Controlled drug release from porous polyelectrolyte multilayers. *Biomacromolecules* 7: 357–364.

Berthelemy, N., H. Kerdjoudj, C. Gaucher, et al. 2008. Polyelectrolyte films boost progenitor cell differentiation into endothelium-like monolayers. *Adv Mater* 20: 2674–2678.

Blacklock, J., H. Handa, D. Soundara Manickam, et al. 2007. Disassembly of layer-by-layer films of plasmid DNA and reducible TAT polypeptide. *Biomaterials* 28: 117–124.

Blacklock, J., Y.Z. You, Q.H. Zhou, G. Mao, and D. Oupicky. 2009. Gene delivery in vitro and in vivo from bioreducible multilayered polyelectrolyte films of plasmid DNA. *Biomaterials* 30: 939–950.

Boudou, T., T. Crouzier, K. Ren, G. Blin, and C. Picart. 2009. Multiple functionalities of polyelectrolyte mulitlayer films: New biomedical applications. *Adv Mater* 21: 1–27.

Boulmedais, F., P. Schwinté, C. Gergely, J.C. Voegel, and P. Schaaf. 2002. Secondary structure of polypeptide multilayer films: An example of locally ordered polyelectrolyte multilayers. *Langmuir* 18: 4523–4525.

Boulmedais, F., M. Bozonnet, P. Schwinté, J.-C. Voegel, and P. Schaaf. 2003. Multilayered polypeptide films: Secondary structures and effect of various stresses. *Langmuir* 19: 9873–9882.

Boulmedais, F., B. Frisch, O. Etienne, et al. 2004. Polyelectrolyte multilayer films with pegylated polypeptides as a new type of anti-microbial protection for biomaterials. *Biomaterials* 25: 2003–2011.

Boura, C., P. Menu, E. Payan, et al. 2003. Endothelial cells grown on thin polyelectrolyte mutlilayered films: An evaluation of a new versatile surface modification. *Biomaterials* 24: 3521–3530.

Boura, C., S. Muller, D. Vautier, et al. 2005. Endothelial cell interactions with polyelectrolyte multilayer films. *Biomaterials* 26: 4568–4575.

Bratskaya, S., D. Marinin, F. Simon, et al. 2007. Adhesion and viability of two enterococcal strains on covalently grafted chitosan and chitosan/kappa-carrageenan multilayers. *Biomacromolecules* 8: 2960–2968.

Brunot, C., L. Ponsonnet, C. Lagneau, et al. 2007. Cytotoxicity of polyethyleneimine (PEI), precursor base layer of polyelectrolyte multilayer films. *Biomaterials* 28: 632–640.

Brunot, C., B. Grosgogeat, C. Picart, et al. 2008. Response of fibroblast activity and polyelectrolyte multilayer films coating titanium. *Dent Mater* 24: 1225–1235.

Burke, S.E., and C.J. Barrett. 2003. pH-responsive properties of multilayered poly(L-lysine)/hyaluronic acid surfaces. *Biomacromolecules* 4: 1773–1783.

Burke, S.E., and C.J. Barrett. 2005. Swelling behavior of hyaluronic acid/polyallylamine hydrochloride multilayer films. *Biomacromolecules* 6: 1419–1428.

Cai, K., A. Rechtenbach, J. Hao, J. Bossert, and K.D. Jandt. 2005. Polysaccharide-protein surface modification of titanium via a layer-by-layer technique: Characterization and cell behaviour aspects. *Biomaterials* 26: 5960–5971.

Cai, K., Y. Hu, Z. Luo, et al. 2008. Cell-specific gene transfection from a gene-functionalized poly(D,L-lactic acid) substrate fabricated by the layer-by-layer assembly technique. *Angew Chem Int Ed Engl* 47: 7479–7481.

Caruso, F., K. Niikura, D.N. Furlong, and Y. Okahata. 1997. Ultrathin multilayer polyelectrolyte films on gold: Construction and thickness determination. *Langmuir* 13: 3422–3426.

Chen, A.M., and M.D. Scott. 2001. Current and future applications of immunological attenuation via pegylation of cells and tissue. *BioDrugs* 15: 833–847.

Chen, J., S.W. Huang, W.H. Lin, and R.X. Zhuo. 2007. Tunable film degradation and sustained release of plasmid DNA from cleavable polycation/plasmid DNA multilayers under reductive conditions. *Small* 3: 636–643.

Chluba, J., J.C. Voegel, G. Decher, et al. 2001. Peptide hormone covalently bound to polyelectrolytes and embedded into multilayer architectures conserving full biological activity. *Biomacromolecules* 2: 800–805.

Cho, J., J.F. Quinn, and F. Caruso. 2004. Fabrication of polyelectrolyte multilayer films comprising nanoblended layers. *J Am Chem Soc* 126: 2270–2271.

Chua, P.H., K.G. Neoh, E.T. Kang, and W. Wang. 2008. Surface functionalization of titanium with hyaluronic acid/chitosan polyelectrolyte multilayers and RGD for promoting osteoblast functions and inhibiting bacterial adhesion. *Biomaterials* 29: 1412–1421.

Collin, D., P. Lavalle, J.M. Garza, et al. 2004. Mechanical properties of cross-linked hyaluronic acid/poly-(L-lysine) multilayer films. *Macromolecules* 37: 10195–10198.

Coviello, T., P. Matricardi, and F. Alhaique. 2006. Drug delivery strategies using polysaccharidic gels. *Expert Opin Drug Deliv* 3: 395–404.

Croll, T.I., A.J. O'Connor, G.W. Stevens, and J.J. Cooper-White. 2006. A blank slate? Layer-by-layer deposition of hyaluronic acid and chitosan onto various surfaces. *Biomacromolecules* 7: 1610–1622.

Crouzier, T., and C. Picart. 2009. Ion pairing and hydration in polyelectrolyte multilayer films containing polysaccharides. *Biomacromolecules* 10: 433–442.

Crouzier, T., K. Ren, C. Nicolas, C. Roy, and C. Picart. 2009. Layer-by-Layer films as a biomimetic reservoir for rhBMP-2 delivery: Controlled differentiation of myoblasts to osteoblasts. *Small* 5: 598–608.

Dai, J., A. Jensen, D. Mohanty, J. Erndt, and M. Bruening. 2001. Controlling the permeability of multilayered polyelectrolyte films through derivatization, cross-linking, and hydrolysis. *Langmuir* 17: 931–937.

Darabi, R., and R.C. Perlingeiro. 2008. Lineage-specific reprogramming as a strategy for cell therapy. *Cell Cycle* 7: 1732–1737.

De Geest, B.G., N.N. Sanders, G.B. Sukhorukov, J. Demeester, and S.C. De Smedt. 2007. Release mechanisms for polyelectrolyte capsules. *Chem Soc Rev* 36: 636–649.

Decher, G., J.D. Hong, and J. Schmitt. 1992. Buildup of ultrathin multilayer films by a self-assembly process: III. Consecutively alternating adsorption of anionic and cationic polyelectrolytes on charged surfaces. *Thin Solid Films* 210–211: 831–835.

Decher, G., and J.B. Schlenoff, *Multilayer thin flms: sequential assembly of nanocomposite materials*. 2003, Weinheim, Germany: Wiley-VCH.

Dierich, A., E. Le Guen, N. Messaddeq, et al. 2007. Bone formation mediated by synergy-acting growth factors embedded in a polyelectrolyte multilayer film. *Adv Mater* 19: 693–697.

Dimitriadis, E.K., F. Horkay, J. Maresca, B. Kachar, and R.S. Chadwick. 2002. Determination of elastic moduli of thin layers of soft material using the atomic force microscope. *Biophys J* 82: 2798–2810.

Dimitrova, M., Y. Arntz, P. Lavalle, et al. 2007. Adenoviral gene delivery from multilayered polyelectrolyte architectures. *Adv Funct Mater* 17: 233–245.

Dimitrova, M., C. Affolter, F. Meyer, et al. 2008. Sustained delivery of siRNAs targeting viral infection by cell-degradable multilayered polyelectrolyte films. *Proc Natl Acad Sci U S A* 105: 16320–16325.

Discher, D.E., P. Janmey, and Y.L. Wang. 2005. Tissue cells feel and respond to the stiffness of their substrate. *Science* 310: 1139–1143.

Dubas, S.T., and J.B. Schlenoff. 1999. Factors controlling the growth of polyelectrolyte multilayers. *Macromolecules* 32: 8153–8160.

Elbert, D.L., C.B. Herbert, and J.A. Hubbell. 1999. Thin polymer layers formed by polyelectrolyte multilayer techniques on biological surfaces. *Langmuir* 15: 5355–5362.

Etienne, O., C. Gasnier, C. Taddei, et al. 2005a. Antifungal coating by biofunctionalized polyelectrolyte multilayered films. *Biomaterials* 26: 6704–6712.

Etienne, O., A. Schneider, C. Taddei, et al. 2005b. Degradability of polysaccharides multilayer films in the oral environment: An in vitro and in vivo study. *Biomacromolecules* 6: 726–733.

Fatisson, J., Y. Merhi, and M. Tabrizian. 2008. Quantifying blood platelet morphological changes by dissipation factor monitoring in multilayer shells. *Langmuir* 24: 3294–3299.

Francius, G., J. Hemmerle, J. Ohayon, et al. 2006. Effect of cross-linking on the elasticity of polyelectrolyte multilayer films measured by colloidal probe AFM. *Micros Res Tech* 69: 84–92.

Francius, G., J. Hemmerle, V. Ball, et al. 2007. Stiffening of soft polyelectrolyte architectures by multilayer capping evidenced by viscoelastic analysis of AFM indentation measurements. *J Phys Chem C* 111: 8299–8306.

Fu, J., J. Ji, W. Yuan, and J. Shen. 2005. Construction of anti-adhesive and antibacterial multilayer films via layer-by-layer assembly of heparin and chitosan. *Biomaterials* 26: 6684–6692.

Fu, J., J. Ji, D. Fan, and J. Shen. 2006. Construction of antibacterial multilayer films containing nanosilver via layer-by-layer assembly of heparin and chitosan-silver ions complex. *J Biomed Mater Res A* 79: 665–674.

Geetha, M., A.K. Singh, R. Asokamani, and A.K. Gogia. 2009. Ti based biomaterials, the ultimate choice for orthopaedic implants—a review. *Prog Mater Sci* 397–425.

Gergely, C., S. Bahi, B. Szalontai, et al. 2004. Human serum albumin self-assembly on weak polyelectrolyte multilayer films structurally modified by pH changes. *Langmuir* 20: 5575–5582.

Gheith, M.K., V.A. Sinani, J.P. Wicksted, R.L. Matts, and N.A. Kotov. 2005. Single-walled carbon nanotube polyelectrolyte multilayers and freestanding films as a biocompatible platformfor neuroprosthetic implants. *Adv Mater* 17: 2663–2667.

Gong, Y., Y. Zhu, Y. Liu, et al. 2007. Layer-by-layer assembly of chondroitin sulfate and collagen on aminolyzed poly(L-lactic acid) porous scaffolds to enhance their chondrogenesis. *Acta Biomater* 3: 677–685.

Guyomard, A., G. Muller, and K. Glinel. 2005. Buildup of multilayers based on amphiphilic polyelectrolytes. *Macromolecules* 38: 5737–5742.

Guyomard, A., E. De, T. Jouenne, et al. 2008. Incorporation of a hydrophobic antibacterial peptide into amphiphilic polyelectrolyte multilayers: A bioinspired approach to prepare biocidal thin coatings. *Adv Funct Mater* 18: 758–765.

Halthur, T.J., P.M. Claesson, and U.M. Elofsson. 2006. Immobilization of enamel matrix derivate protein onto polypeptide multilayers. Comparative in situ measurements using ellipsometry, quartz crystal microbalance with dissipation, and dual-polarization interferometry. *Langmuir* 22: 11065–11071.

Hammond, P.T. 1999. Recent explorations in electrostatic multilayer thin film assembly. *Curr Opin Colloid Interface Sci* 4: 430–442.

Hammond, P.T. 2004. Form and function in multilayer assembly: New applications at the nanoscale. *Adv Mater* 16: 1271–1293.

Hersel, U., C. Dahmen, and H. Kessler. 2003. RGD modified polymers: Biomaterials for stimulated cell adhesion and beyond. *Biomaterials* 24: 4385–4415.

Hillberg, A.L., and M. Tabrizian. 2006. Biorecognition through layer-by-layer polyelectrolyte assembly: In-situ hybridization on living cells. *Biomacromolecules* 7: 2742–2750.

Huang, L.Y., and M.C. Yang. 2006. Hemocompatibility of layer-by-layer hyaluronic acid/heparin nanostructure coating on stainless steel for cardiovascular stents and its use for drug delivery. *J Nanosci Nanotechnol* 6: 3163–3170.

Huang, L.Y., and M.C. Yang. 2008. Surface immobilization of chondroitin 6-sulfate/heparin multilayer on stainless steel for developing drug-eluting coronary stents. *Colloids Surf B Biointerfaces* 61: 43–52.

Hubsch, E., V. Ball, B. Senger, et al. 2004. Controlling the growth regime of polyelectrolyte multilayer films changing from exponential to linear growth by adjusting the composition of polyelectrolyte mixtures. *Langmuir* 20: 1980–1985.

Izquierdo, A., S.S. Ono, J.C. Voegel, P. Schaaf, and G. Decher. 2005. Dipping versus spraying: Exploring the deposition conditions for speeding up layer-by-layer assembly. *Langmuir* 21: 7558–7567.

Jaber, J.A., and J.B. Schlenoff. 2006. Recent developments in the properties and applications of polyelectrolyte multilayers. *Curr Opin Colloid Interface Sci* 11: 324–329.

Jackler, G., C. Czeslik, R. Steitz, and C.A. Royer. 2005. Spatial distribution of protein molecules adsorbed at a polyelectrolyte multilayer. *Phys Rev E Stat Nonlinear Soft Matter Phys* 71: 041912.

Jan, E., and N.A. Kotov. 2007. Successful differentiation of mouse neural stem cells on layer-by-layer assembled single-walled carbon nanotube composite. *Nano Lett* 7: 1123–1128.

Jessel, N., F. Atalar, P. Lavalle, et al. 2003. Bioactive coatings based on polyelectrolyte multilayer architecture functionalised by embedded proteins. *Adv Mater* 15: 692–695.

Jessel, N., P. Schwinté, P. Falvey, et al. 2004. Build-up of polypeptide multilayer coatings with anti-inflammatory properties based on the embedding of piroxicam-cyclodextrin complexes. *Adv Functi Mater* 14: 174–182.

Jessel, N., M. Oulad-Abdelghani, F. Meyer, et al. 2006. Multiple and time-scheduled in situ DNA delivery mediated by beta-cyclodextrin embedded in a polyelectrolyte multilayer. *Proc Natl Acad Sci U S A* 103: 8618–8621.

Jewell, C.M., and D.M. Lynn. 2008. Multilayered polyelectrolyte assemblies as platforms for the delivery of DNA and other nucleic acid-based therapeutics. *Adv Drug Deliv Rev* 60: 979–999.

Ji, J., J.H. Fu, and J.C. Shen. 2006. Fabrication of a superhydrophobic surface from the amplified exponential growth of a multilayer. *Adv Mater* 18: 1444.

Jia, N.Q., Q. Lian, H.B. Shen, et al. 2007. Intracellular delivery of quantum dots tagged antisense oligodeoxynucleotides by functionalized multiwalled carbon nanotubes. *Nano Lett* 7: 2976–2980.

Jiang, C., S. Markutsya, and V.V. Tsukruk. 2004. Compliant, robust, and truly nanoscale free-standing multilayer films fabricated using spin-assisted layer-by-layer assembly. *Adv Mater* 16: 157–161.

Jiang, C., S. Markutsya, and V.V. Tsukruk. 2004. Collective and individual plasmon resonances in nanoparticle films obtained by spin-assisted layer-by-layer assembly. *Langmuir* 20: 882–890.

Johansson, J.A., T. Halthur, M. Herranen, et al. 2005. Buildup of collagen and hyaluronic acid polyelectrolyte multilayers. *Biomacromolecules* 6: 1353–1359.

Kerdjoudj, H., B. Boura, V. Moby, et al. 2007. Re-endothelialization of human umbilical arteries treated with polyelectrolyte multilayers: A tool for damaged vessel replacement. *Adv Funct Mater* 17: 2267–2273.

Kerdjoudj, H., N. Berthelemy, S. Rinckenbach, et al. 2008. Small vessel replacement by human umbilical arteries with polyelectrolyte film-treated arteries: In vivo behavior. *J Am Coll Cardiol* 52: 1589–1597.

Kharlampieva, E., and S.A. Sukhishvili. 2004. Release of a dye from hydrogen-bonded and electrostatically assembled polymer films triggered by adsorption of a polyelectrolyte. *Langmuir* 20: 9677–9685.

Kidambi, S., I. Lee, and C. Chan. 2004. Controlling primary hepatocyte adhesion and spreading on protein-free polyelectrolyte multilayer films. *J Am Chem Soc* 126: 16286–16287.

Kidambi, S., C. Chan, and I. Lee. 2008. Tunable resistive *m*-dPEG acid patterns on polyelectrolyte multilayers at physiological conditions: Template for directed deposition of biomacromolecules. *Langmuir* 24: 224–230.

Kinnane, C.R., K. Wark, G.K. Such, A.P. Johnston, and F. Caruso. 2009. Peptide-functionalized, low-biofouling click multilayers for promoting cell adhesion and growth. *Small* 5: 444–448.

Koktysh, D.S., X. Liang, B.G. Yun, et al. 2002. Biomaterials by design: Layer-by-layer assembled ion-selective and biocompatible films of tio_2 nanoshells for neurochemical monitoring. *Adv Funct Mater* 12: 255–265.

Kreke, M.R., A.S. Badami, J.B. Brady, R.M. Akers, and A.S. Goldstein. 2005. Modulation of protein adsorption and cell adhesion by poly(allylamine hydrochloride) heparin films. *Biomaterials* 26: 2975–2981.

Krol, S., A. Diaspro, R. Magrassi, et al. 2004. Nanocapsules: Coating for living cells. *IEEE Trans Nanobiosci* 3: 32–38.

Krol, S., S. del Guerra, M. Grupillo, et al. 2006. Multilayer nanoencapsulation. New approach for immune protection of human pancreatic islets. *Nano Lett* 6: 1933–1939.

Kujawa, P., P. Moraille, J. Sanchez, A. Badia, and F.M. Winnik. 2005. Effect of molecular weight on the exponential growth and morphology of hyaluronan/chitosan multilayers: a surface plasmon resonance spectroscopy and atomic force microscopy investigation. *J Am Chem Soc* 127: 9224–9234.

Kujawa, P., G. Schmauch, T. Viitala, A. Badia, and F.M. Winnik. 2007. Construction of viscoelastic biocompatible films via the layer-by-layer assembly of hyaluronan and phosphorylcholine-modified chitosan. *Biomacromolecules* 8: 3169–3176.

Kumar, M.N.V.R. 2000. A review of chitin and chitosan applications. *React Funct Polym* 46: 1–27.

Ladam, G., C. Gergely, B. Senger, et al. 2000. Protein interactions with polyelectrolyte multilayers: Interactions between human serum albumin and polystyrene sulfonate/polyallylamine multilayers. *Biomacromolecules* 1: 674–687.

Ladam, G., P. Schaaf, F.G.J. Cuisinier, G. Decher, and J.-C. Voegel. 2001. Protein adsorption onto auto-assembled polyelectrolyte films. *Langmuir* 17: 878–882.

Lapcik, L., L. Lapcik, S. De Smedt, J. Demeester, and P. Chabrecek. 1998. Hyaluronan: Preparation, structure, properties, and applications. *Chem Rev* 98: 2663–2684.

Laugel, N., C. Betscha, M. Winterhalter, et al. 2006. Relationship between the growth regime of polyelectrolyte multilayers and the polyanion/polycation complexation enthalpy. *J Phys Chem B* 110: 19443–19449.

Laurent, T.C., *The chemistry, biology, and medical applications of hyaluronan and its derivatives*. Wenner-Gren International Series, Vol. 72. 1998, Cambridge, U.K.: Cambridge University Press.

Lavalle, P., C. Gergely, F. Cuisinier, et al. 2002. Comparison of the structure of polyelectrolyte multilayer films exhibiting a linear and an exponential growth regime: An in situ atomic force microscopy study. *Macromolecules* 35: 4458–4465.

Lavalle, P., C. Picart, J. Mutterer, et al. 2004. Modeling the buildup of polyelectrolyte multilayer films having exponential growth. *J Phys Chem B* 108: 635–648.

Lee, D., R.E. Cohen, and M.F. Rubner. 2005. Antibacterial properties of Ag nanoparticle loaded multilayers and formation of magnetically directed antibacterial microparticles. *Langmuir* 21: 9651–9659.

Lee, H., Y. Lee, A.R. Statz, et al. 2008. Substrate-independent layer-by-layer assembly by using mussel-adhesive-inspired polymers. *Adv Mater* 20: 1619–1623.

Lee, S.S., J.D. Hong, C.H. Kim, et al. 2001. Layer-by-layer deposited multilayer assemblies of ionene-type polyelectrolytes based on the spin-coating method. *Macromol Rapid Commun* 34: 5358–5360.

Li, B., and D.T. Haynie. 2004. Multilayer biomimetics: Reversible covalent stabilization of a nanostructured biofilm. *Biomacromolecules* 5: 1667–1670.

Li, M., D.K. Mills, T. Cui, and M.J. McShane. 2005. Cellular response to gelatin- and fibronectin-coated multilayer polyelectrolyte nanofilms. *IEEE Trans Nanobiosci* 4: 170–179.

Li, X., J. Xie, X. Yuan, and Y. Xia. 2008. Coating electrospun poly(epsilon-caprolactone) fibers with gelatin and calcium phosphate and their use as biomimetic scaffolds for bone tissue engineering. *Langmuir* 24: 14145–14150.

Li, Z., D. Lee, X. Sheng, R.E. Cohen, and M.F. Rubner. 2006. Two-level antibacterial coating with both release-killing and contact-killing capabilities. *Langmuir* 22: 9820–9833.

Lin, Y.-H., C. Jiang, J. Xu, Z. Lin, and V.V. Tsukruk. 2007. Robust, fluorescent, and nanoscale freestanding conjugated films. *Soft Matter* 3: 432–436.

Lingstrom, R., and L. Wagberg. 2008. Polyelectrolyte multilayers on wood fibers: Influence of molecular weight on layer properties and mechanical properties of papers from treated fibers. *J Colloid Interface Sci* 328: 233–242.

Liu, M., X. Yue, Z. Dai, et al. 2007. Stabilized hemocompatible coating of nitinol devices based on photo-cross-linked alginate/heparin multilayer. *Langmuir* 23: 9378–9385.

Liu, X., C. Gao, J. Shen, and H. Möhwald. 2005a. Multilayer microcapsules as anti-cancer drug delivery vehicle: Deposition, sustained release, and in vitro bioactivity. *Macromol Biosci* 5: 1209–1219.

Liu, X.H., L. Smith, G.B. Wei, Y.J. Won, and P.X. Ma. 2005b. Surface engineering of nano-fibrous poly(L-lactic acid) scaffolds via self-assembly technique for bone tissue engineering. *J Biomed Nanotechnol* 1: 54–60.

Liu, X.H., J.T. Zhang, and D.M. Lynn. 2008. Ultrathin multilayered films that promote the release of two DNA constructs with separate and distinct release profiles. *Adv Mater* 20: 4148–4152.

Liu, Y., T. He, and C. Gao. 2005c. Surface modification of poly(ethylene terephthalate) via hydrolysis and layer-by-layer assembly of chitosan and chondroitin sulfate to construct cytocompatible layer for human endothelial cells. *Colloids Surf B: Biointerfaces* 46: 117–126.
Lu, Z.Z., J. Wu, T.M. Sun, et al. 2008. Biodegradable polycation and plasmid DNA multilayer film for prolonged gene delivery to mouse osteoblasts. *Biomaterials* 29: 733–741.
Lvov, Y., G. Decher, H. Haas, H. Mohwald, and A. Kalachev. 1994. X-ray analysis of ultrathin polymer films self-assembled onto substrates. *Physica B* 198: 89–91.
Lvov, Y., K. Ariga, I. Ichinose, and T. Kunitake. 1995. Assembly of multicomponent protein films by means of electrostatic layer-by-layer adsorption. *J Am Chem Soc* 117: 6117–6123.
Lvov, Y., Z. Lu, X. Xu, J. Schenkman, and J. Rusling. 1998. Direct electrochemistry of myoglobin and cytochrome P450 in alternate layer-by-layer films with DNA and other polyions. *JACS* 120.
Lynn, D.M. 2007. Peeling back the layers: Controlled erosion and triggered disassembly of multilayered polyelectrolyte thin films. *Adv Mater* 19: 4118–4130.
Ma, L., J. Zhou, C. Gao, and J. Shen. 2007. Incorporation of basic fibroblast growth factor by a layer-by-layer assembly technique to produce bioactive substrates. *J Biomed Mater Res Part B: Appl Biomater* 83: 285–292.
Malcher, M., D. Volodkin, B. Heurtault, et al. 2008. Embedded silver ions-containing liposomes in polyelectrolyte multilayers: Cargos films for antibacterial agents. *Langmuir* 24: 10209–10215.
Mao, Z., L. Ma, J. Zhou, C. Gao, and J. Shen. 2005. Bioactive thin film of acidic fibroblast growth factor fabricated by layer-by-layer assembly. *Bioconjug Chem* 16: 1316–1322.
McAloney, R.A., M. Sinyor, V. Dudnik, and M.C. Goh. 2001. Atomic force microscopy studies of salt effects on polyelectrolyte multilayer film morphology. *Langmuir* 17: 6655–6663.
Mehta, G., M.J. Kiel, J.W. Lee, et al. 2007. Polyelectrolyte-clay-protein layer films on microfluidic PDMS bioreactor surfaces for primary murine bone marrow culture. *Adv Funct Mater* 17: 2701–2709.
Mendelsohn, J.D., S.Y. Yang, J. Hiller, A.I. Hochbaum, and M.F. Rubner. 2003. Rational design of cytophilic and cytophobic polyelectrolyte multilayer thin films. *Biomacromolecules* 4: 96–106.
Meng, S., Z. Liu, L. Shen, et al. 2009. The effect of a layer-by-layer chitosan-heparin coating on the endothelialization and coagulation properties of a coronary stent system. *Biomaterials* 30: 2276–2283.
Mermut, O., J. Lefebvre, D.G. Gray, and C.J. Barrett. 2003. Structural and mechanical properties of polyelectrolyte multilayer films studied by AFM. *Macromolecules* 36: 8819–8824.
Meyer, F., M. Dimitrova, J. Jedrzejenska, et al. 2008. Relevance of bi-functionalized polyelectrolyte multilayers for cell transfection. *Biomaterials* 29: 618–624.
Mhamdi, L., C. Picart, C. Lagneau, et al. 2006. Study of the polyelectrolyte multilayer thin films' properties and correlation with the behavior of the human gingival fibroblasts. *Mater Sci Eng C* 26: 273–281.
Moby, V., C. Boura, H. Kerdjoudj, et al. 2007. Poly(styrenesulfonate)/poly(allylamine) multilayers: A route to favor endothelial cell growth on expanded poly(tetrafluoroethylene) vascular grafts. *Biomacromolecules* 8: 2156–2160.
Muller, S., G. Koenig, A. Charpiot, et al. 2008. VEGF-functionalized polyelectrolyte multilayers as proangiogenic prosthetic coatings *Adv Funct Mater* 18: 1767–1775.
Nadiri, A., S. Kuchler-Bopp, H. Mjahed, et al. 2007. Cell apoptosis control using BMP4 and noggin embedded in a polyelectrolyte multilayer film. *Small* 3: 1577–1583.
Nakahara, Y., M. Matsusaki, and M. Akashi. 2007. Fabrication and enzymatic degradation of fibronectin-based ultrathin films. *J Biomater Sci Polym Ed* 18: 1565–1573.
Nichols, J.E., J. Cortiella, J. Lee, et al. 2009. In vitro analog of human bone marrow from 3D scaffolds with biomimetic inverted colloidal crystal geometry. *Biomaterials* 30: 1071–1079.
Olenych, S.G., M.D. Moussallem, D.S. Salloum, J.B. Schlenoff, and T.C. Keller. 2005. Fibronectin and cell attachment to cell and protein resistant polyelectrolyte surfaces. *Biomacromolecules* 6: 3252–3258.

Onda, M., Y. Lvov, K. Ariga, and T. Kunitake. 1996. Sequential actions of glucose oxidase and peroxidase in molecular films assembled by layer-by-layer alternate adsorption. *Biotechnol Bioeng* 51: 163–167.

Ostrander, J.W., A.A. Mamedov, and N.A. Kotov. 2001. Two modes of linear layer-by-layer growth of nanoparticle polylectrolyte multilayers and different interactions in the layer-by-layer deposition. *J Am Chem Soc* 123: 1101–1110.

Park, J., L.D. Fouché, and P.T. Hammond. 2005. Multicomponent patterning of layer-by-layer assembled polyelectrolyte/nanoparticle composite thin films with controlled alignment. *Adv Mater* 17: 2575–2579.

Pastorino, L., F.C. Soumetz, and C. Ruggiero. 2006. Nanofunctionalisation for the treatment of peripheral nervous system injuries. *IEEE Proc Nanobiotechnol* 153: 16–20.

Pavoor, P.V., A. Bellare, A. Strom, D. Yang, and R.E. Cohen. 2004. Mechanical characterization of polyelectrolyte multilayers using quasi-static nanoindentation. *Macromolecules* 37: 4865–4871.

Picart, C., G. Ladam, B. Senger, et al. 2001a. Determination of structural parameters characterizing thin films by optical methods: A comparison between scanning angle reflectometry and optical waveguide lightmode spectroscopy. *J Chem Phys* 115: 1086–1094.

Picart, C., P. Lavalle, P. Hubert, et al. 2001b. Buildup mechanism for poly(L-lysine)/hyaluronic acid films onto a solid surface. *Langmuir* 17: 7414–7424.

Picart, C., J. Mutterer, L. Richert, et al. 2002. Molecular basis for the explanation of the exponential growth of polyelectrolyte multilayers. *Proc Natl Acad Sci U S A* 99: 12531–12535.

Picart, C., R. Elkaim, L. Richert, et al. 2005a. Primary cell adhesion on RGD functionalized and covalently cross-linked polyelectrolyte multilayer thin films. *Adv Funct Mater* 15: 83–94.

Picart, C., A. Schneider, O. Etienne, et al. 2005b. Controlled degradability of polysaccharides multilayer films in vitro and in vivo. *Adv Funct Mater* 15: 1771–1780.

Picart, C., B. Senger, K. Sengupta, F. Dubreuil, and A. Fery. 2007. Measuring mechanical properties of polyelectrolyte multilayer thin films: Novel methods based on AFM and optical techniques. *Colloids Surf A: Physicochem Eng Asp* 303: 30–36.

Podsiadlo, P., Z. Tang, B.S. Shim, and N.A. Kotov. 2007. Counterintuitive effect of molecular strength and role of molecular rigidity on mechanical properties of layer-by-layer assembled nanocomposites. *Nano Lett* 7: 1224–1231.

Podsiadlo, P., M. Michel, J. Lee, et al. 2008. Exponential growth of LBL films with incorporated inorganic sheets. *Nano Lett* 8: 1762–1770.

Porcel, C., P. Lavalle, V. Ball, et al. 2006. From exponential to linear growth in polyelectrolyte multilayers. *Langmuir* 22: 4376–4383.

Porcel, C., P. Lavalle, G. Decher, et al. 2007. Influence of the polyelectrolyte molecular weight on exponentially growing multilayer films in the linear regime. *Langmuir* 2007: 1898–1904.

Pozos-Vazquez, C., T. Boudou, V. Dulong, et al. 2009. Variation of polyelectrolyte film stiffness by photo-cross-linking: a new way to control cell adhesion. *Langmuir* 25: 3556–3563.

Quinn, A., E. Tjipto, A. Yu, T.R. Gengenbach, and F. Caruso. 2007. Polyelectrolyte blend multilayer films: Surface morphology, wettability, and protein adsorption characteristics. *Langmuir* 23: 4944–4949.

Reisch, A., J.C. Voegel, E. Gonthier, et al. 2009. Polyelectrolyte multilayers capped with polyelectrolytes bearing phosphorylcholine and triethylene glycol groups: Parameters influencing antifouling properties. *Langmuir* 25: 3610–3617.

Ren, K., T. Crouzier, C. Roy, and C. Picart. 2008. Polyelectrolyte multilayer films of controlled stiffness modulate myoblast differentiation. *Adv Funct Mater* 18: 1378–1389.

Rhazi, M., J. Desbrieres, A. Tolaimate, et al. 2002. Influence of the nature of the metal ions on the complexation with chitosan. Application to the treatment of liquid waste. *Eur Polym J* 38: 1523–1530.

Richert, L., F. Boulmedais, P. Lavalle, et al. 2004a. Improvement of stability and cell adhesion properties of polyelectrolyte multilayer films by chemical cross-linking. *Biomacromolecules* 5: 284–294.

Richert, L., A.J. Engler, D.E. Discher, and C. Picart. 2004b. Elasticity of native and cross-linked polyelectrolyte multilayers. *Biomacromolecules* 5: 1908–1916.

Richert, L., P. Lavalle, E. Payan, et al. 2004c. Layer-by-layer buildup of polysaccharide films : Physical chemistry and cellular adhesion aspects. *Langmuir* 1: 284–294.

Rinckenbach, S., J. Hemmerle, F. Dieval, et al. 2007. Characterization of polyelectrolyte multilayer films on polyethylene terephtalate vascular prostheses under mechanical stretching. *J Biomed Mater Res A* 84A: 576–588.

Rudra, J.S., K. Dave, and D.T. Haynie. 2006. Antimicrobial polypeptide multilayer nanocoatings. *J Biomater Sci Polym Ed* 17: 1301–1315.

Salloum, D.S., and J.B. Schlenoff. 2004. Protein adsorption modalities on polyelectrolyte multilayers. *Biomacromolecules* 5: 1089–1096.

Salloum, D.S., S.G. Olenych, T.C. Keller, and J.B. Schlenoff. 2005. Vascular smooth muscle cells on polyelectrolyte multilayers: Hydrophobicity-directed adhesion and growth. *Biomacromolecules* 6: 161–167.

Salomaki, M., T. Laiho, and J. Kankare. 2004. Counteranion-controlled properties of polyelectrolyte multilayers. *Macromolecules* 37: 9585–9590.

Salomaki, M., I.A. Vinokurov, and J. Kankare. 2005. Effect of temperature on the buildup of polyelectrolyte multilayers. *Langmuir* 21: 11232–11240.

Salomaki, M., and J. Kankare. 2007. Modeling the growth processes of polyelectrolyte multilayers using a quartz crystal resonator. *J Physi Chem B* 111: 8509–8519.

Salomaki, M., and J. Kankare. 2009. Influence of synthetic polyelectrolytes on the growth and properties of hyaluronan-chitosan multilayers. *Biomacromolecules* 10: 294–301.

Scadden, D.T. 2006. The stem-cell niche as an entity of action. *Nature* 441: 1075–1079.

Schlenoff, J.B., S.T. Dubas, and T. Farhat. 2000. Sprayed polyelectrolyte multilayers. *Langmuir* 16: 9968–9969.

Schneider, A., A.-L. Bolcato-Bellemin, G. Francius, et al. 2006a. Glycated polyelectrolyte multilayer films: Differential adhesion of primary versus tumor cells. *Biomacromolecules* 7: 2882–2889.

Schneider, A., C. Picart, B. Senger, et al. 2007a. Layer-by-Layer films from hyaluronan and amine-modified hyaluronan. *Langmuir* 23: 2655–2662.

Schneider, A., L. Richert, G. Francius, J.-C. Voegel, and C. Picart. 2007b. Elasticity, biodegradability and cell adhesion properties of chitosan/hyaluronan multilayer films. *Biomed Mater Eng* 2: 45–51.

Schneider, A., A. Vodouhê, L. Richert, et al. 2007c. Multi-functional polyelectrolyte multilayer films: Combining mechanical resistance, biodegradability and bioactivity. *Biomacromolecules* 8: 139–145.

Schoeler, B., N. Delorme, I. Doench, et al. 2006. Polyelectrolyte films based on polysaccharides of different conformations: Effects on multilayer structure and mechanical properties. *Biomacromolecules* 7: 2065–2071.

Schönhoff, M., V. Ball, A.R. Bausch, et al. 2007. Hydration and internal properties of polyelectrolyte multilayers. *Colloids Surf A: Physicochem Eng Asp* 303: 14–29.

Schouten, C., J.J. van den Beucken, G.J. Meijer, et al. 2009. In vivo bioactivity of DNA-based coatings: An experimental study in rats. *J Biomed Mater Res A* March 16, ahead of print.

Schuetz, P., and F. Caruso. 2003. Copper-assisted weak polyelectrolyte multilayer formation on microspheres and subsequent film crosslinking. *Adv Funct Mater* 13: 929–937.

Schultz, P., D. Vautier, L. Richert, et al. 2005. Polyelectrolyte multilayers functionalized by a synthetic analogue of an anti-inflammatory peptide, alpha-MSH, for coating a tracheal prosthesis. *Biomaterials* 26: 2621–2630.

Semenov, O.V., A. Malek, A.G. Bittermann, J. Voros, and A. Zisch. 2009. Engineered polyelectrolyte multilayer substrates for adhesion, proliferation and differentiation of human mesenchymal stem cells. *Tissue Eng Part A* 15: 2977–2990.

Serizawa, T., M. Yamaguchi, and M. Akashi. 2002. Alternating bioactivity of polymeric layer-by-layer assemblies: Anticoagulation vs procoagulation of human blood. *Biomacromolecules* 3: 724–731.

Shim, B.S., P. Podsiadlo, D.G. Lilly, et al. 2007. Nanostructured thin films made by dewetting method of layer-by-layer assembly. *Nano Lett* 7: 3266–3273.

Shiratori, S.S., and M.F. Rubner. 2000. pH-dependent thickness behavior of sequentially adsorbed layers of weak polyelectrolytes. *Macromolecules* 33: 4213–4219.
Sinani, V.A., D.S. Koktysh, B.-G. Yun, et al. 2003. Collagen coating promotes biocompatibility of semiconductor nanoparticles in stratified LBL films. *Nano Lett* 3: 1177–1182.
Song, Z., J. Yin, K. Luo, et al. 2009. Layer-by-layer buildup of poly(L-glutamic acid)/chitosan film for biologically active coating. *Macromol Biosci* 9: 268–278.
Sperling, C., M. Houska, E. Brynda, U. Streller, and C. Werner. 2006. In vitro hemocompatibility of albumin-heparin multilayer coatings on polyethersulfone prepared by the layer-by-layer technique. *J Biomed Mater Res A* 76: 681–689.
Srivastava, S., and N.A. Kotov. 2008. Composite Layer-by-layer (LBL) assembly with inorganic nanoparticles and nanowires. *Acc Chem Res* 41: 1831–1841.
Such, G.K., E. Tjipto, A. Postma, A.P. Johnston, and F. Caruso. 2007. Ultrathin, responsive polymer click capsules. *Nano Lett* 7: 1706–1710.
Sui, Z.J., D. Salloum, and J.B. Schlenoff. 2003. Effect of molecular weight on the construction of polyelectrolyte multilayers: Stripping versus sticking. *Langmuir* 19: 2491–2495.
Sukhishvili, S., and S. Granick. 2002. Layered, erasable polymer multilayers formed by hydrogen-bonded sequential self-assembly. *Macromolecules* 35: 301–310.
Sukhishvili, S.A., E. Kharlampieva, and V. Izumrudov. 2006. Where polyelectrolyte multilayers and polyelectrolyte complexes meet. *Macromolecules* 39: 8873–8881.
Sukhorukov, G.B., A.L. Rogach, B. Zebli, et al. 2005. Nanoengineered polymer capsules: Tools for detection, controlled delivery, and site-specific manipulation. *Small* 1(2): 194–200.
Sukhorukov, G.B., A.L. Rogach, M. Garstka, et al. 2007. Multifunctionalized polymer microcapsules: Novel tools for biological and pharmacological applications. *Small* 3: 944–955.
Sun, B., C.M. Jewell, N.J. Fredin, and D.M. Lynn. 2007. Assembly of multilayered films using well-defined, end-labeled poly(acrylic acid): Influence of molecular weight on exponential growth in a synthetic weak polyelectrolyte system. *Langmuir* 23: 8452–8459.
Szyk, L., P. Schaaf, C. Gergely, J.-C. Voegel, and B. Tinland. 2001. Lateral mobility of proteins adsorbed on or embedded in polyelectrolyte multilayers. *Langmuir* 17: 6248–6253.
Tan, Q., J. Ji, M.A. Barbosa, C. Fonseca, and J. Shen. 2003. Constructing thromboresistant surface on biomedical stainless steel via layer-by-layer deposition anticoagulant. *Biomaterials* 24: 4699–4705.
Tang, Z., N.A. Kotov, S. Magonov, and B. Ozturk. 2003. Nanostructured artificial nacre. *Nat Mater* 2: 413–418.
Tang, Z., Y.L. Wang, P. Podsiadlo, and N.A. Kotov. 2006. Biomedical applications of layer-by-layer assembly: From biomimetics to tissue engineering. *Adv Mater* 18: 3203–3224.
Teramura, Y., Y. Kaneda, and H. Iwata. 2007. Islet-encapsulation in ultra-thin layer-by-layer membranes of poly(vinyl alcohol) anchored to poly(ethylene glycol)-lipids in the cell membrane. *Biomaterials* 28: 4818–4825.
Teramura, Y., and H. Iwata. 2008. Islets surface modification prevents blood-mediated inflammatory responses. *Bioconjug Chem* 19: 1389–1395.
Tezcaner, A., D. Hicks, F. Boulmedais, et al. 2006. Polyelectrolyte multilayer films as substrates for photoreceptor cells. *Biomacromolecules* 7: 86–94.
Thevenot, P., W. Hu, and L. Tang. 2008. Surface chemistry influences implant biocompatibility. *Curr Top Med Chem* 8: 270–280.
Thierry, B., F.M. Winnik, Y. Merhi, J. Silver, and M. Tabrizian. 2003. Bioactive coatings of endovascular stents based on polyelectrolyte multilayers. *Biomacromolecules* 4: 1564–1571.
Thompson, M.T., M.C. Berg, I.S. Tobias, M.F. Rubner, and K.J. Van Vliet. 2005. Tuning compliance of nanoscale polyelectrolyte multilayers to modulate cell adhesion. *Biomaterials* 26: 6836–6845.
Thompson, M.T., M.C. Berg, I.S. Tobias, et al. 2006. Biochemical functionalization of polymeric cell substrata can alter mechanical compliance. *Biomacromolecules* 7: 1990–1995.
Thorne, R.G., A. Lakkaraju, E. Rodriguez-Boulan, and C. Nicholson. 2008. In vivo diffusion of lactoferrin in brain extracellular space is regulated by interactions with heparan sulfate. *Proc Natl Acad Sci U S A* 105: 8416–8421.

Tong, W., C. Gao, and H. Möhwald. 2005. Manipulating the properties of polyelectrolyte microcapsules by glutaraldehyde cross-linking. *Chem Mater* 17: 4610–4616.
Tryoen-Toth, P., D. Vautier, Y. Haikel, et al. 2002. Viability, adhesion, and bone phenotype of osteoblast-like cells on polyelectrolyte multilayer films. *J Biomed Mater Res* 60: 657–667.
Turner, R., P. Lin, and M. Cowman. 1988. Self-association of hyaluronante segments in aqueous NaCl solution. *Arch Biochem Biophys* 265: 484–495.
van den Beucken, J.J., X.F. Walboomers, S.C. Leeuwenburgh, et al. 2007a. Multilayered DNA coatings: In vitro bioactivity studies and effects on osteoblast-like cell behavior. *Acta Biomater* 3: 587–596.
van den Beucken, J.J., X.F. Walboomers, M.R. Vos, et al. 2007b. Biological responses to multilayered DNA-coatings. *J Biomed Mater Res B Appl Biomater* 81: 231–238.
Vautier, D., J. Hemmerlé, C. Vodouhe, et al. 2003. 3d surface charges modulate protusive and contractile contacts of chondrosarcoma cells. *Cell Motil Cytoskeleton* 56: 147–158.
Veerabadran, N.G., P.L. Goli, S.S. Stewart-Clark, Y.M. Lvov, and D.K. Mills. 2007. Nanoencapsulation of stem cells within polyelectrolyte multilayer shells. *Macromol Biosci* 7: 877–882.
Vodouhe, C., M. Schmittbuhl, F. Boulmedais, et al. 2005. Effect of functionalization of multilayered polyelectrolyte films on motoneuron growth. *Biomaterials* 26: 545–554.
Vodouhê, C., E.L. Guen, J.M. Garza, et al. 2006. Control of drug accessibility on functional polyelectrolyte multilayer films. *Biomaterials* 27: 4149–4156.
von Klitzing, R. 2006. Internal structure of polyelectrolyte multilayer assemblies. *Phys Chem Chem Phys* 8: 5012–5033.
Wagner, V.E., J.T. Koberstein, and J.D. Bryers. 2004. Protein and bacterial fouling characteristics of peptide and antibody decorated surfaces of PEG-poly(acrylic acid)-*co*-polymers. *Biomaterials* 25: 2247–2263.
Wang, F., N. Ma, Q. Chen, W. Wang, and L. Wang. 2007. Halogen bonding as a new driving force for layer-by-layer assembly. *Langmuir* 23: 9540–9542.
Werner, S., O. Huck, B. Frisch, et al. 2009. The effect of microstructured surfaces and laminin-derived peptide coatings on soft tissue interactions with titanium dental implants. *Biomaterials* 30: 2291–2301.
Wilson, J.T., W. Cui, X.L. Sun, et al. 2007. In vivo biocompatibility and stability of a substrate-supported polymerizable membrane-mimetic film. *Biomaterials* 28: 609–617.
Wilson, J.T., W. Cui, and E.L. Chaikof. 2008. Layer-by-layer assembly of a conformal nanothin PEG coating for intraportal islet transplantation. *Nano Lett* 8: 1940–1948.
Wittmer, C.R., J.A. Phelps, W.M. Saltzman, and P.R. Van Tassel. 2007. Fibronectin terminated multilayer films: Protein adsorption and cell attachment studies. *Biomaterials* 28: 851–860.
Wittmer, C.R., J.A. Phelps, C.M. Lepus, et al. 2008. Multilayer nanofilms as substrates for hepatocellular applications. *Biomaterials* 29: 4082–4090.
Wood, K.C., J.Q. Boedicker, D.M. Lynn, and P.T. Hammond. 2005. Tunable drug release from hydrolytically degradable layer-by-layer thin films. *Langmuir* 21: 1603–1609.
Wu, Z.R., J. Ma, B.F. Liu, Q.Y. Xu, and F.Z. Cui. 2007. Layer-by-layer assembly of polyelectrolyte films improving cytocompatibility to neural cells. *J Biomed Mater Res A* 81: 355–362.
Yang, S.Y., and M.F. Rubner. 2002. Micropatterning of polymer thin films with pH-sensitive and cross-linkable hydrogen-bonded polyelectrolyte multilayers. *J Am Chem Soc* 124: 2100–2101.
Yasui, S., and T. Keigerling. 1986. Vibrational circular-dichroism of polypeptides. Poly(lysine) conformations as a function of pH in aqueous-solution. *J Am Chem Soc* 108: 5576–5581.
Yuan, W., H. Dong, C.M. Li, et al. 2007. pH-controlled construction of chitosan/alginate multilayer film: Characterization and application for antibody immobilization. *Langmuir* 23: 13046–1352.
Zacharia, N.S., D.M. DeLongchamp, M. Modestino, and P.T. Hammond. 2007. Controlling diffusion and exchange in layer-by-layer assemblies. *Macromolecules* 40: 1598–1603.
Zaidel-Bar, R., M. Cohen, L. Addadi, and B. Geiger. 2004. Hierarchical assembly of cell-matrix adhesion complexes. *Biochem Soc Trans* 32: 416–420.
Zhang, J., B. Senger, D. Vautier, et al. 2005. Buildup of collagen and hyaluronic acid polyelectrolyte multilayers. *Biomaterials* 26: 3353–3361.

Zhang, L., W.H. Zhao, J.S. Rudra, and D.T. Haynie. 2007. Context dependence of the assembly, structure, and stability of polypeptide multilayer nonofilms. *ACS Nano* 1: 476–486.
Zhu, H., J. Ji, Q. Tan, M.A. Barbosa, and J. Shen. 2003. Surface engineering of poly(DL-lactide) via electrostatic self-assembly of extracellular matrix-like molecules. *Biomacromolecules* 4: 378–386.
Zhu, H., J. Ji, M.A. Barbosa, and J. Shen. 2004. Protein electrostatic self-assembly on poly(DL-lactide) scaffold to promote osteoblast growth. *J Biomed Mater Res B Appl Biomater* 71: 159–165.

9

Bioactive Glass-Based Coatings and Modified Surfaces: Strategies for the Manufacture, Testing, and Clinical Applications for Regenerative Medicine

Jason Maroothynaden

CONTENTS

Introduction

We are now living in an aging population. It is predicted that in the Western world there will be more people over 65 than under 25 years old by 2015. With the increase in age come the increases in the number of damaged tissues (e.g., fractured bones) that need to be treated. The increased inability of the body to repair tissues and organs is a problem that modern medicine is trying to address. In addition, changes in lifestyle and increased adoption of high-risk sports among people under 30 coupled with increasing life expectancy mean that design lifetime of implanted devices need to be significantly longer. The best treatments currently available are to replace damaged tissues and organs with either transplants or manmade implantable devices, both of which are in limited supply.

In 40 years of research and clinical assessment, many types of biomedical, implantable materials (metals, polymers, ceramics, and glasses) have been developed, tested, and successfully used clinically. As an introduction, these materials will be briefly reviewed. Attention will be given to bioactive glass (calcium phosphate–based) materials. A review of the strategies for their manufacture, testing (in vitro and in vivo), and their possible clinical applications will be presented. In addition, I will introduce the three generational classifications of these glasses based on their intrinsic surface properties.

Tissues are "living" things and as such they respond and adapt to their local biochemical and biomechanical environment. Bioactive coating technologies that facilitate alterations in textural properties of the implant/tissue interface to encourage tissue ingrowth and attachment, limit infection, and host tissue immunological response will be reviewed. Regenerative medicine is an exciting new strategy and emerging commercial market where engineered tissues and organs could potentially address the supply of functional replacement tissues and organs (e.g., bone, cartilage, heart, lung, and kidney).

Finally, a review of nanotechnology-based applications of these bioactive coatings and surface technologies will be briefly introduced, providing food for thought to existing developers of these technologies.

Biomaterials

Since the invention of the first generation of biomedical materials there has been an ever-growing research interest in the development of synthetic biomaterials for use inside the body [1, 2]. The field couples advances in materials with biological sciences to design materials with surface properties that deliberately consider the interactions between living and nonliving materials. As a result, biomaterials ultimately lead to improvements in the quality of human health and quality of life [1]. Materials used as biomaterials include metals, polymers, pyrolitic carbon, polycrystalline materials, glasses, glass–ceramics, and ceramics composites. Their applications in the human body include orthopedics, cardiovascular, ophthalmic, dental, wound-healing, and drug delivery systems (see Figure 9.1).

What Is a Biomaterial?

There have been many attempts to define what a biomaterial is based on inherent mechanical properties and fundamental biological performance.

Black [1] offers a good definition of a biomaterial that is an adaptation of the definition presented by The European Society for Biomaterials:

> A material intended to interface with biological systems to evaluate, treat, augment, or replace any tissue, organ, or function of the body.

The definition reinforces the concept of biological interaction and biodegradation while including biomaterials that incorporate (seeded with) live cells. Biodegradation is defined as the breakdown of a material medicated by a biological system [1].

Implanted biomaterials are foreign objects and will elicit an inflammatory response no matter how bioinert they are. The inflammatory response is known as biocompatibility. In the late 1970s, Osborn [4] attempted to define biocompatibility by segmenting biomaterials via their local host–tissue interface responses as follows: biotolerant, bioinert, or bioactive. Biotolerant has subsequently been dropped and biomaterials are now classified as being bioinert or bioactive. The selecting factor in the use of materials as biomaterials will always be its efficacy at achieving the appropriate biological performance [1].

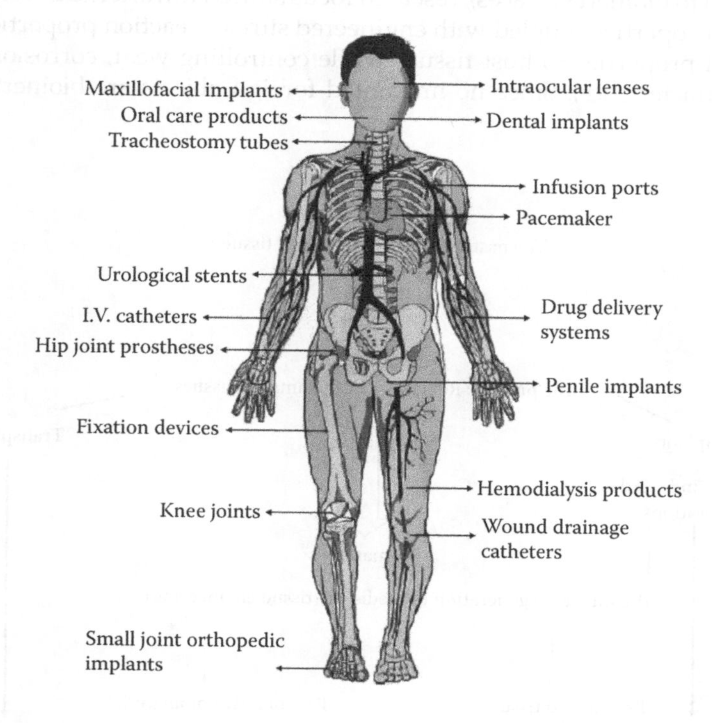

FIGURE 9.1
Schematic showing various applications of biomaterials. (From Balamrugan et al., *Mater. Corros.*, 59(11), 855–869, 2008. With permission [3].)

Clinical Need in Orthopedic Applications

Approximately 40% of the body is bone [1]. It plays an important role, protecting internal organs and enabling body locomotion [5]. Autografts, allografts, xenographs (for periodontal applications only), and biomaterials (synthetic grafts and bone-fillers) have been used to repair bone defects that have damaged surface areas too large for self-repair. Autograph implants (bone material that is transferred from one location to the other in the same patient) have exhibited good clinical performance. However, the surgical procedure is limited by the amount of healthy tissue available coupled with additional damage at the site where bone is harvested. Allograph and xenograph implants (where bone material from another patient is transplanted and where bone material from another species is transplanted) address shortcomings in availability of material but introduce new problems—infections and foreign body reactions [6]. Biomaterials are clinically safe and free from the shortcomings addressed above. Metals, ceramics, and polymers have all been selected and used in orthopedics [7]; however, their discussion is beyond the scope of this chapter, so I recommend the reader consult the excellent review by Navarro et al. [7].

Tissue Engineering Approach to Biomaterials Development

Early biomaterials development was regarded as a means to an end (i.e., materials-focused selection and application driven by appropriate inherent bulk properties matching the host tissue site) solution where suitable materials were chosen or developed to replace absent, damaged, or diseased host tissues. With the discovery of biomaterials, surface reaction responses (even to bioinert surfaces), research focus shifted toward the development of biomaterials bulk properties coupled with engineered surface reaction properties (e.g., matching mechanical properties to host tissues while controlling wear, corrosion, and surface dissolution characteristics). Since no implanted foreign objects are bioinert, biomaterials

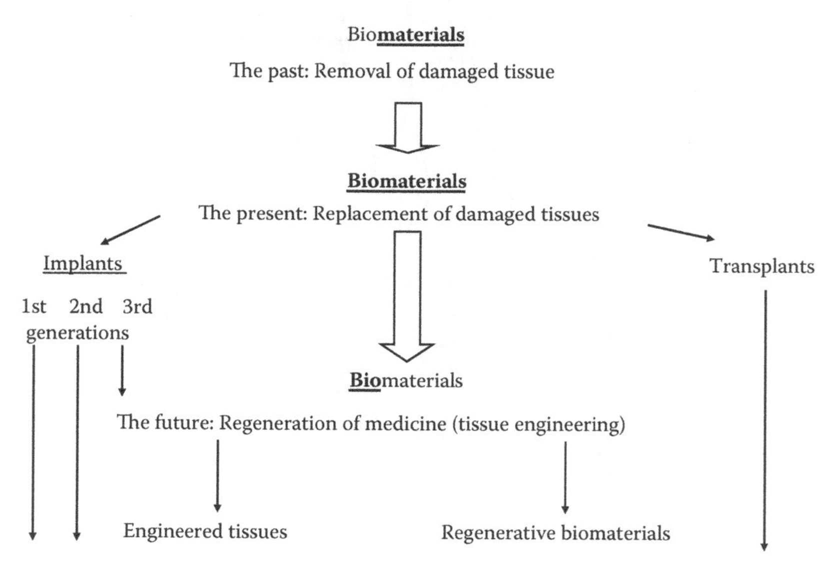

FIGURE 9.2
Shift in biomaterials development over the past 40 years [8].

have had limited implant success lifetimes and often require secondary, revision surgery to either correct or replace them.

Within the past 10 years, tissue engineering has driven biomaterials development toward the understanding and subsequent precise control of the implant material/host–tissue interface, resulting in improved cellular attachment, proliferation, and eventual ingrowth. All these factors are required to prolong implant lifetimes.

Tissue engineered devices consist of an implantable biomaterial scaffold that is resorbed at the implant site and replaced with regenerated, healthy tissue. Often the scaffold is seeded with cells appropriate for biological interaction with the host tissue implant site. This approach requires biomaterials to act as temporary mechanical structures mimicking the host tissue extracellular matrix and eventually being replaced with new, regenerated tissue. It is hoped that this biodriven development focus will result in controlled protein absorption and release, cellular attachment, proliferation, and differentiation resulting in significantly improving implant lifetimes (see Figure 9.2). Recently, much research effort has concentrated on the use of nanotechnology (via morphological and physiochemical approaches) to further mimic extracellular matrix behavior, thus promoting faster rates of tissue ingrowth into the implant surface, prolonged tissue/implant attachment, and subsequent improved implant lifetime.

Bioceramics and Glasses

Ceramics are composed of inorganic and nonmetallic components usually fabricated using traditional pottery processing techniques such as [41]:

1. Ceramic particles suspended in a lubricant or binder solution for shaping and firing
2. Raw materials (e.g., silicates, aluminum silicates, nonsilicates such as alumina) melted to form a liquid and shaped during cooling and solidification

Their mechanical properties (see Table 9.1) coupled with inertness in aqueous environments make them desirable implant material candidates for orthopedic load-bearing applications (see Table 9.2).

Since ceramics have low strength in tension, their application has been limited to compressive loading conditions (see Table 9.2). Readers wanting to know more about bioceramics not classified as either bioactive glass or glass–ceramics should refer to the seminal works by Hench and Wilson [9] and recently by Kokubo [10]. Here, I will refer to them as first-generation bioceramics: they are bioinert and cannot be resorbed or replaced with regenerated host tissue. First-generation ceramics include alumina (Al_2O_3) and zirconia (ZrO_2).

In the late 1960s, Hench discovered and developed the first bioceramics that elicited a specific biological response at the implant/tissue interface, resulting in direct biological bonding into the material and subsequent fixation. Here I will refer to them as second-generation bioceramics. They are commonly termed bioactive ceramics. Although included in many texts as a ceramic, Hench's material was not actually a ceramic but a glass whose composition was based on the $Na_2O–P_2O_5–CaO–SiO_2$ system (45S5 composition). Traded under the name Bioglass, bioceramics research focus shifted from bioinert materials toward a

TABLE 9.1

Typical Mechanical Properties of Bioceramics

Bioceramic	Compressive Strength (MPa)	Tensile (T)/Bending (B) Strength (MPa)	Young's Modulus (GPa)	Fracture Toughness (MPa √m)
First generation (not bioactive)				
Alumina (Al_2O_3)	3000	260–300 (T)	380	3–5
Zirconina (ZrO_2)	2000	248 (T)	200	4–12
Second and third generation (bioactive)				
Bioactive glass (Bioglass®)	~1000	42 (T)	~100	~3
Bioactive glass–ceramic (A/W glass)	1080	215 (B)	118	2
Hydroxyapatite (HA)	~1000	40 (T)	100–200	~ 3
Calcium phosphates	20–900	30–200 (T)	30–103	< 1
Natural tissue				
Cortical bone	130–180	50–151 (T)	12–18	6–8

new paradigm where bioactive ceramics (second-generation bioceramics) elicited a specific biological interfacial bonding responses while maintaining the structural integrity at the host tissue site. In addition, their surfaces could be designed to be either resorbable, where the material interface was replaced with host tissue, or nonresorbable (Figure 9.3). Since the discovery of Hench's composition, various second-generation bioceramics, bioactive glasses, and glass–ceramics have been developed. Resorbable materials include bioactive glass (e.g., 45S5 composition), glass–ceramics (e.g., A–W glass, Ceravital®), bioactive, porous sol–gel glasses (e.g., 58S—see Table 9.5), and calcium phosphates. Hydroxyapatite (HA) is an example of a nonresorbable bioecramic. Recently, biodriven bioactive glass development has focused on engineering surface reaction conditions (including the controlled release of ionic dissolution products into the local interfacial aqueous microenvironment and engineering nanoscopic surface features) that genetically stimulate bone regeneration. These have been termed third-generation bioceramics (Figure 9.3). It is hoped that genetic bases for bone regeneration will represent the next paradigm shift in biomaterials development.

Development of resorbable glasses and glass–ceramics has been limited due to their intrinsic characteristics (e.g., fracture toughness, elastic moduli, and compressive strength lower than cancellous and cortical bone for porous bioactive ceramics) verses specific chemical compositions to be bioactive. However, the nucleation and growth of crystalline phases in glass–ceramics has resulted in improved mechanical properties that are closer to cortical bone (Table 9.2). The advantage of densification of bioactive ceramics results in materials that are much stiffer than bone. However, the disadvantage is that stiffer implanted materials can usually fail due to local implant loosening caused by stress-shielding.

First-Generation Bioceramics

The first total hip replacement was carried out using an ivory implant in 1890. In the 1960s, metals and polymers were used in devices to replace hips (femoral steam and ball;

TABLE 9.2

Uses of Ceramics, Glass, and Composites in Body

Clinical Application/Location	Ceramics, Glass, and Composite Material Used
Head	
Cranial repair	Bioactive glasses
Keratoprosthesis	Alumina
Otolaryngological implants	Alumina, HA, bioactive glasses, bioactive glass–ceramics, bioactive composites
Maxillofacial reconstruction	Alumina, HA, HA–PLA composite, bioactive glasses
Dental implants	Alumina, HA, HA coating, bioactive glasses, bioactive glass–ceramics
Alveolar ride augmentation	Alumina, HA, TCP; HA–autogenous bone composite, HA–PLA composite, bioactive glasses
Periodontal pocket obliteration	HA, HA–PLA composite, calcium phosphate salts, bioactive glasses
Torso and upper limbs	
Percutaneous access devices	Bioactive glasses, bioactive glass–ceramics, bioactive composites, HA, pyrolitic carbon coating
Artificial heart valves	Pyrolitic carbon coating
Spinal surgery	Bioactive glass–ceramics, HA
Iliac crest repair	Bioactive glass–ceramics
Bone space fillers	TCP, calcium phosphate salts, bioactive glasses, bioactive glass–ceramics
Lower limbs	
Orthopedic load-bearing applications	Alumina, zirconia, PE–HA composite, HA coating on metal, bioactive glass, and glass–ceramic coatings on metal
Orthopedic fixation devices	PLA carbon fiber composite, PLS calcium phosphate composite
Artificial tendons	Carbon–fiber composites
Joints	HA

acetabular cups, respectively). Their use continues today in these types of devices. In the past 40 years of research and clinical applications, many types of biomedical materials (ranging from metals, polymers, ceramics, and glasses) have been developed, tested in the laboratory, and used clinically. These first-generation biomaterials all have a fundamental, inherent material-driven design specification—to reduce to a minimum the host tissues' immune response to a foreign body while being mechanically and physically stable.

Tissues are "living" things and as such they respond and adapt to their local biochemical and biomechanical environment. First-generation materials cannot respond to changes in the host tissue environment and as such their useful lifetime is severely limited. Eventually secondary surgery is needed to replace the loosened (e.g., detachment of implant from host tissue and material/tissue interface) or damaged implant (e.g., fracture of the material). Numerous strategies have been employed to enhance the useful lifetime of biomaterials. For total-bone-joint replacement devices, these include altering textural properties of the implant/tissue interface to include voids and other anchor points to encourage tissue ingrowth and attachment and cement fixation at the implant/tissue interface. Their success is limited and survival times (useful lifetime once implanted) are approximately 19 years. Other factors such as infection, host tissue immunological response, and implant fracture can reduce survival times to 5 years or less.

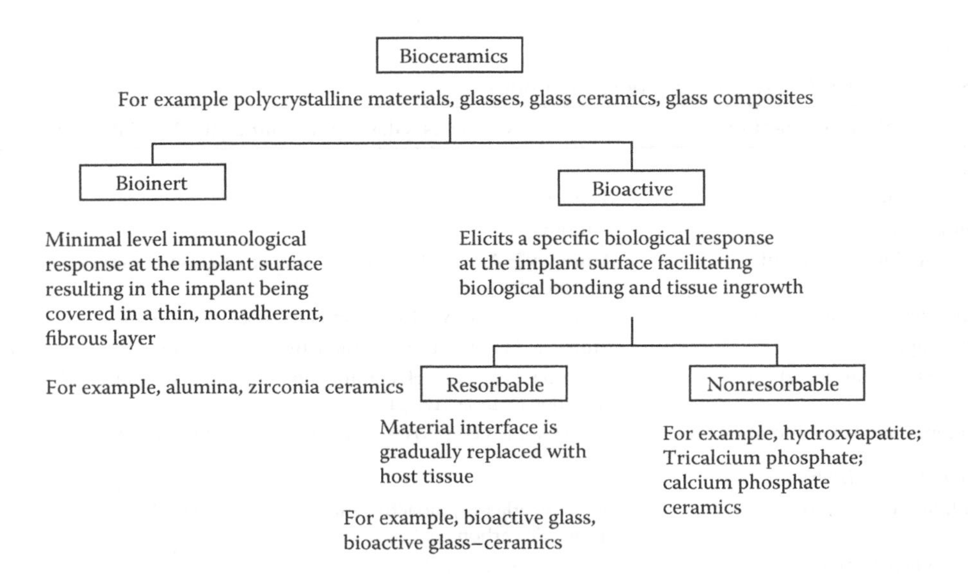

FIGURE 9.3
Classification of bioceramics and bioactive glasses [11].

No first-generation bioactive glasses exist. By definition, bioactivity is a second-generation material property.

Bioactive Glasses

The discovery in the late 1960s that certain compositions of glass could elicit a bioactive response (host tissue responds biologically to implant facilitating tissue growth—osteoproduction—across surface and in some instances tissue growth into the implant surface) initiated a revolutionary paradigm shift. They have been incorporated into implant devices in the form of monoliths, coatings, powders, and composites. Introduction of bioactivity prolongs the lifetime of the device via encouragement of hard tissue (e.g., bone) into and onto the device, forming a mechanically strong and biologically stable interface. Materials compositional changes allow bioactive glasses to bond to soft tissues as well. Another advance of bioactive glasses is their ability to resorb (network degradation facilitating the release of ionic species into the host tissue, allowing biomaterial to be replaced with new host tissue).

45S5 Composition (Bioglass®)

In the late 1960s, Hench demonstrated that interfacial bonding to bone could be achieved with a certain compositional range of glasses that contained SiO_2, Na_2O, CaO, and P_2O_5 in specific proportions. These bioactive glasses differ from traditional SiO_2–Na_2O–CaO glasses in that their SiO_2 content is much lower than 60 mol% and they have a high Na_2O and CaO content and a high CaO/P_2O_5 ratio. These compositional factors directly account for their high surface reaction kinetics and subsequent interfacial bond with bone.

Many melt-derived bioactive glass compositions are based on the 45S5 formula (45 wt.% SiO_2, S as the network former, and a 5:1 molar ratio of Ca to P in the form of CaO and

P_2O_5). For these glasses, no bonding with bone will occur if the ratio of Ca to P is very low (Figure 9.4). There is a compositional dependence (in weight percent) of bonding to bone tissue for the Na_2O–CaO–P_2O_5–SiO_2 glasses (shown in Figure 9.4). All the glasses in Figure 9.4 contain a constant 6 wt.% P_2O_5. Region A represents the bioactive bone-bonding boundary as glasses outside this boundary will not form a bond with bone. Region B glasses include soda–lime–silicate glasses and exhibit first-generation materials responses at their surface. Glasses within region C are resorbable and hence exhibit second-generation materials responses. Region D glasses are not technically feasible using traditional melt-derived glass manufacturing techniques.

Soft tissue bonding occurs within the dashed line of Figure 9.4 via the collagenous constituents strongly adhering to the bioactive silica glasses. For example, in vitro attachment of collagen to 45S5 surfaces occur after 10 days exposure, closely representing that found in vivo. In particular, collagen fibers were woven into the surface by growth of the HCA layer to about 30 to 60 μm of the 100 to 200 μm total interfacial thickness.

Bioactive glasses can be divided into two classes on the basis of their host tissue/material surface interface response. Glass compositions that lie within the region bound by the dashed line in Figure 9.4 have been classified as Class A bioactive glasses. These bioactive glasses bond to both hard and soft tissues. Class B bioactive glasses lie outside the boundaries of the dashed line but within the area of Figure 9.4 described by region A. Class B bioactive glasses bond to hard tissues only.

The 45S5 bioactive glass composition is a Class A biomaterial. It forms a biological bond with bone 20 h after implantation. Upon exposure to a physiological solution, biological proteins and growth factors are absorbed on to the glass surface. The glass structure starts to degrade within 1 h and hydrated silica has leached into solution. At the surface, silanol bonds (Si–OH) form and polycondense to form a stable silica–gel surface layer. Between 1 and 2 h, proteins and growth factors are still being absorbed while amorphous calcium, carbonates, and phosphates migrate from the glass structure and become absorbed into the silica–gel layer, which results in the crystallization of hydroxyapatite (HA). Between 2 and 10 h, proteins and growth factors are still being absorbed while the HA layer crystallizes

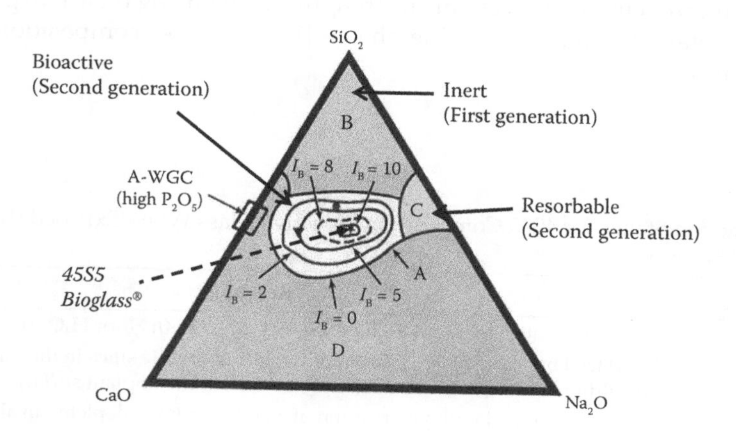

FIGURE 9.4
Compositional dependence (in wt.%) of tissue response with silica-based bioactive glasses. All compositions in region A have constant 6 wt.% of P_2O_5. AW–GSC (apatite wollastonite glass–ceramic) has a higher P_2O_5 content (16.3 wt.%). Soft tissue bonding occurs within the area bounded by the dashed line I_b gives the index of bioactivity [8].

into a high surface area layer on the glass. Between 10 and 20 h, macrophages attach to the surface and then depart. By 100 h, stem cells have attached and are differentiating. After 100 h, bone matrix is generated and crystallized.

Each composition of bioactive glass exhibits specific interfacial reaction kinetics. For materials in the apex of region B (Figure 9.4), surface hydration layer is formed between the implant and the host. Materials in the lower area of region B (i.e., with sufficient SiO_2 in the glass network) form a dense SiO_2 rich film as a result of alkali–proton exchange and repolymerization. This film protects the implant surface from further attack, resulting in an inert tissue response. Region C glasses experience rapid and selective ion exchange of alkaline ions with protons or hydronium ions forming a thick, porous, and subsequently nonprotective SiO_2-rich film. If the local pH rises above 9, the SiO_2-rich film dissolves rapidly allowing bulk network or stoichiometric dissolution to occur. Bioactive glasses in region A form a dual protective film that is rich in Ca and P formed on an alkaline-depleted SiO_2-rich layer.

The interfacial reaction kinetics for 45S5 is well documented. They are summarized below (Table 9.3). There are five reaction stages that include ion exchange (stage 1), silica network dissolution (stage 2), silica repolymerization (stage 3), formation of an amorphous CaP layer (stage 4), followed by crystallization of HA (stage 5).

The index of bioactivity I_b is the inverse of the time required for more than 50% ($t_{0.5bb}$) of the materials' interface to be bonded where the I_b value for 45S5 (Table 9.8) matches bone. In addition, its I_q (qualitative performance ratio; see Section 9.4.1) makes it suitable for cancellous bone replacement. 45S5 can be combined with a polymeric binder (e.g., 0.4% volume fraction of 45S5 plus polysulfone composite) to create a mechanically enhanced composite material with an I_q matching that of cortical bone. In addition, its bioactivity is not compromised.

Bioactive Glass–Ceramics

Referring to Table 9.2, it is clear that the mechanical strength of bioactive glasses does not match human bone. Seminal work by Brömer, Höland, Burger and Miller have all addressed the improvement of mechanical strength by preparing bioactive glass compositions that precipitate different crystalline phases [12, 13]. These compositions are known as glass–ceramics.

TABLE 9.3

The Surface Reaction Stages for 45S5 Composition Bioactive Glass When Exposed/Immersed in an Aqueous-Based Solution

Stage	Reaction
1	Diffusion controlled rapid exchange of Na^+ or K^+ with H^+ or H_3O^+ from solution
2	Interfacial breaking of Si–O–Si bonds, releasing soluble silica in the form of $Si(OH)_4$ resulting in the formation of silanols (Si–OH) at the implant surface
3	Condensation and reploymerization of a SiO_2-rich layer depleted in alkalis and alkaline-earth cations
4	Migration of Ca and P through the SiO_2- rich layer forming a Ca–P rich film, followed by growth of the amorphous Ca–P-rich film by incorporation of soluble Ca and P from solution
5	Crystallization of the amorphous Ca–P film (HA)

TABLE 9.4
Bioactive Glass–Ceramic Compositions [12, 13]

Bioactive Glass–Ceramic System	Comment
Na_2O–K_2O–CaO–SiO_2–P_2O_4	Traded under the name Ceravital®, has enhanced mechanical properties due to apatite precipitation
MgO–CaO–SiO_2–P_2O_5	Known as A–W glass–ceramic, has enhanced mechanical properties due to both apatite and wollastonite precipitation At the time of writing, this composition is the most commonly used glass–ceramic for clinical applications
Na_2O–K_2O–CaO–CaF_2–SiO_2–P_2O_4	Has enhanced mechanical properties due to canasite precipitation
Na_2O–K_2O–MgO–CaO–SiO_2–P_2O_4–CaF_2	Traded as Ilmaplant®, has enhanced mechanical properties due to both apatite and wollastonite precipitation

In an attempt to improve the mechanical properties of bioactive glass compositions, Brohmer and coworkers developed the first bioactive glass–ceramic: Ceravital® [12]. With a composition similar to Hench's 45S5 composition glass, it had half the bioactivity of 45S5. Its mechanical strength was lower than dense HA but higher than 45S5 and as a result used for minimal load-bearing applications such as middle ear ossicular chain replacement. Improvements in mechanical properties were made by Kokubo and coworkers who developed A–W glass–ceramic (commercially traded under the name Cerabone A/W®). Based on the MgO–CaO–SiO_2–P_2O_5 system, thermal treatment lead to the precipitation of apatite (oxfluroapatite-$Ca_{10}(PO_4)_6(OF_2)$) and wollastonite phases (β-$CaSiO_3$) resulting in a fine-grained glass–ceramic with mechanical properties similar to that of human cortical bone. However, its bioactivity was half that of 45S5 composition. Interestingly, unlike 45S5 glass, after 10 days of immersion in simulated body fluid, Ca–P phases were precipitated on the surface of the glass without the prescience of a silica layer, prompting Kokubo to conclude that precipitation of Ca–P and not the formation of a silica layer was the prerequisite for direct implant bonding with bone tissue. Further improvements in bioactivity have lead to compositional modifications resulting in glasses based on Na_2O–K_2O–CaO–CaF_2–SiO_2–P_2O_4 systems and Na_2O–K_2O–MgO–CaO–SiO_2–P_2O_4–CaF_2 systems (see Table 9.4).

However, their inherent precipitation of specific phases has limited their applications as coating materials because it is difficult to precisely control the formation of phases during the coating process. As monoliths, thermal processing steps (i.e., lower temperatures to form nuclei followed by ramping up to higher processing temperatures to grow crystal phases without coarsening) often results in temperature gradients and cracking due to internal stresses. Subsequently, coatings are difficult to produce since they fail due to cracking and delamination before or during in vitro testing.

Sol–Gel Bioactive Glasses

Sol–gel bioactive glasses couple controlled bioactivity with controlled resorbability (facilitating controlled release of ionic dissolution products) to elicit a specific cellular and genetic response capable of improved tissue growth, replacement, and eventual regeneration.

The ideal bioactive glass will degrade at a controlled rate over time and be replaced with natural, healthy host tissue. However this is no easy task because the rate of tissue ingrowth varies with tissue type, tissue age, location, and patient [8].

Bioactive glasses have been developed and applied as coatings, foams, powders, and combined with polymeric binders to form novel composite materials.

Figure 9.4 shows that tissue response is directly related to materials compositions for four-component silicate glasses. For melt-derived glasses, increasing silica content results in decreasing dissolution rates. As silica content reaches 60%, bioactivity is eliminated.

It is now accepted that silica and not Na_2O is the active component of bioactive glasses. Na_2O is a network disrupter. Melt-derived glasses are not inherently porous. Introduction of pores increases surface area, potential bioactivity, and surfaces for tissue ingrowth. Pores have been introduced into melt-derived glasses but with limited success. Monoliths with pore diameters 200 to 300 μm with a total porosity of 21% have been produced; however, the pores were not interconnected. These materials did not mimic trabecular bone [8].

It is possible to extend the compositional range of bioactive glasses beyond 60 mol% silica content via manufacturing the glasses via the sol–gel method.

Sol–gel bioactive glasses (Figure 9.5) have many advantages over melt-derived glass. These are:

- Lower manufacturing temperatures (600–700°C)
- Higher silica and low alkali content (up to 90 mol% silica) compositions that are bioactive
- Better control of bioactivity via changes in composition and or processing temperature
- Inherently porous with porosity content changed via processing temperatures
- Can be foamed resulting in significantly higher surface areas (ranging from 150 to 600 m^2 g 1) ratios, including pore interconnectivity and enhanced bioactivity
- Fewer components required to make bioactive glasses (e.g., SiO_2–CaO–P_2O_5; SiO_2–CaO; pure silica compositions) [8]

Bioactivity is higher because the increased surface area results in more silanol groups on the surface which in turn increases the number of nucleation sites for HCA layer formation. Resorbtion is enhanced and can be controlled via changing porosity.

Sol–gel bioactive glasses follow the same mechanisms of surface dissolution as melt-derived glasses (Table 9.3). The degree of bioactivity and thickness of the tissue boundary layer varies with chemical composition and textural characteristics. For example, for 58S composition, sol–gel glass has significantly faster dissolution rates and faster HA surface layer formation after 6 h of immersion in simulated body fluid (SBF) in vitro. After this time, Si dissolution from the glass network continues and stabilizes after 4 days.

Dissolution rate of Si from glass network exhibits a time-dependent concentration profile response. Dissolution is rapid at short times (e.g., up to 1 h of immersion) and slow after a time t^* (e.g., greater than 6 h of immersion). This can be described by the Douglas and El-Shamy equation:

$$Q = kty \tag{9.1}$$

where Q is the concentration of silicon ions in solution, k is the rate constant, t is time, and y is ½ for first stage (Table 9.3) of silicon dissolution.

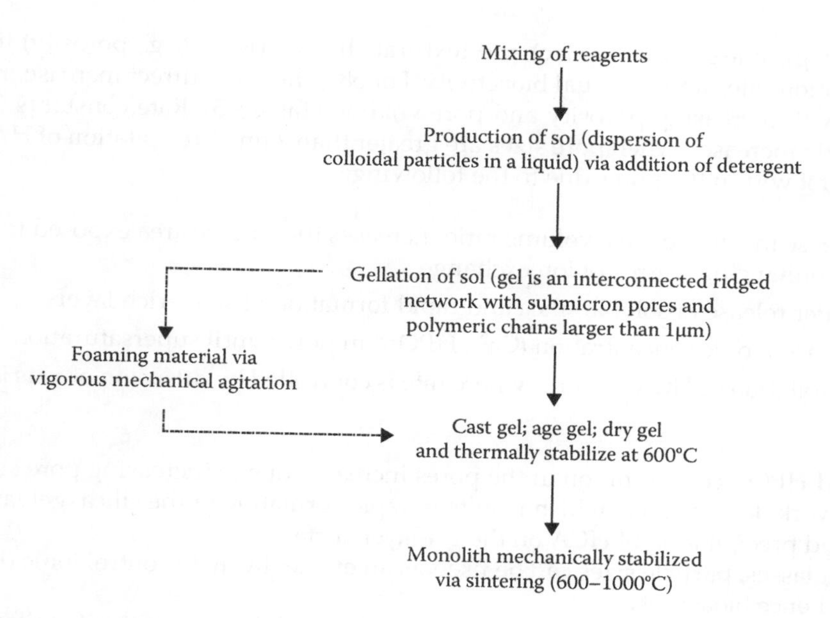

FIGURE 9.5
Schematic showing sol–gel processing of sol–gel glasses [8].

Si dissolution rates can thus be described by (9.2) and (9.3):

$$D[\mathrm{Si}]/\mathrm{d}t = k_1 t^{-1/2} \text{ for } t < t^* \tag{9.2}$$

and

$$D[\mathrm{Si}]/\mathrm{d}t = k_1 t^{-1/2} \text{ for } t > t^* \tag{9.3}$$

These expressions can be used to describe Si dissolution from melt-derived bioactive glasses as well.

TABLE 9.5
Characteristics of 45S5 and 58S Glass Compositions

Material Characteristics	45S5	58S
Bulk composition (mol%)		
SiO_2	46.1	60
CaO	26.1	36
P_2O_5	2.6	4
Na_2O	24.4	–
Powders		
Surface area (m^2g 1)	0.3–2.7	126.5–164.7
Pore volume (cm^3/g)	0.001–0.035	0.213–0.447
Pore diameters (nm)	–	2–5

Morphological (e.g., powder size) and textural characteristics (e.g., porosity) impact on Si degradation rates and eventual bioactivity. For 58S, there is a direct increase in dissolution rate with increasing porosity and pore volume (Table 9.5). Rate constants (*k*) can be significantly increased when pore sizes are greater than 2 nm. Precipitation of HA is likely to occur first within the pores due to the following:

1. Increase in surface area/volume ratio increases the surface area exposed to media thus enhancing degree of ion exchange
2. Greater release of soluble silica and rapid formation of silica-rich layer
3. Increased ionic concentration (Ca^{2+}, HPO^{4-}) in pores until supersaturation
4. Precipitation of HCA in pores where rate is controlled by diffusion of ions into the pores

Ca^{2+} and HPO^{4-} concentration in the pores increases due to increasing pore size (due to glass network degradation), which results in rapid formation of the silica–gel layer on the surface and precipitation of HCA on the gel-layer surface.

For gel glasses, particle sizes can be used as an efficient way to control ionic dissolution rates and hence bioactivity.

The introduction of pores and precise control of materials composition to tailor both bioactive and resorbability offers new applications for regenerative medicine. Tailoring bioactive and resorbability with tissue type and tissue growth rates is an ideal scenario/design requirement for bone tissue regenerative materials. Sol–gel bioactive glasses, in-part, fulfill these requirements but more is being done to improve resorption rates, bioactivity, and even combining with other entities (e.g., macromolecules) to create new novel composite materials that address issues in regenerative medicine and drug delivery.

Development and Selection of Bioactive Glasses (In Vivo and In Vitro Testing)

The human body is a complex biological, chemical, and mechanical system. Bioactivity of a biomaterial is defined as the interaction between the materials and their operational, biological, and cellular microenvironment.

The aim of testing is to identify and minimize the risk of failure in clinical application. Strategies for determining the mechanical, surface chemistry properties (traditional bioactivity testing), and cellular bioactivity of bioactive glasses to assess the suitability of candidate biomaterials for osteogenic tissue regeneration can be tested using the following methods:

1. *Mechanical performance test methods* are screening methods where a detailed database of knowledge of bulk material properties, phase, state, and structure, micro- and nanostructure, surface topology, and coating surface attachment is created [14].
2. *In vitro test methods* are screening methods where the bioactive surface is exposed to (a) cell, tissue, or organ culture to assess the maintenance viable cellular function

on biomaterials surfaces. These tests are used to develop a detailed database of knowledge about cell/biomaterials microenvironment enabling biomaterials surfaces to be screened, characterized, reconstructed, and modified until suitable for in vivo trials, and (b) contact with simulated blood test solutions (e.g., SBF) to quickly assess the rate of bonelike apatite formation (traditionally known as bioactivity testing) on a candidate material surface.

3. *In vivo test methods*, where fully characterized biomaterials are implanted in whole-animal models to initially assess cytotoxicity (site is chosen for nonfunctionality soft-tissue sites such as the peritoneal cavity and subcutaneous "air-pouch" for screening tests, and cortical and corticocancellous bone (e.g., transcortical-femur, tibia, and cranium and intramedullary-femur and tibia) for joint replacement or fracture fixation testing), followed by functional testing in target species/animal models (e.g., load-bearing sites) [1].

Mechanical Performance

For selecting bioactive glasses for load bearing applications, the following specific materials properties are important: bioactivity, tensile strength, fracture toughness, and elastic modulus. These variables can be combined to produce a qualitative performance ratio called the quality index (I_q) (Table 9.6). I_q is described by the following equation:

$$I_q = (k_{IC} I_b \mathrm{UTS})/E \tag{9.4}$$

where k_{IC} is the fracture toughness, I_b is the index of bioactivity, UTS is the ultimate tensile strength, and E is Young's modulus.

The rate of bonding can be used to rank different bioactive compositions according to their index of bioactivity (I_b). I_b is the inverse of the time required for more than 50% ($t_{0.5bb}$) of the materials' interface to be bonded as described by Equation 9.5:

$$I_b = 100/t_{0.5bb} \tag{9.5}$$

TABLE 9.6

Estimated Quality Index (I_q) for Selected Second-Generation Bioactive Glasses [9]

Material	I_q	I_b
Cortical bone	500	13
Cancellous bone	8	13
HA (hydroxyapatite)	3	13
A/W glass ceramic	20	3
Bioglass (45S5)	9	13
HEPAX (45% vol. fraction HA, 55% vol. fraction polyethylene)	42	3
Bioglass 0.4% volume fraction/polysulfone composite	103	13

TABLE 9.7
Five-feature Characterization Approach as Proposed by Hench

Feature	Characterization of Interest	Method of Characterization Technique
1	Chemical composition	SEM-x-ray photoelectron spectroscopy (XPS), Auger electron spectroscopy (AES), Fourier transform spectroscopy (FT-IR), x-ray diffraction (XRD), SIMS.
2	Size, shape, and morphological features of particulate solids and monoliths	Scanning electron microscopy (SEM), wettability, atomic force microscopy (AFM) (incl. Maple technique).
3	Phase state and structure	Thin-film XRD and FT-IR reflection spectra are usually obtained after soaking in SBF solutions.
4	Microstructure	Usually used to determine quality control and assurance. Quantitative microscopy, using either optical or scanning electron microscopy (SEM).
5	Surface behavior (bioactivity testing)	The candidate material is soaked in simulated body fluid (SBF) solutions and degree of apatite formation is investigated.

I_q can be used to select appropriate biomaterials for load-bearing applications that avoid, as much as possible, stress-shielding* of bone.

Standards for Biocompatibility Testing

Biocompatibility is defined as the ability of a material to perform an appropriate host response for a specific application [15]. Biocompatibility testing of materials is based on their potential interactions with cells, muscles and ligaments, bones, fat, and/or organs. Where chemical, mechanical, pharmacological, and surface reaction layer responses are assessed to determine the local toxicity, surface degradation, and mechanical stability.

In the early 1990s, Hench et al. introduced a five-feature approach (see Table 9.7) for the characterization of bioactive glasses that has been widely accepted by the research community as the minimum common denomination for biomaterials characterization [16].

Since bioactive glass surface reaction layer formation is time-dependent, it is useful to use a range of characterization methods (mentioned in Table 9.9) to characterize reaction layer formation with time and depth (see Figure 9.6).

In addition to the above-mentioned methods, contact angle analysis can be performed to estimate surface energies. Sampling depth is very small at 0.3 to 2 nm.

SEM-x-ray photoelectron spectroscopy (SEM-XRD) has proved to be an invaluable tool in characterizing surface coatings. Although it is destructive, its sampling depth is deep enough (greater than 80 μm) to obtain chemical composition profiles spanning from the outer reaction layers through to the silica–gel layers and into the unreacted bulk material.

* Stress-shielding is the redistribution of load (and consequently stress on the bone) that occurs when the host bone tissue is replaced by a corresponding implant component (e.g., replacement of a femoral head by the femoral component of a total hip replacement).

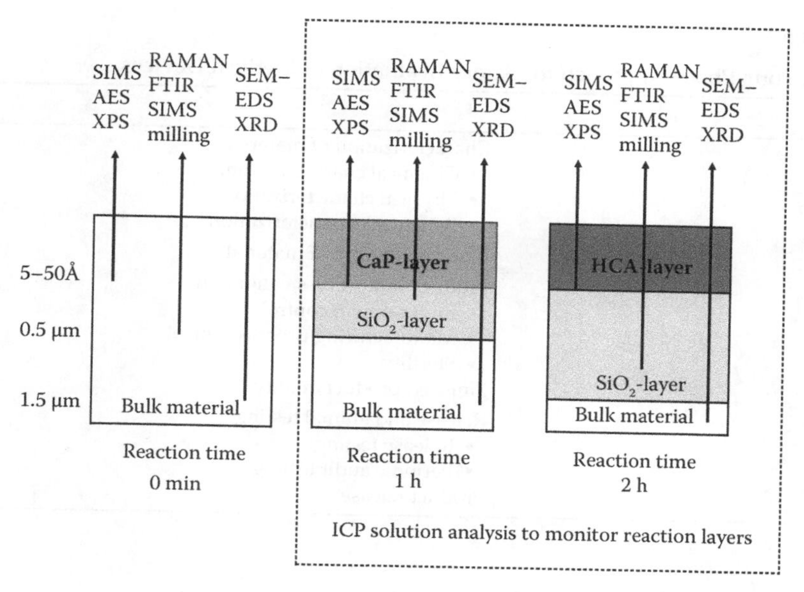

FIGURE 9.6
Methods for surface characterization (with an indication of instrument sampling depth) of bioactive glass surface reaction layers with time [9].

For second- and third-generation materials development, bioactivity was the most important surface response required for selection of candidate biomaterials to be tested in vivo. It was assumed that HA formation on the material's surface, as a result of candidate material immersion in SBS, was a good indicator of potential bone tissue ingrowth and attachment in vivo.

Since bioactive glasses are designed to elicit bone tissue ingrowth and regeneration, cellular-based test methods have been employed to explore these biological interactions. While mirroring the five-feature approach in its phase 1 step, national and international standards for testing regimes such as North American Science Associates (NAMSA) and the International Standardization Organization (ISO) reflect the need to reduce the number of animal experiments while assessing the candidate's potential cytotoxicity, capacity for mutagenesis and carcinogenesis, and its ability to perform with an appropriate host material, extraction conditions, choice of cell lines, and response in a specific application. As such, the NAMSA testing standards include biological characterization in their four-phase approach for safety evaluation of medical devices (see Table 9.8).

It should be noted that Phase 20—biocompatibility evaluation—is based on guidelines provided by ISO (ISO10993).

Bioactivity Testing

Exploration of the materials bioactivity (for bone applications, it is the ability to form an apatite layer) has become an intrinsic part of the biomaterials characterization process for suitability for osseous applications. Kokubo and Takadama give a good reason for this. They state that that the essential requirement for a material to bond to living bone is the

TABLE 9.8

NAMSA Four-Phase Approach for Safety Evaluation of Medical Devices

Phase	
1	Characterization of material • Chemical characterization • Physical characterization • Biological characterization
2	Biocompatibility of material
3	Product and process validation • Environment control • Manufacturing process control • Sterility Finished product quality
4	Release and animal testing • Release testing • Periodic audit testing Product release

formation of bonelike apatite on its surface when implanted in the living body. This in vivo apatite formation can be reproduced in an SBF with ion concentrations nearly equal to those of human blood plasma [17].

A bioactive material is a material on which bonelike hydroxyapatite (apatite) will form selectively after its immersion in a body fluid–like solution, where the rate of bioactivity (I_b) infers the candidates suitability for clinical application.

Typical testing procedures include the following steps:

1. Immersion of candidate material(s) using a defined surface area to volume ratio in an SBF.
2. Soaking is performed at 37°C for 24 h to 4 weeks under either static (no agitation of the SBF solution) conditions or dynamic conditions (agitation of the SBF solution via an orbital shaker).
3. The glass surface after being soaked in the SBF is studied by FT-IR (see Figure 9.8 for an example of a typical profile), thin film x-ray diffraction spectrometry (TF-XRD) and SEM-XPS to assess apatite formation.

Studies by Vallet-Regi and coworkers showed that dynamic conditions can postpone apatite formation [18]. In addition, immersion of smaller particles leads to increase surface area to volume ratios facilitating faster changes in SBF local solution chemistry, resulting in faster apatite formation [21].

FT-IR is the most commonly used tool to assess surface chemistries and has been extensively used to characterize surface reaction kinetics (Figure 9.7). For a detailed review of FT-IR technique, the reader should refer to Hench and Wilson [9].

Soaking times to identify hydroxyapatite precipitation on the surface of the bioactive glasses in SBF solutions is often measured by TF-XRD. Based on the analysis of bioactivity of the glass and the soaking time, a new index to evaluate the bioactivity of materials can be proposed.

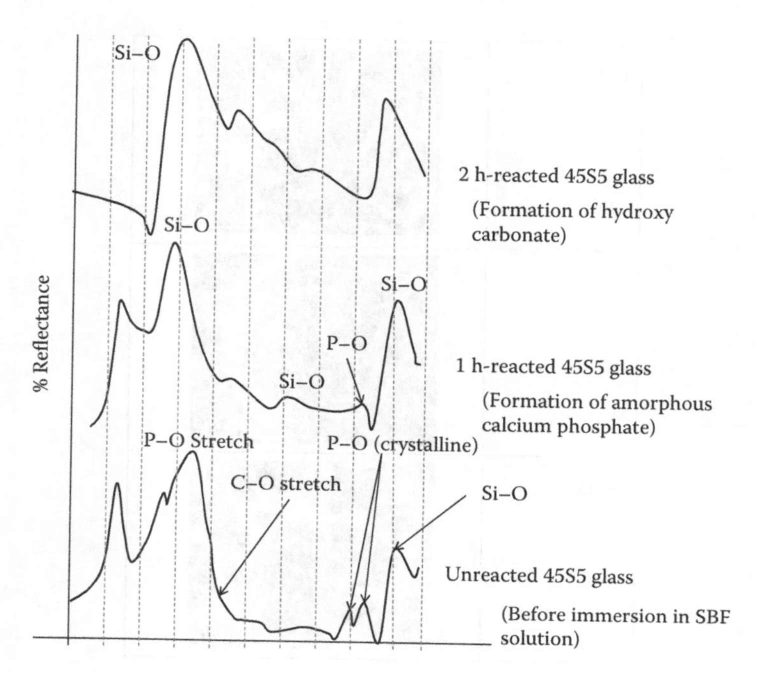

FIGURE 9.7
Typical FT-IR spectra of 45S5 composition glass before and after 1 and 2 h of soaking in SBF [9].

A proposed mechanism for apatite formation on a glass surface that has been immersed in SBF is that the formation of calcium phosphate is preceded by the formation of a hydrated silica layer (Si–O groups) [19]. The hydrated silica layer if formed via ion exchange of Na^+, K^+, and Ca^{2+} with H_3O^+ ions. This results in the formation of specific functional groups leading to nucleation and growth of calcium phosphate.

The use of soaking candidate materials in SBF to induce precipitation of bonelike apatite on bioceramic surfaces (Figure 9.8) has received considerable research interest since its first use by Kokubo and Takadama [17]. Although SBF* was designed to mimic human blood plasma, the following differences with human blood plasma have raised issues regarding its suitability as a test solution:

1. SBF solution has no protein content. It is known that proteins play an essential role in controlling apatite nucleation. In fact, protein absorption into surface reaction layers has been shown to retard the rate of nucleation of apatite [20].
2. TRIS (tris(hydroxymethyl)aminomethane) buffer solution is often added to SBF solutions.
3. Absence of control of carbonate content in SBF solutions even though carbonates act as a pH buffer in human blood serum.

* Kokubo developed simulated body fluid compositions C–SBF2 and C–SBF3. See Table 9.10 for a detailed description of each composition.

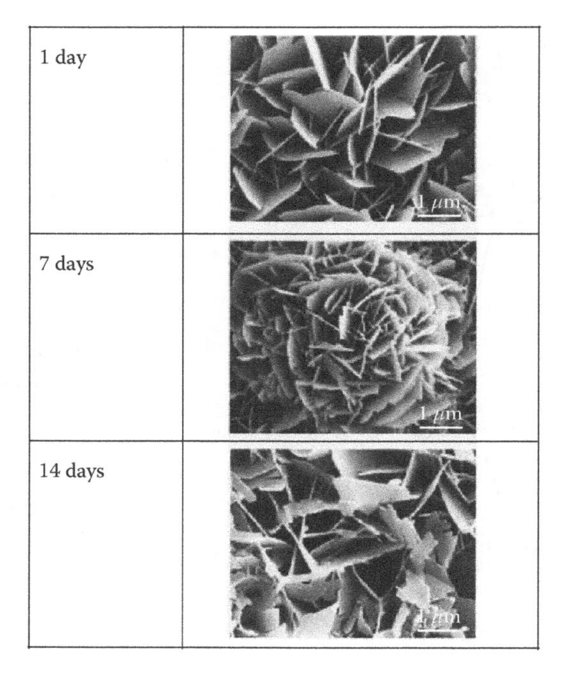

FIGURE 9.8
SEM images typical apatite formation, with time, on bioceramic surfaces during immersion in either SBF.

Research has focused on developing formulations with carbonate contents that are similar to plasma (e.g., R-SBF, I-SBF; see Table 9.9). Oyane and coworkers developed I-SBF that simulated the influence of protein adsorption by including the free ions that were not bound to proteins.

It should be noted that apatite formation on bioceramics/biomaterials surfaces is not an absolute indicator of bone tissue attachment in vivo. For example, immersion of β-TCP

TABLE 9.9
Compositions of Selected Simulated Body Fluids

	Ionic Concentration (mM)						
Ion	Human Blood Plasma [23]	C-SBF2 [21]	C-SBF3 [21]	R-SBF1 [21]	I-SBF5 [21]	SBF-JL1 [21]	SBF-JL2 [23]
Na^+	142.00	142.00	142.00	142.00	142.00	142.00	142.00
K^+	5.00	5.00	5.00	5.00	5.00	–	–
Mg^{2+}	1.50	1.50	1.50	1.00	1.50	–	–
Ca^{2+}	2.50	2.50	2.50	2.50	1.6	2.50	2.31
HCO^{3-}	27.00	4.20	35.23	27.00	27.00	34.90	34.88
HPO_2^{4-}	1.00	1.00	1.00	1.00	1.00	1.00	1.39
SO_2^{4-}	0.50	0.50	0.50	0.50	0.50	–	–
Cl^-	103.00	147.96	117.62	103.00	103.00	111.00	109.90

Note: In addition, solution contains buffer of 11.93 g/L HEPES 2-(4-hydroxyethy1)-1-piperazinyl)ethane surfonic acid.

does not always lead to the formation of apatite in SBF even though it bonds extensively to bone in vivo [18].

Morphological Testing

Scanning electron microscopy (SEM) has been used extensively to give high-resolution surface images of biomaterials [21]. Figure 9.10 shows typical apatite morphologies with increased immersion in SBF solution and human blood serum solution. Even higher-resolution techniques are being employed to image submicron surface features that are being engineered onto the bioactive glass surface reaction layers. Atomic force microscopy (AFM) is the most common technique used.

Atomic Force Microscopy

Invented in 1985 by Gerd Binnig and Christoph Gerber, AFM has become widely used to generate high-resolution* images of surfaces at the nanoscale [22]. One of the advantages of AFM is that it can image the nonconducting surfaces.

In addition to surface roughness characterization, it has been widely adopted as a morphological characterization tool to image microscopic and nanoscopic surface features. AFM has been used to image apatite formation on metallic substrates and even surface peptide adsorption on polymeric substrates. Little sample preparation is required for imaging with the AFM. In most cases it is as simple as drying the sample. In some instances spotting a few microliters of solution on the coating to be tested has been used.

For a detailed explanation of the AFM technique, the reader should refer to the excellent review by Mayer [22].

In Vitro Cellular Testing

Included in the first phase of the NAMSA characterization approach, cell culture allows detailed investigation of early, acute cellular responses at the bioactive glasses interface. Cellular responses under characterization on candidate material surfaces of interest include:

- Degree of surface adhesion and proliferation
- Rate and quality of extracellular matrix produced from test cells
- Enabling the complexity of in vivo interactions to be broken down and investigated as a study of responses to isolated, specific test cell lines

Since bioactive glass surfaces provide a substrate (surface roughness, porosity, etc.) coupled with surface reaction layer chemistries (e.g., controlled release of ionic dissolution products and doped growth factors, adsorption of growth factors added to culture medium) to control cell growth and differentiation, bioactive surfaces, and their dissolution products are tested using either qualitative or quantitative approaches listed in Table 9.10.

* The width of a DNA molecule is loosely used as a measure of resolution, because it has a known diameter of 2.0 nm.

TABLE 9.10

Qualitative or Quantitative Approaches of Cellular Testing

Approach	Test Aim	Test Objectives
Qualitative	To evaluate the possible performance of the test material at a simulated bony site	To assess the: • Morphology and attachments of cells on the surface • Production and subsequent calcification of extracellular matrix
Quantitative	To quantitatively assess cellular physiology/function	To measure: • Cellular viability • Cellular proliferation • Expression of osteoblastic phenotype • Production and subsequent calcification of extracellular matrix • Production of bone specific proteins (e.g., osteoclacin, osteonectin) • Alkaline phosphatase activity • Nucleic activity

Mature, differentiated cells (e.g., fibroblasts, chondrocytes, osteoblasts, and osteoclasts) isolated from connective tissues are usually employed and cultured on bioactive glass surfaces. Cells capable of redifferentiation (e.g., stem cells and marrow stromal cells) have also been cultured either on bioactive surfaces or exposed to their ionic dissolution products to assess their ability to control stem cell growth and differentiation. For specific examples of cellular interactions with bioactive surfaces (bulk, particles, extracts, and composite), see Tables 9.11 to 9.14.

Cell cultures remain simplistic tests in that they do not include the fluid circulation or interactions with multiple cell types and/or proteins. In addition, mechanical loading factors are not taken into account. However, these shortcomings are masked by the significant amount of biological data obtained from traditional qualitative and quantitative testing strategies.

In Vivo Testing

The goal of in vivo testing of a medical device is to determine the safety or biocompatibility of the device in a biological environment. In vivo testing is the final phase in the NAMSA safety evaluation of the medical devices process (see Table 9.8).

As mentioned previously, bioactivity testing via immersion in SBF cannot be taken as a direct indicator that a candidate material with elicit bioactivity in vivo. In addition, bioactivity testing and cellular testing both cannot determine the rate of complex tissue attachment and also the quality/strength of attachment (as indicated by mechanical pull-out tests). Figure 9.9 shows typical in vivo interfacial adherence of Bioglass® composition (BGC) and A/W glass–ceramic (A/W) with bone (B). Due to their compositional related bioactivities, the interfacial strength was shown to be higher than the material strength, resulting in bulk material fracture failure at the implant/tissue interface [24].

Testing protocols designed for in vivo characterization of bioceramics are too numerous to be included in this chapter but in Tables 9.15 and 9.16, I have presented some specific examples. The reader should refer to the excellent review by Hollinger and Citron to find out more about in vivo testing protocols [23].

TABLE 9.11

Cellular Evaluation of Bioactive Glasses

Material	Cell type	Outcome					Remarks	Reference
		Viability/ Adhesion	Growth	Differentiation/ Kept Phenotype	Matrix Synthesis	Mineralization		
BG disks	Chondrocytes	+	+		+	+	Collagen fibril in-growth into surface reaction layers; HA formation on surface	[3]
BG disks	Osteoblasts		+	+	+	+		[4, 5]
BG disks	Osteoblasts	+	+	+	+	+		[29]
BG-P	Osteoblasts	+	+	+	+	+		[29]
BG-E	Osteoblasts	+	+	+	+	+	First indication of genetic influence of BG on cell cycle; critical concentration of ionic products needed for osteostimuation	[6, 29]
BG-E	mFLBs		+			+	Critical concentration of ionic products needed for calcification	[7]
BG powders	Osteoblasts	+	+		+	+		[8]

Note: BG, bioactive glass; BG-E, bioactive glass extract (ionic product solution); BG-P, bioglass particles (90–710 μm); HA, hydroxyapatite.

TABLE 9.12

Cellular Evaluation of Bioactive Glasses

		Outcome						
Material	**Cell Type**	**Viability/ Adhesion**	**Growth**	**Differentiation/ Kept Phenotype**	**Matrix Synthesis**	**Mineralization**	**Remarks**	**References**
BG disks	mFLBs		+			+	BG dissolution products responsible for enhanced mineralization	[31]
BG-E	HMVEC	+	+	+	+	–	↑ VEGF; promoting angiogenesis; ionic concentration critical	[9]

Note: BG, bioactive glass; BG-E, bioactive glass extract (ionic product solution); VEGF, vascular endothelial growth factor; mFLBs, murine fetal long bones; HMVEC, human micro-vascular endothelial cells.

TABLE 9.13

Cellular Evaluation of Bioactive Glasses

		Outcome						
Porous Material	**Cell Type**	**Viability/ Adhesion**	**Growth**	**Differentiation/ Kept Phenotype**	**Matrix Synthesis**	**Mineralization**	**Remarks**	**References**
DAB	BMSC	+	+			+		[10]
BG	Primary OB, human		+		+	+	Mineralization without the addition of growth factors	[11]
58S	Osteoblasts	+	+	+	+	+		[12]
70/30	Osteoblasts	+	+	+	+	+		[36]
58S-E	fHOBs, hES	+	+	+	+	+		[36]
70/30-E	fHOBs, hES	+	+	+	+	+		[36]

Note: BG, bioactive glass; 58S, 58% SiO_2–36%CaO–6%P_2O_5 glass composition; 58S-E, ionic dissolution products extract solution; 70/30, 70% SiO_2–30%CaO glass composition; 70/30-E, ionic dissolution products extract solution; BMSC, bone marrow stromal cells; OB, osteblast; DAB, D-Alk-B (borosilicate glass) glass-based scaffolds; fHOB, fetal human osteoblasts; hES, human embryonic stem cells.

TABLE 9.14
Cellular Evaluation of Bioactive Glasses

Composite Material	Cell Type	Outcome						
		Viability/ Adhesion	Growth	Differentiation/ Kept Phenotype	Matrix Synthesis	Mineralization	Remarks	References
BG + PDLLA	Human osteosarcoma	+	+				Colonization, effect of BG contents	
	Human fetal OB			+	+	+		
	Human primary OB	+	+	+			Effect of BG contents	
BG + PLLA	Human osteosarcoma		+	+			Effect of BG contents	
BG + PLA	Mouse pre-OB cell line	+	+/–	–			P glass —PLA based	

Note: BG, bioactive glass; PLA, polyactic acid; PLLA, poly-(L-lactic) acid; PDLLA, poly-(D/L-lactic) acid; OB, osteoblast.

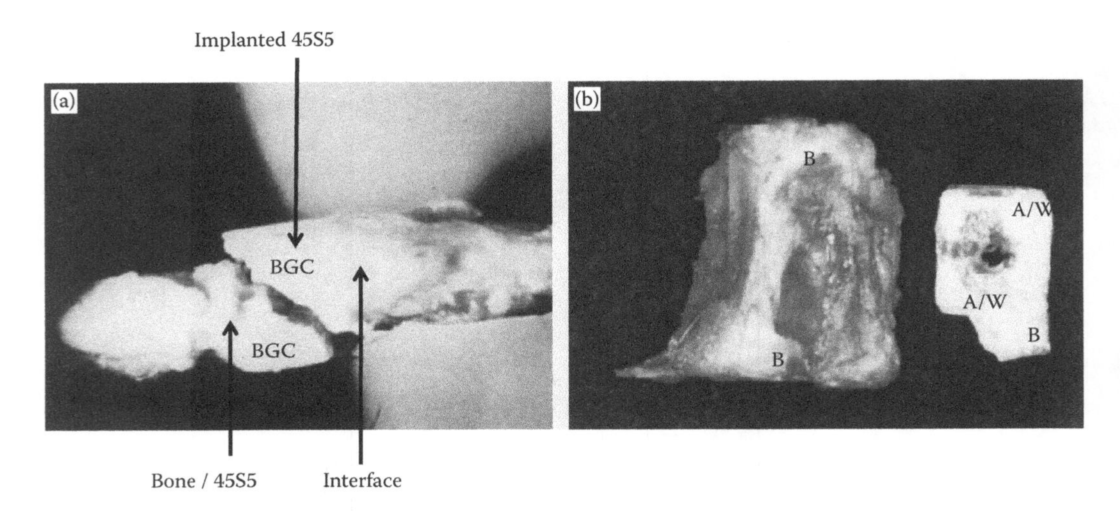

FIGURE 9.9
Example of in vivo interfacial adherence of host bone with (a) 45S5 composition implant and (b) A/W glass–ceramic implant. (From Hench, L.L., *J. Am. Ceramic. Soc.*, 74(7), 1487–1510, 1991. With permission [24].)

Bioactive Glass Coatings on Load-Bearing Implants

Load-bearing metallic prosthesis (e.g., total joint replacement devices) fail due to the reasons stated in Table 9.17.

Strategies for Improved Tissue Attachment

The most common load-bearing implants are total joint replacements of the knee and hip. Composed of either a stainless-steel or titanium alloy femoral stem with a separate articulating surface, these joints need to be mechanically anchored to the host tissue site. After 25 years postimplantation, 24% of cases require secondary surgery due to causes stated in Table 9.17. Biological reactions at the implant/host tissue interface can result in implant encapsulation by fibrous tissue resulting in no direct bonding with host bone tissue. Surgical techniques to fixate implants such as cementation can be sources of wear debris triggering local inflammatory responses reducing implant lifetime. Strategies to encourage direct bone ingrowth in the implant surface have been explored where the bioactivity of metallic surfaces is improved with the aim of minimizing the creation of wear debris and eliminating interfacial micromotion between the implant and host tissue site.

Research has focused on improving implant lifetimes via promoting faster and prolonged tissue growth into the implants surface, resulting in direct mechanical interlocking of the implant with host tissues. Where there is direct apposition of bone on the implant surface without intervening collagen membrane formation, osteointegration is described to have occurred (i.e., new bone has ingrown and formed within/into microscopic surface features on the implant's surface—e.g., pores and groves). Stability of the newly ingrown bone tissue is an issue because after the initial healing phase, a border zone is usually created in response to the implant's functional loading. During implant failure,

TABLE 9.15
Examples of In Vivo Evaluation of Bioactive Glasses and Glass–Ceramics

Material	Animal Model	Outcome: Inflammation/ Encapsulation	Bone Formation	Bone Bridging	Vascularization	Implant Resorption	Remarks	References
BG-P	Monkey jaw		+	+	+		First observation of osteoproduction	[36]
BG-P	Rabbit femoral condyl	+	+	+		+	Enhanced bone formation and mineralization due to BG	[13]

Note: BG, bioactive glass, bioglass particles (90–710 μm); P, phosphate.

TABLE 9.16
Examples of In Vivo Evaluation of Bioactive Glasses and Glass–Ceramics

Composite Material	Animal Model	Outcome: Inflammation/ Encapsulation	Bone Formation	Bone Bridging	Vascularization	Implant Resorption	Remarks	References
BG + PLGA	Mouse—subcutaneous	+			+		Peripheral granulation tissue	[14]
BG + PGA	Rat—subcutaneous				+			
BG + PDLLA	Rabbit—subcutaneous, femur	–	+			+	Rods implanted	
	Nude mice—subcutaneous + BMSC	+	+				Collagen I synthesis	
BG + PDLLA	Sheep—tibia	+/– → +	++			+	Bone inside pores—osteolysis	

Note: BG, bioactive glass; P, phosphate; PLGA, poly-(D/L-lactic-co-glycolic) acid, PGA, polyglycolic acid; PDLLA, poly-(D/L-lactic) acid; BMSC, bone marrow stromal cells.

TABLE 9.17

Major Causes of Failure of Total Joint Replacement Devices

Causes of failure for total joint replacement devices
Biological reaction at implant/tissue interface
Properties of the implant surface
Infection
Surgical technique employed
Dislocation and implant fracture
Host tissue fracture

nonmineralized connective tissue forms in the border zone in contact with the implant, resulting in micromotion at the implant/tissue site and eventual implant failure.

The brittleness of bioactive glasses and glass–ceramics coupled with their limited compositional ranges for bioactivity have limited their possible improvement in mechanical properties. However, there continues to be interest in their development and application as coatings on load-bearing metallic implant surfaces due to their inherent bioactivity and surface reaction layers, which have the potential to significantly retard the rate at which the border zone is converted into nonmineralized connective tissue.

Bioactive glass or glass–ceramic coatings on metallic substrates offer significant improvements in bioactivity but have been difficult to develop due to thermal expansion coefficient (TEC) mismatch, limited coating adhesion, and difficulty in precisely controlling the coating structure (heterogeneous coatings) [25].

Topological Modifications (Surface Roughness)

The development of dental implants from machine-smoothed parts into parts with precisely defined surface roughness provides an indication to possible benefits of topological modifications.

Surface roughness has been attributed to providing better mechanical stability due to higher interfacial surface contact for protein absorption, resulting in enhanced stimulation of bone during the healing process. Surface roughness has also been shown to directly regulate cell–material interactions by effecting cell shape, cellular attachment and resulting proliferation, and ECM production.

Engineered topological (surface roughness) features can be divided into two features of scale:

1. Micron to submicron features (1- to 10-μm-sized grooves, microthreaded designs, and macroporosity; 0.1- to 1.0-μm-sized etched features)
2. Nanofeatures

Nanofeatures have been shown to directly affect adsorption of proteins and will be discussed in Section 9.7.

Bioactive Glass Coatings on Metallic Implants

An approach to introduce surface bioactivity on load-bearing surface of metallic implants (e.g., dental and total joints) has been to apply thick (>100 μm) bioactive glasses as coatings on metallic implant surfaces. These coating can be useful for a number of reasons:

1. They can serve as a protective coating/barrier for corrosion and surface degradation
2. They can protect host tissues from implant corrosion products
3. Bioactive glasses can significantly improve surface bioactivity, resulting in improved tissue in-growth and attachment

Hydroxyapatite is the prevailing bioceramic coating material on metallic substrates. There is an extensive literature database describing the development of hydroxyapatite coatings on titanium implants to improve in vivo implant fixation of artificial teeth and total hip joint prosthesis. There are some reports of CP (β-TCP, $CaHPO_4$) coatings, Y-TZP, and TiO_2 coatings on metallic substrates. In this chapter, I will only describe the application of bioactive glasses as coatings on various substrates.

Regardless of coating material, the literature describes the following shortcomings associated with coatings on metallic implants:

1. Limited adhesion strength of coatings with titanium substrates because of long-term use in the body.
2. Composition of coated layers needs to be adjusted during the application process. As a result, applied coating compositions often deviate from their desired properties.
3. Limited selection of bioactivity of glass coatings due to compositional limitations of the types of glasses that can be coated into metallic substrates while trying to minimize TEC mismatch.

In order to improve the adherence of coatings on metallic substrates, various coating deposition approaches have been explored (Figure 9.10). Starting with bioactive glasses in either gas, solid, or liquid forms, bioactive glass coatings can be applied directly from the gas or liquid state or be further transformed into either liquid (melt or slurry) forms before deposition onto a metallic substrate. Coating methods include: chemical vapor deposition (CVD), physical vapor deposition (PVD), plasma spraying, electrophoretic deposition

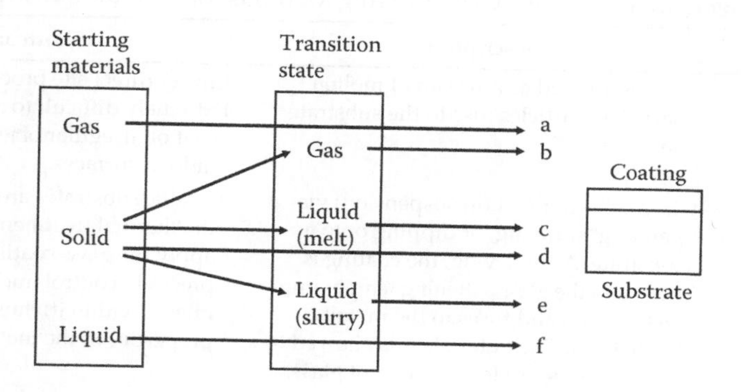

FIGURE 9.10
Various routes (a to f) of coating formation on metallic substrates [26]. Routes: (a) CVD method, (b) PVD method, (c) plasma-spraying method, glazing, and raid immersion, (d) EPD method, (e) sheet formation method and slurry dipping method, and (f) electrodeposition method and sol–gel dipping method.

(EPD), and dipping methods resulting in the production of either thin (<100 μm) or thick (>100 μm) coatings (see Figure 9.10).

Thick Coatings (>100 μm)

Metallic prosthetics (e.g., titanium, Ti_6A1_4V, and chrome cobalt alloys) are widely used as materials for dental and orthopedic implants because of their mechanical properties and nontoxic behavior, but unfortunately, they are bioinert. Much research has been focused on applying bioactive glass and bioceramic coating on metallic substrates in order to introduce surface bioactivity.

Implant failure usually results from the formation of dense fibrous tissue around the site of implantation. Prostheses used in hip and knee replacement surgery often uses cement fixation with acrylic bone cement. However, the use of cements can lead to deterioration of adjacent host tissues. The most common cementless fixation procedure is to use a plasma-sprayed hydroxyapatite coating on the prosthesis. Although bioactivity is potentially improved, the time required for bone ingrowth onto the hydroxyapatite coating remains an issue, resulting in micromotion and reduction in implant lifetime. Bioactive glass coatings have the potential to address this issue due to their high levels of bioactivity, resulting in faster tissue ingrowth and attachment at the host tissue site.

Processes such as thermal spraying (plasma spraying), glazing (enameling) methods, raid immersion, pulsed laser deposition, and electropheric deposition have been used to coat these substrates with second-generation bioactive glasses (see Table 9.18). However, bioactive glass-based coating technologies have been difficult to develop due to:

1. TEC mismatch
2. Minimal chemical bonding, and difficulty in precisely controlling the coating structure (heterogeneous coatings) [24]
3. Negative effect (e.g., loss) on surface reactivity of bioactive glasses due to changes in glass composition during the coating process [27]

TABLE 9.18

Common Second-Generation Bioactive Glass Coating Methods for Metallic Substrates

Method	Description	Shortcoming
Thermal spraying (plasma spraying)	Glass is applied as a stream of molten particles. Particles fuse to the substrate on impact.	Line of direct site process. Extremely difficult to apply a uniform coat on irregular objects; cannot coat hidden surfaces.
Glazing (enameling) methods	Glass frit is applied (in suspension) via painting, spraying, or dipping onto a substrate. After drying, the coating is heated to the glass softening temperature (400–600°C) and fuses to the metallic oxide layer. The outer glass is allowed to sinter together to form a layer of glass.	Metallic substrates are also exposed to the thermal treatments required to apply the glass coating, anneal, and precisely control nucleation of required phases within it, thus affecting physics properties of the metallic substrate.
Rapid immersion	A metallic surface is heated to form an oxide layer of critical thickness and then immersed in molten glass. This results in the oxide layer dissolving in the glass.	This procedure neglects the importance of matching the thermal expansion coefficient of the glass to the metal substrate.

Glass surface reactivity is the biggest problem. Bioactive glasses (less than 60 mol% SiO_2) have a random, sheetlike network that is open for ion transport, resulting in the formation of CaP and HA reaction layers (see Table 9.3). In addition, this open network allows other cations (e.g., Fe, Cr, Ni, Ti, Mo, and Ta) to pass though the glass, thus altering the glasses ability to form either or both the CaP and HA reaction layers. Surface bioactivity is altered and in some cases lost. Only a few percent of migrated cations are needed to make the glass nonbioactive.

Glazing (Enameling)

Early attempts by Hench to directly glaze (see Table 9.18) stainless-steel substrates with bioactive glasses were not successful due to:

1. Rapid diffusion of multications into the glass, resulting in a loss of bioactivity [27]
2. Extensive crystallization in the glass layer, resulting in lack of surface adhesion [28]

Dual layering technique of glass coatings is one strategy that has been investigated to address this problem (see Figure 9.11). Dual glass layers have been applied by either:

1. Creating a preoxidized (TiO_2 layer) first layer on a titanium substrate where the second layer is formed by directly enameling it with liquid glass
2. Directly enameling a metallic substrate with liquid glass with matching thermal expansion coefficients to create the first layer, followed by embedding either hydroxyapatite (HA) or bioglass (BG) particles onto TEC substrate-matching glass coatings [27, 29]

Dual-layer approaches address the limited adhesion strength of coatings with titanium substrates. For example, Hench and Wilson [9] demonstrated that when Co–Cr alloy substrates oxidation temperatures were raised from 350°C to 500°C, glass–metal interfacial

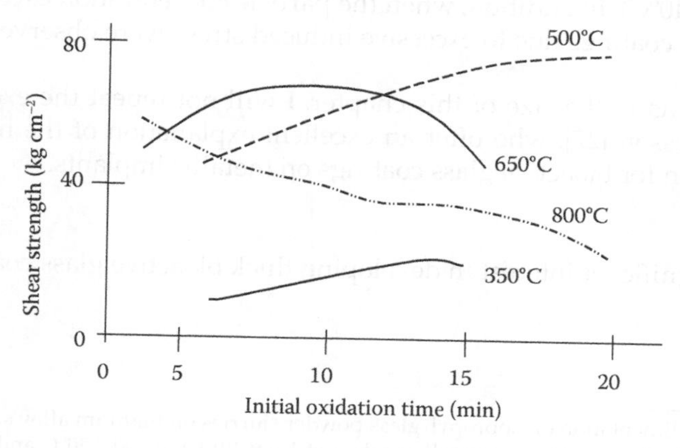

FIGURE 9.11
Glass–metal bond strength as a function of time and temperature of oxidation [9].

TABLE 9.19

Composition and Main Properties Used for Bioactive Particle Embedding Approach

Material	SiO_2 (wt.%)	Na_2O (wt.%)	K_2O (wt.%)	CaO (wt.%)	MgO (wt.%)	P_2O_5 (wt.%)	Thermal Expansion Coefficient (200–400°C)	Young's Modulus (GPa)
Bioglass (45S5)	45.0	24.5	0.0	24.5	0.0	6.0	15.1	70
6P57	56.5	11.0	3.0	15.0	8.5	6.0	10.8	80–90
6P68	67.7	8.3	2.2	10.1	5.7	6.0	8.8	80–90

strengths could be doubled (Figure 9.11). In addition, interfacial strengths could be increased with time of oxidation. However, they found that there was a critical oxidation temperature where higher than 650°C, glass layers were created with decreasing shear strength with increasing oxidation time.

Hench describes a two-layer glass coatings approach where the first glass layer provides a direct interfacial bond with the metallic substrate (the glass has substrate-matching thermal expansion coefficients coupled with a low T_g). The second glass layer is composed of a bioactive glass fused to the first layer (again with a matching thermal coefficients of expansion coupled with slightly lower T_g).

An alternative to making the second bioactive glass coating is the embedding approach developed by Gomez-Vega and coworkers [30] and is interesting because:

1. Substrates were first coated* with specially formulated glass compositions (6P57, 6P58; see Table 9.19) with thermal expansion coefficients matched to the titanium substrates.
2. Coating bioactivity was introduced via embedded HA or BG particles on the coating. They found that HA particles were immersed partially during heating and remained firmly embedded on the coating after cooling, whereas the BG particles softened and some infiltration into the glass coating took place during heat treatment (800–840°C). In addition, when the particle concentration exceeded 20% surface, cracked coatings due to excessive induced stress were observed.

Due to limitations in the size of this chapter, I will not repeat the excellent review by Hench and Andersson [27], who offer an excellent explanation of the need for compositional optimization for bioactive glass coatings on metallic implants.

Ideal Thick Coating

There remains significant interest in developing thick bioactive glass coatings on metallic implants.

* Coating was via sedimentation of isopropyl/glass powder slurries on titanium alloy substrates, followed by firing at 600°C. Coatings were then thermally soaked at 1.3×10^4 Pa at 700–820°C and then allowed to cool to room temperature [45]. Since Bloyer and coworkers classify this coating method as enameling, it has been included in this section.

Recently, Hill and coworkers stated the following material requirements for the ideal thick bioactive glass coating [31]:

1. Matching thermal expansion coefficient (TEC) between the bioactive glass and that of the alloy.
2. The coating can sinter at 750°C or lower (to prevent crystallization and inhibit oxidation of the alloy at the surface).
3. The glass composition has a network connectivity (NC) value close to 2.0, in order to maintain bioactivity, where NC is a measure of the average number of bridging bonds per network forming element in the glass structure. NC determines glass properties such as viscosity, crystallization rate, and degradability.

Thin Coatings (<100 μm)

Under fatigue tensile loading conditions, thick coatings fail due to delamination and fragmentation. Compared with thick coatings, thinner coatings (<100 μm) have been found to enhance interfacial stability and in some cases exhibit stronger biological fixation.

Pulsed Laser Deposition

Pulsed laser deposition (PLD) is a PVD method where a high-power pulsed laser is focused, inside a vacuum chamber, on a target of the material that is to be deposited [32]. Referring to Figure 9.12, a plasma plume, the vaporized material is deposited as a thin film on a substrate. PLD usually occurs in ultrahigh vacuum or in the presence of a background gas such as oxygen that is commonly used when depositing oxides to fully oxygenate the deposited films. The advantage of PLD method is that a thin coating can be precisely deposited at rates of 1 μm cm^{-2} s^{-1}. For further detail, the reader is referred to the text by Eason [33].

Figure 9.12 shows a bioactive glass (BG) thin film coating that has been deposited on titanium substrates using the PLD method [35]. A UV laser KrF (λ = 248 nm, τ = 25 ns) was used for the multipulse irradiation of the BG targets with 57 wt.% or 61 wt.% SiO_2 content (and Na_2O–K_2O–CaO–MgO–P_2O_5 oxides). The depositions were performed in oxygen atmosphere at 13 Pa and for substrates temperature of 400°C. The PLD films displayed typical BG of 2 to 5 μm particulates nucleated on the film surface or embedded in. The PLD films stoichiometry was found to be the same as the targets. After 3 to 7 days immersion in SBF, the Si content substantially decreases in the coatings and PO_4^{3-} maxima start to increase in FTIR spectra. After 14 to 21 days the XRD peaks show a crystallized fraction of the carbonated hydroxyapatite. The SEM micrographs show also significant changes in the films' surface morphology.

Laser Cladding

Laser cladding is a method of depositing material onto a substrate via powered injection where the material is melted and consolidated by use of a laser in order to coat a substrate (see Figure 9.13). The application of this technique to create bioactive coatings was first presented in the literature by Lusquiños and coworkers [36]. They used laser cladding to apply a CaP coating on a Ti alloy substrate.

Recently, Comesañaa and coworkers [37] used this method to clad bioactive glass onto titanium alloy (Ti_6Al_4V) substrates. A homogeneous deposition of the coating with limited Ti migration over the substrate was achieved using 45S5 composition glass. In addition,

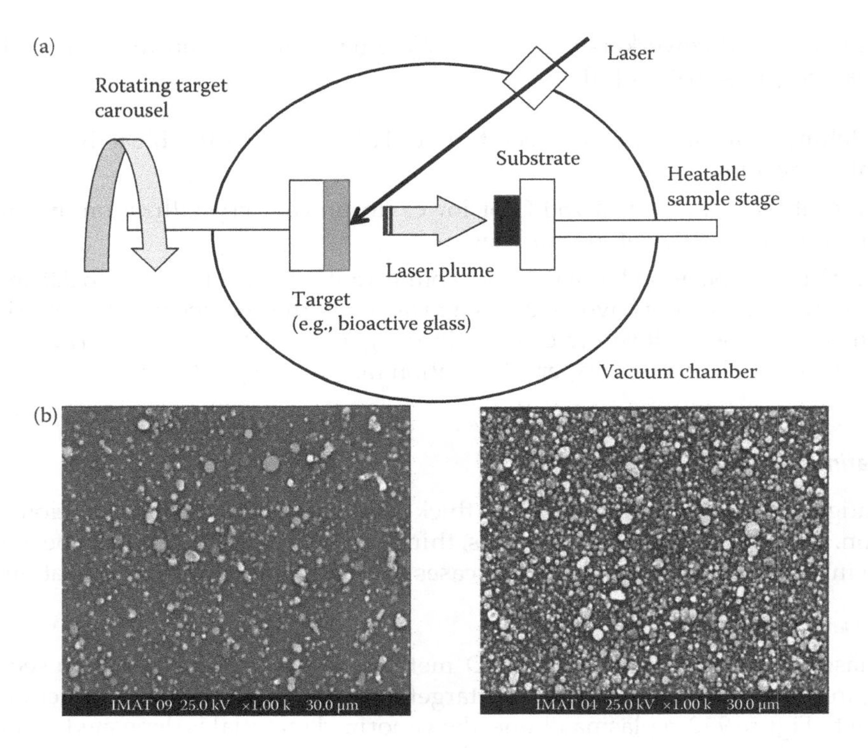

FIGURE 9.12
(a) Pulsed laser deposition (PLD) method. (b) Typical glass coating (31% SiO_2; 26.7% MgO; 31.7% CaO; 10.6% P_2O_5) morphologies on Ti substrates using a KrF laser. Left image shows coating produced at low pressure (10^{-7} bar); right image shows coating produced at high pressure (10^{-2} bar). (From Joanni et al., *Mater. Res.*, 7 (3), 2004. [34].)

bioactivity testing showed no loss in bioactivity as a result of the coating process (see Figure 9.13). Using the technique, they were also able to precisely control glass layer thickness by reraster scanning the substrates surface.

Sol–Gel Coating/Dipping

The use of sol–gel compositions offers the developer the ability to extend the compositional range of bioactive glass coatings beyond 60 mol% silica. In addition, sols have the ability to form films on substrates introduced onto them. Dip-coating technology has proved useful in creating sol–gel-derived bioactive coatings with good interface mechanical properties, precise control of microstructure, and composition. Precise control of extraction velocity of the metallic substrate coupled with sol viscosity is the most important parameter to manufacture good-quality coatings. Extraction velocities must be less than, or equal to, the gelling rate of the film to avoid flocculation processes and maximize adhesion to the substrate.

Gomez and coworkers were able to apply glass coatings with thermal expansion coefficients close to Ti_6Al_4V substrates using sol–gel dipping. Their glass compositions (see Table 9.19) exhibited limited capacity to induce apatite formation in SBF immersion (bioactivity testing). To improve bioactivity, they applied an additional thin (approximately 50 μm) film of mesoporous silica by spin-coating a sol–gel solution [30]. Improved bioactivity was observed via apatite formation after 7 days immersion in SBF. In addition,

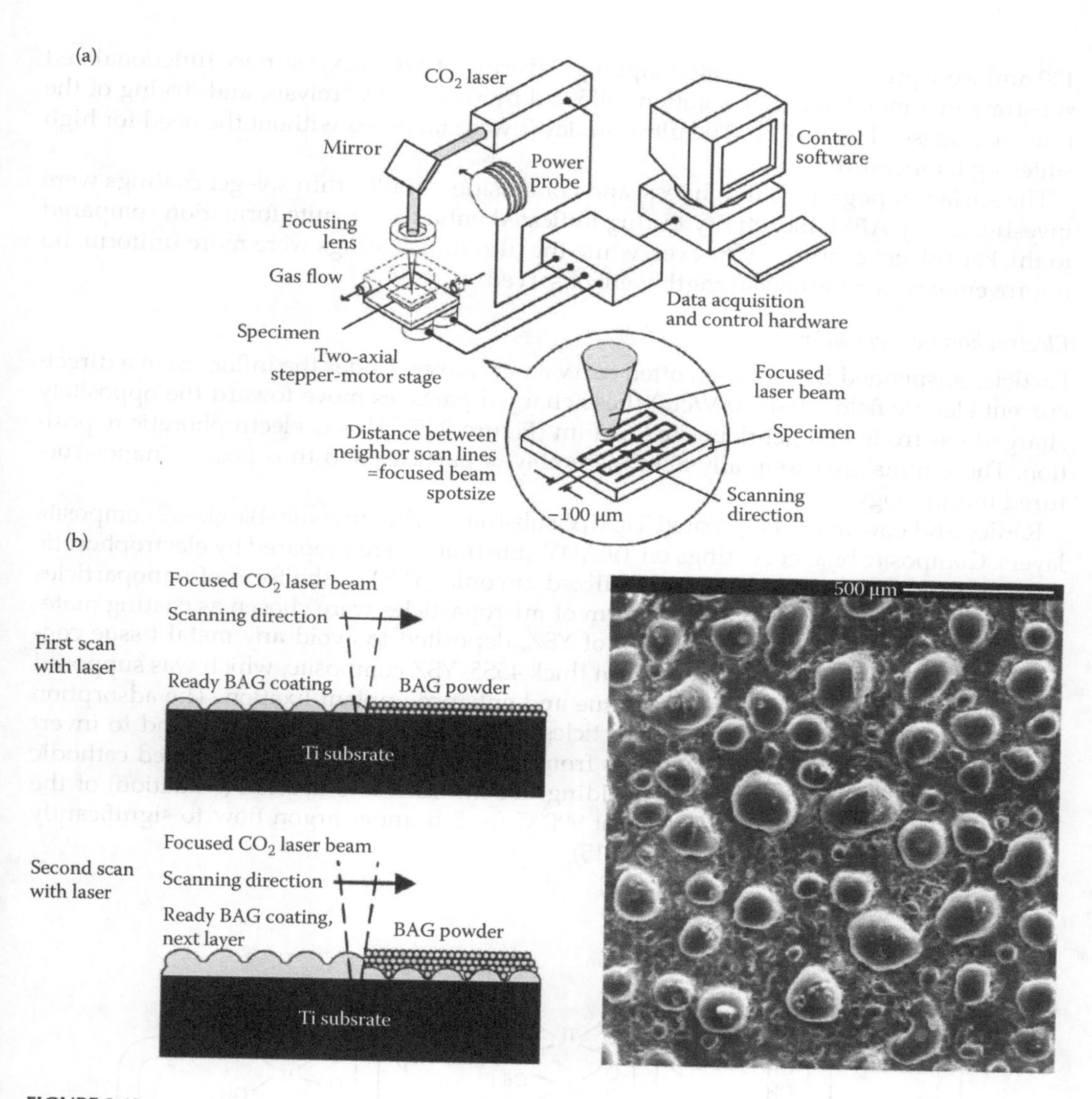

FIGURE 9.13
(a) Laser cladding process setup using power injection of the coating material where (b) a CO_2 laser sweeps across the bioactive glass (BAG) powders melting them and forming a coating either composited of amorphous glass, which is then built up by recoating the surface with powder followed by the BAG particles with the CO_2 laser. (b) Typical coating morphology. (From Moritz et al., *J. Mater Sci. Mater. Med.*, 15(7), 787–794, 2004. With permission [38].)

precise control of pore diameter was achieved via changing the size of the directing agent.

The advantage of this technique is that substrate dipping can be performed at low temperatures. However, the disadvantage is that the sintering temperatures required to stabilize the coating are high (400°C), which often results in poor coating adhesion and nonuniform coverage [39]. To address the issue of high sintering temperatures, Advincula and coworkers [39] developed a dual-layer approach. Ultrathin sol–gel films (approximately

100 nm) were produced by repeated dipping/layering of a hydroxyl surface functionalized substrate in a metal alkoxide solution followed by rinsing, hydrolysis, and drying of the film coating (see Figure 9.14). The ultrathin layer was stabilized without the need for high sintering temperatures.

The surface topography, roughness, and composition of ultrathin sol–gel coatings were investigated by AFM. Bioactivity testing indicated enhanced apatite formation compared to thicker sol–gel coatings. However, while the ultrathin coatings were more uniform, no improvements in adhesion strength were observed.

Electrophoretic Deposition

Particles suspended in a solution often carry a net charge. Under the influence of a direct-current electric field (20–1000 V/cm) these charged particles move toward the oppositely charged electrode and get deposited as film (Figure 9.15). This is electrophoretic deposition. These films are essentially a 3-D assembly of particles and thus possess nanostructured morphology.

Radice and coworkers [40] coated Ti_6Al_4V substrates with zirconia–Bioglass® composite layers. Composite bilayer coatings on Ti6Al4V substrates were prepared by electrophoretic deposition. Biocompatible yttrium-stabilized zirconia (YSZ) in the form of nanoparticles and bioactive Bioglass® (45S5) in the form of microparticles were chosen as coating materials. The first layer consisted of 5 μm of YSZ, deposited to avoid any metal tissue contact. The second layer consisted of 15 μm thick 45S5–YSZ composite, which was supposed to react with the surrounding bone tissue and enhance implant fixation. The adsorption of YSZ nanoparticles on 45S5 microparticles in organic suspension was found to invert the surface charge of the 45S5 particles from negative to positive. This enabled cathodic electrophoretic deposition of 45S5, avoiding uncontrolled anodization (oxidation) of the substrate. The coatings were sintered at 900°C for 2 h under argon flow to significantly improve coating adhesion (see Figure 9.15).

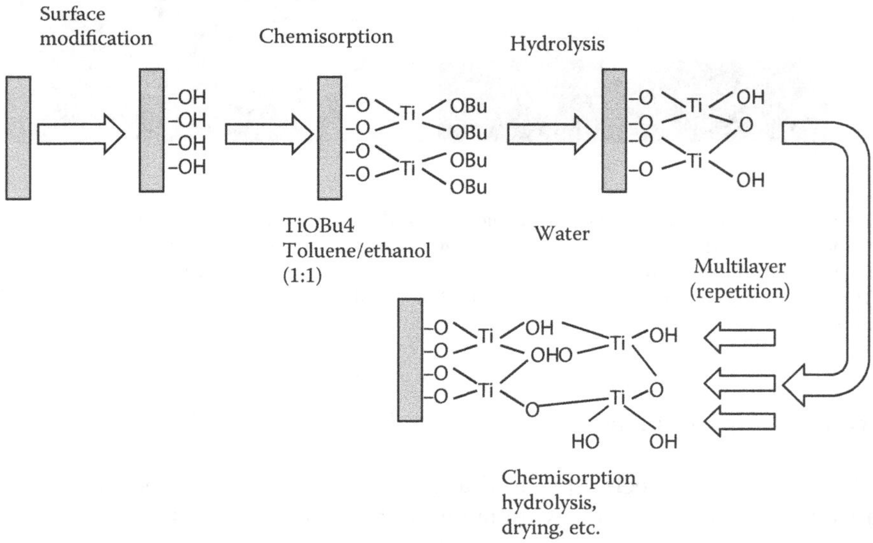

FIGURE 9.14
Chemisorption layering of sol–gel to produce an ultrathin bioactive glass film on titanium alloy substrates [39].

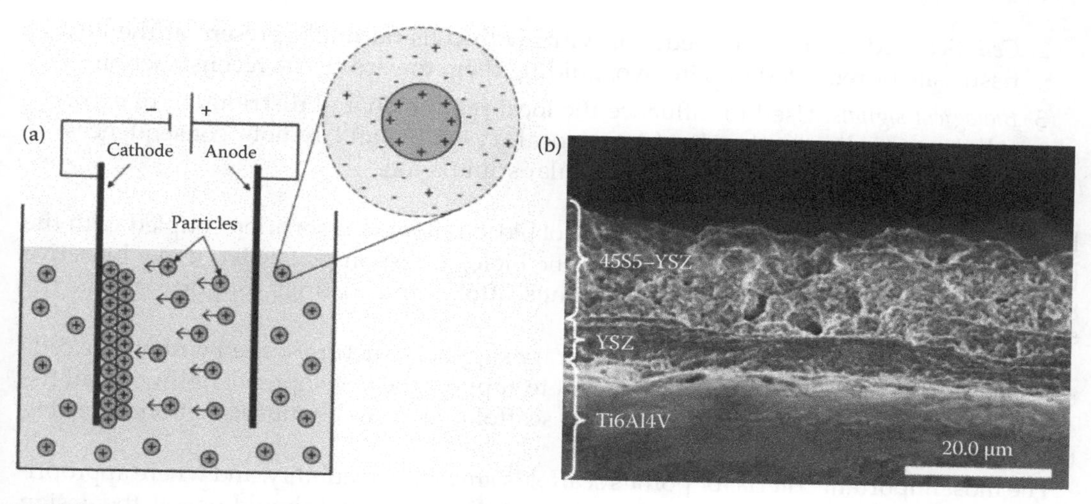

FIGURE 9.15
(a) Double-layer EPD process with a magnification of the particle and its double layer. (b) SEM of Ti_6Al_4V substrates with zirconia–Bioglass® composite layers. (From Radice et al., *J. Biomed. Mater. Res.* A, 82A(2), 436–444, 2007. With permission [40].)

Bioactive Glass Coatings for Tissue Engineering Applications

Tissue engineering is defined as the design and manufacture, in the laboratory, of living, functional tissue components that can be used for the repair and regeneration of malfunctioning tissues [8]. The field is an interdisciplinary one, bringing together engineering, science, and medicine. Initially, tissue-engineered devices consisted of two functional groups: cells and scaffolds. In the early 1990s, much effort was focused on engineering complete functional tissues and organs. Host tissue structural complexity coupled with difficulties in perfusion of large tissue constructs have, in part, limited the development of engineered tissues. In the past 10 years, research has focused on engineering specific genetic/bimolecular/nanoscopic process to regenerate host tissue sections as opposed to organs. This has mainly been due to the fact it is currently not possible to create a fully vascularized tissue. Ideally the biomaterial devices used would be resorbed away and replaced with regenerate healthy tissue. Based on recent data from both in vivo studies and limited clinical trials, it has become clear that biomaterial scaffolds need be designed to include nanoscopic features to mimic the form and function of the host tissue extracellular matrix (ECM) regulating, in part to achieve precise cellular immobilization and function at the host tissue site.

The development of implantable devices for tissue engineering applications is considered as the marriage of three functional design components:

1. *Scaffold*. A temporary structure, via controlled degradation, that mimics the extracellular matrix (ECM) providing appropriate mechanical integrity, porosity, and pore interconnectivity, and favorable surface conditions (e.g., geometric surface features, hydrophobicity, surface roughness, and surface attachment of proteins) for cellular growth and regulation of intracellular signaling molecules

2. *Cell.* Scaffolds can be preseeded in vitro with cells normally present at the host tissue site or recruited into in vivo, guiding them toward tissue reconstruction
3. *Biological signals.* Used to influence the local regulation and distribution of extracellular signaling molecules (at the local, systemic, and remote consequences) required for specifically designed cellular stimulation.

For regeneration of bone, the ability to control bioactivity and resorption coupled with the potential of mimicking ECM to elicit specific biologic responses in vivo make bioactive glasses ideal potential candidates for implant scaffolds and coatings supporting bone tissue regeneration.

Salih [41] states that "A scaffold is a temporary support structure seeded with viable cells coupled with a suitable culture environment to support the development of functional tissue." For tissue-engineering applications, a scaffold needs to be multifunctional serving the considerations stated in Table 9.20.

The most important criteria for porous scaffolds are biocompatibility, and where appropriate, vascularization [42]. For bone regeneration, the ideal scaffold should posses the design requirements stated in Table 9.21 in order to address the tissue characteristics not addressed by current bone replacement materials.

Coatings on Tissue-Engineering Scaffolds

Coating with bioactive glasses can functionalize scaffold surfaces, thus significantly improving, and in some cases introducing, bioactivity.

Polymeric Scaffolds

The choice of scaffold material is very important. For bone applications, it must serve all the required design criteria stated in Table 9.21. Scaffolds are currently utilized in the following two ways:

TABLE 9.20

Design Considerations for Scaffolds to Be Used in Tissue Engineering Applications

Before Implantation	At/During Implantation	During Implant Lifetime
Host the cells of interest plus biological molecules (e.g., extracellular matrices, growth factors, and differentiation agents)	Be permanently implanted in vivo Have a three-dimentional, porous structure Have the appropriate host-site mechanical stability Be biocompatible at the host tissue site resulting in tissue regeneration and growth Try to mimic the ECM by exhibiting suitable physical and chemical properties to facilitate cell immobilization, migration, proliferation, and differentiation into a mature phenotype coupled with production and maintenance of extracellular matrix	Be able to mature while maintaining viability Allow adequate perfusion of nutrients and waste Possibly support appropriate vascularization (depending on implant site)

TABLE 9.21
Ideal Scaffold Design Requirements

Design Requirement	Description
1	Act as a template for tissue growth, while maintaining 3-dimensional structure of host tissue during tissue regeneration.
2	Should not elicit scar tissue formation.
3	Have a porous structure (similar to trabecullar bone) with interconnected pore network allowing tissue growth in 3-D.
4	Pore interconnects should have apertures greater than 100 μm to allow cells to migrate throughout the scaffold, in addition to allowing the fluid flow throughout the scaffold.
5	Pores' surface textures should mimic ECM form and function: support cell attachment, growth, and generation of extracellular matrix.
6	Resorbability matching host tissue growth/replacement rates.
7	Act as a delivery system for time release of chemical species (e.g., ions, growth factors) enhancing bioactive response.
8	Capable of being mass-produced for clinical application.

1. Acellular scaffolds have been used to initiate repair of host tissues in situ. Scaffolds have consisted of a biomaterial matrix coupled with biomolecules.
2. Cellular scaffolds have been preseeded/loaded with either stem cells or differentiated cells before implantation. These scaffolds mature in vivo.

Synthetic polymers have received considerable research focus as scaffold materials because their chemistries can be precisely controlled resulting in their ability to biodegrade at rates determined by their surface chemistries [43]. However, they are not bioactive. Strategies to introduce bioactivity in porous polymeric scaffolds have included:

1. Polymer-based scaffolds coated with ceramic (glass) particles
2. Ceramic (glass) scaffolds coated with a polymer

Polymers lack osteoconductivity [44]. The incorporation of bioactive ceramics and glasses (e.g., hydroxyapatite, calcium phosphates, and Bioglass) in combination with biodegradable polymers (e.g., poly(DL-lactic acid) (PDLLA)/bioglass, collagen/hydroxyapatite, poly(hydroxybutyrate-*co*-hydroxyvalerate)/wollastonite, poly(lactic-*co*-glycolic acid)/HA, polycaprolactone/calcium phosphate) have been explored to develop composite scaffolds [44]. Strategies used to functionalize polymeric surfaces via the introduction of bioactive glasses include cold pressing and slurry dipping.

Cold Pressing

The use of cold pressing was first reported by Stamboulis and coworkers [45]. By cold pressing at 100 to 160 mPa, Bioglass powders (less than 5 μm) onto the surface of Polyglactin 910 (Vicryl®) sutures, they were able to coat the sutures. Although the coatings were not uniform, the effect of Bioglass coating did not significantly alter the tensile properties of the suture.

Ross and coworkers [46] developed a method for coating silicone tubing (with peritoneal dialysis catheters) bioactive glasses using prewashing of the silicone tubing. Catheter surface modification was achieved by washing in a hexane solution followed by immersion in a silicone solution further diluted with hexane. BG particles were then applied by cold pressing, by hand, onto the tubing circumferentially in BG powders. The tubes were air dried and then placed in an oven at 65°C at ambient humidity for approximately 12 h. Tubes were then washed in a 1% solution of Triton-X 100 and then gas-sterilized using ethylene oxide. In vivo testing via subcutaneous implantation in a rat model was performed. No in vivo toxicity was observed. The BG coating demonstrated good bioactivity in vivo, inducing soft tissue adhesion without the formation of a fibrous tissue coating (Figure 9.16).

Slurry Dipping

In this technique, coatings have been applied using a suspension of bioactive glass particles in either a diluted binder or water prior to either:

1. No surface processing of the polymeric material
2. Surface functionalization, via washing with ethanol, of the polymeric material

Without pretreating the scaffold, polyurethane (PUR) foam scaffolds were coated with bioactive glass (SiO_2–P_2O_5–CaO–MgO–Na_2O–K_2O system) particles using slurry dipping followed by drying at room temperature (see Figure 9.17). PVA (6% polyvinyl alcohol (PVA), 64% water) was used to bind the bioactive glass particles to the scaffold. The glass coating increased the scaffold stiffness while no statistically significant differences in terms of failure strength were observed between uncoated and coated scaffold. HA was observed on scaffold surface after 7 days of soaking in SBS solution.

Using a slurry dipping method including pretreatment with ethanol to reduce substrate hydrophobicity, macroporous poly(DL-lactide) (PDLLA) foams have been coated with 45S5 Bioglass® particles [48, 49]. Slurry dipping technique was used in conjunction with pretreatment of the foam with ethanol to produce bioactive glass coatings of uniform thickness on the internal and external surfaces of the foams. The coating exhibited good adhesion.

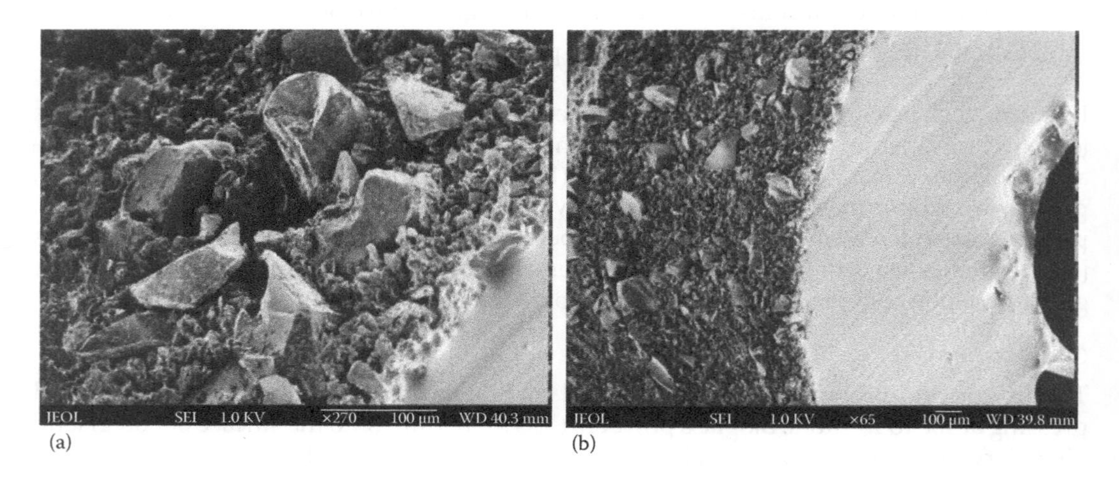

FIGURE 9.16
Scanning electron micrographs of the bioactive glass-coated silicone tubing segment in (a) the outer surface, magnification times 270, and (b) cross section, magnification times 65. (Ross et al., *Kidney Int.*, 63, 702–708, 2003. With permission [46].)

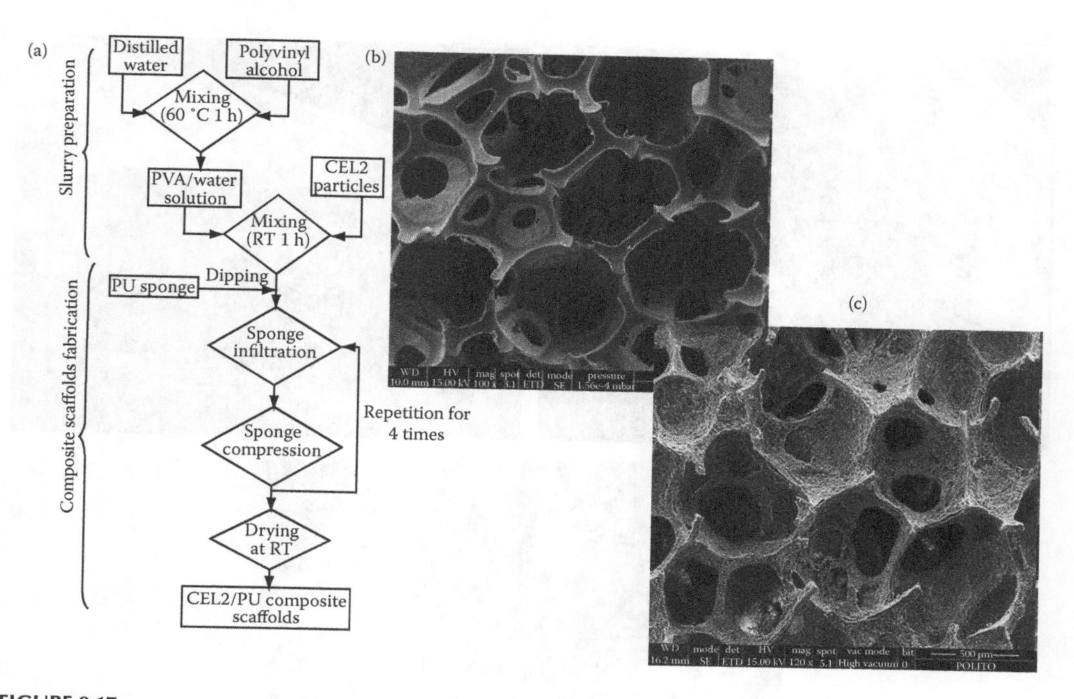

FIGURE 9.17
Example of a slurry dipping method used to coat PUR foam scaffolds. (a) Processing flow chart. (b) Uncoated PUR. (c) Bioactive glass (CEL2 composition–molar composition: 45% SiO_2, 3% P_2O_5, 26% CaO, 7% MgO, 15% Na_2O, 4% K_2O) coated PUR foam scaffold. (From Baino et al., *J. Mater. Sci. Mater. Med.*, 20(11), 2189–2195, 2009. With permission [47].)

However, human osteoblast cell cultures indicated that cell attachment and spreading was slower compared with both Bioglass and Thermanox substrates, which was likely due to surface roughness and morphology.

45S5 Bioglass® and antibacterial AgBG* glass powders have been coated onto Mersilk® sutures using the slurry (glass particles suspended in deionized water) dipping process described by Roether et al. [49] (see Figure 9.18). In vitro experiments were carried out using *Staphylococcus epidermidis* under both batch and flow conditions. While the traditional batch culture testing was used to determine the number of viable cells adhered to the surface, the flow cell was used to visualize attachment and detachment over time. Under batch conditions of up to 180 min, statistically significant differences were observed in the colony forming units (CFU) per suture for both the coated and uncoated Mersilk® sutures. The results showed that the AgBG coating had the greatest effect on limiting bacterial attachment (8×10^2 CFU) when compared to the 45S5 Bioglass® coating (3.2×10^3 CFU) and the uncoated Mersilk® (1.2×10^4 CFU). Under flow conditions, differences were also seen between the coated and uncoated sutures.

* The ability of silver-doped bioactive glass (AgBG) coatings to prevent bacterial colonization on surgical sutures was investigated.

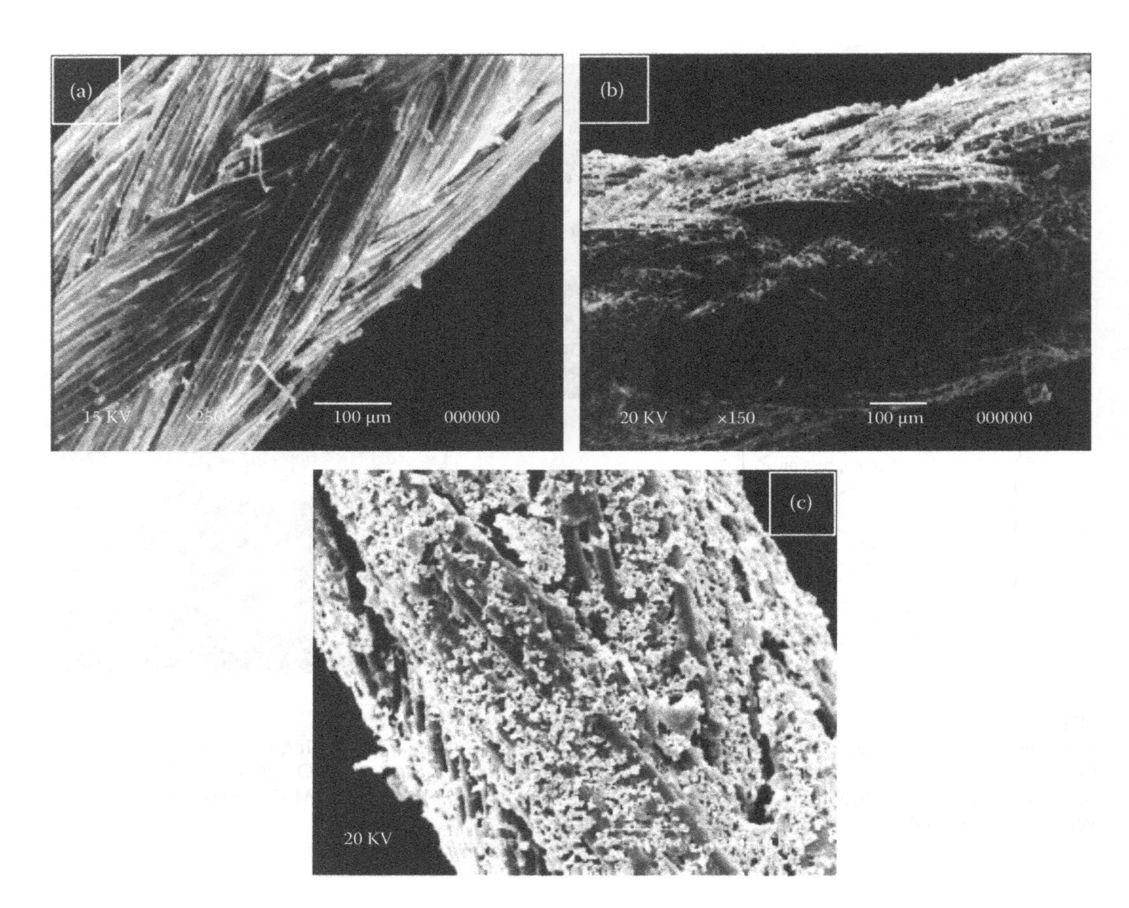

FIGURE 9.18
SEM of Mersilk® sutures (a) uncoated, (b) slurry-dip-coated with AgBG glass powders and (c) 45S5 Bioglass® powders. (From Pratten et al., *J. Biomater. Appl.*, 19(1), 47–57, 2004. With permission [50].)

Nanoscopic Surface Modification of Bioactive Glasses

Materials composed of one or more engineering nanocomponents/surface features (1–100 nm) are called nanomaterials [41]. They offer an exciting new possibility for medical device technology development. Possible applications include imaging and diagnosis, anticancer therapies, drug delivery platforms, and gene therapy. It is expected that nanotechnology will revolutionize tissue engineering.

Nanotechnology can be used to engineer surfaces to:

- Significantly improve/control rates of bioactivity (I_b), resulting in faster tissue integration/growth
- Create bioinspired nanoarchitectures mimicking ECM form and function

Bioinspired nanotechnological engineering coupled with bioactivity presents a new and exciting strategy to potentially and significantly improve the in vivo performance of implants to last the lifetime of the patient.

TABLE 9.22
Possible Surface Fictionalization Strategies for Bioactive Glass Surfaces

Modification	Example Technique
Morphological modifications	The introduction of pores, gratings, columns, dots, pits, and random surface roughness
Physiochemical modifications	Glow discharge, ion implantation
Biological modifications	Adsorption, entrapment, and covalent attachment of biomolecules on glass surfaces

Strategies to Mimic Extracellular Matrix

Strategies currently include the introduction of pores, gratings, columns, dots, pits, and random surface roughness (morphological modifications); glow discharge and ion implantation (physiochemical modifications); adsorption, entrapment, and covalent attachment of biomolecules on glass surfaces (biological modifications) (Table 9.22).

Complex, spatiotemporally regulated interactions between cells and their extracellular matrix (ECM) regulate many crucial cellular processes in our tissues [51–53]. "Biodriven" developments in biomaterials research have the potential to generate smart synthetic bioactive glasses that mimic some of the key structural and biochemical characteristics of the host tissue ECM [52, 53]. It should be noted that the mechanisms required for bone tissue attachment and regeneration at the implant interface are still not well understood. As a result, the importance of ECM structure and function remains controversial but should not be ignored in developing the next generation of bioactive glass coatings (see Table 9.23).

Surface engineering strategies (see Table 9.22) that mimic ECM form include creating morphologies, physiochemically engineered surfaces, and biological modification strategies. The precise entrapment, absorbtion, and covalent attachment of biomolecules (e.g., peptides, proteins, and other functional groups) have been used to mimic the chemical clues for cellular differentiation and proliferation.

Physiochemical modifications are aimed at changing surface properties such as surface energy, surface charge, and surface composition to precisely control initial protein absorption, production, and cellular differentiation. Due to limited size of the chapter, their description has not been included.

Morphological Approach

Morphological modifications are aimed at creating three-dimensional features (nanofeatures) in the form of pores, gratings, columns, dots, pits, and random surface roughness (see Table 9.24). These modifications are aimed at mimicking the ECM morphology. It should be noted that the sole effect of nanofeatures on cellular activity (bioreactivity) remains unresolved.

TABLE 9.23
Biomaterials Design Requirements to Mimic ECM Structure and Function

	Biomaterials Design Requirements Mimic ECM Structure and Function
1	Provide chemical clues to control cellular activity
2	Provide mechanical and surface morphological clues to control cellular activity
3	Controlled delivery of soluble factors directly from the material

TABLE 9.24
Range of Cellular Reactions to Nanomorphology

Cell Property	Cell Type	Topographical Feature	Cellular Reaction
Adhesion	Fibroblasts	Nanopits	Decrease
		27-nm high nanoislands	Increase
		Nanopillar	Depends on spacing
	Osteoblasts	Nanopits (near-square) on PMMA and silica	Decreased
		Pyramids on Ti	Decreased
Activation	Platelets and monocytes	Nanodeep grooves	Increase
		Random hills	Increase
Movement	Smooth muscle cells	Nanodeep grooves	Increase
	Fibroblasts	Nanopillar	Depends on spacing
Morphology	Smooth muscle cells	Nanodeep grooves	Alignment
	Epithelia	Nanodeep grooves on silica oxide	Alignment
	Fibroblasts	Nanoprojections (pores, gratings, columns, dots, pits)	Alignment
Shape	Fibroblasts	Random surface roughness	Spreading
Proliferation	Fibroblasts (corneal)	Nanodeep grooves	Little effect
	Fibroblasts	Nanoprojections	Lower
Osteogenesis	Osteoblasts	Random nanoislands	Raised
		Nanopits	Raised
		Nanogrooves	Raised

Nanofeatures can be created using either top-down or bottom-up manufacturing process. Top-down methods include electron beam lithography (via e-beam, x-ray beam, ion beams) and holographic writing methods, while bottom-up methods include colloidal lithography and polymer demixing.

There are limited reports of top-down methods being applied to bioceramic substrates as these techniques have been developed for metallic substrates. In the bottom-up approach, the nanofeatures are assembled from nanometric-sized components, for example nanopowders and nanofibers. The powders and fibers can themselves be used as the topological features coated on an implant surface [55–57, 59].

Nanoparticles

The work by Watari and coworkers [58] gives an indication of possible effects of engineered nano-sized features on biological activity. Using various-sized particles (range 500 nm–150 μm) of pure Ti, Fe, Ni, TiO_2, and carbon nanotubes (CNTs), they investigated the effect of material nanosizing on cell proliferation and animal implantation testing. They found:

- Increase in specific surface area caused the enhanced release of ionic dissolution products resulting in local toxicity.
- For nonresorbable particles, there was a critical size for the transition of cellular behavior at approximately 100 μm, 10 μm, and 200 nm. Below 100 μm, the particles

were not surrounded by fibrous connective tissue and no inflammation was observed in vivo. They exhibit biologically stimulating properties. Below 10 μm, in vitro phagocytosis and in vivo tissue inflammation was observed. Below 200 nm, bioactivity decreased and particles diffused into internal organs of an animal model and collected in both the respiratory and digestive systems.

Bioactive glass–ceramic nanoparticles (nBGC) have been prepared by the sol–gel technique based on polymerization reactions of metal alkoxide precursors (TEOS and/or TEP mixture). The precursors are dissolved in a solvent, and a gel is formed by hydrolysis and condensation reactions. Prior to hydrolysis calcium phosphate and/or antibacterial compounds (e.g., silver nitrate) are added. The gel is subjected to a controlled thermal process to strengthen the gel by drying (aging temperature of 120°C for 24 h) any liquid by-products followed by thermal stabilization (500–800°C for less than 6 h) to remove any organic species from the surface of the material. Attractive forces between nanoparticles can cause agglomeration of particles, resulting in porosity among the particles (Figure 9.19).

Nanofibers

Nanofiber-based scaffolds show great promise for tissue engineering applications due to their inherent high porosities and surface-area-to-volume ratios. In addition, fiber diameters

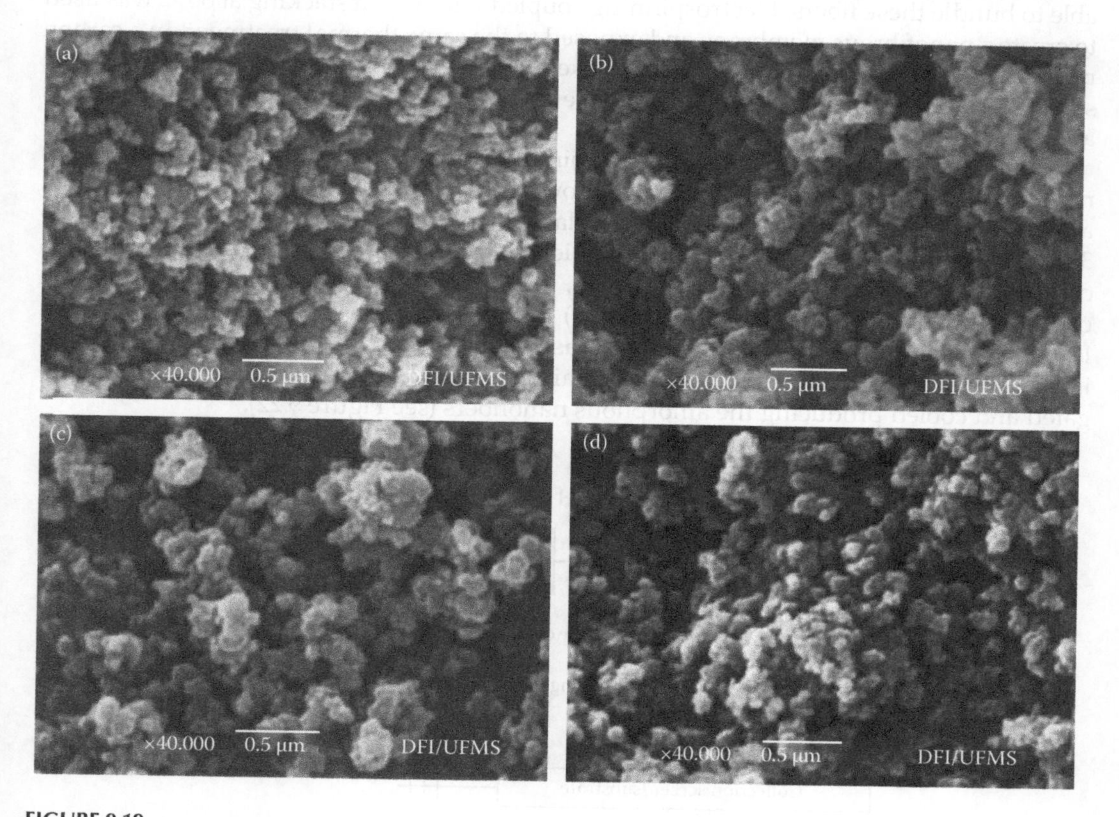

FIGURE 9.19
Coatings composed of bioactive glass nanoparticles doped with (a) 0%, (b) 1%, (c) 3%, and (d) 5% silver to make them antibacterial. (From Delben et al., *J. Therm. Anal. Calorim.*, 97(2), 433–436, 2009. With permission [59].)

and other topological features can be precisely controlled to encourage cellular adhesion, migration, and proliferation. Research exploring this technique has focused on electrospinning of polymeric solutions to produce nonwoven fiber mats [65]. Over the past 5 years there has been continued interest in producing bioactive nanofibers using sol–gel derived glasses, where the charged sol is ejected onto a charged collection substrate (see Figure 9.20) [60–62, 64]. As the metal capillary is charged by the high voltage bias, the sol–gel solution is ejected from the tip, forming a Taylor cone. The sol–gel spirals downward, bending and stretching to produce ultrathin fibers. Factors such as capillary/collection substrate distance, voltage, and solution viscosity can be altered to produce fibers of various diameters. Fiber orientation is changed by changing the orientation of the collection substrate (e.g., dual rings or rotating drums).

Kim and coworkers [64] were the first to describe the production of potential sol–gel-derived bioactive glass nanofibers using electrospinning. Limiting sol concentrations to 1 to 0.25 M, continuous and uniform fibers were produced. Thermal stabilization of the fibers resulted in a reduction (by a factor of 2–3) in fiber diameter due to burnout of polymeric precursors. They were able to produce average fibers diameters of 630 to 84 nm (see Figure 9.21).

Apatite formation was observed after 3 days of immersion in SBF coupled with dramatic changes in surface morphology.

Interestingly, using fiber compaction followed by thermal treatment (700°C), they were able to bundle these fibers. Electrospinning coupled with warm stacking at 80°C was used to create a nanofibrous membrane and exposed to the same thermal treatment. In a carbon mold, the membrane and bundles were stacked to produce 3-D constructs followed by the same thermal treatment. To further stabilize the scaffold, it was impregnated with PLA and pressed at 120°C.

In 2009, a completely new method (laser spinning method) for producing bioactive glass nanofibers was presented by Quintero and coworkers [65]. Using a laser spinning method, a mesh of disordered intertwined fibers (glass fibers in diameters ranging from 200 to 300 nm) were produced from melt-derived bioactive glasses (45S5 composition and 52S4.6 composition). Laser spinning is an exciting, simple method because it does not rely on chemical processing (e.g., sol–gel formation) and does not need any chemical additives. It involves melting, via high powered CO_2 laser, a glass substrate, where the melt droplet is blown off the substrate via a compressed airflow. During this stage, the droplet is elongated and cooled producing the amorphous nanofibers (see Figure 9.22).

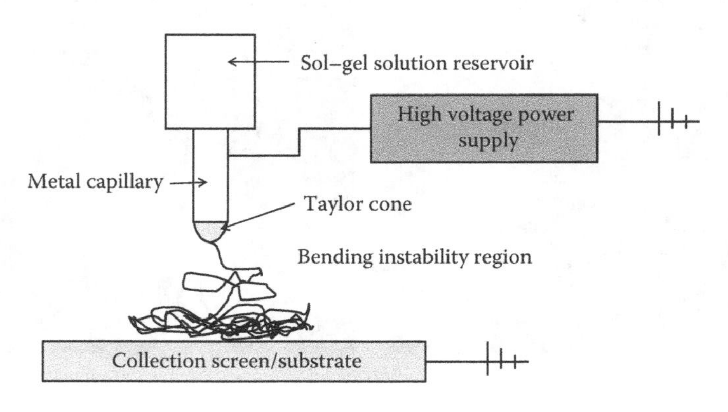

FIGURE 9.20
Schematic of electrospinning method [63].

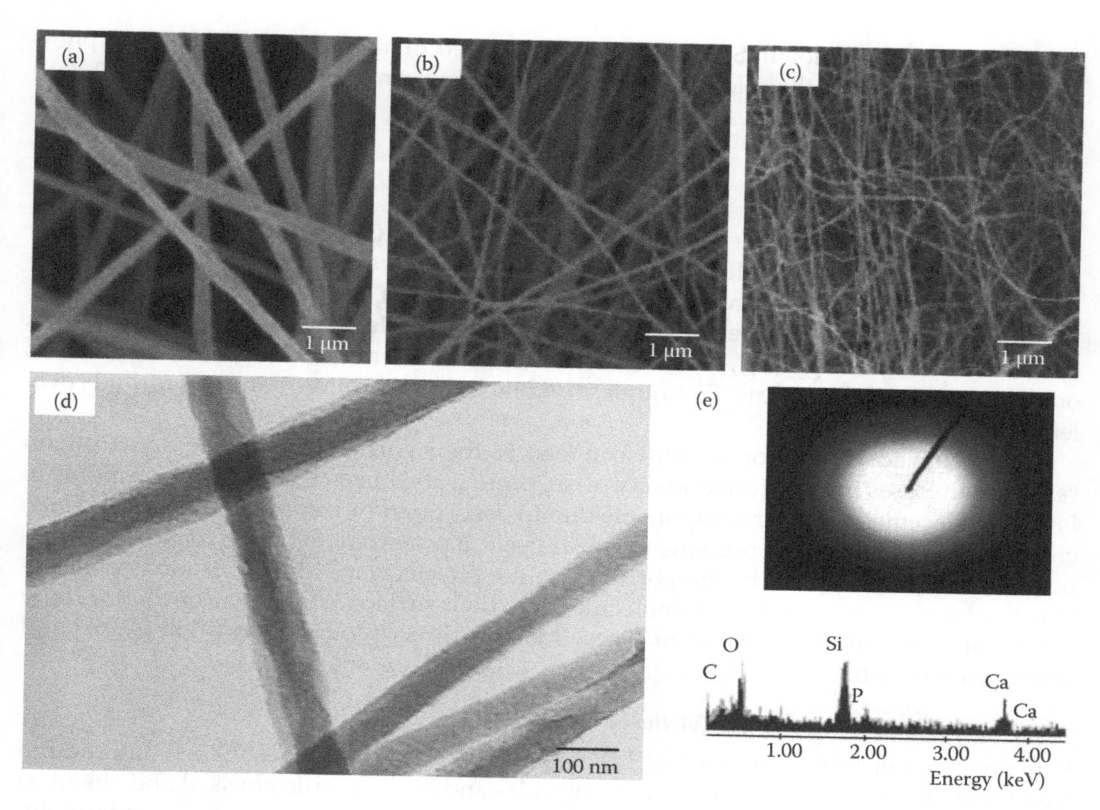

FIGURE 9.21
Bioactive glass fibers produced by electrospinning and heat treatment at 700°C. (From Kim et al., *Adv. Funct. Mater.*, 16(12), 1529–1535, 2006. With permission [64].) (a–c) SEM of nanofibers made from varying sol concentration (1, 0.5, and 0.25m, respectively). (d) TEM of nanofiber, where diameter has been measured to be approximately 84 nm. (e) EDS profile of a nanofiber.

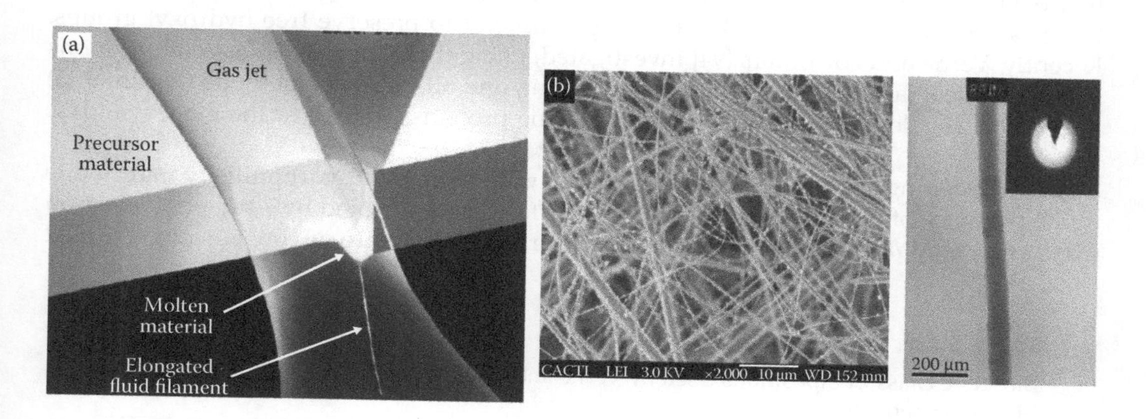

FIGURE 9.22
(a) Laser spinning fabrication of melt-derived bioactive glasses (45S5 composition and 52S4.6 composition). (b) Left image shows the FESEM of as produced glass fibers; right image shows TEM of nanofiber with inset SAED image showing amorphous structure. (From Quintero et al., *Adv. Funct. Mater.*, 19(19), 3084–3090, 2009. With permission [65].)

After 12 h of immersion in SBF, the fibers were coated in undense, porous calcium phosphate. Densification of the calcium phosphate coating was not observed even after 2 days of immersion in SBF solution.

Biological Approach

In addition to providing a structural support, scaffolds must also provide biological signals. They are therefore usually loaded with growth factors, antibiotics, and bone morphogenic proteins or used as delivery vehicles for the release of drugs/proteins or genes [66].

Biological modifications are aimed at mimicking the molecular biological mechanisms of the ECM morphology (e.g., structure and function) by immobilizing bimolecular cues on the surface of biomaterials. Techniques used include adsorption, entrapment, and covalent attachment.

Nonspecific adsorption of proteins can lead to their partial or complete denaturation resulting in losses in their functionality. Also, protein absorbed coatings are susceptible to loss or replacement of their components due to desorption or competitive binding. Thus, covalent attachment of the proteins to substrates is a preferred approach for surface engineering. Little is stated in the literature regarding physiochemical modifications of bioactive glass surfaces via grafting biomolecules onto their surface. At the time of writing, only two techniques have been reported. These include: direct protein absorption [67, 68] and silanization methods.

Silanization (Silane Modification) Methods

Functional groups (e.g., methyl ($-CH_3$), hydroxyl ($-OH$), carboxyl ($-COOH$), and amino ($-NH_2$)) are present in many biological molecules and have specific physical and chemical properties that influence cellular processes. Silanization offers the possibility of immobilization of biological molecules on biomaterial surfaces via –OH groups activated on the biomaterials surface that facilitate grafting of biomolecules due to free unbound, amino terminal groups [69, 70, 94]. The surface reaction stages responsible for bioactivity of bioactive glass make them ideal substrates for protein immobilization due to their inherent surface hydroxylation [71]. However, the reaction layer kinetics, including cation migration from the glass network, occurs, quickly making it difficult to preserve free hydroxyl groups. Recently, Verne and coworkers [94] investigated, using three bioactive glass compositions substrates (see Table 9.25), and different cleaning and silanization methods (Figure 9.23) in order to covalently bond bone morphogenetic proteins (BMP-2) to the bioactive glass surfaces.

All the cleaning methods produced surfaces with increased hydrophilicity nature due to the presence of hydroxyl groups on their surfaces as confirmed by x-ray photoelectron (XPS) analyses. Washing in acids, bases, and SBF resulted in hydroxyl condensation coupled

TABLE 9.25

Bioactive Glass Compositions Used by Verne and Coworkers to Covalently Bond Bone Morphogenetic Proteins

Material	SiO_2	P_2O_5	Al_2O_3	MgO	CaO	Na_2O	K_2O
SCNA	57	–	9	–	34	6	–
4.5 A	47.5	2.5	–	–	30	10	10
CEL2	45	3	–	7	26	15	4

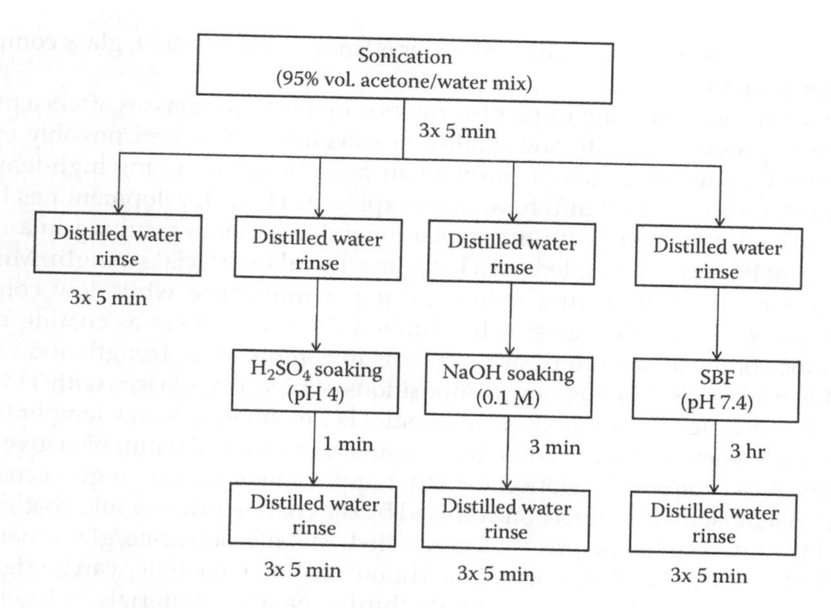

FIGURE 9.23
Cleaning methods investigated [71].

with complex ionic exchange resulting in few free –OH groups. The cleaned glasses were then functionalized using 3-amino-propyl-triethoxysilane (APTS). Not surprisingly, acid-, base-, and SBF-washed glasses exhibited poor functionalization with APTS. Washing the glasses with acetone/water mixture resulted in high numbers of free hydroxyl groups coupled with poor condensation, resulting in higher APTS functionalization. Finally, human BMP-2 protein was grafted onto all the functionalized substrates and protein immobilization tracked via determining N/Si ratios using XPS spectra. As expected, N/Si ratios indicated successful grafting of BMP-2 on all silanized surfaces.

Summary

Bioactive glasses offer new concepts for both loading-bearing implant applications and regenerative medicine devices. For all generations of biomaterials, bioactive glasses show the highest levels of bioactivity.

First-generation bone replacement biomaterials were bioinert and were selected because they mechanically matched host tissues. These materials were designed as a means to an end to replace host tissue and interact, to a minimum, with the hosts' immune system. The discovery that certain compositions of glasses could elicit in vivo biological responses with bone and soft tissues (bioactivity) revolutionized biomaterials research. Second-generation materials are bioactive or resorbable. Silica has been shown to be the active component for bioactivity via the formation of a silica–gel layer on/in which HA precipitation occurs and subsequent tissue bonding. Precipitation of HA is believed to be crucial for bioactivity. Varying silica content directly correlates to the materials bonding ability to hard (e.g., bone) and soft tissues (e.g., collagen). After 60 mol% silica content, glass compositions are no longer bioactive.

Coating metallic load-bearing implant surfaces with bioactive glasses offers a promising approach to improving the rate and quality of osteointegration and possibly extending implant lifetime by making metallic implant surfaces bioactive. Using high-temperature methods, thick coatings (>100 μm) have been explored. Their development has been limited due to glass interactions with the implant metallic surfaces resulting in a reduction and even loss of bioactivity coupled with low glass/metal interfacial strength. Mismatches in TECs have resulted in coating failure during manufacture while low compressive strength of second-generation glasses has limited their usefulness as coating materials. Glass–ceramic compositions offer improvements in compressive strength and research is currently focused on developing new compositions of bioactive glasses with TECs matching metallic substrates. In an attempt to avoid TEC mismatch, lower temperature coating process have been explored. These have resulted in thin (<100 μm) bioactive coatings. Based on PVD techniques developed for other applications, bioactive glass coatings are superior in that bioactivity is not compromised by the coating process, and coating compositions and thicknesses can be precisely controlled. Metallic substrate/glass coating interfacial strength are also much stronger. In addition, coating bioactivity can be significantly increased by coating metallic substrates with third-generation materials. Sol–gel bioactive glasses exhibit bioactivity with compositions that are much simpler (three-component systems) and ingredients that are purer than melt-derived bioactive glasses. Inherent porosity offers surface areas that are significantly higher than melt-derived bioactive glasses accounting, in part, for their significantly higher bioactivity rates resulting in faster tissue ingrowth and mechanical bonding. For regenerative medicine applications, bioactive glass coatings can transform polymeric bioinert scaffolds into bioactive scaffolds without compromising scaffold degradation rates.

Nanotechnology offers an exciting new strategy to further improve the bioactivity of implant surfaces by allowing materials to mimic host tissue extracellular matrix form and function (third-generation biomaterials), thus providing a genetic stimulus for bone tissue regeneration. Although the fundamental mechanisms by which cell functions are regulated by nanoscopic features remain unresolved, research has recently focused on creating nanoscopic bioactive glass-powder–based coatings and nanoscopically modified bioactive glass surfaces. It is too early to predict what the clinical impact of these materials will be, but it is almost certain that third-generation bioactive glasses that elicit specific genetic responses will be the next generation.

References

[1] Black, J. 2006. *Biological Performance of Materials. Fundamentals of Biocompatibility*, 4th edn. CRC Press, Boca Raton, FL.

[2] Paital, S.R., Dahotre, N.B. 2009. Calcium phosphate coatings for bio-implant applications: material, performance factors and methodologies. *Mater. Sci. Eng. R* 66, 1–70.

[3] Balamrugan, A., Rajeswari, S., Balossier, G., Rebelo, A.H.S., Ferreira, J.M.F. 2008. Corrosion aspects of metallic ceramics—an overview. *Mater. Corros.* 59(11), 855–869.

[4] Osborn, J.F. 1979. Biomaterials and their use in implants. *Schweiz. Mschr. Zahnheilk.* 89, 1138.

[5] Ohtsuki, C., Kamitahara, M., Miyazaki, T. 2009. Bioceramic based materials with designed reactivity for bone regeneration. *J. R. Soc. Interface* 6, S349–S360.
[6] Stavropoulos, A. 2008. Deproteinized bovine bone xenograft. In: Pietrzak, W.S. (ed.), *Musculoskeletal Tissue Regeneration. Orthopedic Biology and Medicine*. Humana Press, Totowa, New Jersey, USA.
[7] Navarro, M., Michiradi, A., Castano, O., Planell, J.A. 2008. Biomaterials in orthopaedics. *J. R. Soc. Interface* 5, 1137–1158.
[8] Maroothynaden, J. 2008. Bioactive glasses—new opportunities for regenerative medicine. In *Biomaterials and Biomedical Engineering*. TTP Trans Tech Publications, Switzerland.
[9] Hench, L.L., Wilson, J. (eds.) 1993. *An Introduction To Bioceramics*. World Scientific Press, Singapore.
[10] Kukobo, T. 2008. *Bioceramics and Their Clinical Applications*. Woodhead Publishing and Maney Publishing, on behalf of the Institute of Materials, Minerals & Mining, Cambridge, UK.
[11] Best, S.M. 2008. Bioceramics, past, present and future. *J. Eur. Ceram. Soc.* 28, 1319–1327.
[12] Donglu, S. (ed.). 2004. *Biomaterials and Tissue Engineering*. Springer, Berlin Heidelberg, Germany.
[13] Höland, W., Vogel, W., Nauman, K. 1985. Interface reactions between machinable bioactive glass-ceramic and bone. *J. Biomed. Mater. Res.* 19, 303–312.
[14] Hench, L.L. 1993. Characterisation of bioceramics. In: Hench, L.L., Wilson, J. (eds.), *Advanced Series in Ceramics*, vol. 1. *An introduction to Bioceramics*, 319–334. World Scientific, Singapore.
[15] William, D.F. 1987. Tissue–biomaterials interactions. *J. Sci.* 22, 3421–3445.
[16] Inayat-Hussain, S., Rajab, N.F. 2009. In vitro testing of biomaterials toxicity and biocompatibility. In: Di Silvio, L. (ed.), *Cellular Responses to Biomaterials*, 508–537. CRC Press, Woodhead publishing Ltd, Cambridge, UK.
[17] Kokubo, T., Takadama, H. 2006. How useful is SBF in predicting in vivo bioactivity? *Biomaterials* 27, 2907–2915.
[18] Bohner, M., Lemaitre, J. 2009. Can bioactivity be tested in vitro with SBF solution? *Biomaterials* 30(12), 2175–2179. Epub 2009 Jan 26. Review.
[19] Lee, K.Y., Park, M., Lim, Y.J., Chun, H.J., Kim, H., Moon, S.H. 2006. Ceramic bioactivity: progress, challenges and perspectives. *Biomed. Mater.* 1, R31–R37.
[20] Juhasz, J.A., Best, S.M., Auffret, A.D., Bonfield, W. 2008. Biological control of apatite growth in simulated body fluid and human blood serum. *J. Mater. Sci: Mater Med.* 19, 1823–1829.
[21] Kirk, S.E., Skepper, J,N., Donald, A.M. 2009. Application of environmental scanning electron microscopy to determine biological surface structure. *J. Microsc.* 233(2), 205–224.
[22] Mayer, E. 1992. *Atomic Force Microscopy. Progress in Surface Sciences*. Vol. 42, 3–49. Pergamon Press, New York, USA.
[23] Hollinger, J.O., Citron, M. 2006. Considerations for in-vivo testing of biomaterials. In: Guelcher, S.A., and Hollinger. J.O. (eds.), An *Introduction to Biomaterials*, 81–104. CRC Press, USA.
[24] Hench, L.L. 1991. Bioceramics: from concept to clinic. *J. Am. Ceram. Soc.* 74(7), 1487–1510.
[25] Park, J. 2009. *Bioceramics—Properties, Characterization and Applications*. Springer, New York, NY.
[26] Tanaka, Y., Yamashita, K., 2008. Fabrication processes for bioceramics. In: Kukobo, T. (ed.) *Bioceramics and Their Clinical Applications*. Woodhead Publishing and Maney Publishing, on behalf of the Institute of Materials, Minerals & Mining, Cambridge, UK.
[27] Hench, L.L., and Andersson, O. 1993. Bioactive glass coatings. In: Hench, L.L., and Wilson, J. (eds.), *An Introduction to Bioceramics*, 239–259. World Scientific Press, Singapore.
[28] Pazo, A., Saiz, E., Tomsai, A.P., 1998. Silicate coatings on titanium based implants. *Acta Mater.* 46, 2551–2558.
[29] Van Landuyt, P., Streydio, J.M., Delannay, F., Munting, E. 1994. Synthesis of bioactive coatings on Ti substrates using glass enamel. *Clin Mater.* 17(1), 29–33.
[30] Gomez-Vega, J.M., Hozumi, E., Saiz, E., Tomsia, A.P., Sugimura, H., Takai, O. 2001. Bioactive glass-mesoporous silica coatings on Ti6Al4V through enamelling and triblock-copolymer-templated sol–gel processing. *J. Biomed. Mater. Res.* 56(3), 382–389.
[31] Hill, R.G., Stevens, M.M., O'Donnell, M. 2009. WO=2009081120.

[32] Venkatesan, T., Green, S.M. 1996. Pulsed laser deposition: thin films in a flash. The American Institute of Physics. *Ind. Physicists Mag.*, 22–24.
[33] Eason, R. 2007. Pulsed laser deposition of thin films. In: Eason, R. (ed.), *Applications-Led Growth of Functional Materials*. John Wiley & Sons, Hoboken, New Jersey, USA.
[34] Joanni, E., Ferro, M.C., Mardare, C.C., Mardare, A.I., Fernandes, J.R.A., de Almeida, S.C. 2004. Pulsed laser deposition of SiO_2–P_2O_5–CaO–MgO glass coatings on titanium substrates. *Mater. Res.* 7(3).
[35] Berbecarua, C., Alexandrua, H.V., Ianculescub, A., Popescuc, A., Socolc, G., Simac, F., Mihailescuc, I. 2009. Bioglass thin films for biomimetic implants. *Appl. Surf. Sci.* 255(10), 5476–5479.
[36] Lusquiños, F., De Carlos, A., Pou, J., Arias, J.L., Boutinguiza, M., León, B., Pérez-Amor, M., Driessens, F.C.M., Hing, K., Gibson, I., Best, S., Bonfield, W. 2003. Calcium phosphate coatings obtained by Nd:YAG laser cladding: physicochemical and biologic properties. *J. Biomed. Mater. Res. A* 64A(4), 630–637.
[37] Comesañaa, R., Quinteroa, F., Lusquiñosa, F., Pascualb, M.J., Boutinguizaa, M., Duránb, A., Pou, J. 2010. Laser cladding of bioactive glass coatings. *Acta Biomater*. 6(3), 953–961.
[38] Moritz, N., Vedel, E., Ylanen, H., Jokinen, M., Hupa, M., Yli-Urpo, A. 2004. Characterisation of bioactive glass coatings on titanium substrates produced using a CO_2 laser. *J. Mater. Sci. Mater. Med.* 15(7), 787–794.
[39] Advincula, M.C., Petersen, D., Rahemtulla, F., Advincula, R., Lemons, J.E. 2007. surface analysis and biocorrosion properties of nanostructured surface sol–gel coatings on Ti6Al4V titanium alloy implants. *J. Biomed. Mater. Res. Part B: Appl. Biomater.* 80B, 107–120.
[40] Radice, S., Kern, P., Bürki, G., Michler, J., Texto, M. 2007. Electrophoretic deposition of zirconia-Bioglass® composite coatings for biomedical implants. *J. Biomed. Mater. Res. A* 82A(2), 436–444.
[41] Salih, V. 2009. Biodegradable scaffolds for tissue engineering. In: Di Silvio, L. (ed.), *Cellular Response to Biomaterials*, 185–211. Woodhead Publishing in Materials, CRC Press, Cambridge.
[42] Hutmacher, D.W., Schantz, J.T., Lam, C.X.F., Tan, K.C., Lim, T.C. 2007. State of the art and future directions of scaffold-based bone engineering from a biomaterials perspective. *J. Tissue Eng. Regen. Med.* 1(4), 245–260.
[43] Tuzlakoglu, K., Reis, R.L. 2008. Biodegradable polymeric fibre structures in tissue engineering. *Tissue Eng. Part B Rev* 15, 17–25.
[44] Misra, S.K., Philip, S.E., Chrzanowski, W., Nazhat, S.N., Roy, I., Knowles, J.C., Salih, V., Boccaccini, A.R. 2008. Incorporation of vitamin E in poly(3hydroxybutyrate)/bioglass composite films: effect on surface properties and cell attachment. *J. R. Soc, Interface* 2, 1–9.
[45] Stamboulis, L., Hench, L., Boccaccini, A.R. 2002. Mechanical properties of biodegradable polymer sutures coated with bioactive glass. *J. Mater. Sci.: Mater. Med.* 13(9).
[46] Ross, E.A., Batich, C.D., Clapp, W.L., Sallustio, J.E., Lee, N.C. 2003. Tissue adhesion to bioactive glass-coated silicone tubing in a rat model of peritoneal dialysis catheters and catheter tunnels. *Kidney Int.* 63, 702–708.
[47] Baino, F., Verné, E., Vitale-Brovarone, C. 2009. Feasibility, tailoring and properties of polyurethane/bioactive glass composite scaffolds for tissue engineering. Feasibility, tailoring and properties of polyurethane/bioactive glass composite scaffolds for tissue engineering. *J. Mater. Sci. Mater. Med.* 20(11) 2189–2195.
[48] Zhang, K., Wang, Y.B., Hillmyer, M.A., Francis, L.F. 2004. Processing and properties of porous poly(Image-lactide)/bioactive glass composites. *Biomaterials* 25(13), 2489–2500.
[49] Roether, J.A., Gough, J.E., Boccaccini, A.R., Hench, L.L., Maquetand, V., Jérôme, R. 2002. Novel bioresorbable and bioactive composites based on bioactive glass and polylactide foams for bone tissue engineering. *J. Mater. Sci. Mater. Med.* 13(12), 1207–1214.
[50] Pratten, J., Nazhat, S.N., Blaker, J.J., Boccaccini, A.R. 2004. In vitro attachment of *Staphylococcus epidermidis* to surgical sutures with and without Ag-containing bioactive glass coating. *J. Biomater. Appl.* 19(1), 47–57.
[51] Lutolf, M.P. 2009. Integration column: artificial ECM: expanding the cell biology toolbox in 3D. *Integr. Biol.* 1, 235–241.

[52] Badylak, S.F., Freytes, D.O., Gilbert, T.W. 2009. Extracellular matrix as a biological scaffold material: structure and function. *Acta Biomater*. 5(1), 1–13.
[53] Liao, S., Chan, C., Ramakrishna, S. 2008. Stem cells and biomimetic materials strategies for tissue engineering. *Mater. Sci. Eng. C* 28, 1189–1202.
[54] Curtis, A., Dalby, A. 2009. Cell response to nanofeatures in biomaterials. In: Di Silvio, L. (ed.) *Cellular Response to Biomaterials*. Woodhead Publishing in Materials, 429–461. CRC Press, Cambridge.
[55] Nishimura, I., Huang, Y., Butz, F., Ogawa, T., Lin, A., Wang, C.J. 2007. Discrete deposition of hydroxyapatite nanoparticles on a titanium implant with predisposing substrate microtopography accelerated osseointegration. *Nanotechnology* 18(24), 1–9.
[56] Ballarre, J., Pellice, SA., Schreiner, WH., et al. 2008. Coatings containing silica nanoparticles and glass ceramic particles applied onto surgical grade stainless steel. 21st International Symposium on Ceramics in Medicine, Oct 21–24, 2008, Buzios, Brazil. *Bioceramics* 21, 396–398, 311–314.
[57] Li, X., Huang, J., Edirisinghe, M.J., 2008. Novel patterning of nano-bioceramics: template-assisted electrohydrodynamic atomization spraying. *J. R. Soc. Interface* 5(19) 253–257.
[58] Watari, F., Takashi, N., Yokoyama, A., Uo, M., Akasaka, T., Sato, Y., Abe, S., Totsuka, Y., Thoji, K. 2009. Material nanosizing effect on living organisms: non-specific, biointeractive, physical size effects. *J. R. Soc. Interface* 6, S371–S388.
[59] Delben, J.R.J., Pimentel, O.M., Coelho, M.B., Candelorio, P.D., Furini, L.N., dos Santos, F.A., de Vicente, F.S., Delben, A.A.S.T. 2009. Synthesis and thermal properties of nanoparticles of bioactive glasses containing silver. *J. Therm. Anal. Calorim*. 97(2) 433–436.
[60] Lu, H., Zhang, T., Wang, X.P., Fang, Q.F. 2009. Electrospun submicron bioactive glass fibers for bone tissue scaffold. *J. Mater. Sci. Mater. Med*. 20(3), 793–798.
[61] Kim, H.W., Lee, H.H., Chun, G.S. 2008. Bioactivity and osteoblast responses of novel biomedical nanocomposites of bioactive glass nanofiber filled poly(lactic acid). *J. Biomed. Mater. Res. A* 85A(3) 651–663.
[62] Xia, W., Zhang, D.M., Chang, J. 2007. Fabrication and in vitro biomineralization of bioactive glass (BG) nanofibres. *Nanotechnology* 18(13), Article number: 135601.
[63] Hutmacher, D.W., Ekaputra, A.K. 2008. Design and fabrication of electrospinning of scaffolds. In: Chu, P.K., and Liu, X. (eds.), *Biomaterials Fabrication and Processing Handbook*, 115–139. CRC Press, Boca Raton, FL.
[64] Kim, H.W., Kim, H.E., Knowles, J.C. 2006. Production and potential of bioactive glass nanofibers as a next-generation biomaterial. *Adv. Funct. Mater*. 16(12), 1529–1535.
[65] Quintero, F., Pou, J., Comesaña, R., Lusquiños, F., Riveiro, A., Mann, A.B., Hill, R.G., Wu, Z.Y., Jones, J.R. 2009. Laser spinning of bioactive glass nanofibers. *Adv. Funct. Mater*. 19(19), 3084–3090.
[66] Gittens, S.A., Uludag, H. 2001. Growth factor delivery for bone tissue engineering. *J. Drug Target*. 9(6), 407–429.
[67] Kaufmann, E.A., Ducheyne, P., Radin, S., Bonnell, D.A., Composto, R. 2000. Initial events at the bioactive glass surface in contact with protein-containing solutions. *J. Biomed. Mater. Res*. 15, 52(4), 825–830.
[68] Lobel, K.D., Hench, L.L. 1996. In-vitro protein interactions with a bioactive gel-glass. *J. Sol–Gel Sci. Technol*. 7(1–2), 69–76.
[69] Wan, J.D., Thomas, M.S., Guthrie, S., Vullev, V.I. 2009. Surface-bound proteins with preserved functionality. *Ann. Biomed. Eng*. 37(6), 1190–1205.
[70] Verné, E., Ferraris, S., Vitale-Brovarone, C., Spriano, S., Bianchi, C.L., Naldoni, A., Morra, M., Cassinelli, C. 2010, Alkaline phosphatase grafting on bioactive glasses and glass ceramics. *Acta Biomater*. 6(1), 229–240.
[71] Verne, E., Vitale-Brovarone, C., Bui, E., et al. 2009. Surface functionalization of bioactive glasses. *J. Biomed. Mater. Res. A* 90A(4), 981–992.

Index

Note: Page numbers with italicized f's and t's refer to figures and tables.

P

Q

R

S

T